2014
YEAR BOOK OF
PEDIATRICS®

The 2014 Year Book Series

Year Book of Endocrinology®: Drs Schott, Apovian, Clarke, Eugster, Meikle, Oetgen, Ovalle, Schteingart, and Toth

Year Book of Hand and Upper Limb Surgery®: Drs Yao, Adams, Isaacs, and Rizzo

Year Book of Medicine®: Drs Barker, Garrick, Gersh, Khardori, LeRoith, Panush, Talley, and Thigpen

Year Book of Neonatal and Perinatal Medicine®: Drs Fanaroff, Benitz, Donn, Neu, Papile, and Van Marter

Year Book of Ophthalmology®: Drs Rapuano, Cohen, Flanders, Hammersmith, Milman, Myers, Nagra, Nelson, Penne, Pyfer, Sergott, Shields, Talekar, and Vander

Year Book of Orthopedics®: Drs Morrey, Huddleston, Rose, Swiontkowski, and Trigg

Year Book of Pathology and Laboratory Medicine®: Drs Raab and Bissell

Year Book of Pediatrics®: Dr Stockman

Year Book of Plastic and Aesthetic Surgery™: Drs Miller, Boehmler, Gosman, Gutowski, Ruberg, Salisbury, and Smith

Year Book of Pulmonary Disease®: Drs Barker, Jones, Maurer, Spradley, Tanoue, and Willsie

Year Book of Surgery®: Drs Behrns, Daly, Fahey, Hines, Howe, Huber, Klodell, Mozingo, and Pruett

Year Book of Urology®: Drs Andriole and Coplen

Year Book of Vascular Surgery®: Drs Gillespie, Bush, Passman, Starnes, and Watkins

2014

The Year Book of
PEDIATRICS®

Editor
James A. Stockman III, MD
Clinical Professor of Pediatrics, University of North Carolina Medical School at
Chapel Hill, and Duke University Medical Center, Durham, North Carolina

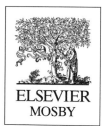

ELSEVIER
MOSBY

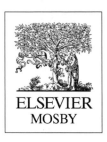

Senior Vice President, Content: Linda Belfus
Editor: Kerry Holland
Production Supervisor, Electronic Year Books: Donna M. Skelton
Electronic Article Manager: Mike Sheets
Illustrations and Permissions Coordinator: Dawn Vohsen

2014 EDITION

Printed in the United States of America
Composition by TNQ Books and Journals Pvt Ltd, India
Printing/binding by Sheridan Books, Inc.

Editorial Office:
Elsevier
Suite 1800
1600 John F. Kennedy Blvd.
Philadelphia, PA 19103-2899

International Standard Serial Number: 0084-3954
International Standard Book Number: 978-0-323-26526-3

Table of Contents

Journals Represented

Journals represented in this YEAR BOOK are listed below.

Acta Paediatrica
Annals of Internal Medicine
Archives of Disease in Childhood
Archives of Disease in Childhood Fetal and Neonatal Edition
Archives of Pediatrics & Adolescent Medicine
Blood
British Medical Journal
Clinical Pediatrics
Hospital Pediatrics
Journal of Adolescent Health
Journal of Pediatric Gastroenterology and Nutrition
Journal of Pediatric Hematology/Oncology
Journal of Pediatric Orthopaedics (Part B)
Journal of Pediatric Orthopedics
Journal of Pediatrics
Journal of the American Academy of Child & Adolescent Psychiatry
Journal of the American Medical Association
Journal of the American Medical Association Pediatrics
Lancet
Nature Medicine
New England Journal of Medicine
Pediatric Cardiology
Pediatric Emergency Care
Pediatric Infectious Disease Journal
Pediatric Research
Pediatrics

STANDARD ABBREVIATIONS

The following terms are abbreviated in this edition: acquired immunodeficiency syndrome (AIDS), cardiopulmonary resuscitation (CPR), central nervous system (CNS), cerebrospinal fluid (CSF), computed tomography (CT), deoxyribonucleic acid (DNA), electrocardiography (ECG), health maintenance organization (HMO), human immunodeficiency virus (HIV), intensive care unit (ICU), intramuscular (IM), intravenous (IV), magnetic resonance (MR) imaging (MRI), ribonucleic acid (RNA), ultrasound (US), and ultraviolet (UV).

NOTE

The YEAR BOOK OF PEDIATRICS® is a literature survey service providing abstracts of articles published in the professional literature. Every effort is made to assure the accuracy of the information presented in these pages. Neither the editors nor the publisher of the YEAR BOOK OF PEDIATRICS® can be responsible for errors in the original materials. The editors' comments are their own opinions. Mention of specific products within this publication does not constitute endorsement.

To facilitate the use of the YEAR BOOK OF PEDIATRICS® as a reference tool, all illustrations and tables included in this publication are now identified as they appear in the original article. This change is meant to help the reader recognize that any illustration or table appearing in the YEAR BOOK OF PEDIATRICS® may be only one of many in the original article. For this reason, figure and table numbers will often appear to be out of sequence within the YEAR BOOK OF PEDIATRICS.®

Introduction

Across the road from the Accademia Nazionale Dei Lincei in Rome is the *Villa Farnesina*, completed in 1509 by the renowned architect Baldassarre Peruzzi. In the garden of the Villa is a marble plaque that reads:

Quisquis huc accedis: quod tibi horridum videtur mihi amoenum est;
si placet, maneas, si taedet abeas, utrumque gratum.

The words on this plaque give warning to those entering the Villa Farnesina garden. Translation. "Whoever enters here: What seems horrid to you is pleasant to me. If you like it, stay; if it bores you, go away; both are equally pleasing to me." The words could also be provided somewhat irreverently by this editor to those opening the pages of this 2014 edition of YEAR BOOK OF PEDIATRICS, the editor's 36th, and last.

A bit of history on the transitions of prior editors of YEAR BOOK OF PEDIATRICS seems in order. In a publisher's note to the 1979 edition of the YEAR BOOK, it was remarked that Dr Sydney Gellis had relinquished his role as editor of the YEAR BOOK after 27 years. Dr Gellis was known for commentaries that were thoughtful, instructive, and often humorous. He was always able to keep new knowledge in perspective. Previous editions of the YEAR BOOK had been edited by individuals equally prominent in medicine and pediatrics: Drs Isaac Abt, Henry Poncher, and Julius Richmond. With the need to pass the editorial torch at that time, the publishers looked to someone with similar pluck to Dr Gellis. The word "pluck" is little used today, but in earlier years it was the preferred term for heroes and heroines who displayed a combination of resourcefulness, dash, and spirited courage to take on challenges that others often neglect. They did not have to look very far to find someone with pluck. There was Dr Frank Oski, unrivaled in his acumen as a pediatrician with trenchant wit. At the time, Frank was professor and chair of the Department of Pediatrics at the State University of New York Medical School in Syracuse. He was a world class generalist and a subspecialist in pediatric hematology. In his first introduction to the YEAR BOOK, Frank wrote that he had gladly accepted his new role, but with some trepidation. He quoted the Arabic proverb: "When fate arrives the physician becomes a fool." He was referring to the fact that it was a next-to-impossible task to take on the solo editorship of a comprehensive annual review of pediatrics. It was Frank's intent to do exactly that, at least until the quickly looming deadline for the 1979 YEAR BOOK manuscript necessitated a different strategy. That is how I became an "accidental" associate editor of the 1979 YEAR BOOK. I was less than a handful of years out of a pediatric fellowship and somewhat of an Oski "protégé" (there were actually quite a number). Frank threw in the towel at the solo writing and asked if I would be willing to finish 4 of the 19 chapters of the 1979 YEAR BOOK. He didn't have to ask twice. I jumped at the chance. From the 1980 edition onward we were equally splitting the writing and were co-editors until Frank's resignation in 1991. It's been a solo effort since then.

It has been an honor to prepare the YEAR BOOK OF PEDIATRICS, and while the honor has been executed with continuing irreverence from time to time, it's hard to match the pluck of Drs Oski and Gellis. As an example, in his very first attempt at editing the 1979 YEAR BOOK, Frank wrote a commentary on the topic of smoking in pregnancy. The commentary (p.71) read:

> "Pregnant women should not drink. Pregnant women should not smoke. If you give up drinking, it should be easier to give up smoking. Pregnant women should not take drugs. Shouldn't we ask fathers to make the same sacrifices as well?

> "Every time I hear about the dangers of drinking and smoking, I am reminded of the following story of two old men: First man: 'I have never made love to women, I have never smoked and I have never had a drink. Tomorrow I am going to celebrate my 90th birthday. Second man: 'How?'"

So it is not with a joke, but with some irreverence and a modest degree of celebratory crapulence,* that I close this episode in the history of editing the YEAR BOOK OF PEDIATRICS and turn over the honor to another. Last episodes are often poignant moments in history. The very last TV episode of *St Elsewhere* (younger readers will need to check with Wikipedia on the origins of a fictional hospital in Boston called St Eligius) is a favorite and ended with the tale of a rather corpulent female opera singer, in full Wagnerian regalia, including an armored breast plate and helmet with horns. She was experiencing aphonia, secondary to a bad case of laryngitis. In the closing scene of the series, Howie Mandel (in his days with hair and playing an intern at St Eligius) looked straight into the cameras and uttered the not-so-PC Yogi Berra-ism: "It ain't over till the fat lady sings."

She did ... *camera fade*. So does this introduction and this era.

...Adipem domina cecinisse

There are many who have assisted in the preparation of the YEAR BOOK OF PEDIATRICS over the past three and a half decades. It would be hard to thank all of you (you know who you are), but three have been most important in keeping everything working right and on time: Marge Gillette in Syracuse, Linda Groble in Chicago, and Dylo Mitchell here in Chapel Hill. Special thanks also to Drs Rich Strauss and Alvin Eden, who seemed to have read every word of every edition of this book over the decades and

---

*Crap-u-lence (*n*): The correct medical term for sickness or indisposition resulting from an excess of drinking (or eating). Crapulence is an almost exact synonym for a <u>hangover</u>. From the Latin *crapulentus*, very drunk.

who have consistently written me with their well-framed critiques of the work. I thank you all.

J. A. Stockman III, MD
"Accidental" Editor, Year Book of Pediatrics

Dedication

The 2014 YEAR BOOK OF PEDIATRICS is dedicated to those family members whose medical encounters have been referred to within these pages over the last several decades.

To my wife, Lee, who has also proofed in excess of 20,000 pages of the YEAR BOOK OF PEDIATRICS and who knows more about pediatrics as a mother of four than most of the rest of us ever will
To my children, Jennifer (aka Jenny), James IV (aka Jamie), Samantha (aka Sam), and Meredith (aka Merry)
To my grandchildren, Taylor, Logan, Michael, Greyson, Avery, Jameson, and Ashley

Last, but not least, long-time readers of the YEAR BOOK will likely recall learning of the travails of our more extended canine family members, past and present, whose medical conditions have been related from time to time (with full HIPPA compliance). To them and their disorders, this edition of the YEAR BOOK OF PEDIATRICS is also dedicated.

Gwinevere and her age-related renal failure
Winston and his lymphoid malignancy and grand mal seizures (auditorically evoked by Sam's clarinet practice)
Murphy and her DSM-IV-TR #296.0–296.89 — bipolar disorder
Jordan and her diabetes mellitus secondary to Cushing syndrome with its related metabolic syndrome and liver failure
Spike and his transitional cell carcinoma of the prostate
Riley and her Familial Sharpei Fever (the animal model of Familial Mediterranean Fever), with its secondary amyloidosis and systemic mastocytosis
Theo and his congenital deafness and sudden death from long QT interval (pugs can inherit the canine equivalent of the human Jervell Lang-Neilson syndrome)
Fritz and his congenital hip dysplasia and non-EBV related nasopharyngeal carcinoma
Oliver and his blindness, a complication of diabetes mellitus secondary to pancreatitis, secondary to biliary tract obstruction
Jackson ... aka "Jack" (Sam's dog who domiciled periodically in the editor's home) and his cervical cord compression secondary to a herniated disc
Duke, a guy who is amazingly fit as a fiddle, but certainly no Antonio Stradivari

Special gratitude is given to all these four-legged friends who have taught us the following baker's dozen of life's lessons:

That you don't need a bunch of toys or treats to make you happy. Lots of love and a stick are just as good, if not better.

To stop and play every once in awhile, even if you think you are too busy.

How to be completely single-minded in pursuit of a treat.

That it's fun to just run around like a crazy person sometimes.

To leap for joy for everything you get!

That you should always greet someone when they walk in the door.

To stop and say hello to strangers, but not to automatically sniff them from nose to tail.

That if at first you don't succeed, try, try again … and then if all else fails, take a nap.

That life's too short to be cranky.

To never leave cash on the coffee table … Dalmatian puppies will eat anything!

That if you make enough noise, people will give you what you want.

To always be yourself, even when everyone's watching!

And finally, to recognize the value of turning around three times before going potty.

1 Adolescent Medicine

Trends of Sexual and Violent Content by Gender in Top-Grossing U.S. Films, 1950–2006

Bleakley A, Jamieson PE, Romer D (Univ of Pennsylvania, Philadelphia)

J Adolesc Health 51:73-79, 2012

Purpose.—Because popular media such as movies can both reflect and contribute to changes in cultural norms and values, we examined gender differences and trends in the portrayal of sexual and violent content in top-grossing films from 1950 to 2006.

Methods.—The sample included 855 of the top-grossing films released over 57 years, from 1950 to 2006. The number of female and male main characters and their involvement in sexual and violent behavior were coded and analyzed over time. The relationships between sexual and violent behavior within films were also assessed.

Results.—The average number of male and female main characters in films has remained stable over time, with male characters outnumbering female characters by more than two to one. Female characters were twice as likely as male characters to be involved in sex, with differences in more explicit sex growing over time. Violence has steadily increased for both male and female characters.

Conclusions.—Although women continue to be underrepresented in films, their disproportionate portrayal in more explicit sexual content has grown over time. Their portrayal in violent roles has also grown, but at the same rate as men. Implications of exposure to these trends among young movie-going men and women are discussed.

▶ Bet you were not aware that youth are the largest movie consumers per capita in the United States. Thus it is important to examine the movie content to which they are exposed and therefore the importance of the report of Bleakley et al. Studies from the Kaiser Family Foundation on youth media consumption note that on any given day about 12% of 8- to 18-year-olds report watching a film in a theater where they spend a little more than 3 hours.[1] In addition to this, time spent watching movies on DVDs or videos account for, on average, about 30 minutes of daily screen time among 8- to 18-year-old subjects.

What Bleakley et al have done is to study a sample of top-grossing films for more than a half a century (1950–2006), examining changes over time in the differences in sexual and violent behavior among female and male characters. Films were chosen from *Variety Magazine*'s annual top-selling US films during the period of study. The top 30 movies for each year were selected. The films were chosen by selecting every other film, starting from the movie that ranked either number 1 or number 2 on a random basis. The resulting sample therefore was 15 movies for each year from 1950 through 2006, 855 in total. Movie lengths ran from 1 hour 12 minutes to 3 hours 45 minutes with an average length of 2 hours across most films. Coders assessed the presence or absence of sexual content for each segment. Sexual content was defined as including kissing (on the lips), nudity, sexual behavior, or sexual intercourse (implicitly or explicitly shown). Violent content was defined as "intentional acts (e.g., to cause harm, to coerce, or for fun) where the aggressor makes or attempts to make some physical contact that has potential to inflict injury or harm."

The results of this study included the fact that 31% of the main characters in the films were women. The findings underscore the fact that popular films since the 1950s have featured sexual and violent behavior in a way that is inextricably linked with gender stereotypes and roles. The roles of women in movies were more constrained than roles for men: there were significantly fewer female main characters in films, but when they did appear, they were more likely to be involved in sexual content and had, over time, become involved in more onscreen violence. Male main characters were consistently involved in more violence than female characters, no surprise. For the five and a half decades represented in the sample, women were more continually underrepresented in top-grossing box office movies. The average number of female main characters in films remained consistent for more than half a century and unchanged despite women having increased political, cultural, and social influence and comprising more than half of the US population by a slight margin. In contrast to women being disproportionately involved in sexual content, male characters were overwhelmingly perpetrators of violence.

The findings from this report add to the literature regarding sexual and violent content in films and how the gender of main characters relates to such content. Substantial research evidence suggests that entertainment media are an important public health issue and that the effects of exposure to sexual and violent content on adolescent health do require the attention of health practitioners, parents, researchers, and policy makers.

J. A. Stockman III, MD

Reference

1. Rideout V, Foehr U, Roberts D. *Generation M2: Media in the Lives of 8–18 Year Olds*. Menlo Park, CA: Kaiser Family Foundation; 2010.

Sexting Among Young Adults
Gordon-Messer D, Bauermeister JA, Grodzinski A, et al (Univ of Michigan School of Public Health, Ann Arbor)
J Adolesc Health 52:301-306, 2013

Purpose.—Sexting has stirred debate over its legality and safety, but few researchers have documented the relationship between sexting and health.

We describe the sexting behavior of young adults in the United States, and examine its association with sexual behavior and psychological well-being.

Methods.—Using an adapted Web version of respondent-driven sampling, we recruited a sample of U.S. young adults (aged 18—24 years, N − 3,447). We examined participant sexting behavior using four categories of sexting: (1) nonsexters, (2) receivers, (3) senders, and (4) two-way sexters. We then assessed the relationships between sexting categories and sociodemographic characteristics, sexual behavior, and psychological well-being.

Results.—More than half (57%) of the respondents were nonsexters, 28.2% were two-way sexters, 12.6% were receivers, and 2% were senders. Male respondents were more likely to be receivers than their female counterparts. Sexually active respondents were more likely to be two-way sexters than non-sexually active ones. Among participants who were sexually active in the past 30 days, we found no differences across sexting groups in the number of sexual partners or the number of unprotected sex partners in the past 30 days. We also found no relationship between sexting and psychological well-being.

Conclusions.—Our results suggest that sexting is not related to sexual risk behavior or psychological well-being. We discuss the findings of this study and propose directions for further research on sexting.

▶ *Sexting* is defined as the act of sending sexually explicit messages or images between cell phones or other mobile media. It is the modern equivalent to what used to be called phone sex. Sexting is a combination of the words *sex* and *texting* and traces its origins back to the early 2000s as teens became increasingly equipped with camera phones. Unlike phone sex of the 1990s and earlier, sexting leaves very little to the imagination.

Gordon-Messer et al note that a significant percentage of those in the teen years have sent sexually suggestive nude or seminude images via cell phones and an even larger percentage receive such messages. Sexually active youth much more commonly have shared sexually explicit images compared with nonsexually active peers. Investigators have suggested that mental health is connected with a youth's motivation to engage in sexting. Some researchers have indicated that sexting may lead to risky behaviors such as sexual initiation and less contraceptive use, whereas others say sexting may be a safer sex behavior if it is used in lieu of physical contact. Still others say that sexting may reflect a new medium for the long-standing evidence of photo sharing and romantic and sexual relationships and has no association with safer or riskier sex behaviors.

Gordon-Messer et al designed this study with 3 objectives. The first was to describe the prevalence of sexting in a large sample of 18- to 24-year-olds in the United States. In this report, sexting was divided into 4 categories: nonsexters, senders (sent, but never received a sext), receivers (receive, but never sent a sext), and 2-way sexters (both sent and received a sext). Second, the investigators examined whether participants who engaged in different sexting behaviors differ in their sociodemographic characteristics. Finally, the investigators tested the association between sexting behaviors, sexual behavior, and psychological well-being. The methodology used included surveys delivered via the Web.

The data from this report showed that among young adults (18 to 24 years), 30% had sent a sext and 41% had received a sext. The number of people sending photos or videos via cell phone had increased dramatically over a recent several-year period. Men in this report were more likely than young women to receive a sext without sending one.

The most important finding in this report is that sexting does not appear to be correlated with riskier or safer behavior. The study did find that young adults who are sexually active are more likely to sext than those who are not sexually active. The findings from this report suggest that sexting is not associated with depression, anxiety, or self-esteem issues.

It should be noted that this study included young adults only as young as 18 years of age. In the same issue of the *Journal of Adolescent Health*, Bennotsch et al examining the same age group (18 through 24 years) do suggest that sexting is robustly associated with high-risk sexual behavior.[1] An editorial by Levine attempts to reconcile these 2 very disparate conclusions about sexting.[2] Levine notes that the researchers in both of these studies posed a number of reasons young adults might be engaging in sexting with the primary 3 being sexting is a standalone safer practice, sexting is a risky (and risqué) sexual behavior, and sexting is part of the repertoire of sexually active young adults in a relationship. Levine notes that future research is needed to tell us whether sexting in fact does represent high-risk behavior or is perhaps merely a part of this millennium's adaptation to developmental sexuality. It is important for primary care providers to be aware of the issues related to sexting and also to know a little bit about the common sexting slang terms that are being used these days. The following list includes some of the less worrisome, but not altogether acceptable, terms that teens are using.

8, Oral Sex
143, I Love You
cu46, See You For Sex
GNOC, Get Naked On Cam
IWS, I Want Sex
TDTM, Talk Dirty To Me
S2R, Send To Receive
NIFOC, Naked In Front Of Computer
SorG, Straight Or Gay?
PAW, Parents Are Watching
PIR, Parent In Room
POS, Parent Over Shoulder
YWS, You Want Sex
WYCM, Will You Call Me?
RU18, Are You 18?

CD9/Code 9, Parent/Adult around
NALOPKT, Not A Lot Of People Know This

J. A. Stockman III, MD

References

1. Benotsch EG, Snipes DJ, Martin AM, Bull SS. Sexting, substance use, and sexual risk behavior in young adults. *J Adolesc Health*. 2013;52:307-313.
2. Levine D. Sexting: a terrifying health risk...or the new normal for young adults? *J Adolesc Health*. 2013;52:257-258.

The Association Between Sequences of Sexual Initiation and the Likelihood of Teenage Pregnancy
Reese BM, Haydon AA, Herring AH, et al (Univ of North Carolina at Chapel Hill; Natl Insts of Health, Bethesda, MD)
J Adolesc Health 52:228-233, 2013

Purpose.—Few studies have examined the health and developmental consequences, including unintended pregnancy, of different sexual behavior initiation sequences. Some work suggests that engaging in oral—genital sex first may slow the transition to coital activity and lead to more consistent contraception among adolescents.

Methods.—Using logistic regression analysis, we investigated the association between sequences of sexual initiation (i.e., initiating oral—genital or vaginal sex first based on reported age of first experience) and the likelihood of subsequent teenage pregnancy among 6,069 female respondents who reported vaginal sex before age 20 years and participated in waves I and IV of the National Longitudinal Study of Adolescent Health.

Results.—Among female respondents initiating vaginal sex first, 31.4% reported a teen pregnancy. Among female respondents initiating two behaviors at the same age, 20.5% reported a teen pregnancy. Among female respondents initiating oral—genital sex first, 7.9% reported a teen pregnancy. In multivariate models, initiating oral—genital sex first, with a delay of at least 1 year to vaginal sex, and initiating two behaviors within the same year were each associated with a lower likelihood of adolescent pregnancy relative to teens who initiated vaginal sex first (odds ratio = .23, 95% confidence interval: .15−.37; and odds ratio = .78, 95% confidence interval: .60−.92, respectively).

Conclusions.—How adolescents begin their sexual lives may be differentially related to positive and negative health outcomes. To develop effective pregnancy prevention efforts for teens and ensure programs are relevant to youths' needs, it is important to consider multiple facets of sexual initiation and their implications for adolescent sexual health and fertility.

▶ This report reminds us how serious the consequences are of early sexual initiation during teen years. There are approximately 750 000 pregnancies annually in the United States in women younger than 20 years. This represents a pregnancy rate of about 7% in the teen population annually. Teen pregnancy brings significant social and economic costs with both immediate and long-term impacts on teen parents and their children. Data suggest that only about 50% of teen mothers ever achieve a high school diploma, whereas 90% of teen girls who do not give birth have at least a high school degree.[1] Data also show that teen childbearing costs US tax payers about $9 billion each year, costs related to health care, child welfare, and lost tax revenue.[2]

The authors of this report note that there are few studies that have examined the order and timing of initiating different types of sex among adolescents and even fewer that have explored whether these have health implications. Most data suggest that most adolescents, especially white teens, progress from less intimate (eg, kissing) to more intimate (eg, coitus) behavior. In most instances, sexually active adolescents move quickly from oral-genital contact to vaginal sex within a 6-month period with oral sex typically occurring first.

The study abstracted by Reese et al looks at whether there is an association between sequences of sexual initiation among adolescence (defined here as initiating oral-genital sex or vaginal intercourse first) and the likelihood of subsequent teenage pregnancy using a large national representative sample from the National Longitudinal Study of Adolescent Health. This is a prospective cohort study that has followed a national representative sample of US adolescents into adulthood over many years. The study found that initiating vaginal sex first and waiting at least a year until initiating oral-genital sex was the most prevalent sequence in the database of female adolescents, followed by initiating 2 behaviors in the same year, and finally initiating oral-genital sex first. The investigators found a significantly lower likelihood of pregnancy among female respondents who initiated oral-genital sex first and waited at least a year to progress to other behaviors, relative to teens who initiated vaginal sex first. Initiating 2 behaviors in the same year versus initiating vaginal sex first also significantly lowered the odds of teen pregnancy; however, the weaker association suggests that it is not only important to consider which type of sex is initiated first but also the pace of moving to new experiences.

The reasons underlying the associations observed in this study are not entirely clear. Initiating oral-genital sex first, negating the risk of pregnancy, and waiting at least a year to move to other behaviors may allow adolescents time to develop better skills related to planning sexual encounters and negotiating contraception decisions with partners when they progress to vaginal intercourse. Starting with oral-genital experiences may also give adolescents more time to experiment and clarify their own desires and preferences, perhaps thereby increasing their sexual self-confidence. It is also possible that certain teens "select into" the group that begins their sexual experience with oral-genital sex. Although they may be underestimating some risks, adolescents may perceive fewer negative health consequences from oral versus vaginal sex. Adolescents who are motivated to avoid pregnancy and exposure to sexually transmitted diseases (eg, because of social and educational aspirations) may opt to engage in sexual activity that is perceived as safer and to proceed at a slower rate to protect their future.

This study is among the first to investigate the association between sequences of sexual initiation and the likelihood of teen pregnancy. How adolescents begin their sexual lives may have important implications for reproductive health outcomes. The information from this report probably should be read by anyone taking care of teenagers so that they understand what is going on within the social context of this age group to provide meaningful advice during office visits.

This commentary closes with a bit of good news, this having to do with pregnancy rates in teens. According to a report from the Guttmacher Institute, fewer woman aged 15-19 years in 2008 became pregnant in the USA than ever recorded in the previous 40 years. Seven percent became pregnant that year, a substantial decline from a peak in the 1990s, but large differences between ethnic groups are still reported. The overall drop is attributed to improved contraceptive use.[3]

J. A. Stockman III, MD

References

1. Centers for Disease Control and Prevention. *CDC Vital Statistics 2011*. Atlanta, GA: Office of Surveillance Epidemiology and Laboratory Services; 2011.
2. Hoffman SD. By the Numbers: the Public Cost of Teen Childbearing. http://www. thenationalcampaign.org/resources/pdf/pubs/btn_full.pdf. Accessed March 5, 2011.
3. Editorial comment. Teen pregnancy USA. *Lancet*. 2012;379.

Prime Time: Sexual Health Outcomes at 24 Months for a Clinic-Linked Intervention to Prevent Pregnancy Risk Behaviors
Sieving RE, McRee A-L, McMorris BJ, et al (Univ of Minnesota, Minneapolis; et al)
JAMA Pediatr 167:333-340, 2013

Importance.—Preventing early pregnancy among vulnerable adolescents requires innovative and sustained approaches. Prime Time, a youth development intervention, aims to reduce pregnancy risk among adolescent girls seeking clinic services who are at high risk for pregnancy.

Objective.—To evaluate sexual risk behaviors and related outcomes with a 24-month postbaseline survey, 6 months after the conclusion of the Prime Time intervention.

Design.—Randomized controlled trial.

Setting.—Community and school-based primary care clinics.

Participants.—Of 253 sexually active 13- to 17-yearold girls meeting specified risk criteria, 236 (93.3%) completed the 24-month follow-up survey.

Intervention.—Offered during an 18-month period, Prime Time includes case management and youth leadership programs.

Main Outcome Measures.—Self-reported consistency of condom, hormonal, and dual-method contraceptive use with most recent male sex partner and number of male sex partners in the past 6 months.

Results.—At 24-month follow-up, the intervention group reported significantly more consistent use of condoms, hormonal contraception, and dual-method contraception than the control group. Intervention participants also reported improvements in family connectedness and self-efficacy to refuse unwanted sex, and reductions in the perceived importance of having sex. No between-group differences were found in the number of recent male sex partners.

Conclusions and Relevance.—This study contributes to what has been a dearth of evidence regarding youth development interventions offered through clinic settings, where access to high-risk adolescents is plentiful but few efforts have emphasized a dual approach of strengthening sexual and nonsexual protective factors while addressing risk. Findings suggest that health services grounded in a youth development framework can lead to long-term reductions in sexual risk among vulnerable youth.

▶ This report reminds us how far we have to go with teen pregnancies. The report tells us that more than three-quarters of a million young women age 15 to 19 years become pregnant annually in the United States and deliver more than 400 000 births. Such pregnancies are higher than average for teens as a whole among adolescents of color, with non-Hispanic black and Hispanic teenagers experiencing twice the rate of pregnancy as their non-Hispanic white counterparts. To date, limited evidence exists regarding outcomes of health services grounded in a youth development framework, especially from studies using vigorous evaluation designs.

Prime Time is a multicomponent youth development intervention for girls at high risk for pregnancy. Designed for primary care clinics, this 18-month intervention aims to reduce precursors of teen pregnancy, including sexual risk behaviors, violence involvement, and school disconnection. The report of Sieving et al tells us about a study that evaluates sexual risk behaviors and related outcomes with a 24-month post-baseline survey, 6 months after the conclusion of a Prime Time intervention program. The Prime Time case management program establishes a trusting relationship in which a teenager and her case manager work together to address attributes targeted by the intervention. One-on-one visits focus on core topics, including healthy relationships, responsible sexual behaviors (eg, contraceptive use), and positive family and school involvement. In addition, peer educator groups address interpersonal skills, expectations and skills for healthy relationships, social influences on sexual behavior, sexual decision making, and contraceptive skills.

At 24 months of follow-up, it was clear that the intervention group more consistently used condoms, hormonal contraception, and dual methods of contraception compared with a control group. Findings of sustained Prime Time Program impact add to a growing body of evidence supporting multicomponent youth development approaches for reducing sexual risk among adolescent girls at high risk for pregnancy.

To read more about nonoral hormonal contraception, including the use of transdermal patches, vaginal rings, and long-acting reversible methods such as the levonorgestrel intrauterine system and the single rod, progestogen-only implant, see the excellent review by Bateson et al.[1]

J. A. Stockman III, MD

Reference

1. Bateson D, McNamee K, Briggs P. Newer non-oral hormonal contraception. *BMJ.* 2013;346:f341.

Effectiveness of Long-Acting Reversible Contraception

Winner B, Peipert JF, Zhao Q, et al (Washington Univ School of Medicine, St Louis, MO)

N Engl J Med 366:1998-2007, 2012

Background.—The rate of unintended pregnancy in the United States is much higher than in other developed nations. Approximately half of unintended pregnancies are due to contraceptive failure, largely owing to inconsistent or incorrect use.

Methods.—We designed a large prospective cohort study to promote the use of long-acting reversible contraceptive methods as a means of reducing unintended pregnancies in our region. Participants were provided with reversible contraception of their choice at no cost. We compared the rate of failure of long-acting reversible contraception (intrauterine devices [IUDs] and implants) with other commonly prescribed contraceptive methods (oral contraceptive pills, transdermal patch, contraceptive vaginal ring, and depot medroxyprogesterone acetate [DMPA] injection) in the overall cohort and in groups stratified according to age (less than 21 years of age vs. 21 years or older).

Results.—Among the 7486 participants included in this analysis, we identified 334 unintended pregnancies. The contraceptive failure rate among participants using pills, patch, or ring was 4.55 per 100 participant-years, as compared with 0.27 among participants using long-acting reversible contraception (hazard ratio after adjustment for age, educational level, and history with respect to unintended pregnancy, 21.8; 95% confidence interval, 13.7 to 34.9). Among participants who used pills, patch, or ring, those who were less than 21 years of age had a risk of unintended pregnancy that was almost twice as high as the risk among older participants. Rates of unintended pregnancy were similarly low among participants using DMPA injection and those using an IUD or implant, regardless of age.

Conclusions.—The effectiveness of long-acting reversible contraception is superior to that of contraceptive pills, patch, or ring and is not altered in adolescents and young women. (Funded by the Susan Thompson Buffet Foundation.)

▶ In the United States, the most commonly used contraceptive method for teenagers and women of reproductive age is the oral contraceptive pill. Unfortunately, because the pill requires daily compliance, failure rates calculated on the basis of "perfect use" differ from real-world failure rates calculated on the basis of typical use. It is estimated that annual failure rates with typical use of oral contraceptives run about 9% for the general population, 13% for teenagers, and 30% or higher for some high-risk subgroups. On the other hand, long-acting reversible contraceptive methods, including intrauterine devices and subdermal implants, are not user dependent and have failure rates of less than 1%. This rivals the rate seen with sterilization. Despite the proven safety in adolescents and in women of all ages, intrauterine devices are used in only about 5.5% of women who use contraception in the United States. This is unlike the rest of the developed world including the United Kingdom and France, where intrauterine devices are used more frequently and are associated with rates of unintended pregnancy that are much lower than those in the United States.

Prior estimates of the failure rates with typical oral contraceptive use have relied mostly on retrospective survey information. These authors have designed a large prospective study examining the outcomes related to the promotion of the use of long-acting reversible contraceptive methods as a means of reducing unintended pregnancy. This study was carried out in the Midwest. From August 2007 through September 2011, the investigators enrolled 9256 participants at risk for unintended pregnancy. All participants chose a contraceptive method and received it at no cost. The subjects were offered long-acting reversible contraceptive methods, including intrauterine devices and subdermal implants. Participants were then followed prospectively.

The study results document that participants using oral contraceptive pills, a transdermal patch, or a vaginal ring had a risk of contraceptive failure that was 20 times as great as the risk among those using long-acting reversible contraception. The failure rate among participants who used pills, patch, or ring was 4.55 per 100 participant years, as compared with 0.22 for those who used depot medroxyprogesterone acetate injection and 0.27 for those who used an intrauterine device or a subdermal implant. Participants less than 21 years of age who used pills, patch, or ring had almost twice the risk of unintended pregnancy as older women who used the same methods. There appear to be few contraindications to the use of long-acting reversible contraception. Almost all women were eligible for an intrauterine device or implant. Modern intrauterine devices do not carry an increased risk of pelvic inflammatory disease after the first 20 days following insertion. Women who are at average risk for sexually transmitted infections appear to be good candidates for intrauterine devices, as long as they do not have cervicitis at the time of insertion. Intrauterine devices and implants are also associated with acceptable adverse event rates among adolescents and nulliparous women.

Half of all pregnancies in the United States are unintended, and half of those result from contraceptive failure. Seventy percent of women using a contraceptive are using pills or condoms, and 1 in every 8 users of reversible methods will have a contraceptive failure in the first year. Such statistics underscore the importance of the results of this article. Figs 1 and 2 in the original article illustrate the cumulative percentage of participants who have contraceptive failure.

All those caring for teenagers should be familiar with the data from this report as they provide the most up-to-date information on this topic.

J. A. Stockman III, MD

Sexual Dysfunctions Among Young Men: Prevalence and Associated Factors

Mialon A, Berchtold A, Michaud P-A, et al (Centre Hospitalier Universitaire Vaudois and University of Lausanne, Switzerland; et al)
J Adolesc Health 51:25-31, 2012

Purpose.—The purposes of this study are to measure the prevalence of premature ejaculation (PE) and erectile dysfunction (ED) among a population of Swiss young men and to assess which factors are associated with these sexual dysfunctions in this age-group.

Methods.—For each condition (PE and ED), we performed separate analyses comparing young men suffering from the condition with those who were not. Groups were compared for substance use (tobacco, alcohol, cannabis, other illegal drugs, and medication without a prescription), self-reported body mass index, sexual orientation, physical activity, professional activity, sexual experience (sexual life length and age at first intercourse), depression status, mental health, and physical health in a bivariate analysis. We then used a log-linear analysis to consider all significant variables simultaneously.

Results.—Prevalence rates for PE and ED were 11% and 30%, respectively. Poor mental health was the only variable to have a direct association with both conditions after controlling for potential confounders. In addition, PE was directly associated with tobacco, illegal drugs, professional activity, and physical activity, whereas ED was directly linked with medication without a prescription, length of sexual life, and physical health.

Conclusions.—In Switzerland, one-third of young men suffer from at least one sexual dysfunction. Multiple health-compromising factors are associated with these dysfunctions. These should act as red flags for health professionals to encourage them to take any opportunity to talk about sexuality with their young male patients.

▶ This report reminds us of an interesting finding, which is that some aspects of sexual dysfunction are more common among young men. The report of Mialon et al was designed to measure the prevalence of something we do not think a whole lot about, and that is how often young men, including those in the older teenage population, suffer from sexual dysfunction including premature ejaculation (PE) and erectile dysfunction (ED). The investigators looked at men in Switzerland age 18 to 25 years, a captive audience who are routinely called up for a 2-day evaluation prior to military service. The study only involved men who were sexually active and divided the group into those who had and did not have PE or ED. PE was characterized when control over ejaculation was self-evaluated as fair or poor. ED was assessed by a standard scoring system that many investigators have used over the years. The average age of the men studied in this report was 19.5 years.

The results of this study showed a prevalence rate of PE in this young adult population to be 11%, somewhat lower than has been suggested from previously published reports. Concerning ED, its prevalence among the young male population in Switzerland was almost 30%, also consistent with the results of a previously published study. Among the associated factors examined, mental health was the only variable to be directly associated with both PE and ED. There seemed to be an association between depression and both forms of sexual dysfunction. The literature has described that sexual dysfunction may cause some degree of depression and that depressed young men may experience sexual dysfunction as a side effect of their mental difficulties. Nonetheless, whatever this association cause is, those caring for these fellows should be aware of the link between sexual dysfunction and mental status.

There are other associations related to PE. One is tobacco use. The association between tobacco use and sexual dysfunction has been previously noted in the literature. Curiously, those who are consistent tobacco users actually have less PE than those who occasionally smoke. It is possible that those who are occasional users have the more anxious personalities that smoke from time to time to relax, perhaps increasing their propensity for PE. PE is also associated with the use of illegal drugs and low physical activity. One final additional link with PE appears to be professional activity. Students, for example, report PE twice as frequently as same age working young men. Presumably the link is increased physical activity associated with being part of the labor force.

With respect to ED, there were also several associations noted. Medication without a prescription appears to be more frequent among young men with ED. Also, almost half of young men in the ED group report a sexual lifespan of less than 2 years compared with only 30% in the non-ED group. As expected, experience seems then to have an important impact on ED in this age category. Physical health also appears to be directly associated with ED. ED has been associated with chronic physical conditions and this finding may reflect that chronic conditions can affect a young man's sexual health. Interestingly, neither ED nor PE was linked with body mass index, presumably related to the absence of obesity-associated vascular lesions at this young age.

This study is the first to estimate the prevalence of sexual dysfunction among young men, at least in Switzerland. The report highlights that 1 young man out of 3 suffers from 1 of the 2 most frequent forms of sexual dysfunction. The data from Switzerland do correlate with what little is known about the same problem in the United States in this age group. Given that many young patients generally will not talk about sexual topics such as PE and ED, these conditions are likely underappreciated. However, because these conditions may be markers of other issues as well as being embarrassing in and of themselves, they are worth paying attention to when evaluating the older teen. We should take any opportunity to talk about sexuality with these young adult males.

J. A. Stockman III, MD

Health Risks of Oregon Eighth-Grade Participants in the "Choking Game": Results From a Population-Based Survey

Ramowski SK, Nystrom RJ, Rosenberg KD, et al (Oregon Health Authority, Portland; et al)
Pediatrics 129:846-851, 2012

Objective.—To examine the risk behaviors associated with participation in the "choking game" by eighth-graders in Oregon.

Methods.—We obtained data from the 2009 Oregon Healthy Teens survey, a cross-sectional weighted survey of 5348 eighth-graders that questioned lifetime prevalence and frequency of choking game participation. The survey also included questions about physical and mental health, gambling, sexual activity, nutrition, physical activity/body image, exposure to violence, and substance use.

Results.—Lifetime prevalence of choking game participation was 6.1% for Oregon eighth-graders, with no differences between males and females. Of the eighth-grade choking game participants, 64% had engaged in the activity more than once and 26.6% >5 times. Among males, black youth were more likely to participate than white youth. Among both females and males, Pacific Islander youth were much more likely to participate than white youth. Multivariate logistic regression revealed that sexual activity and substance use were significantly associated with choking game participation for both males and females.

Conclusions.—At >6%, the prevalence of choking game participation among Oregon youth is consistent with previous findings. However, we found that most of those who participate will put themselves at risk more than once. Participants also have other associated health risk behaviors. The comprehensive adolescent well visit, as recommended by the American Academy of Pediatrics, is a good opportunity for providers to conduct a health behavior risk assessment and, if appropriate, discuss the dangers of engaging in this activity.

▶ Most everyone in the medical community is now familiar with the term "choking game." This refers to an activity in which pressure is applied to the neck/carotid artery to limit oxygen and blood flow. Once the pressure is released, a high or euphoric feeling may be achieved as blood and oxygen rush back to the brain. This is a nonsexual activity and therefore is distinct from auto-erotic asphyxiation in its underlying motivation. Needless to say, participation in a choking game can lead to serious injury or death.

Little has been written about the choking game in terms of its prevalence. Some have suggested that there is an increased likelihood of participation among boys, older youth, and those living in rural areas. Over a recent 12-year period (1995—2007), there were 82 deaths reported in children ages 6 to 19 years as a result of participation in the choking game as identified through newspaper and other media reports.[1] As one might suspect, such numbers are likely to be a significant underestimation because only those deaths covered by media were included in these statistics.

In the state of Oregon, there is an ongoing survey known as the Oregon Healthy Teens (OHT) Survey of teen activities. Ramowski et al collected data on choking game awareness, lifetime prevalence, and participation frequency by using the 2009 OHT Survey on a population of 8th and 11th graders. The survey was designed to measure adolescent health and wellbeing in general. All Oregon public secondary schools were a part of the sampling for the survey. A total of 5348 8th graders completed the survey; of these, 96.6% answered the choking game lifetime prevalence question. Overall, 22% of 8th graders said they had heard of someone participating in the choking game. Only 1.2% indicated they have helped someone participate. Actual participation prevalence related to gender, race, and ethnicity. Among males, black students, and Pacific Islanders, there was a significantly higher rate of participation than among whites (respective odds ratios 3.47, 3.47, and 4.95). Among females, Pacific Islander youth had significantly higher participation rates (odds ratio 5.77) than white females. The lifetime prevalence of choking game participation was 6.1% for Oregon 8th graders. Of these, two-thirds had engaged in the activity more than once and 1 in 4 more than 5 times. For 11th graders, the lifetime prevalence was 7.6%.

The findings from this article show that choking game participation clusters with other risk-taking behaviors and is not an activity among those who are high achievers and otherwise low-risk takers. The authors of this article did not provide specific recommendations as to the types of prevention messages or screening tools that may be most effective in preventing and/or curbing participation in the choking game. Unfortunately, many pediatricians and family practitioners have limited awareness of this activity. It is suggested, however, that questions about the choking game be included with questions related to substance use and sexual activity as well as violence prevention at the time of routine visits of teens.

We should be grateful to these investigators for sharing concrete information about the prevalence of the choking game, at least in Oregon and presumably elsewhere. Anticipatory guidance may be the first step toward reducing youth participation and its associated risk of injury and death.

J. A. Stockman III, MD

Reference

1. Centers for Disease Control and Prevention (CDC). Unintentional strangulation deaths from the "choking game" among youths aged 6–19 years–United States, 1995–2007. *MMWR Morb Mortal Wkly Rep.* 2008;57:141-144.

Internet Alcohol Sales to Minors
Williams RS, Ribisl KM (Univ of North Carolina at Chapel Hill)
Arch Pediatr Adolesc Med 166:808-813, 2012

Objectives.—To determine whether minors can successfully purchase alcohol online and to examine age verification procedures at the points of order and delivery.

Design.—A cross-sectional study evaluated underage alcohol purchase attempts from 100 popular Internet vendors.

Setting.—The study was conducted at the University of North Carolina at Chapel Hill, July 14-27, 2011.

Participants.—Eight 18- to 20-year-old individuals participated.

Outcome Measures.—Rates of successful sales to minors and use of age verification procedures at order and delivery were determined.

Results.—Of the 100 orders placed by the underage buyers, 45% were successfully received; 28% were rejected as the result of age verification. Most vendors (59%) used weak, if any, age verification at the point of order, and, of 45 successful orders, 23 (51%) used none. Age verification at delivery was inconsistently conducted and, when attempted, failed about half of the time.

Conclusions.—Age verification procedures used by Internet alcohol vendors do not adequately prevent online sales to minors. Shipping companies should work with their staff to improve administration of age verification at delivery, and vendors should use rigorous age verification at order and delivery. Further research should determine the proportion of minors who buy alcohol online and test purchases from more vendors to inform enforcement of existing policies and creation of new policies to reduce youth access to alcohol online.

▶ Prior to this report, no peer-reviewed studies have examined the sales and age verification practices of Internet alcohol vendors, nor have they assessed the ability to purchase alcohol online. Williams and Ribisl did research on Internet alcohol vendors and found an industry with sales of more than $2.4 billion per year. Their methodology for ferreting out alcohol vendors was identical to those previously used to identify online tobacco vendors. The authors were able to readily identify more than 5000 Internet alcohol vendors and performed "underage" purchases at various web sites. Forty-five of 100 attempts at alcohol purchases by a "minor" were successful. There was very little use of age verification at the point of order. Most vendors (59%) used weak age verification methods, if any at all, relying on check boxes or buttons (31%) or spurious claims that by merely submitting an order, users were legally certifying their age (23%). Forty-one percent of vendors did not address age verification at the point of order. Of alcohol orders successfully received, 71% did not use rigorous age verification at the point of order, and 51% used none. Some vendors requested age verification at the time of delivery of the alcohol, but when used, such verification techniques failed about half of the time. It appeared that FedEx did a poorer job than UPS in verifying age at delivery. About one-third of each company's deliveries labeled with a requirement for age verification were returned to the sender after the delivery was refused on the basis of age verification. However, in cases in which delivery staff attempted to perform age verification, FedEx packages were significantly more likely to be delivered to an underaged buyer.

This study was limited to the 100 most popular Internet alcohol providers, which were disproportionately wine vendors (vs beer, liquor, or other alcohol, which are more frequently used by youth). This study provides important evidence that Internet alcohol vendors do a poor job of preventing youth access to Internet-delivered alcohol.

The authors of this report suggest that states should apply similar approaches that have been quite effective at regulating Internet cigarette vendors. There are well over 5000 alcohol vendors, and now fewer than 400 cigarette vendors online. For more on who is minding the virtual alcohol store, see the excellent editorial by Jernigan.[1]

J. A. Stockman III, MD

Reference

1. Jernigan DH. Who is minding the virtual alcohol store? *Arch Pediatr Adolesc Med.* 2012;166:866-867.

Adolescent Males' Awareness of and Willingness to Try Electronic Cigarettes

Pepper JK, Reiter PL, McRee A-L, et al (Univ of North Carolina at Chapel Hill; The Ohio State Univ, Columbus; Univ of Minnesota, Minneapolis; et al)
J Adolesc Health 52:144-150, 2013

Purpose.—Electronic cigarettes (e-cigarettes) are a new type of device that delivers vaporized nicotine without the tobacco combustion of regular cigarettes. We sought to understand awareness of and willingness to try e-cigarettes among adolescent males, a group that is at risk for smoking initiation and may use e-cigarettes as a "gateway" to smoking.

Methods.—A national sample of 11−19-year-old males ($n = 228$) completed an online survey in November 2011. We recruited participants through their parents, who were members of a panel of U.S. households constructed using random-digit dialing and addressed-based sampling.

Results.—Only two participants (< 1%) had previously tried e-cigarettes. Among those who had not tried e-cigarettes, most (67%) had heard of them. Awareness was higher among older and non-Hispanic adolescents. Nearly 1 in 5 (18%) participants were willing to try either a plain or flavored e-cigarette, but willingness to try plain versus flavored varieties did not differ. Smokers were more willing to try any e-cigarette than nonsmokers (74% vs. 13%; OR 10.25, 95% CI 2.88, 36.46). Nonsmokers who had more negative beliefs about the typical smoker were less willing to try e-cigarettes (OR.58, 95% CI.43, .79).

Conclusions.—Most adolescent males were aware of e-cigarettes, and a substantial minority were willing to try them. Given that even experimentation with e-cigarettes could lead to nicotine dependence and subsequent use of other tobacco products, regulatory and behavioral interventions are needed to prevent "gateway" use by adolescent nonsmokers. Campaigns promoting negative images of smokers or FDA bans on sales to youth may help deter use.

▶ Electronic cigarettes have been around for a while now. They are also known as e-cigarettes. They first came onto the market in the United States 7 years ago.

E-cigarettes, of course, are battery-powered devices that look like cigarettes and deliver a nicotine vapor to the user. Advertisements present them as advanced and healthier alternatives to tobacco-containing cigarettes. E-cigarettes are sold everywhere these days and available to teens who can get them at virtually any shopping mall kiosk.

These authors provide the only data currently available regarding adolescents' awareness, use, and susceptibility to using e-cigarettes. In a study of several hundred adolescents, awareness of e-cigarettes was high (67%), but fewer than 1% of teens had actually tried them. The same study showed that 40% of adults were aware of e-cigarettes. The higher awareness of adolescents versus adults (67% vs 40%) calls into question whether these nicotine products are being marketed solely to existing adult tobacco smokers.

E-cigarettes should not be considered entirely safe. The Food and Drug Administration has found, for example, tobacco-specific impurities and contaminants, such as diethylene glycol in e-cigarette cartridges, and the nicotine content in e-cigarette products often does not match the advertised or labeled content. Administration of an addictive drug such as nicotine at levels that are unintended may harm users and possibly encourage addiction. It should be noted that e-cigarette cartridges may leak, creating the potential for dermal nicotine exposure and potential poisoning. Studies examining the toxicity of exhaled e-cigarette vapors show them to contain volatile organic compounds and fine particulate matter, although at levels well below secondhand tobacco cigarette smoke.[1]

This article is important given the dearth of empirical research on e-cigarette products and who may be using them. The major issue is whether e-cigarettes will become the newest gateway to addiction for millions of youths. Many states and localities have passed laws restricting e-cigarette sales to minors and include e-cigarettes in their smoke-free policies as all states and localities should.

J. A. Stockman III, MD

Reference

1. Schripp T, Markewitz D, Uhde E, Salthammer T. Does e-cigarette consumption cause passive vaping? *Indoor Air*. 2013;23:25-31.

Attentional Bias and Disinhibition Toward Gaming Cues Are Related to Problem Gaming in Male Adolescents
van Holst RJ, Lemmens JS, Valkenburg PM, et al (Univ of Amsterdam, The Netherlands)
J Adolesc Health 50:541-546, 2012

Purpose.—The aim of this study was to examine whether behavioral tendencies commonly related to addictive behaviors are also related to problematic computer and video game playing in adolescents. The study of attentional bias and response inhibition, characteristic for addictive disorders, is relevant to the ongoing discussion on whether problematic gaming should be classified as an addictive disorder.

Methods.—We tested the relation between self-reported levels of problem gaming and two behavioral domains: attentional bias and response inhibition. Ninety-two male adolescents performed two attentional bias tasks (addiction-Stroop, dot-probe) and a behavioral inhibition task (go/no-go). Self-reported problem gaming was measured by the game addiction scale, based on the Diagnostic and Statistical Manual of Mental Disorders-fourth edition criteria for pathological gambling and time spent on computer and/or video games.

Results.—Male adolescents with higher levels of self-reported problem gaming displayed signs of error-related attentional bias to game cues. Higher levels of problem gaming were also related to more errors on response inhibition, but only when game cues were presented.

Conclusions.—These findings are in line with the findings of attentional bias reported in clinically recognized addictive disorders, such as substance dependence and pathological gambling, and contribute to the discussion on the proposed concept of "Addiction and Related Disorders" (which may include non-substance-related addictive behaviors) in the Diagnostic and Statistical Manual of Mental Disorders-fourth edition.

▶ It should come as no surprise that teens gamble. In the past 10 years, there has been a virtual explosion of internet gambling, currently one of the most popular activities on the internet. Nonmonetary gambling games, including poker, are routinely available on social media sites, regardless of a member's age. Although these virtual games are currently only offered for points rather than for cash, these are indications that Apple, Facebook, and Google are interested in eventually offering games for actual money. There is clear evidence that adolescents are gaming and gambling on the Internet. A survey performed for the Pew Internet and American Life Project found that teens age 12 to 17 years are most likely to play online games.[1] About one-third of adolescents 12 to 17 years play gambling type games on the Internet. This is likely to be an underestimate.

van Holst et al have studied the question of whether excessive gaming can be conceptualized as a behavior addiction similar to pathological gaming. They have observed that excessive gaming and pathological gambling share certain commonalities, such as craving, loss of control, and withdrawal symptoms. They have been able to identify distinct behavior patterns among problem gamers, similar to those of pathological gamblers. These investigators even go so far as to suggest that teens may begin to exhibit behavioral addictions that fit within the psychiatric taxonomy of mental disorders.

In a commentary that accompanied this report, Volberg tells us that online gambling is here to stay and will continue to evolve as competition among Internet gambling sites aggressively heats up, new demographic groups enter the market, and a growing number of jurisdictions legalize and regulate online gambling activities.[2] Teens are a specifically vulnerable group in terms of the future development of gambling problems at a pathological level. It is likely that we are setting up our teenage population for a form of addiction that most

were not exposed to until well into adulthood. All of us should pay careful attention to this problem. You can bet that we will see more and more literature on the
topic in the near future.

J. A. Stockman III, MD

References

1. Zickhr K. *Generations 2010*. Washington, DC: Pew Research Center; 2010.
2. Volberg RA. Still not on the radar: adolescent risk and gambling, revisited. *J Adolesc Health*. 2012;50:539-540.

Factors Associated With Adolescents' Propensity to Drive With Multiple Passengers and to Engage in Risky Driving Behaviors
Mirman JH, Albert D, Jacobsohn LS, et al (The Children's Hosp of Philadelphia, PA; Univ of North Carolina at Chapel Hill)
J Adolesc Health 50:634-640, 2012

Purpose.—Research shows that parenting factors and individual difference variables, such as sensation seeking (SS) and risk perceptions (RPs),
are associated with increased motor vehicle crash risk for young drivers.
The presence of peer passengers is also known to be associated with
increased crash risk. However, as previous studies did not study these factors
concurrently, less is known about the factors that are associated with driving
with peer passengers and if peer passengers may mediate the effect of
parenting and individual difference variables on adolescents' engagement
in risky driving behavior.

Methods.—We examined predictors of driving with multiple passengers
(DWMPs) and explored it as a potential mediator of pathways from three
factors: (1) SS, (2) RPs, and (3) Parental monitoring and rule-setting to
risky driving behaviors in a convenience sample of 198 adolescent drivers
using a cross-sectional Web-based survey.

Results.—Findings indicate that both stronger RPs and perceiving
parents as strong monitors and rule setters were associated with less engagement in risky driving, whereas greater SS was associated with more engagement in risky driving; RPs, monitoring, and SS were also significantly
associated with DWMPs in these same directions. DWMPs partially medi-
ated the effect of these risk factors on risky driving behavior.

Conclusions.—Results inform theory and policy by examining factors
associated with risk taking in the context of adolescent driving. Interventions can be developed to complement graduated driver licensing laws by
targeting individual difference variables and decreasing opportunities for
peer passenger carriage.

▶ Until this report appeared, I was not aware of the astounding statistics associated with the risky driving behaviors of teens. In one recent year, a total of 3118
adolescent drivers (age 15 to 19 years) and their passengers were killed when an

adolescent driver was behind the wheel. Furthermore, in that same year, more than 1000 other drivers, pedestrians, and bicyclists were killed and more than 40 000 people were severely injured (eg, brain or spinal cord injury, fractures, concussions) because of adolescent driver motor vehicle crashes.[1] Motor vehicle accidents by adolescent drivers are the single greatest source of morbidity and mortality during the adolescent period. One in three adolescent deaths is the result of motor vehicle accidents.

Mirman et al have undertaken a study that focuses on how peer presence may contribute to engaging in risky driving behaviors. It is not surprising that the influence of peer passengers affects how young drivers perform. The study was undertaken as part of the Young Driver Research Initiative, a collaborative research program between the Center for Injury Research and Prevention at the Children's Hospital of Philadelphia and State Farm Insurance Company. From motor vehicle department and insurance company databases, the perception of risk by a teen driver was shown to be inversely associated with having one or more passengers in an automobile. Although this is no surprise, the findings do represent an important documentation underpinning many state laws that do not permit the naïve learner driver to have multiple passengers in the car. It is also clear that parents cannot defer to graduated driver licensing laws or rely on police enforcement to protect their young teen drivers. Parents need to be part of the process of educating their progeny even though adolescents tend to view passenger carriage as a personal behavior and not safety-related behavior and are less likely to be supportive of parent attempts to regulate their behavior in this regard. Sometimes it is necessary to set down firm rules.

In another report that accompanied this one, it was shown exactly how passengers affect male teen drivers.[2] Analyzing data from the National Motor Vehicle Crash Causation Survey, a study was performed with a nationally representative sample of 677 drivers ages 16 to 18 years involved in serious crashes, comparing the risk of specific distraction-related and risk-taking—related precrash factors documented via on-scene crash investigation for teens driving with peer passengers and teens driving alone. The study showed that those with peer passengers were more likely to perform an aggressive act or an illegal maneuver just before crashing. This risk increased regardless of the gender of the passenger. Interestingly, girls with passengers were more often engaged in at least one interior nondriving activity other than conversing with passengers, particularly when driving with opposite-gender passengers. Female drivers, both with and without passengers, drove aggressively or performed an illegal maneuver before crashing. With passengers in the car, teens were more likely to report focusing on some object within the car, eating or drinking as well as retrieving an object from the floor and/or seat. For male drivers, having male passengers produced more risky behavior than having a female passenger.

Few studies in the past have evaluated the role of peer passengers in the context of crash involvement. The contributions of investigators at the Children's Hospital of Philadelphia provide us with specific ways in which peer—driver interactions contribute to crashes, especially in the case of distraction.

J. A. Stockman III, MD

References

1. Curry A, Garcia-Espana J, Winston F, et al. Miles to go: establishing benchmarks for teen driver safety. http://www.teendriversource.org/tools/researcher/detail/122. Accessed September 10, 2012.
2. Curry AE, Mirman JH, Kallan MJ, Winston FK, Durbin DR. Peer passengers: how do they affect teen crashes? *J Adolesc Health*. 2012;50:588-594.

The Relative Odds of Involvement in Seven Crash Configurations by Driver Age and Sex

Bingham CR, Ehsani JP (Univ of Michigan Transportation Res Inst, Ann Arbor)
J Adolesc Health 51:484-490, 2012

Introduction.—Much is known about sex and age differences in collision types, but most studies have examined the effect of declining physical and mental capabilities on older drivers' performance. Fewer studies have focused on the relationship between younger driver's sex and crash type, and these studies have largely ignored the multidimensionality of crashes, have not consistently examined sex differences, and are based on outdated data. This study addressed these issues by examining differences in the likelihood of involvement in seven crash configurations between adolescent and adult male and female drivers.

Method.—Fatal crash data from the Fatality Analysis Reporting System and nonfatal crash data from the General Estimation System for years 2005–2009 were used. Crash configurations were identified using point of initial impact, manner of collision, and vehicle action (i.e., striking or struck). Logistic regression estimated relative odds ratios among four driver groups: male and female drivers aged 15–19 years, and male and female drivers aged 45–64 years.

Results.—Crash likelihood varied dramatically by driver age and sex across crash configuration. Adolescent male drivers were most likely to be in single-vehicle and fatal head-on crashes; adolescent drivers had a higher likelihood of front-to-rear crashes; adults had the highest likelihood of rear-end crashes; and female drivers had higher likelihoods of left- and right-side crashes.

Conclusions.—These findings may result from differences in driving experience, driving styles, or cognitive spatial abilities. Future research is needed to identify contributors to different crash configurations so that they can be directly addressed through tailored interventions and programs.

▶ There have been a lot of studies examining the effects of declining physical and mental capacities that can reduce an older adult's driving performance, but little has been written about the crash characteristics of adolescent male and female drivers and how they differ from their adult counterparts. Such information is essential before the introduction of effective interventions and policies that reduce the risk of crashes involving adolescent drivers.

This study was designed to use a combination of crash characteristics in the identification of commonly occurring fatal and nonfatal crash configurations to determine which configurations are more likely to involve adolescent male and female drivers relative to their adult counterparts. The study used 5 years of data on fatal and nonfatal crashes from the Fatality Analysis Reporting System (FARS) and the General Estimates System (GES), respectively. FARS contains all police-reported fatal crashes occurring on public roadways in the United States. GES is a nationally representative probability sample of police-reported crash records collected from approximately 400 agencies throughout the United States. It includes crashes ranging in severity from property-damage only to fatal crashes. The fatal crashes recorded in GES are a subset of those reported in FARS.

Adolescent drivers in this study were 15 to 19 years old and were compared with adult drivers 45 to 64 years old. The latter provided a comparison group for which crash characteristics were at their lowest. Point of impact, manner of collision (ie, vehicle's orientation to each other), and vehicle role (ie, striking or being struck) were combined to create crash configurations. The data from this study show that adolescent female drivers were 1.92 times more likely than adult women drivers to be in nonfatal front-to-rear crashes but did not differ from adolescent male drivers. Similarly, adult men and women drivers did not differ significantly from each other, indicating a general age difference in the likelihood of nonfatal front-to-rear crashes. Adolescent male drivers had the lowest likelihood of rear-end crashes, suggesting that adolescent female drivers were more distractible for whatever reason, such as cell phone use. Adolescent male drivers had the highest likelihood of fatal single-vehicle crashes, whereas adult female drivers had the lowest likelihood. Adolescent female drivers had the lowest likelihood of fatal front-to-rear crashes, and adult male drivers had a greater than 2-fold likelihood of crashes of this configuration and had the highest likelihood of any group.

This study had some interesting conclusions. The study yielded new information demonstrating that although adolescent drivers have the highest relative odds of involvement in some configuration of crashes, they have the lowest odds of others. Adolescents do have more crashes than adults, and adolescent male drivers have especially high crash rate involvement. Several factors may contribute to adolescent male drivers' greater involvement in single-vehicle and head-on crashes. Compared with female drivers, adolescent male drivers are more likely to speed, which increases their risk of speed-related loss of control resulting from rapidly developing roadway events and curves. This risk is probably exacerbated by young drivers' lack of driving experience. Moreover, evidence suggests that compared with driving alone, adolescents of both sexes drive more slowly with longer following distances when riding with a female passenger. A possible implication of these 2 influences is that a greater proportion of adolescent female drivers' total trips are made either driving alone or with female passengers, both of which are associated with lower speed and longer following distances. In contrast, male adolescents when alone or with male passengers drive in a riskier manner relative to female drivers in similar situations. The net result could be that female adolescents spend more time as drivers in relatively lower-risk conditions than do male adolescents. The authors also suggest that male adolescents' greater risk of single-vehicle and head-on crashes might result from hegemonic masculinity, identity exploration, differing cognitive development, or other social and psychological factors that elevate injury risk. To say this differently, macho male teens tend to be even more macho when they drive.

It is clear that driver education can be redesigned to produce better outcomes.[1] The data from this article should be incorporated into our teachings as part of driver education. Some of the data are not exactly intuitive, thus, data speak more loudly than intuition in such circumstances.

This commentary closes with a couple of questions on teen driving. Based on current survey data, what percentage of those eligible to have a driver's license aged 14 32 do in fact have a driver's license?

A. 6.5%

B. 13%

C. 19.5%

D. 26%

Is this percentage increasing over a recent 8-year period?

A. No, has remained approximately the same

B. Yes

C. No

The answers come from a report in Motor Trend.[2] It appears that the economy or social trends have significantly affected the interest or ability of young people to want to drive. The numbers cycling and walking have dramatically increased. According to the National Household Travel Survey, from 2001 to 2009, the annual number of vehicle miles traveled by young people (16- to 34-year-olds) decreased from 10 300 miles to 7900 miles per capita, a drop of 23 percent. In 2009, 16- to 34-year-olds as a whole took 24 percent more bike trips than they took in 2001, despite the age group actually shrinking in size by 2 percent. In 2009, 16- to 34-year-olds walked to destinations 16 percent more frequently than did 16- to 34-year-olds living in 2001. From 2001 to 2009, the number of passenger-miles traveled by 16- to 34-year-olds on public transit increased by 40 percent.

According to the Federal Highway Administration, from 2000 to 2010, the share of 14- to 34-year-olds without a driver's license increased from 21 percent to 26 percent.

J. A. Stockman III, MD

References

1. Mayhew DR, Simpson HM. The safety value of driver education and training. *Inj Prev.* 2002;8:ii3-ii7.
2. Lassa T. Is the automobile over? *Motor Trend.* 2012;8:20.

2 Allergy and Dermatology

Acupuncture in Patients With Seasonal Allergic Rhinitis: A Randomized Trial

Brinkhaus B, Ortiz M, Witt CM, et al (Charité Univ Med Ctr, Berlin, Germany; et al)
Ann Intern Med 158.225-234, 2013

Background.—Acupuncture is frequently used to treat seasonal allergic rhinitis (SAR) despite limited scientific evidence.

Objective.—To evaluate the effects of acupuncture in patients with SAR.

Design.—Randomized, controlled multicenter trial. (ClinicalTrials.gov: NCT00610584)

Setting.—46 specialized physicians in 6 hospital clinics and 32 private outpatient clinics.

Patients.—422 persons with SAR and IgE sensitization to birch and grass pollen.

Intervention.—Acupuncture plus rescue medication (RM) (cetirizine) ($n = 212$), sham acupuncture plus RM ($n = 102$), or RM alone ($n = 108$). Twelve treatments were provided over 8 weeks in the first year.

Measurements.—Changes in the Rhinitis Quality of Life Questionnaire (RQLQ) overall score and the RM score (RMS) from baseline to weeks 7 and 8 and week 16 in the first year and week 8 in the second year after randomization, with predefined noninferiority margins of -0.5 point (RQLQ) and -1.5 points (RMS).

Results.—Compared with sham acupuncture and with RM, acupuncture was associated with improvement in RQLQ score (sham vs. acupuncture mean difference, 0.5 point [97.5% CI, 0.2 to 0.8 point; $P < 0.001$]; RM vs. acupuncture mean difference, 0.7 point [97.5% CI, 0.4 to 1.0 point; $P < 0.001$]) and RMS (sham vs. acupuncture mean difference, 1.1 points [97.5% CI, 0.4 to 1.9 points; $P < 0.001$]; RM vs. acupuncture mean difference, 1.5 points [97.5% CI, 0.8 to 2.2 points; $P < 0.001$]). There were no differences after 16 weeks in the first year. After the 8-week follow-up phase in the second year, small improvements favoring real acupuncture over the sham procedure were noted (RQLQ mean difference, 0.3 point [95% CI, 0.03 to 0.6 point; $P = 0.032$]; RMS mean difference, 1.0 point [95% CI, 0.2 to 1.9 points; $P = 0.018$]).

Limitation.—The study was not powered to detect rare adverse events, and the RQLQ and RMS values were low at baseline.

Conclusion.—Acupuncture led to statistically significant improvements in disease-specific quality of life and antihistamine use measures after 8 weeks of treatment compared with sham acupuncture and with RM alone, but the improvements may not be clinically significant.

▶ If you suffer from allergic rhinitis, join the rest of the millions the United States who also do. Also join the millions who spend our good money trying to find the best cure for this annoying, at best, problem.

These authors report on the evidence for the efficacy of acupuncture for allergic rhinitis. Before this article appeared, there was relatively little in the literature on this topic. These authors have designed a trial to assess the short-term, midterm, and long-term effects of acupuncture on disease-specific quality of life and the need for antihistamine medication in patients with seasonal allergic rhinitis. The investigators designed a multicenter trial that randomly assigned patients to 8 weeks of acupuncture plus the use of cetirizine or just cetirizine alone. Assessment was made of outcomes at the end of treatment (7-8 weeks), 8 weeks after treatment (at 16 weeks), and after an 8-week period starting at the onset of birch pollen flow in the year after randomization. Patients initially randomly assigned to cetirizine alone received 12 sessions of real acupuncture between 8 and 16 weeks so that all trial groups would receive some form of acupuncture. The study was carried out in Germany. You will need to read the report in detail to see exactly how the acupuncture was performed.

This study found that acupuncture led to statistically significant improvements in disease-specific quality of life and histamine use after 8 weeks of treatment compared with a control acupuncture with cetirizine alone, but the clinical significance of the findings was sufficiently borderline to remain uncertain. It is also possible that individual patient's beliefs about the value of acupuncture could have influenced some of the outcomes in this study, and it was difficult for the investigators to tease this point out.

You will have to be the judge of what marginal clinical significance is. If you suffer from allergic rhinitis, any improvement in your itchy eyes and runny nose might be considered a major improvement.

J. A. Stockman III, MD

Omalizumab for the Treatment Of Chronic Idiopathic or Spontaneous Urticaria

Maurer M, Rosén K, Hsieh H-J, et al (Charité-Universitätsmedizin, Berlin; Genentech, South San Francisco, CA; et al)
N Engl J Med 368:924-935, 2013

Background.—Many patients with chronic idiopathic urticaria (also called chronic spontaneous urticaria) do not have a response to therapy with H_1-antihistamines, even at high doses. In phase 2 trials, omalizumab, an IgE monoclonal antibody that targets IgE and affects mast-cell and basophil function, has shown efficacy in such patients.

Methods.—In this phase 3, multicenter, randomized, double-blind study, we evaluated the efficacy and safety of omalizumab in patients with moderate-to-severe chronic idiopathic urticaria who remained symptomatic despite H_1-antihistamine therapy (licensed doses). We randomly assigned 323 patients to receive three subcutaneous injections, spaced 4 weeks apart, of omalizumab at doses of 75 mg, 150 mg, or 300 mg or placebo, followed by a 16-week observation period. The primary efficacy outcome was the change from baseline in a weekly itch-severity score (ranging from 0 to 21, with higher scores indicating more severe itching).

Results.—The baseline weekly itch-severity score was approximately 14 in all four study groups. At week 12, the mean ($\pm$ SD) change from baseline in the weekly itch-severity score was -5.1 ± 5.6 in the placebo group, -5.9 ± 6.5 in the 75-mg group ($P = 0.46$), -8.1 ± 6.4 in the 150-mg group ($P = 0.001$), and -9.8 ± 6.0 in the 300-mg group ($P < 0.001$). Most prespecified secondary outcomes at week 12 showed similar dose-dependent effects. The frequency of adverse events was similar across groups. The frequency of serious adverse events was low, although the rate was higher in the 300-mg group (6%) than in the placebo group (3%) or in either the 75-mg or 150-mg group (1% for each).

Conclusions.—Omalizumab diminished clinical symptoms and signs of chronic idiopathic urticaria in patients who had remained symptomatic despite the use of approved doses of H_1-antihistamines. (Funded by Genentech and Novartis Pharma; ClinicalTrials.gov number, NCT01292473.)

▶ Both children and adults can suffer from chronic idiopathic or spontaneous urticaria. The terms chronic idiopathic urticaria and chronic spontaneous urticaria are interchangeable and are defined as itchy hives that last for at least 6 weeks, with or without angioedema, and that have no apparent external trigger. Those unfortunate enough to develop this problem generally have it for a lengthy period of time, on average 1 to 5 years. Somewhere between 10% and 15% of patients have persistent chronic urticaria for longer than half a decade. The disorder is associated with a number of other symptomatologies, including lack of energy, emotional upheaval, and often social isolation. Treatment of the disorder has been largely unsatisfactory, although nonsedating H_1 antihistamines may provide some relief. These are the only agents licensed for use in patients with chronic idiopathic urticaria. Most data suggest that the majority of patients do not have a sustained or even immediate response to such antihistamines, however. Alternatives to treatment failure with H_1 antihistamines include the use of H_2 antihistamines, leukotriene-receptor antagonist, systemic steroids, cyclosporine, hydroxychloroquine, dapsone, methotrexate, sulfasalazine, and intravenous immunoglobulin. None of these agents have been approved for use for this purpose, however.

These authors explore the potential of an agent that uses a completely different pathway to manage patients with chronic idiopathic urticaria. It is known that histamine release from skin mast cells is part of the pathogenesis of urticaria. In patients with chronic idiopathic urticaria, basophils and immuno-globulin-E (IgE) may also play an important role. This is where omalizumab comes in. Omalizumab is a recombinant humanized monoclonal antibody approved as an additional therapy for moderate to severe persistent allergic asthma. It reduces the levels of free IgE in the high-affinity receptor for the Fc region of IgE, essential for mast cell and basophil activation. This recombinant agent can suppress allergic-mediated skin reactions through reduction of the high-affinity receptor in basophils and mast cells.

To study the potential benefits of omalizumab for the treatment of chronic idiopathic urticaria, these authors undertook an international, multicenter, randomized, double-blind, placebo-controlled study to examine the efficacy and safety of omalizumab over a 7-month period in adult and adolescent patients (the latter were aged 12 years and older) with chronic idiopathic urticaria who remained symptomatic despite the use of approved H_1 antihistamines. All patients had a history of at least 6 months of chronic idiopathic urticaria that included the presence of hives associated with itching for at least 8 consecutive weeks at any time before enrollment, despite the use of H_1 antihistamines. Three hundred twenty-three patients were randomly assigned to receive 3 subcutaneous injections spaced 4 weeks apart of omalizumab at varying doses.

This study found that omalizumab administered as 3 doses of 150 or 300 mg at 4-week intervals significantly reduced symptoms as compared with placebo. The agent had an onset of action within 1 week after initiation in this patient population. There did not appear to be a rebound increase in symptoms back to baseline during the course of the study once omalizumab was discontinued. The observation that symptoms gradually recurred after discontinuation suggests that the drug in fact was effective by controlling the disorder as long as it was being administered.

The actual mechanism by which omalizumab works to improve urticaria has not been fully elucidated. The mechanism of action is, however, most likely by diminution in the binding of circulating IgE by its receptors. It should be noted that in this study, the number of patients who were treated was too small to draw any definitive conclusions about safety, but no serious problems were found in this trial. Without question, if further evaluation shows that the initial study results with this new recombinant agent hold up, this novel approach to chronic urticaria will be a blessing for affected individuals.

J. A. Stockman III, MD

Oral Immunotherapy for Treatment of Egg Allergy in Children
Burks AW, for the Consortium of Food Allergy Research (CoFAR) (Duke Univ Med Ctr, Durham, NC; et al)
N Engl J Med 367:233-243, 2012

Background.—For egg allergy, dietary avoidance is the only currently approved treatment. We evaluated oral immunotherapy using egg-white powder for the treatment of children with egg allergy.

Methods.—In this double-blind, randomized, placebo-controlled study, 55 children, 5 to 11 years of age, with egg allergy received oral immunotherapy (40 children) or placebo (15). Initial dose-escalation, build-up, and maintenance phases were followed by an oral food challenge with egg-white powder at 10 months and at 22 months. Children who successfully passed the challenge at 22 months discontinued oral immunotherapy and avoided all egg consumption for 4 to 6 weeks. At 24 months, these children underwent an oral food challenge with egg-white powder and a cooked egg to test for sustained unresponsiveness. Children who passed this challenge at 24 months were placed on a diet with ad libitum egg consumption and were evaluated for continuation of sustained unresponsiveness at 30 months and 36 months.

Results.—After 10 months of therapy, none of the children who received placebo and 55% of those who received oral immunotherapy passed the oral food challenge and were considered to be desensitized; after 22 months, 75% of children in the oral-immunotherapy group were desensitized. In the oral-immunotherapy group, 28% (11 of 40 children) passed the oral food challenge at 24 months and were considered to have sustained unresponsiveness. At 30 months and 36 months, all children who had passed the oral food challenge at 24 months were consuming egg. Of the immune markers measured, small wheal diameters on skin-prick testing and increases in egg-specific IgG4 antibody levels were associated with passing the oral food challenge at 24 months.

Conclusions.—These results show that oral immunotherapy can desensitize a high proportion of children with egg allergy and induce sustained unresponsiveness in a clinically significant subset. (Funded by the National Institutes of Health; ClinicalTrials.gov number, NCT00461097.)

▶ The senior author of this report and his colleagues have been leaders in the United States in the area of food allergy desensitization. Food allergies are a common problem in children. Data suggest that egg allergy prevalence runs almost 3% by 2 to 3 years of age, with allergic reactions varying quite a bit in affected individuals. Some may have mild urticaria and others might experience anaphylaxis. Severe allergic reactions can occur with a single bite of a cooked egg (approximately 70 mg of egg protein). Treatment of egg allergy historically has been to restrict the diet so that it is egg free. Needless to say, in American society, such avoidance of eggs is difficult if not impossible.

Alternatives to avoidance diets are being actively investigated. One such approach is allergen immunotherapy designed to produce desensitization and immune tolerance to various allergens. Desensitization, a state in which the threshold dose of food that triggers an allergic reaction is increased during therapy, is more easily achieved. Traditional subcutaneous immunotherapy, effective against certain airborne allergens, is risky for the treatment of food allergy. Oral immunotherapy appears to be safer than subcutaneous immunotherapy for food allergies and is capable of inducing desensitization. Immune tolerance is a much more difficult goal to achieve than desensitization.

The authors of this report did not study the induction of immune tolerance but assessed what they called "sustained unresponsiveness" defined as the ability, after 22 months of oral immunotherapy and subsequent avoidance of egg consumption for 4 to 6 weeks, to consume 10 g of egg white powder and a whole cooked egg without clinically significant symptoms. In addition, children who passed the oral food challenge at 24 months were then placed on an ad libitum diet and were followed up for 12 more months. The study undertaken was a multicenter, double-blind, randomized, placebo-controlled trial of the effectiveness and safety of oral immunotherapy, including its capacity to induce sustained unresponsiveness in children with egg allergy. Eligible participants were 5 to 18 years of age and had a convincing clinical history of egg allergy as shown by the development of allergic symptoms within minutes to hours after ingesting egg and a serum egg-specific IgE antibody level of more than 5 kU/L in children 6 years of age or older or 12 kU/L or more for those 5 years old. Children with a history of severe anaphylaxis after egg consumption were excluded. The levels of IgE antibody chosen for inclusion were selected to exclude children who were likely to outgrow the allergy during the course of the study. The protocol for oral immunotherapy consisted of 3 phases: an initial-day dose escalation, a build-up phase, and a maintenance phase during which participants ingested up to 2 g of egg white powder per day, which is the approximate equivalent of one-third of an egg. The children and their families were instructed that the child should avoid egg consumption other than oral immunotherapy. The severity of allergic reactions was reported with the use of a customized grading system with scores ranging from 1 (transient or mild discomfort) to 5 (death)! The average age of enrollment was 7 years. A total of 91% report at least 1 additional food allergy.

The results of this study were impressive. Unlike previous studies, these investigators enrolled a substantial number of children at multiple sites across the United States and observed sustained unresponsiveness in a double-blind, randomized, controlled study design that included long-term follow-up. As expected, none of the children with egg allergy who received placebo showed improvement, whereas more than half of those who received oral immunotherapy passed the oral food challenge and were considered to be desensitized. At 30 months and 36 months, all children who had passed the oral food challenge at 24 months were able to consume egg without difficulty. The study results clearly indicated that oral immunotherapy is capable of desensitizing a fair percentage of children with egg allergy and can do so with sustained effectiveness. It is not known whether children who had good responses would maintain these responses if ad libitum egg consumption was discontinued. It is not likely that those participating in this study had spontaneously outgrown egg allergy, because the control group did not. It should be noted that some patients did have allergic reactions during the course of the study. The reactions were of such significant clinical consequences that 15% of children who received oral immunotherapy did not complete the therapy, in most cases because of the allergic reactions. The mechanisms underlying the success of oral immunotherapy in some and failure in others remain unknown.

The authors of this report, although pleased with the results, do say that for oral immunotherapy to be recommended as a standard of care, it is important to better define the risks of this approach versus allergen avoidance, determine the dosing effects with the most favorable outcomes, identify patients who are most likely to benefit from oral immunotherapy, and develop postdesensitization strategies that promote long-term immune tolerance.

J. A. Stockman III, MD

Eczema Herpeticum in Children: Clinical Features and Factors Predictive of Hospitalization

Luca NJC, Lara-Corrales I, Pope E (Univ of Toronto, Ontario, Canada)

J Pediatr 161:671 675, 2012

Objective.—To describe the clinical characteristics of pediatric patients with eczema herpeticum and to determine the predictors of hospitalization, and recurrence and repeat episodes.

Study Design.—A retrospective cohort study of patients 0-18 years of age diagnosed with eczema herpeticum between May 2000 and April 2009 was carried out at a tertiary pediatric care center in Canada. Seventy-nine patients were included. The primary outcome was hospitalization; secondary outcomes were recurrent and repeat episodes of eczema herpeticum.

Results.—At presentation, 76% of 79 patients with eczema herpeticum had a generalized eruption, 56% had fever, 37% had systemic symptoms, and 10% had eye involvement (keratoconjunctivitis). Forty-five patients (57%) were hospitalized. Predictors for hospitalization included male sex (OR = 3.09; 95% CI, 1.20-7.95, P = .017), fever (OR = 5.75; 95% CI, 2.17-15.26, P < .001), systemic symptoms (OR = 2.84; 95% CI, 1.06-7.62, P = .035), and age < 1 year (OR = 7.17; 95% CI, 2.17-23.72, P = .001). Recurrence rate (< 1 month) was 8.9% and rate of repeat episodes (> 1 month) was 16%. Hospitalized patients were more likely to have a repeat episode (OR = 8.25; 95% CI, 0.99-68.69, P = .05). Patients with a previous history of eczema herpeticum had increased likelihood of early recurrence (OR = 6.80; 95% CI, 0.99-46.62, P = .05) and repeat episodes (OR = 9.43; 95% CI, 1.52-55.9, P = .01).

Conclusions.—Predictors of hospitalization in this cohort included male sex, age < 1 year, fever, and systemic symptoms at presentation. Hospitalized patients may be at risk for repeat episodes of eczema herpeticum.

▶ Most pediatric care providers do not see much in the way of eczema herpeticum these days. One wonders why, because atopic dermatitis is such a common dermatologic condition in children. Eczema herpeticum itself refers to herpes simplex virus (HSV) 1 or 2 infection superimposed on the skin of a child with atopic dermatitis. The disorder is not really all that rare and is said to have an incidence of 3% to 6% of patients with atopic dermatitis. Most of the cases involve youngsters who are younger than 3 years of age. The presentation is that of a distinct monomorphic eruption of dome-shaped vesicles that are generally found in the setting of fever, malaise, and lymphadenopathy. The disorder usually starts in areas affected by atopic dermatitis (the head, neck, and trunk), but lesions subsequently spread over many other parts of the body that had previously normal skin. The spread occurs for a week to 10 days. The skin manifestations can linger for many weeks, with vesicles beginning to crust and then forming eroded pits that fortunately heal without scarring unless there is serious bacterial superinfection, particularly that caused by *Staphylococcus aureus*, *Streptococcus pyogenes*, and *Pseudomonas aeruginosa*. The eye can be involved, causing a serious problem. The worst cases occur when the HSV infection results in multiple organ involvement, meningitis, and/or encephalitis. Mortality rates of close to 10% have been described, although management with antiviral agents has reduced complication rates significantly. Acyclovir is the treatment of choice. This drug can be given orally or intravenously.

Luca et al tell us about a retrospective cohort study of pediatric age patients (0 to 18 years) diagnosed with eczema herpeticum. The data from this report tell us a lot more about the presentation and course of eczema herpeticum than many previous reports have. It is no surprise that we learn that hospitalization rates are much higher in patients 1 year of age and younger as well as in those with fever and/or systemic symptoms at presentation. The average age of patients in this report was 0.6 years. One-third of patients presented before 1 year of age. In this study, one-third of patients with eczema herpeticum already had a personal history of HSV or known contact with a caregiver with HSV prior to the clinical presentation of eczema herpeticum.

There has been a lot of speculation about risk factors for the development of eczema herpeticum including that of a relationship between the topical treatment of atopic dermatitis with either corticosteroids or calcineurin inhibitors. The authors of this report found no evidence that the use of topical steroids in any potency or of calcineurin inhibitors was associated with more severe disease requiring hospitalization. In general, however, it seems wise not to use steroids or calcineurin inhibitors after a diagnosis has been made of eczema herpeticum. Other interesting findings from this report are a rate of recurrence (within 1 month) of eczema herpeticum of 8.9% and a rate of repeated episodes (after 1 month) of 16%. Thus youngsters who seem to be out of the woods with their first bout of eczema herpeticum may wind up coming back to haunt a care provider with 1 or more recurrences.

J. A. Stockman III, MD

Fish Consumption in Infancy and Asthma-like Symptoms at Preschool Age
Kiefte-de Jong JC, de Vries JH, Franco OH, et al (Erasmus Med Ctr, Rotterdam; Dept of Human Nutrition, Wageningen, Netherlands)
Pediatrics 130:1060-1068, 2012

Objective.—To assess whether timing of introduction of fish and the amount of fish consumption in infancy were associated with asthmalike symptoms at preschool age.

Methods.—This study was embedded in the Generation R study (a population-based birth cohort in Rotterdam, Netherlands). At the age of 12 and 14 months, timing of introduction of fish into the infant's diet was assessed. The amount of fish consumption at 14 months was assessed by a semiquantitative food frequency questionnaire. Presence of asthma-like symptoms in the past year was assessed at the child's age of 36 and 48 months.

Results.—Relative to no introduction in the first year of life, introduction between age 6 and 12 months was significantly associated with a lower risk of wheezing at 48 months (odds ratio [OR]: 0.64; 95% CI: 0.43—0.94). When compared with introduction between 6 and 12 months, no introduction in the first year and introduction between 0 and 6 months were associated with an increased risk of wheezing at 48 months (OR: 1.57; 95% CI: 1.07—2.31 and OR: 1.53; 95% CI: 1.07—2.19, respectively). The amount of fish at age 14 months was not associated with asthmalike symptoms (*P* > .15).

Conclusions.—Introduction of fish between 6 and 12 months but not fish consumption afterward is associated with a lower prevalence of wheezing. A window of exposure between the age of 6 and 12 months might exist in which fish might be associated with a reduced risk of asthma.

▶ There has been much written about the impact of early diet and its composition on the subsequent development of reactive airway disease. It has been suggested that the increasing widespread use of a Western diet in young children can be one of the reasons related to the increased prevalence of asthma.

These authors are from the Netherlands, where there is an interesting ongoing study looking at a number of life characteristics from birth through early adulthood, including the impact of diet on health. These authors use data from the Generation R study to determine whether the timing of introduction of fish in the first year of life, as well as fish consumption afterward, might be associated with the development of asthma-like symptoms at preschool age. The study shows that introduction of fish between 6 and 12 months, but not the amount of fish servings later in life, was associated with a lower prevalence of wheezing in preschool children. Absence of fish in the diet in the first year of life, or introduction between 0 and 6 months of age, was in fact associated with an increased prevalence of asthma-like symptoms.

There are studies to suggest that there are protective effects of fish and fish-related fatty acids during pregnancy on the development of asthma in children, so the findings in this article are somewhat consistent with earlier data. The study itself suggests that appropriate timing of introduction of fish, rather than the amount of fish servings after 12 months, is important in the association with wheezing. Underlying mechanisms why fish may protect against asthma are at best speculative.

Obviously fish is a great source of polyunsaturated fatty acids. Several studies have suggested that polyunsaturated fatty acids can have an immunoregulatory or anti-inflammatory set of properties. Unfortunately, the optimal intake of polyunsaturated fatty acids in children remains controversial. More than 10 years ago, the Institute of Medicine concluded that there was insufficient evidence to provide clear recommendations on polyunsaturated fatty acid intake in children, although the Technical Committee on Dietary Lipids of the International

Life Sciences Institute of North America made a recommendation in 2009 that the daily intake of specific polyunsaturated fatty acids be between 250 and 500 mg per day to reduce the risk of coronary heart disease later in life.[1]

There may be a specific window of opportunity between the ages of 6 and 12 months in which fish consumption might protect against the later development of asthma. The data from this study suggest a 36% lower prevalence of asthma in those preschool children who had begun to consume fish in the second half of the first year of life. These authors are to be congratulated for mining data from the Generation R study, which is a prospective cohort study from fetal life until young adulthood in a multiethnic urban population in the Netherlands. The study is designed to identify early environmental and genetic causes of normal and abnormal growth and development and overall health from fetal life until young adulthood. The results will be forthcoming from the Generation R study, and they will contribute to the creation of strategies for optimizing health and health care for pregnant women and children.

Many may not be familiar with the various alphabets that have been used with the term "generation." It all started with generation X. The latter term was coined by the Magnum photographer Robert Capa in the early 1950s to describe young men and women growing up immediately somewhat after World War II. Generation Xers are also known as "baby busters" because of the drop in the birth rate following the baby boom immediately after World War II. By the way, generation Y, also known as the millennial generation, is the demographic cohort immediately following generation X. This usually involves those born from the early 1980s to the early 2000s. Generation Z is the generation that grew up as young children during the post-9/11 period and also during the wars in Afghanistan and Iraq. It is generally accepted that the current generation R refers to a term coined to describe frustrated professionals who have survived the recent recession and who have progressed faster than usual during the recession by taking on the work of more senior X colleagues and are now pushing for higher pay and recognition to match. Is there no end to the alphabet?

J. A. Stockman III, MD

Reference

1. Harris WS, Mozaffarian D, Lefevre M, et al. Towards establishing dietary reference intakes for eicosapentaenoic and docosahexaenoic acids. *J Nutr.* 2009;139: 804S-819S.

Breastfeeding Protects against Current Asthma up to 6 Years of Age
Silvers KM, on behalf of the New Zealand Asthma and Allergy Cohort Study Group (Univ of Otago Christchurch, New Zealand; et al)
J Pediatr 160:991-996.e1, 2012

Objective.—To investigate the effects of breastfeeding on wheezing and current asthma in children 2 to 6 years of age.

Study Design.—Infants (n = 1105) were enrolled in a prospective birth cohort in New Zealand. Detailed information about infant feeding was collected using questionnaires administered at birth and at 3, 6, and 15 months. From this, durations of exclusive and any breastfeeding were calculated. Information about wheezing and current asthma was collected at 2, 3, 4, 5, and 6 years. Logistic regression was used to model associations between breastfeeding and outcomes with and without adjustment for confounders.

Results.—After adjustment for confounders, each month of exclusive breastfeeding was associated with significant reductions in current asthma from 2 to 6 years (all, $P < .03$). Current asthma at 2, 3, and 4 years was also reduced by each month of any breastfeeding (all, $P < .005$). In atopic children, exclusive breastfeeding for ≥ 3 months reduced current asthma at ages 4, 5, and 6 by 62%, 55%, and 59%, respectively.

Conclusion.—Breastfeeding, particularly exclusive breastfeeding, protects against current asthma up to 6 years. Although exclusive breastfeeding reduced risk of current asthma in all children to age 6, the degree of protection beyond 3 years was more pronounced in atopic children.

▶ There has been a lot written about the potential relationship of breastfeeding and the development of asthma. The literature unfortunately gives a mixed message in that the data appear to be conflicting. The literature tends to support the fact that breastfeeding will protect against wheezing in infancy and early childhood, but the effect of breastfeeding on asthma in older children remains a bit murky. Some studies have suggested breastfeeding does protect against asthma, whereas others have shown little or no effect at any age. A meta-analysis observed that breastfeeding did reduce the risk of asthma in young children and that the protective effect was larger in children with a family history of atopy.[1] Silvers et al[2] abstracted a previously published study showing a strong protective effect of breastfeeding on adverse respiratory outcomes, including asthma, in New Zealand children aged 15 months using comprehensive breastfeeding data. In this article, investigators studied whether breastfeeding continues to protect against current asthma and wheezing in children up to 6 years of age. In addition, these investigators explored the relationships in children with and without atopy and a family history of allergic disease. The results of the study showed that breastfeeding, particularly exclusive breastfeeding, continues to protect against current asthma between the ages of 2 and 6 years. Although the degree of protection for each month of exclusive breastfeeding across the whole group decreased from 21% at 15 months to around 9% at 6 years, it is important to note the magnitude of these findings. If every infant in this study cohort had been exclusively breastfed for 6 months, as is the current recommendation of the World Health Organization, current asthma rates would have been reduced by 50% at 2 years, 42% at 3 years, 30% at 4 years, 42% at 5 years, and 32% at 6 years. Despite finding no association between breastfeeding and atopy, children with atopy were much more likely than nonatopic children to have current asthma at 4, 5, and 6 years, but if they had been exclusively breastfed for at least 3 months, their risk would have been reduced to approximately that of nonatopic children.

This study was well done. The data collection was prospective, and there were good retention rates and sufficient statistical power. The breastfeeding information collected was comprehensive and the definition of exclusive breastfeeding was rigorous. Although it is possible that the strong protective effect of breast-feeding is seen only in populations where there is a high prevalence of asthma and allergy, it is likely that breastfeeding would be protective where the preva-lence of a positive family history is relatively low. The data do not appear to support the hypothesis that breastfeeding only protects the infant against virus-induced wheezing episode in early life.

It is fair to say that breastfeeding, particularly exclusive breastfeeding, will protect against current asthma up to 6 years of age in a high proportion of chil-dren. The degree of protection after 3 years of age will be expected to be more pronounced in atopic children.

J. A. Stockman III, MD

References

1. Gdalevich M, Mimouni D, Mimouni M. Breast-feeding and the risk of bronchial asthma in children: a systematic review with meta-analysis of prospective studies. *J Pediatr.* 2001;139:261-266.
2. Silvers KM, Frampton CM, Wickens K, et al. Breastfeeding protects against adverse respiratory outcomes at 15 months of age. *Matern Child Nutr.* 2009;5: 243-250.

Efficacy and Safety of Vismodegib in Advanced Basal-Cell Carcinoma
Sekulic A, Migden MR, Oro AE, et al (Mayo Clinic, Scottsdale, AZ; M.D. Anderson Cancer Ctr, Houston, TX; Stanford Univ School of Medicine, CA; et al)
N Engl J Med 366:2171-2179, 2012

Background.—Alterations in hedgehog signaling are implicated in the pathogenesis of basal-cell carcinoma. Although most basal-cell carci-nomas are treated surgically, no effective therapy exists for locally advanced or metastatic basal-cell carcinoma. A phase 1 study of vismode-gib (GDC-0449), a first-in-class, small-molecule inhibitor of the hedgehog pathway, showed a 58% response rate among patients with advanced basal-cell carcinoma.

Methods.—In this multicenter, international, two-cohort, nonrandom-ized study, we enrolled patients with metastatic basal-cell carcinoma and those with locally advanced basal-cell carcinoma who had inoperable disease or for whom surgery was inappropriate (because of multiple recur-rences and a low likelihood of surgical cure, or substantial anticipated disfigurement). All patients received 150 mg of oral vismodegib daily. The primary end point was the independently assessed objective response rate; the primary hypotheses were that the response rate would be greater than 20% for patients with locally advanced basal-cell carcinoma and greater than 10% for those with metastatic basal-cell carcinoma.

Results.—In 33 patients with metastatic basal-cell carcinoma, the independently assessed response rate was 30% (95% confidence interval [CI], 16 to 48; $P = 0.001$). In 63 patients with locally advanced basal-cell carcinoma, the independently assessed response rate was 43% (95% CI, 31 to 56; $P < 0.001$), with complete responses in 13 patients (21%). The median duration of response was 7.6 months in both cohorts. Adverse events occurring in more than 30% of patients were muscle spasms, alopecia, dysgeusia (taste disturbance), weight loss, and fatigue. Serious adverse events were reported in 25% of patients; seven deaths due to adverse events were noted.

Conclusions.—Vismodegib is associated with tumor responses in patients with locally advanced or metastatic basal-cell carcinoma. (Funded by Genentech; Erivance BCC ClinicalTrials.gov number, NCT00833417.)

▶ This article about basal cell carcinoma may seem out of place in a pediatric review, but in fact, children can inherit what is known as the heritable basal cell nevus syndrome (Gorlin syndrome; Online Mendelian Inheritance in Man 10 940). Children carrying this genetic aberration may eventually become adults who have hundreds to thousands of basal cell carcinomas on their bodies. Those affected with this syndrome are at increased risk for medulloblastomas and rhabdomyosarcomas.[1] Patients with basal cell nevus syndrome inherit 1 defective copy of the tumor-suppressor gene encoding patched 1 (*PTCH1*), which acts as a primary inhibitor of what is known as the hedgehog signaling pathway. *PTCH1* mutations and loss of the remaining wild type allele can also occur in sporadic basal cell carcinomas. Essentially all basal cell carcinomas, whether or not they are associated with identifiable mutations, demonstrate enhanced hedgehog signaling. Currently, no pharmacologic therapy is consistently efficacious for basal cell carcinomas, and the quality of life for patients with basal cell nevus syndrome is severely diminished by the need for frequent, repetitive, and scarring surgical procedures. In 2006, more than 2 million new cases of nonmelanoma skin cancer were treated in the United States, the majority of which were basal cell carcinomas, although only a few of these occurred in patients with Gorlin syndrome. Basal cell carcinomas can, on rare occurrence, become metastatic.

These authors report on the effects of a new agent, vismodegib, in basal cell carcinoma. This agent is a low-molecular-weight systemic inhibitor of the hedgehog signaling pathway that was approved by the Food and Drug Administration in January 2012 for the treatment of locally advanced or metastatic basal cell carcinomas. The drug is particularly suitable for patients with basal cell nevus syndrome, whose large numbers of basal cell carcinomas represent a substantial physical and psychological burden. The investigators tested the anti—basal cell carcinoma efficacy and safety of vismodegib in patients with basal cell nevus syndrome, reporting results from a phase II trial. Among 33 patients with metastatic basal cell carcinoma, the response rate was 30%. Among 63 patients with locally advanced basal cell carcinoma, the response rate was 43%, with 13 complete responses (21%). Adverse events were seen in more than 30% of patients, including muscle spasms, alopecia, and taste disturbance. The agent reduced the rate of new basal cell carcinomas by almost 90%.

The remarkable effects of vismodegib, particularly in patients with basal cell nevus syndrome, document that this therapy is tailor-made for patients with basal cell nevus syndrome. However, the side effects are considerable and frequent, resulting in high rates of drug discontinuation, and these rates will probably be even higher in clinical practice. Furthermore, there is the question of whether inhibition of the hedgehog pathway truly clears basal cell carcinomas or whether it leaves clones of resistant cells with the potential for recurrence or rebound. There are a number of other hedgehog pathway inhibitors under investigation, and it will be interesting to see what the differences are that emerge, particularly with respect to side effects. Nonetheless, in patients who have large locally advanced basal cell carcinomas, the usefulness of local control and improving quality of life should not be underestimated. One of the questions to be resolved is whether early institution in the natural history of basal cell nevus syndrome will make any difference on the long term. Hopefully this study signals good news for children with the affected mutation so they can grow to be adults without the current problems affected patients have as a result of inheriting Gorlin syndrome.

J. A. Stockman III, MD

Reference

1. Gorlin RJ. Nevoid basal-cell carcinoma syndrome. *Medicine*. 1987;66:98-113.

Petechiae/Purpura in Well-Appearing Infants
Lee MH, Barnett PL (Royal Children's Hosp, Victoria, Australia)
Pediatr Emerg Care 28:503-505, 2012

Background.—Well infants with petechiae and/or purpura can present to emergency departments, and their management can be difficult. Many will have extensive investigations and treatment that may not be necessary.

Methods.—This was a retrospective and descriptive audit investigating well infants (< 8 months of age) presenting with petechiae or purpura in the absence of fever to a pediatric emergency department over a 9½-year period. All presenting problems of petechiae or purpura were reviewed. Patients were excluded if they appeared unwell, were febrile or have a history of fever, or had eccyhmoses on presentation.

Results.—Thirty-six babies were identified. The average age was 3.8 months (range, 1−7 months). The majority of the infants had localized purpura/petechiae to the lower limbs (92%) with two thirds of these patients having bilateral signs. None had generalized signs. Most infants had a full blood count (94%), coagulation profile (59%) and C-reactive protein (59%), and blood cultures (59%), with all being normal (except for mild elevation in platelets). Nine patients were admitted for observation, with only 1 patient having progression of signs. This patient had a diagnosis of acute hemorrhagic edema of infancy. The rest of the patients were thought to have either a mechanical reason for their petechiae/purpura (tourniquet phenomena) or a formal diagnosis was not specified.

Conclusions.—Well infants with localized purpura and/or petechiae with an absence of fever are more likely to have a benign etiology. Further study is required to determine if a full blood count and coagulation profile is necessary, or a period of observation (4 hours) is all that is required. If there is no progression of signs, it is likely that they can be safely discharged. The likely cause may be due to a tourniquet phenomenon (eg, diaper) (Table 2).

▶ The clinical finding of petechiae and/or purpura will put chills down the spines of many care providers given the concern about the association of these findings with meningococcal disease. There are, however, many other causes of petechiae or purpura in children including immune thrombocytopenic purpura and Henoch-Schoenlein purpura. Localized petechiae or purpura may also be related to accidental or self-inflicted injury or child abuse. Generally speaking, in nonmobile infants, especially those younger than 8 months, petechiae or purpura caused by accidental injury should be considered extremely uncommon.

Lee et al describe infants younger than 8 months of age who presented to the emergency room at the Royal Children's Hospital in Victoria, Australia, with petechiae or purpura without fever. Their review was a retrospective one in which the researchers gathered data by searching electronic medical records for the words petechiae, bruising, purpura, and nonblanching rash. The investigators were able to find a total of 36 well appearing babies who had evidence of petechiae and/or purpura. Ninety-two percent of these infants presented with petechiae or purpura in a lower-limb distribution, with the majority (58%) presenting with bilateral findings. Most patients (61%) presented with a petechial rash and 12% presented with mixed petechial and purpuric lesions. Virtually all the patients had a complete blood count and none showed abnormalities in the platelet count. In addition, almost 70% had a coagulation screen. All results were normal except for 2 patients with increased fibrinogen levels. Most patients also had blood cultures taken. All of these were negative. Three patients had extensive platelet function testing. These were normal. One third of the infants were reported by their parents to have current symptoms consistent with a viral illness or recently had such an illness. The most common symptoms were respiratory.

TABLE 2.—Provisional Diagnoses

Diagnosis	No. Babies (%)
Mechanical cause	10 (28)
Viral illness	9 (25)
Either mechanical or viral	3 (8)
No diagnosis	11 (31)
Other	3 (8)

Children younger than 8 months were specifically targeted in this study as the age group presents the greatest diagnostic difficulty and also has the highest mortality from meningococcal septicemia. The authors suggest that well-appearing infants with normal laboratory studies can be observed for a minimum of 4 hours and then discharged home after reassessment. The authors do note that although meningococcal disease usually presents with a generalized petechial rash, isolated petechiae can occur.

The authors of this report conclude that conservative management seems appropriate if an infant with petechiae/purpura appears well and if the lesions are localized to a single limb. It is unclear from this report whether patients should have a comprehensive testing for clotting disorders such as mild von Willebrand disease. Obviously this decision can be deferred to a recurrence of symptoms. Table 2 provides the provisional diagnoses that appeared on patients' charts. The major mechanical cause listed was a tourniquet effect resulting from a tight diaper—presumably the elasticized area around each leg.

J. A. Stockman III, MD

Anti−Interleukin-17 Monoclonal Antibody Ixekizumab in Chronic Plaque Psoriasis

Leonardi C, Matheson R, Zachariae C, et al (Saint Louis Univ School of Medicine, MO; Oregon Med Res Ctr PC, Portland; Univ Hosp of Copenhagen Gentofte, Hellerup; et al)

N Engl J Med 366:1190-1199, 2012

Background.—Type 17 helper T cells have been suggested to play a pathological role in psoriasis. They secrete several proinflammatory cytokines, including interleukin-17A (also known as interleukin-17). We evaluated the safety and efficacy of ixekizumab (LY2439821), a humanized anti−interleukin-17 monoclonal antibody, for psoriasis treatment.

Methods.—In our phase 2, double-blind, placebo-controlled trial, we randomly assigned 142 patients with chronic moderate-to-severe plaque psoriasis to receive subcutaneous injections of 10, 25, 75, or 150 mg of ixekizumab or placebo at 0, 2, 4, 8, 12, and 16 weeks. The primary end point was the proportion of patients with reduction in the psoriasis area-and-severity index (PASI) score by at least 75% at 12 weeks. Secondary end points included the proportion of patients with reduction in the PASI score by at least 90% or by 100%.

Results.—At 12 weeks, the percentage of patients with a reduction in the PASI score by at least 75% was significantly greater with ixekizumab (except with the lowest, 10-mg dose) — 150 mg (82.1%), 75 mg (82.8%), and 25 mg (76.7%) — than with placebo (7.7%, $P < 0.001$ for each comparison), as was the percentage of patients with a reduction in the PASI score by at least 90%: 150 mg (71.4%), 75 mg (58.6%), and 25 mg (50.0%) versus placebo (0%, $P < 0.001$ for each comparison). Similarly, a 100% reduction in the PASI score was achieved in significantly more patients in the 150-mg group (39.3%) and the 75-mg group (37.9%) than in the placebo group

(0%) ($P < 0.001$ for both comparisons). Significant differences occurred at as early as 1 week and were sustained through 20 weeks. Adverse events occurred in 63% of patients in both the combined ixekizumab groups and in the placebo group. No serious adverse events or major cardiovascular events were observed.

Conclusions.—Use of a humanized anti–interleukin-17 monoclonal antibody, ixekizumab, improved the clinical symptoms of psoriasis. Further studies are needed to establish its long-term safety and efficacy in patients with psoriasis. (Funded by Eli Lilly; ClinicalTrials.gov number, NCT01107457.)

▶ These authors have reported on the results of 2 phase II clinical trials in which patients with psoriasis were treated with antibodies directed against interleukin-17 or its receptor. Included were patients 18 years of age and older as well as young and middle-age adults. The investigators used a humanized anti-interleukin 17 monoclonal antibody. In a related article, Papp et al[1] used a humanized monoclonal antibody directed against interleukin-17RA, another of the 6 members of the interleukin-17A through interleukin-17F family. Papp et al also treated older teenagers and adults with psoriasis. The 2 studies are quite similar in design. After 12 weeks on protocol, the results of both trials showed that patients receiving either antibody had marked improvements in clinical scores used to rate the severity of psoriasis. Few adverse effects were observed, and very few patients had to withdraw from the trials.

Interleukin-17 is a cytokine that belongs to a family of interleukins that bind a total of 5 receptors. The first of these interleukins was identified in 1993 as a cytokine that had the ability to mediate the production of chemokines and subsequently the recruitment of neutrophils to sites of inflammation. The main physiologic function of this cytokine is to provide protection against infectious disease. Mice that are deficient in interleukin-17 are highly susceptible to infection by certain bacterial and fungal organisms. Similarly, mice that lack the expression of the receptor for interleukin have severe host defense deficiencies against both bacteria and fungi. Interleukin-17 induces a broad tissue response, leading to neutrophil trafficking to the sites of inflammation. Interleukin itself can be produced by a variety of cells but is produced in the greatest amounts by type 17 helper T cells and gamma-delta T cells. Interleukin-17 can be suppressed by administration of antibodies against it or its receptor. These have been used recently in a number of protocols as part of the management of autoimmune diseases.

One particular interleukin, interleukin-22, will result in an inflammatory response that mimics psoriasis. It has been shown that psoriasis can be prevented by the administration of antibodies targeting interleukin-22. Most likely, psoriasis is a disorder that depends not solely on either interleukin-17 signaling or interleukin-22, but on both. Targeting interleukin-17 signaling also affects interleukin-22, because both need to work in concert for full-blown psoriasis to develop.

Chances are we will be seeing more and more use of cytokine inhibitors as part of the management of immune-mediated disorders, including those of the skin, such as psoriasis. Needless to say, further studies are required to determine the long-term safety and efficacy of such inhibitors.

J. A. Stockman III, MD

Reference

1. Papp KA, Leonardi C, Menter A, et al. Brodalumab, an anti-interleukin-17-receptor antibody for psoriasis. N Engl J Med. 2012;366:1181-1189.

Topical 0.5% Ivermectin Lotion for Treatment of Head Lice

Pariser DM, Meinking TL, Bell M, et al (Eastern Virginia Med School, Norfolk, VA; Global Health Association of Miami, Coral Gables, FL; Clin-Data Services, Fort Collins, CO; et al)

N Engl J Med 367:1687-1693, 2012

Background.—The emergence of resistance to treatment complicates the public health problem of head-louse infestations and drives the need for continuing development of new treatments. There are limited data on the activity of ivermectin as a topical lousicide.

Methods.—In two multisite, randomized, double-blind studies, we compared a single application of 0.5% ivermectin lotion with vehicle control for the elimination of infestations without nit combing in patients 6 months of age or older. A tube of topical ivermectin or vehicle control was dispensed on day 1, to be applied to dry hair, left for 10 minutes, then rinsed with water. The primary end point was the percentage of index patients (youngest household member with ≥3 live lice) in the intention-to-treat population who were louse-free 1 day after treatment (day 2) and remained so through days 8 and 15.

Results.—A total of 765 patients completed the studies. In the intention-to-treat population, significantly more patients receiving ivermectin than patients receiving vehicle control were louse-free on day 2 (94.9% vs. 31.3%), day 8 (85.2% vs. 20.8%), and day 15 (73.8% vs. 17.6%) ($P < 0.001$ for each comparison). The frequency and severity of adverse events were similar in the two groups.

Conclusions.—A single, 10-minute, at-home application of ivermectin was more effective than vehicle control in eliminating head-louse infestations at 1, 7, and 14 days after treatment. (Funded by Topaz Pharmaceuticals [now Sanofi Pasteur]; ClinicalTrials.gov numbers, NCT01066585 and NCT01068158.)

▶ Any study that is able to round up 765 patients with head lice is a study to be paid attention to. Infestation with Pediculus humanus capitis is no laughing matter, stigmatizing hundreds of millions of people worldwide, mostly children in the preschool and middle school age. Every socioeconomic class is affected, even though head lice are commonly considered to be a sign of poor hygiene. The medical consequences of such an infestation often involve more than itching and scratching. The latter can lead to bacterial superinfection resulting in a pyoderma or impetigo. Recall that Bartonella quintana, the organism causing trench-fever, is also transmitted by body lice. The annual overall cost of head louse infestation in our country is more than the budget of a number of emerging nations.

If you are not familiar with the head louse, it is an obligate, blood-sucking ectoparasite that feeds 3 to 6 times daily. The female louse lays up to 300 eggs during her lifespan (approximately 1 month). An egg, once laid, hatches and releases nymphs that become adults in a week to 10 days. Transmission is usually direct head-to-head contact, and for this reason the ideal treatment is simultaneous management of all infested contacts (eg, household members and classmates). Failure to achieve such group treatment is the most frequent cause of head lice infestation treatment failure. It is additionally possible to become infected via indirect transmission via fomites such as bed linens, but this is a rare occurrence and is easily preventable because the female louse dies within hours after being separated from her host and machine laundering at a temperature of 122°F will kill all lice and nits.

Since the 1980s, the most commonly available treatment formulations to treat head lice include 1% permethrin and pyrethrins plus piperonyl butoxide. These agents have up to 95% effectiveness. In the 1990s, 0.5% malathion lotion was shown to achieve a better louse-free rate than previously used agents. It should be noted that pyrethroids are neurotoxins in that they modify louse voltage-gated sodium channels causing spastic paralysis and death. These agents have a rapid immobilizing effect, called knockdown, which often precedes lethality. The louse has developed a knockdown resistance ranging from 0% to 100%, depending on regions where the lice are found. For example, in Florida, California, and Texas, knockdown resistance is almost 100%. Genetic resistance, however, is not totally predictive of clinical or parasitologic failure. This resistance is one of the reasons why malathion use became more popular starting about 12 years ago. Other potential topical agents now include iver-mectin, an agent initially used to treat onchocerciasis and lymphatic filariasis.

Pariser et al describe 2 randomized, controlled trials comparing a single appli-cation of 0.5% ivermectin lotion with a control vehicle in patients 6 months of age or older. The louse-free rate at day 15 was 73.8% among index patients (vs 17.6% among control vehicle recipients). Patients were deloused rapidly (94.9% on day 2). The topical drug formulation is considered to have less risk of systemic adverse events in comparison with oral ivermectin. The lotion fórmulation is convenient, applied to dry hair, left for 10 minutes, and then rinsed with water. Notably, a randomized controlled trial in which malathion lotion was applied for 8 to 10 hours on parent and child volunteers achieved a compliance rate of just 50%, meaning that ivermectin is much more likely to achieve full compliance.

In 2010, the American Academy of Pediatrics made a recommendation to use 1% permethrin or pyrethrin insecticide as first-line therapy for head lice.[1] This recommendation also includes the observation that if resistance in a community that is proven or if live lice are present one day after completion of treatment, malathion may be necessary. Other options include wet combing or treatment with dimethicone or other topical agents. Nit removal has been proven to be useful.

In an editorial that accompanied the report of Pariser et al, Chosidow and Giraudeau suggest that ivermectin should be used last in the treatment of head lice employing topical lotions for still-infested persons or oral therapy for mass treatment.[2] Management should also include frequent checking for head louse infestation in families and in schools. These recommendations seem to make sense.

J. A. Stockman III, MD

References

1. Frankowski BL, Bocchini JA Jr, Council on School Health and Committee on Infectious Diseases. Head lice. *Pediatrics*. 2010;126:392-403.
2. Chosidow O, Giraudeau B. Topical ivermectin—a step toward making head lice dead lice? *N Engl J Med*. 2012;367:1750-1752.

Tedizolid Phosphate vs Linezolid for Treatment of Acute Bacterial Skin and Skin Structure Infections: The ESTABLISH-1 Randomized Trial
Prokocimer P, De Anda C, Fang E, et al (Trius Therapeutics Inc, San Diego, CA; et al)
JAMA 309:559-569, 2013

Importance.—Acute bacterial skin and skin structure infections (ABSSSIs), including cellulitis or erysipelas, major cutaneous abscesses, and wound infections, can be life-threatening and may require surgery and hospitalization. Increasingly, ABSSSIs are associated with drug-resistant pathogens, and many antimicrobial agents have adverse effects restricting their use. Tedizolid phosphate is a novel oxazolidinone in development for the treatment of ABSSSIs.

Objectives.—To establish the noninferiority of tedizolid phosphate vs linezolid in treating ABSSSIs and compare the safety of the 2 agents.

Design, Setting, and Patients.—The Efficacy and Safety of 6-day Oral Tedizolid in Acute Bacterial Skin and Skin Structure Infections vs 10-day Oral Linezolid Therapy (ESTABLISH-1) was a phase 3, randomized, double-blind, noninferiority trial that was conducted from August 2010 through September 2011 at 81 study centers in North America, Latin America, and Europe. The intent-to-treat analysis set consisted of data from 667 adults aged 18 years or older with ABSSSIs treated with tedizolid phosphate (n = 332) or linezolid (n = 335).

Interventions.—A 200 mg once daily dose of oral tedizolid phosphate for 6 days or 600 mg of oral linezolid every 12 hours for 10 days.

Main Outcome Measures.—The primary efficacy outcome was early clinical response at the 48- to 72-hour assessment (no increase in lesion surface area from baseline and oral temperature of $\leq 37.6°C$, confirmed by a second temperature measurement within 24 hours). A 10% noninferiority margin was predefined.

Results.—In the intent-to-treat analysis set, the early clinical treatment response rates were 79.5% (95% CI, 74.8% to 83.7%) of 332 patients in the tedizolid phosphate group and 79.4% (95% CI, 74.7% to 83.6%) of 335 patients in the linezolid group (a treatment difference of 0.1% [95% CI, −6.1% to 6.2%]). The sustained clinical treatment response rates at the end of treatment (day 11) were 69.3% (95% CI, 64.0% to 74.2%) in the tedizolid phosphate group and 71.9% (95% CI, 66.8% to 76.7%) in the linezolid group (a treatment difference of −2.6% [95% CI, −9.6% to 4.2%]). Results of investigator-assessed clinical treatment success rates at a posttherapy evaluation visit (1-2 weeks after the end-of-treatment visit) were 85.5% (95% CI, 81.3% to 89.1%) in the tedizolid phosphate group and 86.0% (95% CI, 81.8% to 89.5%) in the linezolid group (a treatment difference of −0.5% [95% CI, −5.8% to 4.9%), and were similar for 178 patients with methicillin-resistant *Staphylococcus aureus* isolated from the primary lesion.

Conclusions and Relevance.—Tedizolid phosphate was a statistically noninferior treatment to linezolid in early clinical response at 48 to 72 hours after initiating therapy for an ABSSSI. Tedizolid phosphate may be a reasonable alternative to linezolid for treating ABSSSI.

Trial Registration.—clinicaltrials.gov Identifier: NCT01170221.

▶ Probably the most complicated skin structure infection these days is that caused by methicillin-resistant *Staphylococcus aureus* (MRSA). Many antimicrobials are effective in the management of bacterial skin infections, including those caused by MRSA, but each has substantial limitations as a result of toxicity, antibiotic resistance, or the lack of an oral formulation. In 2010, the Food and Drug Administration issued draft guidelines for the development of systemic drugs to treat acute bacterial skin and skin structural infections.

The drugs reported in this article are among the new agents developed according to these guidelines. Tedizolid phosphate (also known as TR-701) is a novel, potent agent rapidly converted in vivo into microbiologically active substances. Tedizolid interacts with the bacterial 23S ribosome initiation complex to inhibit translation and is active against all clinically relevant grampositive pathogens, including MRSA, which is resistant to linezolid, a drug proven to treat MRSA in 2000.

These authors tell us about a study using a 6-day course of oral tedizolid in the management of acute bacterial skin and skin structure infections vs a 10-day oral linezolid treatment (the standard therapy these days). The study was an international, multicenter, double-blind study that showed comparability between the 2 antibiotics.

If there is an advantage to the new agent tedizolid, it is that it can be as effective when given in a shorter course than with standard antibiotic therapy over 10 days. Shorter courses of antibiotics are helpful in the prevention of collateral damage attributable to their use, including the development of colonization or infection from multiresistant organisms, such as *Clostridium difficile*. Thus, tedizolid does appear as efficacious as standard antibiotic therapy for serious skin infections, but it can be given over a shorter period of time and therefore may have a better safety profile. It is extremely important that safe and effective drugs be developed for this serious skin problem and to avoid bacterial resistance with its own set of difficulties.

J. A. Stockman III, MD

Effect of Daily Chlorhexidine Bathing on Hospital-Acquired Infection

Climo MW, Yokoe DS, Warren DK, et al (Hunter Holmes McGuire Veterans Affairs Med Ctr, Richmond, VA; Brigham and Women's Hosp and Harvard Med School, Boston; Washington Univ School of Medicine, St Louis; et al)
N Engl J Med 368:533-542, 2013

Background.—Results of previous single-center, observational studies suggest that daily bathing of patients with chlorhexidine may prevent hospital-acquired bloodstream infections and the acquisition of multidrug-resistant organisms (MDROs).

Methods.—We conducted a multicenter, cluster-randomized, nonblinded crossover trial to evaluate the effect of daily bathing with chlorhexidine-impregnated washcloths on the acquisition of MDROs and the incidence of hospital-acquired bloodstream infections. Nine intensive care and bone marrow transplantation units in six hospitals were randomly assigned to bathe patients either with no-rinse 2% chlorhexidine-impregnated wash-cloths or with nonantimicrobial washcloths for a 6-month period, exchanged for the alternate product during the subsequent 6 months. The incidence rates of acquisition of MDROs and the rates of hospital-acquired bloodstream infections were compared between the two periods by means of Poisson regression analysis.

Results.—A total of 7727 patients were enrolled during the study. The overall rate of MDRO acquisition was 5.10 cases per 1000 patient-days with chlorhexidine bathing versus 6.60 cases per 1000 patient-days with nonantimicrobial washcloths ($P = 0.03$), the equivalent of a 23% lower rate with chlorhexidine bathing. The overall rate of hospital-acquired bloodstream infections was 4.78 cases per 1000 patient-days with chlorhexidine bathing versus 6.60 cases per 1000 patient-days with nonantimicrobial washcloths ($P = 0.007$), a 28% lower rate with chlorhexidine-impregnated washcloths. No serious skin reactions were noted during either study period.

Conclusions.—Daily bathing with chlorhexidine-impregnated wash-cloths significantly reduced the risks of acquisition of MDROs and development of hospital-acquired bloodstream infections. (Funded by the Centers for Disease Control and Prevention and Sage Products; ClinicalTrials.gov number, NCT00502476.)

▶ This study was carried out with adults. It will be important for a similar study to be implemented in the care of hospitalized children. Before the latter occurs, however, we can assume that a bacterial organism is a bacterial organism, and that it is likely that the findings from this study apply to at least the older age pediatric population, if not the entire pediatric age population. Multidrug resistant organisms, including methicillin-resistant *Staphylococcus aureus* (MRSA) and vancomycin-resistant *Enterococcus*, have become staples in the causation of hospital-acquired infections. Infections with these 2 organisms are extremely difficult to treat because fewer and fewer antimicrobials are effective in their management. For these and other reasons, targeted interventions, particularly in patients who are hospitalized for longer-than-average periods of time, could theoretically substantially reduce the risk of hospital-acquired bloodstream infections associated, for example, with use of central venous catheters. Studies have suggested that careful attention to catheter-insertion processes, including standardizing insertion-site antisepsis with the use of chlorhexidine-containing products, can decrease the risk of infection. What has been more controversial, at least in the care of adults, is the role of patient bathing and the use of antiseptic agents for this purpose in reducing such types of infections.

These authors have studied the value of bathing with chlorhexidine gluconate in the prevention of infections related to *S aureus* and *Aerococcus* species. This agent has shown historical effectiveness for these purposes. Unlike many other antiseptics, chlorhexidine has residual antibacterial activity, which may decrease the microbial load on a patient's skin and prevent secondary environmental contamination as well. Prior studies, such as that of Bleasdale et al,[1] have found that daily bathing with 2% chlorhexidine-impregnated washcloths reduces the incidence of primary bloodstream infections by as much as 60%.

These authors, based on prior studies, designed a multicenter, randomized trial to evaluate the usefulness of bathing with chlorhexidine to reduce the risks of multiresistant organism acquisition and hospital-acquired bloodstream infections in patients at high risk for health care—associated infections. The study was carried out in 6 intensive care and bone marrow transplantation units. The units themselves were randomly assigned to perform daily bathing of patients with either nonantimicrobial washcloths or washcloths impregnated with 2% chlorhexidine gluconate. Washcloths were used in sequential order to rinse all body surfaces, with the exception of the face, during bathing with the 2% chlorhexidine-impregnated cloths to avoid exposure of the mucous membranes of the eyes and mouth. The occurrence of drug-resistant infections and the presence of resistant organisms were documented. The findings from this study support the results of previous single-center trials suggesting that bathing with chlorhexidine will reduce the transmission of resistant organisms and the risk of hospital-acquired bloodstream infections, at least in patients in intensive care units and bone marrow transplantation units. This approach seems to be highly effective in reducing the risk of bloodstream infections. Bathing with chlorhexidine was associated with lower rates of central-catheter associated fungal bloodstream infections as well. This is the first article on the reduced rates of fungemia with such washings. Chlorhexidine does have fungicidal activity, but topical use has not been suggested as a possible intervention to reduce the incidence of fungemia among patients with indwelling central catheters.

No serious adverse effects of daily bathing with chlorhexidine-impregnated washcloths were observed in this study. There have been prior reports of serious allergic reactions with the topical use of chlorhexidine, but such reactions appear to be quite rare. There did not appear to be any emergence of resistance to chlorhexidine. It can be concluded that the daily use of chlorhexidine-impregnated washcloths is a cost-effective and safe strategy for the prevention of health care—associated infections in hospitalized patients. As noted earlier, it would be important to see this study redone with children, with particular emphasis on side effects as well as benefits.

J. A. Stockman III, MD

Reference

1. Bleasdale SC, Trick WE, Gonzalez IM, Lyles RD, Hayden MK, Weinstein RA. Effectiveness of chlorhexidine bathing to reduce catheter-associated bloodstream infections in medical intensive care unit patients. *Arch Intern Med.* 2007;167: 2073-2079.

Outbreak of *Mycobacterium chelonae* Infection Associated with Tattoo Ink
Kennedy BS, Bedard B, Younge M, et al (Monroe County Dept of Public Health, Rochester, NY; et al)
N Engl J Med 367:1020-1024, 2012

Background.—In January 2012, on the basis of an initial report from a dermatologist, we began to investigate an outbreak of tattoo-associated *Mycobacterium chelonae* skin and soft-tissue infections in Rochester, New York. The main goals were to identify the extent, cause, and form of transmission of the outbreak and to prevent further cases of infection.

Methods.—We analyzed data from structured interviews with the patients, histopathological testing of skin-biopsy specimens, acid-fast bacilli smears, and microbial cultures and antimicrobial susceptibility testing. We also performed DNA sequencing, pulsed-field gel electrophoresis (PFGE), cultures of the ink and ingredients used in the preparation and packaging of the ink, assessment of source water and faucets at tattoo parlors, and investigation of the ink manufacturer.

Results.—Between October and December 2011, a persistent, raised, erythematous rash in the tattoo area developed in 19 persons (13 men and 6 women) within 3 weeks after they received a tattoo from a single artist who used premixed gray ink; the highest occurrence of tattooing and rash onset was in November (accounting for 15 and 12 patients, respectively). The average age of the patients was 35 years (range, 18 to 48). Skin-biopsy specimens, obtained from 17 patients, showed abnormalities in all 17, with *M. chelonae* isolated from 14 and confirmed by means of DNA sequencing. PFGE analysis showed indistinguishable patterns in 11 clinical isolates and one of three unopened bottles of premixed ink. Eighteen of the 19 patients were treated with appropriate antibiotics, and their condition improved.

Conclusions.—The premixed ink was the common source of infection in this outbreak. These findings led to a recall by the manufacturer.

▶ The information reported here reminds us that tattoos are getting a lot of bad ink in the press these days (pardon the pun). In August 2012, the Centers for Disease Control noted that earlier that year, the Monroe County (New York) Department of Public Health began an outbreak investigation after receiving a report of a person with a persistent papular rash beginning 1 week after being tattooed by an artist in October 2011. *Mycobacterium chelonae* was isolated from a skin biopsy. The tattoo artist had begun using a particular company's prediluted gray ink earlier that year. Using a list of customers provided by the artist, a total of 19 infections was identified, including 14 confirmed with *M chelonae*. All infected persons had been tattooed with the same company's prediluted gray ink. This same organism was able to be isolated from the tattoo ink. Cases were also discovered elsewhere where infection related to the tattoo ink had occurred.

The frequency of nontuberculous mycobacterial (NTM) skin infections and soft tissue infections occurring subsequent to tattooing is not known but has been reported previously. In most cases, these have been the result of dilution of inks with nonsterile water during tattooing procedures. These infections can range from mild inflammation (eg, rash, papules, or nodules) to severe abscesses requiring extensive and multiple surgical debridements. NTM infections tend to be very difficult to treat and can require a minimum of 4 months of therapy with a combination of 2 or more antibiotics. All physicians who encounter persistent rashes of this type or nodules localized to newly tattooed areas should consider the possibility of NTM infection.

Chances are that the contaminated inks that were the cause of this problem were the result of the addition of nonsterilized water to the ink during the manufacturing of the product. Under the Federal Food, Drug, and Cosmetic Act, tattoo inks are considered cosmetics, and the pigments used in inks are color additives requiring premarket approval. No specific US Food and Drug Administration regulatory requirement explicitly provides that tattoo inks must be sterile. This is despite the fact that such inks do pose a health risk and a public health concern.

The Centers for Disease Control and Prevention have made a number of recommendations to minimize or eliminate the risk of NTM infections resulting from tattooing.[1] It should be noted that a Harris poll performed in 2012 found that by the time one reaches adulthood, 21% of US adults will have at least one tattoo, up from 14% in 2008.[2] This increase is quite remarkable despite the widely published acknowledgment about the increased risk of hepatitis and other diseases associated with tattooing. Fig 2 in the original article shows the typical rash associated with *Mycobacterium chelonae* infection. Any teen who gets a tattoo should seek medical attention quickly if red papules or a diffuse macular rash develops at the tattoo site.

J. A. Stockman III, MD

References

1. Editorial comment Centers for Disease Control and Prevention (CDC). Tattoo-associated nontuberculous mycobacterial skin infections—multiple states, 2011–2012. *MMWR Morb Mortal Wkly Rep.* 2012;61:653-656.
2. Seppa N. Tattoo infections connected to ink. *Sci News.* September 22, 2012.

3 Blood

Anemia, Apnea of Prematurity, and Blood Transfusions

Zagol K, Lake DE, Vergales B, et al (Univ of Virginia, Charlottesville; et al)
J Pediatr 161:417-421.e1, 2012

Objective.—To compare the frequency and severity of apneic events in very low birth weight (VLBW) infants before and after blood transfusions using continuous electronic waveform analysis.

Study Design.—We continuously collected waveform, heart rate, and oxygen saturation data from patients in all 45 neonatal intensive care unit beds at the University of Virginia for 120 weeks. Central apneas were detected using continuous computer processing of chest impedance, electro-cardiographic, and oximetry signals. Apnea was defined as respiratory pauses of >10, >20, and >30 seconds when accompanied by bradycardia (<100 beats per minute) and hypoxemia (<80% oxyhemoglobin saturation as detected by pulse oximetry). Times of packed red blood cell transfusions were determined from bedside charts. Two cohorts were analyzed. In the transfusion cohort, waveforms were analyzed for 3 days before and after the transfusion for all VLBW infants who received a blood transfusion while also breathing spontaneously. Mean apnea rates for the previous 12 hours were quantified and differences for 12 hours before and after transfusion were compared. In the hematocrit cohort, 1453 hematocrit values from all VLBW infants admitted and breathing spontaneously during the time period were retrieved, and the association of hematocrit and apnea in the next 12 hours was tested using logistic regression.

Results.—Sixty-seven infants had 110 blood transfusions during times when complete monitoring data were available. Transfusion was associated with fewer computer-detected apneic events ($P < .01$). Probability of future apnea occurring within 12 hours increased with decreasing hematocrit values ($P < .001$).

Conclusions.—Blood transfusions are associated with decreased apnea in VLBW infants, and apneas are less frequent at higher hematocrits (Fig 2).

▶ There have been a number of studies over the past several decades that have analyzed the association between anemia seen in preterm infants (the physiologic anemia of prematurity and/or blood loss associated with laboratory studies) and bradycardic apnea in the newborn. Some studies have shown that volume expansion from transfusion plays an important role in alleviating apneic episodes independent of the additional oxygen carrying capacity provided by a transfusion. At the same time, some studies have shown no decrease in the frequency of apnea

51

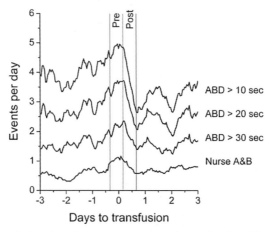

Days to transfusion

FIGURE 2.—Transfusion cohort. Apnea rate, as events per day, as a function of time until and following transfusion for VLBW infants not receiving mechanical ventilation. The *top 3 lines* are the average numbers of events lasting >10, >20, and >30 seconds, respectively. The *bottom line* is the rate of events recorded on the bedside apnea and bradycardia sheets. The values at the *vertical lines* are the average of the event rates measured during two 12-hour periods: 8 hours before to 4 hours after the transfusion, and 4 hours after to 16 hours after the transfusion, respectively. (Reprinted from Journal of Pediatrics, Zagol K, Lake DE, Vergales B, et al. Anemia, apnea of prematurity, and blood transfusions. *J Pediatr.* 2012;161:417-421.e1. Copyright 2012 with permission from Elsevier.)

following transfusions. It is fair to say that the literature regarding the role of transfusions for the management of apnea of prematurity has been somewhat muddy. This is why the report of Zagol is so important: it compares the frequency and severity of apneic episodes in very low-birth-weight infants immediately before and after blood transfusions using a computer algorithm to objectively detect apnea—bradycardia desaturation events. A method employing continuous electronic waveform analysis was used for this purpose.

In this report, all infants with birth weights ≤1500 g admitted to the neonatal intensive care unit or intermediate care unit at the University of Virginia between January 2009 and June 2011 were studied. Electrocardiographic waveforms and pulse oximetry were used to detect periods of apnea. Of 323 very low-birth-weight infants discharged during the study period, 67 had received 110 blood transfusions while not on a ventilator and therefore otherwise met inclusion criteria for this study. The study quantified apneic events using a computer analysis of waveforms continuously collected from the bedside monitors of the infants studied. The analysis did allow accurate measurement of the frequency, duration, and timing of apnea events before and after blood transfusion. The authors identified a strong statistical relationship of blood transfusion and a decrease in the frequency of central apnea events for very low-birth-weight infants. The presumption was that the effect was due to some response on central apnea, not obstructive apnea. If there was a weakness to this study, it was that infants were not randomized to transfusion or no transfusion, perhaps for obvious reasons. Also, the authors did not determine the indication for blood transfusion in this retrospective review of the patients enrolled in the study. They did, however, conclude that there is a correlation between transfusions and decreased frequency of apnea and that the probability of future apnea is inversely related to the patient's hematocrit. Fig 2 shows the effects of transfusion on apnea rates as events per day.

J. A. Stockman III, MD

Effect of Fresh Red Blood Cell Transfusions on Clinical Outcomes in Premature, Very Low-Birth-Weight Infants: The ARIPI Randomized Trial
Fergusson DA, Hébert P, Hogan DL, et al (Univ of Ottawa Ontario, Canada; et al)
JAMA 308:1443-1451, 2012

Context.—Even though red blood cells (RBCs) are lifesaving in neonatal intensive care, transfusing older RBCs may result in higher rates of organ dysfunction, nosocomial infection, and length of hospital stay.

Objective.—To determine if RBCs stored for 7 days or less compared with usual standards decreased rates of major nosocomial infection and organ dysfunction in neonatal intensive care unit patients requiring at least 1 RBC transfusion.

Design, Setting, and Participants.—Double-blind, randomized controlled trial in 377 premature infants with birth weights less than 1250 g admitted to 6 Canadian tertiary neonatal intensive care units between May 2006 and June 2011.

Intervention.—Patients were randomly assigned to receive transfusion of RBCs stored 7 days or less (n = 188) vs standard-issue RBCs in accordance with standard blood bank practice (n = 189).

Main Outcome Measures.—The primary outcome was a composite measure of major neonatal morbidities, including necrotizing enterocolitis, retinopathy of prematurity, bronchopulmonary dysplasia, and intraventricular hemorrhage, as well as death. The primary outcome was measured within the entire period of neonatal intensive care unit stay up to 90 days after randomization. The rate of nosocomial infection was a secondary outcome.

Results.—The mean age of transfused blood was 5.1 (SD, 2.0) days in the fresh RBC group and 14.6 (SD, 8.3) days in the standard group. Among neonates in the fresh RBC group, 99 (52.7%) had the primary outcome compared with 100 (52.9%) in the standard RBC group (relative risk, 1.00; 95% CI, 0.82-1.21). The rate of clinically suspected infection in the fresh RBC group was 77.7% (n = 146) compared with 77.2% (n = 146) in the standard RBC group (relative risk, 1.01; 95% CI, 0.90-1.12), and the rate of positive cultures was 67.5% (n = 127) in the fresh RBC group compared with 64.0% (n = 121) in the standard RBC group (relative risk, 1.06; 95% CI, 0.91-1.22).

Conclusion.—In this trial, the use of fresh RBCs compared with standard blood bank practice did not improve outcomes in premature, very low-birth-weight infants requiring a transfusion.

Trial Registration.—clinicaltrials.gov Identifier: NCT00326924; Current Controlled Trials Identifier: ISRCTN65939658.

▶ One would think that after so many years of studying the role of blood transfusions in the nursery, we would have little remaining topic to study. Au contraire. This report of Fergusson et al adds to our basic understanding of transfusion therapy in the neonatal intensive care unit in a number of ways. The report looks at the advantages or lack of advantages of using fresh red blood cell transfusions as opposed to red cells that have been stored for varying periods. This is an important issue that needed to be addressed.

Red cells that have been stored for a length of time have been reported to have certain defects, presumably as a result of the generation of cytokines in the storage medium. Stored red blood cells become less deformable and have an inability to scavenge nitric oxide. Over time, stored blood also has lesser ability to unload oxygen because of changes in the levels of red cell 2, 3 diphosphoglycerate. It has been suspected that in vulnerable patients, such as critically ill immature infants, transfusing older red blood cells may result in higher rates of organ dysfunction and morbidity because of the deleterious oxygen deficits or the proinflammatory effects of bioactive materials that accumulate during red blood cell storage. Data from adults show that prolonged red blood cell storage is associated with increased rates of infection, organ failure, death, and increased lengths of hospital stay. There are a few studies dealing with this in infants, however.

The use of older red blood cells is particularly common in neonatal units. Premature infants requiring multiple transfusions are routinely exposed to older red blood cells because of a dedicated donor policy introduced back in the 1980s to decrease the risk of viral transmission through transfusions of blood from multiple donors. The dedicated donor policy designates a specific unit of donated red blood cells for use by 1 infant exclusively over the course of his or her transfusion needs up to the expiration date of a particular unit of blood. Despite the inherent significant decrease in the risk of viral transmission with dedicated units, this approach increases rates of transfusion of older red blood cells. The policy remains a standard of practice in most neonatal care units in the United States and Canada. Fergusson et al carried out a double-blind randomized controlled trial in several hundred premature infants weighing less than 1250 g admitted to half a dozen Canadian neonatal intensive care units in order to determine if red blood cells stored for less than 7 days decreased rates of major infection or organ dysfunction in neonatal intensive care patients. The mean age of the transfused blood was just 5.1 days in the modified new program versus 14.6 days when using the standard approaches. There were no differences in the rates of infection in either group and no other adverse effects were seen with the use of aged blood compared with use of young red blood cells. Among critically ill premature infants, fresh red blood cell transfusions compared with standard red blood cell transfusions did not decrease or increase rates of complications or death in this study. The authors could not recommend any changes to storage time practices for the provision of red blood cells to infants admitted to a neonatal intensive care unit.

Thus it is that the dedicated transfusion program so commonly in place here in North America is likely to continue. It does minimize the risk of transfusion-associated infection by exposing neonates to fewer units of blood from different donors.

This commentary in the Blood chapter closes with a question. You are asked to consult on a 6-year-old child who experienced anaphylactic reactions while receiving a transfusion as part of the management of acute lymphoblastic leukemia. During transfusion, rash, angioedema, hypotension, and difficulty breathing occurred requiring resuscitation. No conventional mechanism could explain the reaction. Interestingly, however, the mother related a similar though less serious reaction occurring at one year of age after eating peanuts. Your diagnosis?

If you guessed that this was an allergic reaction to something the blood donor had in his blood, you would be correct. The blood donor was contacted and recalled eating several handfuls of peanuts the evening before his blood donation. It is known that peanut protein can be detected in blood up to 24 hours post ingestion. This case highlights the need to consider peanut allergy in any patient experiencing an anaphylactic reaction post transfusion.[1]

J. A. Stockman III, MD

Reference

1. Jacobs JFM, Baumert JL, Brons PP, et al. Anaphylaxis from passive transfer of peanut allergen in a blood product. *N Eng J Med.* 2011;364:20.

Hepcidin Concentrations in Serum and Urine Correlate with Iron Homeostasis in Preterm Infants

Müller KF, Lorenz L, Poets CF, et al (Univ of Tuebingen, Germany; et al)
J Pediatr 160:949-953.e2, 2012

Objectives.—To evaluate whether hepcidin concentrations in serum ($Hep_{(S)}$) and urine ($Hep_{(U)}$) correlate with iron metabolism, erythropoiesis, and inflammation in preterm infants.

Study Design.—Thirty-one preterm infants (23-32 weeks gestational age) were included. The concentration of the mature, 25 amino-acid form of hepcidin was determined by enzyme-linked immunosorbent assay in serum, urine, blood counts, reticulocytes, and iron measurements.

Results.—Median (IQR) $Hep_{(S)}$ was 52.4 (27.9-91.9) ng/mL. The highest values were measured in patients with systemic inflammation. $Hep_{(S)}$ and $Hep_{(U)}$ correlated strongly ($P = .0007$). $Hep_{(S)}$ and $Hep_{(U)}$ also correlated positively with ferritin ($P = .005$ and $P = .0002$) and with reticulocyte hemoglobin content ($P = .015$ and $P = .015$). $Hep_{(S)}$ and $Hep_{(U)}$ correlated negatively with soluble transferrin receptor/ferritin-ratio ($P = .005$ and $P = .003$). Infants with lower hemoglobin concentrations and higher reticulocyte counts had lower $Hep_{(S)}$ ($P = .0016$ and $P = .0089$).

Conclusion.—In sick preterm infants, iron status, erythropoiesis, anemia, and inflammation correlated with the mature 25 amino-acid form of hepcidin. Further evaluation of Hep$_{(U)}$ for non-invasive monitoring of iron status in preterm infants appears justified.

▶ We have written previously about hepcidin. You will recall that hepcidin is a key regulator of iron balance. It is a 25-amino-acid peptide that is synthesized mainly in the liver and is excreted by the kidneys. This peptide functions as a negative feedback regulator of iron homeostasis binding to the sole known cellular iron exporter, ferroportin, which is expressed in enterocytes, macrophages, hepatocytes, and syncytiotrophoblast cells in the placenta and initiates internalization and degradation of ferroportin, thus blocking further iron export from these tissues. To say this differently, elevated levels of hepcidin concentrations reduce intestinal iron absorption and systemic iron availability to the bone marrow. Low hepcidin levels lead to enhanced activity of ferroportin and increased iron availability in the plasma. Currently, the regulation of hepcidin is not fully understood, but seems to be regulated by the amount of iron stored in the body, inflammation and hypoxia, and red cell production rates.

Because hepcidin is a key factor in regulating iron balance beyond the pediatric age group, its biologic regulation and role in pregnancy in preterm infants has become of great interest in recent years. This is because hepcidin, particularly that found in the urine, could very well be a suitable biomarker for monitoring iron supplementation in preterm infants given that other studies of iron balance usually require access to blood and that is a lot more difficult to obtain than a sample of urine.

Müller et al designed a study to determine whether there is any correlation between serum levels of hepcidin and urine levels of hepcidin and whether these in any way correlate with indices of iron status such as serum ferritin and reticulocyte hemoglobin content. The authors also attempted to correlate hemoglobin and reticulocyte count as markers of anemia and activity of erythropoiesis with serum and urine hepcidin levels while attempting also to establish correlations with signs of inflammation. Thirty-one preterm infants with a gestational age at birth between 23 weeks and 31 weeks were enrolled.

Findings from this study included the observation that the median concentration of serum hepcidin as measured in preterm infants was 52.4 ng/mL. This figure was approximately 30% lower than hepcidin concentrations measured in full-term infants in cord blood as determined in previous studies. The authors suggest that lower serum hepcidin concentrations in preterm infants are likely caused by total iron stores being lower in these infants compared with full-term infants who were in utero longer and had an accessible iron supply for many weeks longer and who had not been exposed to repeated blood sampling during neonatal intensive care. It should also be noted that serum hepcidin concentrations in preterm and term infants are lower than those reported in healthy adult men and women (median 112 ng/mL and 65 ng/mL, respectively), possibly reflecting the increased demand for iron availability in growing newborn infants. This study also showed that ferritin values correlated positively with serum hepcidin levels. Reticulocyte hemoglobin content also correlated with hepcidin levels in serum.

Although the numbers of preterm infants reported on in this study are small, there is an interesting finding related to the presence of inflammation in 2 infants. In this study, the 2 highest serum hepcidin concentrations were observed in infants with probable infection and systemic inflammatory responses indicated by increased C-reactive protein concentration and leukocyte counts. The literature suggests that there is an important role of hepcidin in the innate immune system in which hepcidin reduces the amount of iron available for microbes. Indeed, a study using adult volunteers has shown that hepcidin excretion in urine increases by 7.5-fold within 2 hours of the injection of interleukin-6, an acute inflammatory mediator.[1] It should also be noted that the data from this report do suggest that urinary hepcidin might be a useful noninvasive biomarker, at least in the absence of inflammation, to assess iron availability and to adjust iron supplementation in preterm infants.

J. A. Stockman III, MD

Reference

1. Nemeth E, Rivera S, Gabayan V, et al. IL-6 mediates hypoferremia of inflammation by inducing the synthesis of the iron regulatory hormone hepcidin. *J Clin Invest.* 2004;113:1271-1276.

Effect of Micronutrient Sprinkles on Reducing Anemia: A Cluster-Randomized Effectiveness Trial

Jack SJ, Ou K, Chea M, et al (World Health Organization, Phnom Penh, Cambodia; Natl Maternal and Child Health Centre, Phnom Penh, Cambodia; et al)

Arch Pediatr Adolesc Med 166:842-850, 2012

Objective.—To evaluate the effectiveness of Sprinkles alongside infant and young child feeding (IYCF) education compared with IYCF education alone on anemia, deficiencies in iron, vitamin A, and zinc, and growth in Cambodian infants.

Design.—Cluster-randomized effectiveness study.

Setting.—Cambodian rural health district.

Participants.—Among 3112 infants aged 6 months, a random subsample (n = 1350) was surveyed at baseline and 6-month intervals to age 24 months.

Intervention.—Daily micronutrient Sprinkles alongside IYCF education vs IYCF education alone for 6 months from ages 6 to 11 months.

Main Outcome Measures.—Prevalence of anemia; iron, vitamin A, and zinc deficiencies; and growth via biomarkers and anthropometry.

Results.—Anemia prevalence (hemoglobin level < 11.0 g/dL [to convert to grams per liter, multiply by 10.0]) was reduced in the intervention arm compared with the control arm by 20.6% at 12 months (95% CI, 9.4-30.2; $P = .001$), and the prevalence of moderate anemia (hemoglobin level < 10.0 g/dL) was reduced by 27.1% (95% CI, 21.0-31.8; $P < .001$).

At 12 and 18 months, iron deficiency prevalence was reduced by 23.5% (95% CI, 15.6-29.1; $P < .001$) and 11.6% (95% CI, 2.6-17.9; $P = .02$), respectively. The mean serum zinc concentration was increased at 12 months (2.88 μg/dL [to convert to micromoles per liter, multiply by 0.153]; 95% CI, 0.26-5.42; $P = .03$). There was no statistically significant difference in the prevalence of zinc and vitamin A deficiencies or in growth at any time.

Conclusions.—Sprinkles reduced anemia and iron deficiency and increased the mean serum zinc concentration in Cambodian infants. Anemia and zinc effects did not persist beyond the intervention period.

Trial Registration.—anzctr.org.au Identifier: ACTRN12608000069358.

▶ Both in the United States and in Cambodia, the site of this clinical trial, anemia remains fairly common, although it is obviously greater in prevalence in Southeast Asia. In Cambodia, 55% of Cambodian children younger than age 5 years are anemic, and 40% have altered growth as a result. Those ages 6 to 23 months are at highest risk for anemia that can be associated with impairments in both growth and immune function as well as with cognitive and learning disabilities. The authors of this report undertook a study in which families received monthly a supply of sprinkles that contained a variety of micronutrients, including daily requirements for iron, zinc, vitamin A, iodine, vitamins B1, B2, B6, B12, niacin, folic acid, vitamin C, copper, vitamin D, and vitamin E. These sprinkles were mixed with an infant's or child's food immediately before serving. Each "dose" of sprinkles contained 12.5 mg iron as microencapsulated ferrous fumarate. The presence of anemia defined as a hemoglobin < 11.0 g/dL was 84%. Anemia prevalence at 12 months was reduced by 20.6% in the intervention group compared with the control group. The prevalence of moderate anemia (hemoglobin level < 10.0 g/dL) at 12 months was reduced by 27.1%. The overall mean baseline hemoglobin was 10.3 g/dL and did not differ between treatment groups and placebo-treated groups. The sprinkles had a similar proportional effect in decreasing anemia whether the child had a hemoglobinopathy disorder or not.

This trial undertaken in Cambodia included intensive nutrition education that took the form of verbal and written instructions, pictures, and cooking demonstrations. The study was unique in that it was the first to isolate the impact of iron fortification in a population with a high prevalence of genetic hemoglobin disorders (the latter is seen in 30% to 70% of Cambodian infants). Obviously, individuals with genetic hemoglobin disorders tend to have varying degrees of anemia from mild to quite severe. For an individual patient, it is often difficult to distinguish between a genetic hemoglobin disorder and iron deficiency without specific testing. In the current study, there was about a 20% decline in the rate of anemia among those without a genetic hemoglobin disorder compared with a 17% decline in those with a disorder, a difference that was not significant. This implies that in an environment in which the dietary iron intake is predicted to be low and rates of anemia high, the presence of a genetic hemoglobin disorder should not preclude programs that aim to increase the amount of iron in the diet.

In an editorial that accompanied this report, Zlotkin noted that there are important public health lessons to be learned from this study, perhaps the most important being that the typical cereal-based diets, even when combined with breast milk, cannot meet the iron needs of rapidly growing infants between 6 months and 24 months of age, thus the need for iron fortification.[1] Also, the use of home diet fortification at 6 months may not be in and of itself adequate. If feasible, home fortification should be continued well into the second year of life.

Micronutrient supplements given in the form of sprinkles can and do help alleviate the problem of multiple nutritional deficiencies in the growing infant and toddler. They are easy to use, and one wonders if more widespread consideration of their use in the United States is appropriate.

J. A. Stockman III, MD

Reference

1. Zlotkin S. More proof that home fortification is of value in children with iron deficiency anemia. *Arch Pediatr Adolesc Med.* 2012;166:869-870.

Incidence of neoplasia in Diamond Blackfan anemia: a report from the Diamond Blackfan Anemia Registry

Vlachos A, Rosenberg PS, Atsidaftos E, et al (Steven and Alexandra Cohen Children's Med Ctr of New York; Natl Cancer Inst, Rockville, MD)
Blood 119:3815-3819, 2012

Diamond Blackfan anemia (DBA) is an inherited bone marrow failure syndrome characterized by red cell aplasia and congenital anomalies. A predisposition to cancer has been suggested but not quantified by case reports. The DBA Registry of North America (DBAR) is the largest established DBA patient cohort, with prospective follow-up since 1991. This report presents the first quantitative assessment of cancer incidence in DBA. Among 608 patients with 9458 person-years of follow-up, 15 solid tumors, 2 acute myeloid leukemias, and 2 cases of myelodysplastic syndrome were diagnosed at a median age of 41 years in patients who had not received a bone marrow transplant. Cancer incidence in DBA was significantly elevated. The observed-to-expected ratio for all cancers combined was 5.4 ($P < .05$); significant observed-to-expected ratios were 287 for myelodysplastic syndrome, 28 for acute myeloid leukemia, 36 for colon carcinoma, 33 for osteogenic sarcoma, and 12 for female genital cancers. The median survival was 56 years, and the cumulative incidence of solid tumor/leukemia was approximately 20% by age 46 years. As in Fanconi anemia and dyskeratosis congenita, DBA is both an inherited bone marrow failure syndrome and a cancer predisposition syndrome; cancer risks appear lower in DBA than in Fanconi anemia or dyskeratosis congenita. This trial was registered at www.clinicaltrials.gov as #NCT00106015.

▶ There have been individual case reports describing Diamond Blackfan anemia (DBA) patients as having a predisposition to cancer, particularly acute myeloid leukemia and myelodysplastic syndrome. Unfortunately, the literature does not make it possible to quantify specific cancer risks because reporting of neoplastic events may be biased and the denominator representing the total DBA population at risk is not available from case reports or small series. What has been helpful in that regard is the establishment of the Diamond Blackfan Anemia Registry of North America, the largest known source of Diamond Blackfan patients with more than 600 patients enrolled and over 20 years of follow-up. It was this database that Vlachos et al used to systematically classify the types of cancer and patient ages in an attempt to quantify the cumulative incidence and hazard rates of malignancy development in patients with DBA.

The data from this report provide, for the first time, specific information on the spectrum and incidence of cancer in DBA, incorporating approximately 20 years of patient accrual and prospective follow-up from the DBA Registry. Overall, the investigators identified that the rate of any solid tumor or leukemia developing in a patient with DBA was 5.4-fold higher than expected in a demographically matched comparison with the general population. Furthermore, significantly elevated incidence ratios were noted for myelodysplastic syndrome, acute myeloid leukemia, adenocarcinoma of the colon, osteogenic sarcoma, and female genital cancer. There were more solid tumors developing in DBA patients than hematologic malignancies. Patients with DBA who developed a subsequent malignancy had a much poorer survival than might otherwise have been expected.

The information from this report shows that DBA now joins 2 other inherited bone marrow failure syndromes that have cancer predisposition: Fanconi anemia and dyskeratosis congenita. The cumulative incidence of solid tumors and the development of acute myelogenous leukemia in DBA was approximately 20% by age mid-40s compared with 30% in Fanconi anemia and dyskeratosis congenita. The present data strongly suggest that patients with DBA should receive appropriate counseling and surveillance for neoplastic complications beginning much earlier than the general population.

J. A. Stockman III, MD

Stroke With Transfusions Changing to Hydroxyurea (SWiTCH)
Ware RE, for the SWiTCH Investigators (Baylor College of Medicine, Houston, TX; et al)
Blood 119:3925-3932, 2012

Stroke is a devastating complication of sickle cell anemia (SCA) with high recurrence if untreated. Chronic transfusions reduce recurrent strokes but have associated morbidities including iron overload. Stroke With Transfusions Changing to Hydroxyurea (SWiTCH) was a multicenter phase 3 randomized trial comparing standard treatment (transfusions/chelation) to alternative treatment (hydroxyurea/phlebotomy) for children with SCA, stroke, and iron overload. SWiTCH was a noninferiority trial with a composite primary end point, allowing an increased stroke risk but requiring superiority for removing iron. Subjects on standard treatment received monthly transfusions plus daily deferasirox iron chelation. Subjects on alternative treatment received hydroxyurea plus overlap transfusions during dose escalation to maximum tolerated dose (MTD), followed by monthly phlebotomy. Subjects on standard treatment (N = 66) maintained 30% sickle hemoglobin (HbS) and tolerated deferasirox at 28.2 ± 6.0 mg/kg/d. Subjects on alternative treatment (N = 67) initiated hydroxyurea and 60 (90%) reached MTD at 26.2 ± 4.9 mg/kg/d with 29.1% ± 6.7% fetal hemoglobin (HbF). Adjudication documented no strokes on transfusions/ chelation but 7 (10%) on hydroxyurea/phlebotomy, still within the noninferiority stroke margin. The National Heart, Lung, and Blood Institute closed SWiTCH after interim analysis revealed equivalent liver iron content, indicating futility for the composite primary end point. Transfusions and chelation remain a better way to manage children with SCA, stroke, and iron overload.

▶ Stroke remains the most devastating neurologic manifestation of sickle cell anemia. The incidence of primary stroke in children with sickle cell anemia runs on the order of 0.6 events to 0.8 events per 100 patient years with a cumulative incidence of 7.8% by 14 years and 11% by 20 years. Once a stroke has occurred, the incidence of recurrent stroke ranges from 47% to 93% in untreated patients. Thus every patient who has experienced a stroke in association with sickle cell anemia will need some form of management to prevent recurrence. Chronic red blood cell transfusions have been the therapy of choice to prevent secondary stroke. Blood transfused every 3 to 4 weeks raises the hemoglobin concentration, reduces sickle hemoglobin, improves blood flow with non-sickled red blood cells, and suppresses endogenous sickle red blood cell production. Most transfusions centers target a 30% hemoglobin S to manage problems needing transfusion therapy. This reduces the risk of secondary stroke to somewhere in the neighborhood of 15% to 20% and an event rate of 2.2 to 6.4 recurrent strokes per 100 patient-years.

The rub with prophylactic transfusions as part of the prevention of recurrent stroke is the development of iron overload, which in itself can result in organ dysfunction and death. When used as the sole prophylactic therapy, transfusions are given for the individual's lifetime. Based on anecdotal experiences, hydroxyurea might be an alternative to chronic transfusion therapy in sickle cell disease anemia patients who have had a stroke. Hydroxyurea raises the level of erythrocyte hemoglobin F, protecting that red cell against sickling. Ware et al report on a study known as Stroke With Transfusion Changing to Hydroxyurea (SWiTCH). This study was designed to determine whether children with sickle cell anemia who are on transfusion therapy for stroke might be able to be successfully transitioned to an oral therapy to reduce the risk of iron overload. Chelation therapy to reduce the burden of iron from transfusions could be undertaken as well.

The results of this trial were not encouraging. Based on the SWiTCH trial results, standard transfusion therapy and chelation remain the better way to manage children with sickle cell anemia, stroke, and iron overload. Nonetheless, management of existing cerebrovascular disease in patients with sickle cell anemia is still an extremely difficult clinical problem, and the prevention of vasculopathy and stroke is the preferred goal. Studies are ongoing to determine whether one can use hydroxyurea instead of transfusion for children who have evidence of abnormal blood vessels, but no primary stroke as yet, but once a stroke has occurred, transfusion therapy remains the way to go. Obviously, early initiation of hydroxyurea, perhaps in all patients with sickle cell anemia, could help prevent or retard the development of cerebrovascular disease in this vulnerable patient population while simultaneously avoiding serious complications of transfusions including iron overload and auto/alloimmunization. The rub is that we do not know as yet what the truly long-term side effects of hydroxyurea are, particularly when started at a very young age.

J. A. Stockman III, MD

Outcomes 5 years after response to rituximab therapy in children and adults with immune thrombocytopenia

Patel VL, Mahévas M, Lee SY, et al (Weill Med College of Cornell Univ, NY; Université Paris Est, Créteil, France; et al)
Blood 119:5989-5995, 2012

Treatments for immune thrombocytopenic purpura (ITP) providing durable platelet responses without continued dosing are limited. Whereas complete responses (CRs) to B-cell depletion in ITP usually last for 1 year in adults, partial responses (PRs) are less durable. Comparable data do not exist for children and 5-year outcomes are unavailable. Patients with ITP treated with rituximab who achieved CRs and PRs (platelets > 150 × 10^9/L or 50-150 × 10^9/L, respectively) were selected to be assessed for duration of their response; 72 adults whose response lasted at least 1 year and 66 children with response of any duration were included. Patients had baseline platelet counts < 30 × 10^9/L; 95% had ITP of > 6 months in duration. Adults and children each had initial overall response rates of 57% and similar 5-year estimates of persisting response (21% and 26%, respectively). Children did not relapse after 2 years from initial treatment whereas adults did. Initial CR and prolonged B-cell depletion predicted sustained responses whereas prior splenectomy, age, sex, and duration of ITP did not. No novel or substantial long-term clinical toxicity was observed. In summary, 21% to 26% of adults and children with chronic ITP treated with standard-dose rituximab maintained a treatment-free response for at least 5 years without major toxicity. These results can inform clinical decision-making.

▶ In recent years, rituximab has come to the rescue of many children and adults with otherwise refractory immune thrombocytopenia (ITP). Rituximab is a chimeric monoclonal antibody directed against CD20, an antigen expressed on the surface of B lymphocytes but not on most plasma cells. This agent was initially developed to treat non-Hodgkin B-cell lymphoma in the early 1990s and was licensed for this indication in 1997 in the United States. Since that time, it has been widely used in the treatment of autoantibody-mediated disorders. The initial hypothesis for this effect was that removal of autoreactive B-cell clones would lead to amelioration of clinical disease by reducing the levels of or even eliminating circulating autoantibody. The autoimmune disorders treated with rituximab, in addition to ITP, include systemic lupus erythematosus, vasculitis, rheumatoid arthritis, autoimmune hemolytic anemia, cryoglobulinemia, acquired factor VIII antibodies, immunoglobulin-M polyneuropathies, and thrombotic thrombocytopenic purpura. Studies undertaken as part of the management of ITP in both children and adults suggest a response rate to rituximab of about 60%. Of these responses, two-thirds are complete and one-third partial. Among those who respond, about 50% will have a sustained response over a period of a year.

These authors report on the duration of response in patients who had already demonstrated initial responses to rituximab. Using a relatively large cohort of 130 responders (both children and adults), a relapse-free 5-year sustained response rate in both children and adults with refractory ITP was projected, and clinical and immunologic correlates of long-term response were assessed. Needless to say, treatment of patients with chronic ITP that provides a curative effect without untoward toxicity or poor tolerability would be highly desirable. Data in this article show that adults and children each have initial overall response rates of 57% to rituximab treatment, and both groups have similar 5-year estimates of persisting response (21% and 26%, respectively). Children do not relapse after 2 years from initial treatment, whereas adults will. No significant long-term clinical toxicity was uncovered in either group. Other studies have reported toxicities of rituximab use in ITP that include neutropenia, long-term infections, hematologic malignancies, and other isolated conditions. Fortunately these were not observed in this article.

Needless to say, rituximab is not a perfect drug. Nonetheless, when it works, it works fairly well, and although the majority of patients will not have sustained long-term responses to it, it can be life-saving and can reduce significant morbidity in an otherwise difficult disorder to treat, namely chronic ITP.

J. A. Stockman III, MD

Association Between Physical Activity and Risk of Bleeding in Children With Hemophilia

Broderick CR, Herbert RD, Latimer J, et al (Univ of Sydney, Australia; Neuroscience Res Australia, Randwick; et al)
JAMA 308:1452-1459, 2012

Context.—Vigorous physical activity is thought to increase risk of bleeds in children with hemophilia, but the magnitude of the risk is unknown.

Objective.—To quantify the transient increase in risk of bleeds associated with physical activity in children with hemophilia.

Design, Setting, and Participants.—A case-crossover study nested within a prospective cohort study was conducted at 3 pediatric hemophilia centers in Australia between July 2008 and October 2010. A total of 104 children and adolescent boys aged 4 through 18 years with moderate or severe hemophilia A or B were monitored for bleeds for up to 1 year. Following each bleed, the child or parent was interviewed to ascertain exposures to physical activity preceding the bleed. Physical activity was categorized according to expected frequency and severity of collisions. The risk of bleeds associated with physical activity was estimated by contrasting exposure to physical activity in the 8 hours before the bleed with exposures in two 8-hour control windows, controlling for levels of clotting factor in the blood.

Main Outcome Measures.—Association of physical activity and factor level with risk of bleeding.

Results.—The participants were observed for 4839 person-weeks during which time 436 bleeds occurred. Of these, 336 bleeds occurred more than 2 weeks after the preceding bleed and were used in the primary analysis of risk. Compared with inactivity and category 1 activities (eg, swimming), category 2 activities (eg, basketball) were associated with a transient increase in the risk of bleeding (30.6% of bleed windows vs 24.8% of first control windows; odds ratio, 2.7; 95% CI, 1.7-4.8, $P < .001$). Category 3 activities (eg, wrestling) were associated with a greater transient increase in risk (7.0% of bleed windows vs 3.4% of first control windows; odds ratio, 3.7; 95% CI, 2.3-7.3, $P < .001$). To illustrate absolute risk increase, for a child who bleeds 5 times annually and is exposed on average to category 2 activities twice weekly and to category 3 activities once weekly, exposure to these activities was associated with only 1 of the 5 annual bleeds. For every 1% increase in clotting factor level, bleeding incidence was lower by 2% (95% CI, 1%-3%; $P = .004$).

Conclusions.—In children and adolescents with hemophilia, vigorous physical activity was transiently associated with a moderate relative increase in risk of bleeding. Because the increased relative risk is transient, the absolute increase in risk of bleeds associated with physical activity is likely to be small.

▶ One of the most common questions parents of a newly diagnosed hemophiliac will ask is whether their son (this is an X-linked disorder) will ever be able to lead a normal life including participating in sporting activities. Broderick et al report results of a study of the association between vigorous sports and bleeding rates in 104 children and adolescents with moderate or severe hemophilia. Most of the participants in the study were actively receiving prophylactic infusions of replacement clotting factor. The investigators scored the physical activities as category 1, 2, or 3 depending on the expected trauma related to frequency and severity of collisions associated with the activity. Category 2 and 3 activities are collision sports.

The data from this report indicate that the risk of bleeding requiring acute factor replacement was increased after collision sports with an odds ratio of 2.7 for category 2 activities (such as basketball or baseball) and 3.7 for category 3 activities (such as wrestling or US football). Because exposure time to the higher risk activities was a small percentage of total life hours and because the annual rate of bleeding was low, the absolute increase in risk was in fact low. The math also showed that each 1% increase in plasma factor activity of factor VIII was associated with a 2% lower bleeding risk, thus suggesting therapeutic strategies that might reduce the bleeding risk associated with collision sports. Fig 2 in the original article shows the odds ratio for bleeds by clotting factor level and activity. Based on these figures, one could design a prophylactic treatment that could minimize the risk of bleeding depending on what sporting activity one was engaged in. The safest sporting activity looked at in this report was swimming.

With respect to details of this report, in the patients looked at there were 436 bleeds examined as part of the study. The mean incidence of bleeds per year was 4.9 for participants with moderate hemophilia and 3.0 for those with severe hemophilia. The most frequent sites of bleeding were the knee (15%), ankle (14%), and elbow (10%). Less frequent sites were the hand, foot, arm, thigh, leg, shoulder, head, trunk, wrist, forearm, nose, and hip. There was no evidence that the rate of bleeds varied by week of the year or day of the week, but there were large variations with time of the day. The frequency of bleeds was highest between 7:00 AM and 8:00 AM and 3:00 PM and 4:00 PM, coinciding with the periods immediately before and after school.

This report may seem counterintuitive to the average care provider in that participation in collision sports does not worsen the outcome of severe hemophilia. In fact, the conclusions are not inconsistent with conventional wisdom in that the data from the report suggest that a factor level below a critical threshold actually is much more important as a determinant of bleeding risk than modest exposure to vigorous activities. This is important information because all children need to feel part of their peer group. Participation in desired, but possibly higher-risk sports, may be a strong motivator for positive health promoting activities such as self-infusion of prophylactic factor replacement, year-round conduct of strengthening exercise, and increased body awareness with early blood recognition. It is clear that a higher factor level at the time of a collision is preventative of most injuries. The risk of bleeding is mitigated by prophylaxis to the extent that clotting factor levels of around 50% or higher will reduce the risk of bleeds to below the risk experienced during periods of inactivity with no exogenous clotting factor administration. With typical prophylactic regimens (doses of 35 IU/kg to 50 IU/kg), peak factor concentrations of 70% to 100% are achieved, which, given a factor VIII half-life of 10.7 hours, is sufficient to maintain levels greater than 50% for between approximately 6 and 12 hours. Because exposure to physical activity of the sort described in this report is quite transient, one could expect that one can readily prepare a youngster for the type of physical activity described in the report.

Yes, in children and adolescents with hemophilia, vigorous physical activity will be associated with an increased risk of bleeding. Nevertheless, the absolute increased risk with physical activity is small and to the extent reasonable, largely a risk that can be modified downward by proper factor prophylactic replacement.

J. A. Stockman III, MD

Management of bleeding in acquired hemophilia A: results from the European Acquired Haemophilia (EACH2) Registry

Baudo F, on behalf of the EACH2 registry contributors (Ospedale Niguarda, Milan, Italy; et al)
Blood 120:39-46, 2012

Acquired hemophilia A is a rare bleeding disorder caused by autoantibodies to coagulation FVIII. Bleeding episodes at presentation are spontaneous and severe in most cases. Optimal hemostatic therapy is controversial, and available data are from observational and retrospective studies only. The EACH2 registry, a multicenter, pan-European, Web-based database, reports current patient management. The aim was to assess the control of first bleeding episodes treated with a bypassing agent (rFVIIa or aPCC), FVIII, or DDAVP among 501 registered patients. Of 482 patients with one or more bleeding episodes, 144 (30%) received no treatment for bleeding; 31 were treated with symptomatic therapy only. Among 307 patients treated with a first-line hemostatic agent, 174 (56.7%) received rFVIIa, 63 (20.5%) aPCC, 56 (18.2%) FVIII, and 14 (4.6%) DDAVP. Bleeding was controlled in 269 of 338 (79.6%) patients treated with a first-line hemostatic agent or ancillary therapy alone. Propensity score matching was applied to allow unbiased comparison between treatment groups. Bleeding control was significantly higher in patients treated with bypassing agents versus FVIII/DDAVP (93.3% vs 68.3%; $P = .003$). Bleeding control was similar between rFVIIa and aPCC (93.0%; $P = 1$). Thrombotic events were reported in 3.6% of treated patients with a similar incidence between rFVIIa (2.9%) and aPCC (4.8%).

▶ Most everyone is familiar with congenital factor VIII deficiency, better known as hemophilia A. What most are not familiar with is that there is an acquired form of hemophilia A. This too is a hemorrhagic disorder, but one characterized by a deficiency of coagulation factor VIII resulting from autoantibodies targeting specific epitopes that cause neutralization and/or accelerated clearance of factor VIII from plasma. This disorder is rare, but when it does occur it is difficult to manage. It is commonly associated with a variety of clinical conditions, including autoimmune disorders, solid tumors, lymphoproliferative diseases, and pregnancy. Teens have been affected, although most patients afflicted with acquired hemophilia A are adults. In half the cases, no underlying condition is identified.

Acquired hemophilia A presents without a family or personal history of bleeding and most often with sudden onset. The affected individual has a spontaneous bleeding episode without a significant history of trauma. About 1 in 4 cases occurs after trauma or is identified when a surgical procedure is performed. All too often the bleeding is at a site that is silent initially, but ultimately presents with serious problems. For example, retroperitoneal and large intramuscular hematomas may compress nervous and vascular structures leading to compartment syndromes. In most cases, the bleeding presentation is usually severe.

The European Acquired Hemophilia Registry was established in 2003 to collect information on the current management of patients with acquired hemophilia

A. Baudo et al provide information from this worldwide registry that does not recommend any specific treatment. The information from this report simply catalogs what others are doing locally to manage this disorder. The registry shows that hemostatic agents most frequently used to control bleeding in patients with acquired hemophilia A are bypassing agents (recombinant activated factor VII and activated prothrombin complex concentrate) or factor VIII replacement therapy with concentrates or induction of factor VIII release using 1-desamino-8-D-arginine-vasopressin. In many respects, these same agents are the agents of choice for management of hemophilia A under certain circumstances. It appears that worldwide, bypassing agents are recommended as first-line therapy because of their rapid action and high level of effectiveness. Prospective randomized trials comparing the efficacy of these agents have not been carried out to date, however, and it is very unlikely that an adequately powered studied will ever be feasible given the rarity of acquired hemophilia A.

This report also provides a fair amount of new information about acquired hemophilia A. In the European registry, clinical bleeding at presentation was observed in 96.2% of patients and was severe in 69.5% of patients. However, a few patients may not require hemostatic treatment for most bleeding emergencies.

The European registry represents the largest collection of bleeding episodes recorded ever in acquired hemophilia A and certainly is also the most rigorous analysis of treatment outcomes. The data seem to underscore that the optimal treatment of bleeding in this disorder is composed of bypassing agents that can be expected to resolve bleeding in more than 90% of cases. Alternative therapies are just not predictable enough to be used as first-line treatments. Although bypassing agents do seem to be the treatment of choice, they are associated with a risk of both arterial and venous thrombotic events because they directly stimulate clotting bypassing a number of the regulatory steps of thrombus formation.

There is 1 alternative therapy recently reported for acquired hemophilia, and that is the use of immunosuppressants including steroids alone or steroids combined with cyclophosphamide rituximab. Combinations of these agents seem to improve the clinical situations in between 50% and 70% of patients.[1]

J. A. Stockman III, MD

Reference

1. Collins P, Baudo F, Knoebl P, et al. Immunosuppression for acquired hemophilia A: results from the European Acquired Haemophilia Registry (EACH2). *Blood*. 2012;120:47-55.

A bispecific antibody to factors IXa and X restores factor VIII hemostatic activity in a hemophilia A model
Kitazawa T, Igawa T, Sampei Z, et al (Fuji-Gotemba Res Laboratories, Gotemba, Shizuoka, Japan; et al)
Nat Med 18:1570-1574, 2012

Hemophilia A is a bleeding disorder resulting from coagulation factor VIII (FVIII) deficiency. Exogenously provided FVIII effectively reduces bleeding complications in patients with severe hemophilia A. In approximately 30% of such patients, however, the 'foreignness' of the FVIII molecule causes them to develop inhibitory antibodies against FVIII (inhibitors), precluding FVIII treatment in this set of patients. Moreover, the poor pharmacokinetics of FVIII, attributed to low subcutaneous bioavailability and a short half-life of 0.5 d, necessitates frequent intravenous injections. To overcome these drawbacks, we generated a humanized bispecific antibody to factor IXa (FIXa) and factor X (FX), termed hBS23, that places these two factors into spatially appropriate positions and mimics the cofactor function of FVIII. hBS23 exerted coagulation activity in FVIII-deficient plasma, even in the presence of inhibitors, and showed *in vivo* hemostatic activity in a nonhuman primate model of acquired hemophilia A. Notably, hBS23 had high subcutaneous bioavailability and a 2-week half-life and would not be expected to elicit the development of FVIII-specific inhibitory antibodies, as its molecular structure, and hence antigenicity, differs from that of FVIII. A long-acting, subcutaneously injectable agent that is unaffected by the presence of inhibitors could markedly reduce the burden of care for the treatment of hemophilia A.

▶ Although not the most common of blood disorders, hemophilia A does affect 1 in 10 000 boys born in the United States. Half of these youngsters will be classified as having severe disease (less than 1% of normal factor VIII activity without replacement). Patients with moderate hemophilia A (1%–5% of normal activity) will experience far fewer bleeding episodes. In either group of patients, replacement therapy effectively reduces joint bleeding leading to a better quality of life and better joint status. Nonetheless, despite these advantages, routine supplementation with factor VIII has 2 major drawbacks aside from its expense: the development of inhibitors and the need for frequent venous access for factor VIII injection. The most worrisome problem is of course the development of inhibitors that preclude the use of factor VIII or make it difficult to control hemorrhaging. This may result in the use of alternative treatment agents such as recombinant activated factor VII and activated prothrombin complex concentrates. These have shorter half-lives and cost significantly more than routine factor VIII replacement. Management of inhibitors with high doses of factor VIII is currently being attempted, but the process is very expensive and does not always work. Also, the need for frequent venous access is problematic, particularly when treating younger patients at home. It negatively affects the implementation of and adherence to the supplementation routine.

Because of the problems described in the abstract, a new agent that resolves the 2 major drawbacks in the management of hemophiliacs would have the potential to markedly improve the treatment possibilities for individuals with hemophilia A. The authors of this report have created a humanized bispecific antibody to factor IXa (FIXa) and factor X (FX), termed *hBs23*. This product is unique in that it places these 2 factors into spatially appropriate positions that mimic the cofactor function of factor VIII. The authors have shown that the humanized bispecific antibody, hBs23, will actually exert coagulation activity in factor VIII–deficient plasma, even in the absence of inhibitors, and show in vivo hemostatic activity in an animal model (a nonhuman primate model of acquired hemophilia A). The beauty of hBs23 is that it can be administered subcutaneously and has a long half-life (2 weeks). It would not be expected to elicit the development of factor VIII–specific antibodies.

Although hBs23 was shown by these authors to have efficacy in an animal study, the molecular structure of the antibody would require further optimization in several ways before clinical use of such an agent in humans. One of the important things that needs to be done is to engineer the product further to reduce the immunogenicity of the humanized antibody. Even though humanized or fully human antibodies generally have low immunogenicity, they can be immunogenic.

We just may be seeing the first glimpse of a way to treat hemophiliacs that does not require the rigorous use of intravenous factor VIII concentrate. Needless to say, it will be some time before the story regarding the use of antibodies factors IXa and X used as part of the management of hemophilia A will play out, but a long-acting subcutaneously injectable agent that is unaffected by the presence of inhibitors could markedly reduce the burden of care in these patients.

J. A. Stockman III, MD

The efficacy and the risk of immunogenicity of FIX Padua (R338L) in hemophilia B dogs treated by AAV muscle gene therapy

Finn JD, Nichols TC, Svoronos N, et al (Children's Hosp of Philadelphia, PA; Univ of North Carolina at Chapel Hill; et al)
Blood 120:4521-4523, 2012

Studies on gene therapy for hemophilia B (HB) using adeno-associated viral (AAV) vectors showed that the safety of a given strategy is directly related to the vector dose. To overcome this limitation, we sought to test the efficacy and the risk of immunogenicity of a novel factor IX (FIX) R338L associated with ~ 8-fold increased specific activity. Muscle-directed expression of canine FIX-R338L by AAV vectors was carried out in HB dogs. Therapeutic levels of circulating canine FIX activity (3.5%-8%) showed 8- to 9-fold increased specific activity, similar to humans with FIX-R338L. Phenotypic improvement was documented by the lack of bleeding episodes for a cumulative 5-year observation. No antibody formation and T-cell responses to FIX-R338L were observed, even on challenges with FIX wild-type protein. Moreover, no adverse vascular thrombotic complications were noted. Thus, FIX-R338L provides an attractive strategy to safely enhance the efficacy of gene therapy for HB.

▶ This article points out how far we have come and how far we have yet to go with respect to gene therapy for the management of a fairly common form of hemophilia, hemophilia B, also known as factor IX deficiency. The long-standing goal of continuous expression of a clotting factor gene after a single administration of a viral vector carrying that gene has now been achieved in men with severe hemophilia B. The obvious question that has followed is how quickly and even whether this can become a widely available treatment option for those with hemophilia, and if so, how it will fit into the evolving therapeutic landscape of the disease, as the long-acting clotting factor concentrates are now entering the market.

The most promising clinical trials in hemophilia currently are for hemophilia B, where the continuous infusion of an adeno-associated viral vector encoding factor IX has resulted in expression of functional factor IX levels ranging from 1% to 6% for periods of more than 2 years in a number of adult males with severe hemophilia B. These patients who had been receiving twice-weekly prophylactic infusions of factor IX concentrates have been able to discontinue routine prophylaxis, reserving factor IX infusion for surgery or trauma. The majority of patients so managed with gene therapy have achieved excellent results. Most have successfully ceased using prophylaxis. The safety of the approach to date has been excellent with the only adverse effect being a rise in liver enzymes in a few patients, which resolved after tapering of associated steroid use.

The delicate problem here is the applicability of gene therapy as part of the much more common hemophilia A (factor VIII deficiency). It appears that much larger amounts of vector genes must be given, and these produce a profound immunologic response requiring steroid therapy. To say this differently, we are not there yet when it comes to factor VIII deficiency, not even close. One of the problems with the vectors that are being used is that the proteins expressed are gradually lost over time if the vector is injected into a growing animal, so we would expect much more limited success in young children.

It is good news that gene therapy seems to be able to convert severe hemophilia B to a more mild form of hemophilia B. At this point, this demonstration has occurred in a relatively restricted subset of hemophilia patient populations: adults who are human immunodeficiency virus (HIV) negative, hepatitis V virus RNA viral load negative, and those lacking neutralizing antibodies to the viral vector used. Studies over the next few years will demonstrate whether this patient population can be safely and effectively expanded and whether the same approach will ultimately be effective for hemophilia A. The journey from proof of concept in humans to commercial availability can be long. For example, it was a 14-year effort to move from the first convincing use of purified factor VIIa in a patient with an inhibitor to factor VIII (in 1982) to the licensing of this recombinant product in 1996. On the other hand, under the pressure of the HIV epidemic, recombinant factor VIII went from first infusion in a human in 1987 to a licensed product by 1992, just a 5-year period. What the pace of product development will be for gene therapy remains unknown, but hopefully it will be rapid.

J. A. Stockman III, MD

Recombinant factor XIII: a safe and novel treatment for congenital factor XIII deficiency

Inbal A, Oldenburg J, Carcao M, et al (Tel Aviv Univ, Israel; Univ Clinic, Bonn, Germany; Hosp for Sick Children, Toronto, Ontario, Canada; et al)
Blood 119:5111-5117, 2012

Congenital factor XIII (FXIII) deficiency is a rare, autosomal-recessive disorder, with most patients having an A-subunit (FXIII-A) deficiency. Patients experience life-threatening bleeds, impaired wound healing, and spontaneous abortions. In many countries, only plasma or cryoprecipitate treatments are available, but these carry a risk for allergic reactions and infection with blood-borne pathogens. The present study was a multinational, open-label, single-arm, phase 3 prophylaxis trial evaluating the efficacy and safety of a novel recombinant FXIII (rFXIII) in congenital FXIII A subunit deficiency. Forty-one patients ≥ 6 years of age (mean, 26.4; range, 7-60) with congenital FXIII-A subunit deficiency were enrolled. Throughout the rFXIII prophylaxis, only 5 bleeding episodes (all trauma induced) in 4 patients were treated with FXIII-containing products. The crude mean bleeding rate was significantly lower than the historic bleeding rate (0.138 vs 2.91 bleeds/patient/year, respectively) for on-demand treatment. Transient, non-neutralizing, low-titer anti-rFXIII Abs developed in 4 patients, none of whom experienced allergic reactions, any bleeds requiring treatment, or changes in FXIII pharmacokinetics during the trial or follow-up. These non-neutralizing Abs declined below detection limits in all 4 patients despite further exposure to rFXIII or other FXIII-containing products. We conclude that rFXIII is safe and effective in preventing bleeding episodes in patients with congenital FXIII-A subunit deficiency. This study is registered at http://www.clinicaltrials.gov as number NCT00713648.

▶ It was back in 1960 that the first clinical case of congenital factor XIII deficiency was described in a young Swiss boy presenting with severe bleeding associated with slow and poor wound healing but normal routine coagulation tests. This youngster was not able to form tightly linked clots. When treated with fresh frozen plasma, his bleeding symptoms improved. It is interesting that the first patient described with factor XIII deficiency, otherwise known as fibrin stabilizing factor deficiency, actually took part in a genetic study 45 years later in which the gene abnormality was sequenced.

Those affected with congenital factor XIII deficiency need prophylactic treatment to avoid fatal or seriously disabling bleeding from minor trauma or spontaneous intracranial hemorrhage. As shown in 1960, the usual screening tests for coagulation disorders such as prothrombin time, activated partial thromboplastin time, and thrombin time do not show any abnormalities in factor XIII deficiency. Specific tests must be performed that detect this deficiency. The deficiency itself results in a severe bleeding disorder that is transmitted in an autosomal-recessive manner. Typical bleeding manifestations include umbilical stump bleeding during the first few days of life, postoperative bleeding, and intracranial hemorrhage. The latter is observed more frequently in factor XIII deficiency than in any other inherited bleeding disorder. In addition, factor XIII deficiency is associated with recurrent pregnancy losses and delayed wound healing. Most congenital factor XIII deficiencies are caused by a factor XIII-A subunit deficiency which occurs at a frequency of approximately 1 in 2 million.

The severity of bleeding in congenital factor XIII deficiency is the main reason for regular replacement therapy. Prophylaxis is highly efficient and successful because of the prolonged half-life of factor XIII. To date, only plasma-derived sources of factor XIII have been available including fresh frozen plasma, cryoprecipitate, and a plasma-derived, virally inactivated factor XIII concentrate. All these products carry the usual risks associated with human-derived blood products. Because of the prolonged half-life of factor XIII, administration of these products every 4 to 6 weeks at a dosage ranging from 10 to 35 U/kg will suffice. When prophylactic treatment is available, the prognosis is very good, although the life-long risk of bleeding remains.

Inbal et al have now taken the treatment of factor XIII deficiency a step further in eliminating the risks of infection with bloodborne pathogens from standard replacement therapy products by showing in a multinational, open-label, phase III prophylaxis trial that a new recombinant factor XIII product works amazingly well for these patients. Although a cost-effectiveness profile needs to be established for this product, its introduction is a blessing for affected patients.

J. A. Stockman III, MD

Unexpected frequency of Upshaw-Schulman syndrome in pregnancy-onset thrombotic thrombocytopenic purpura

Moatti-Cohen M, on behalf of the French Reference Center for Thrombotic Microangiopathies (Hôpital Antoine Béclère, Clamart, France; et al)
Blood 119:5888-5897, 2012

Pregnancy may be complicated by a rare but life-threatening disease called thrombotic thrombocytopenic purpura (TTP). Most cases of TTP are due to an acquired autoimmune or hereditary (Upshaw-Schulman syndrome [USS]) severe deficiency of a disintegrin and metalloprotease with thrombospondin type 1 repeats, member 13 (ADAMTS13). In the present study, we performed a cross-sectional analysis of the national registry of the French Reference Center for Thrombotic Microangiopathies from 2000-2010 to identify all women who were pregnant at their initial TTP presentation. Among 592 adulthood-onset TTP patients with a severe ADAMTS13 deficiency, 42 patients with a pregnancy-onset TTP were included. Surprisingly, the proportion of USS patients (n = 10 of 42 patients [24%]; confidence interval, 13%-39%) with pregnancy-onset TTP was much higher than that in adulthood-onset TTP in general (less than 5%) and was mostly related to a cluster of *ADAMTS13* variants. In the present study, subsequent pregnancies in USS patients not given prophylaxis were associated with very high TTP relapse and abortion rates, whereas prophylactic plasmatherapy was beneficial for both the mother and the baby. Pregnancy-onset TTP defines a specific subgroup of patients with a strong genetic background. This study was registered at www.clinicaltrials.gov as number NCT00426686 and at the Health Authority, French Ministry of Health, as number P051064.

▶ Approximately 1 in 25 000 to 1 in 100 000 pregnancies are complicated by a rare, but life-threatening group of disorders called thrombotic microangiopathies (TMAs). These disorders are life-threatening not just to the mother but also to the fetus and newborn. Some TMAs, such as preeclampsia and HELLP (hemolysis, elevated liver enzymes, low platelet count) syndrome, are pregnancy specific, whereas others such as hemolytic uremic syndrome and thrombotic thrombocytopenic purpura (TTP) are not. TTP is defined by the association of thrombocytopenia, mechanical hemolytic anemia, and multivisceral ischemia that occur by recurrent bouts often triggered by infections and pregnancy. The incidence of TTP itself runs 4 to 10 cases per 1 million people per year, and the global mortality rate is estimated at 20%, despite plasma therapy, which remains the standard treatment. The specific pathophysiology for most cases of TTP was defined about 15 years ago and includes a severe functional deficiency of a disintegrin and metalloprotease, the specific von Willebrand factor cleaving protease. This causes an accumulation of platelet-hyperadhesive molecules that leads to the spontaneous formation of microthrombi within the microcirculation. In the large majority of cases, TTP is an adult-onset disease characterized by a female predominance (2:1). More than 95% of cases are in the acquired form.

With respect to obstetrical issues, TTP may be particularly challenging because of the difficulty differentiating it from other TMAs, its dramatic effects on the fetus, and its specific therapeutic management. Pregnancy-associated TTP is reported to represent approximately 10% to 30% of all adult TTP cases.

This article is based on a prospective study of pregnancy-associated TTP patients addressing the epidemiologic and management issues of the differential diagnosis between the acquired and hereditary forms of TTP. The major finding of the article was new information to assist in the differentiation between hereditary and acquired TTP. The study identified a very high rate of adult-onset Upshaw-Schulman syndrome linked to a cluster of a certain genetic set of mutations in a gene known as *ADAMTS13*. Most cases of TTP arise from inhibition of the enzyme ADAMTS13, the metalloprotease responsible for cleaving large multimers of von Willebrand factor into smaller units. The rarest of all TTPs is Upshaw-Schulman syndrome, the genetically inherited version of TTP that is the result of dysfunction of the *ADAMTS13* gene. The problem resulting from this inherited gene abnormality may not show up until pregnancy.

The authors conclude that pregnancy-associated TTP defines a specific subgroup of patients among female adult onset TTP patients who manifest a severe form of *ADAMTS13* deficiency. Thus pregnancy-associated TTP has a strong genetic background in many instances.

The differential diagnosis between hereditary and acquired *ADAMTS13* deficiency in pregnancy-onset TTP remains difficult at presentation, although some clinical and biologic criteria may be more in favor of Upshaw-Schulman syndrome. However, making the differential diagnosis between the inherited form (Upshaw-Schulman syndrome) and acquired TTP after remission is of major importance for several reasons. First, it allows care providers to give specific information to patients in terms of definitive diagnosis (ie, genetic disease vs acquired autoimmune disease) and specific related consequences. Second, it determines a specific therapeutic approach to subsequent pregnancies in the genetically affected patient and improves outcomes in both mother and baby. Third, it allows familial inquiry into the asymptomatic nulliparous sisters of affected patients in order to forestall future problems with their pregnancies. Finally, the results of this study also confirm that any subsequent pregnancy in a TTP patient requires careful clinical monitoring (ideally as soon as the patient becomes pregnant) and that this early care should be supported by a multidisciplinary team involving obstetricians, hematologists, apheresis specialists, and genetic experts.

J. A. Stockman III, MD

Residual plasmatic activity of ADAMTS13 is correlated with phenotype severity in congenital thrombotic thrombocytopenic purpura
Lotta LA, Wu HM, Mackie IJ, et al (Università degli Studi di Milano and Luigi Villa Foundation, Milan, Italy; The Ohio State Univ, Columbus; Univ College London, UK; et al)
Blood 120:440-448, 2012

The quantification of residual plasmatic ADAMTS13 activity in congenital thrombotic thrombocytopenic purpura (TTP) patients is constrained by limitations in sensitivity and reproducibility of commonly used assays at low levels of ADAMTS13 activity, blunting efforts to establish genotype-phenotype correlations. In the present study, the residual plasmatic activity of ADAMTS13 was measured centrally by surface-enhanced laser desorption/ionization time-of-flight mass spectrometry (limit of detection = 0.5%) in 29 congenital TTP patients. The results were used to study correlations among *ADAMTS13* genotype, residual plasmatic activity, and clinical phenotype severity. An ADAMTS13 activity above 0.5% was measured in 26 (90%) patients and lower levels of activity were associated with earlier age at first TTP episode requiring plasma infusion, more frequent recurrences, and prescription of fresh-frozen plasma prophylaxis. Receiver operating characteristic curve analysis showed that activity levels of less than 2.74% and 1.61% were discriminative of age at first TTP episode requiring plasma infusion < 18 years, annual rate of TTP episodes > 1, and use of prophylaxis. Mutations affecting the highly conserved N-terminal domains of the protein were associated with lower residual ADAMTS13 activity and a more severe phenotype in an allelic-dose dependent manner. The results of the present study show that residual ADAMTS13 activity is associated with the severity of clinical phenotype in congenital TTP and provide insights into genotype-phenotype correlations.

▶ Congenital thrombotic thrombocytopenic purpura (TTP) is an uncommon recessively inherited thrombotic microangiopathy. The disease is characterized by the severe congenital deficiency of ADAMTS13 plasma activity caused by mutations in the ADAMTS13 gene. Aficionados of the disorder also know that it is called the Upshaw-Schulman syndrome. It was back in 1960 that Irving Schulman and others reported an 8-year-old girl who had repeated episodes of thrombocytopenia that responded to plasma infusions. They concluded that the child had a "congenital deficiency of a platelet-stimulating factor."[1] Later Upshaw reported a 29-year-old woman who had repeated episodes of TTP. These 2 patients were among the 4 patients with chronic relapsing TTP studied in much greater depth showing the presence of unusually large von Willebrand factor (VWF) multimers. This led to the theory of a missing factor required for VWF cleavage. Ultimately, the missing factor was identified initially as a VWF-cleaving protease. This protease is now called ADAMTS13. For those who really love hematology, this 50-year journey that takes us to our current understandings is a fascinating saga.

Unfortunately, there is little known about what actually happens to people who have a lifetime deficiency of ADAMTS13. The observations of Lotta et al help us in this regard. Lotta et al describe 29 patients born with hereditary TTP in 25 families from 4 centers across Europe. The severity of the deficiency of ADAMTS13 activity correlated with younger age of the first TTP episode, a higher frequency of TTP episodes, and the use of regular plasma prophylaxis. Certain mutations in the affected gene are associated with lower residual enzyme activity and more severe clinical features. Thus this report provides the basis for understanding the genetic heterogeneity of hereditary TTP.

Unfortunately, little is indeed known about the long-term outcome of children with hereditary TTP other than the fact that, if left alone, those affected will have recurrent episodes of thrombocytopenia and the development of a microangiopathy resulting in thrombotic episodes. These can be life-threatening, particularly when associated with neurologic symptoms. Until recently, it was thought that hereditary TTP was too rare for clinicians to care about. Many pediatric hematologists have never seen the disorder, although we read about it all the time. Plasma infusions are the treatment of choice to replace the missing enzyme. Other than for treatment during pregnancy, it is not known whether plasma infusion should only be given when there is actually evidence of active TTP. Pregnancy requires prophylaxis. The relative benefits and risks of regular prophylactic plasma transfusions are unknown. The risk of the development of kidney disease, hypertension, and cardiovascular disease remains unknown. The patient initially reported by Schulman et al did develop chronic renal failure and became dialysis-dependent. There are data to suggest that ADAMTS13 deficiency can accelerate the development of atherosclerosis.

To answer questions about the future of patients with hereditary TTP, systematic lifetime follow-up of many patients is required. To achieve this, an international hereditary TTP registry (www.TTPRegistry.net) was established in 2009. Currently, 83 patients from 74 families in 18 countries have been enrolled with more patients being added as they are diagnosed. The study is looking at long-term outcomes as well as attempting to determine appropriate management. In an editorial that accompanied this report, George notes that hematologists are increasingly convinced that hereditary TTP is an important, albeit rare, problem for patients and clinicians. Patients can be readily diagnosed by measurement of ADAMTS13 plasma activity. The disease should be thought of any time there is the occurrence of thrombocytopenia and hemolytic anemia in a newborn infant for which there is no ready cause identifiable. The disease should also be thought of in any youngster with recurrent episodes of acute thrombocytopenia. If classic TTP occurs during a pregnancy, it may be the first manifestation of a hereditary form of TTP. Once suspected, the definitive genetic diagnosis of TTP is available. The next step is to determine the appropriate management. Regular plasma infusions have logistical problems and potential risks that could be minimized by future availability of recombinant ADAMTS13 enzyme. Unfortunately, this is an orphan disease and, as of now, no one has produced a recombinant form of the enzyme for routine use.

J. A. Stockman III, MD

Reference

1. Schulman I, Pierce M, Lukens A, Currimbhoy Z. Studies on thrombopoiesis. I. A factor in normal human plasma required for platelet production; chronic thrombocytopenia due to its deficiency. *Blood*. 1960;16:943-957.

Treatment, Survival, and Thromboembolic Outcomes of Thrombotic Storm in Children

Manco-Johnson MJ, Wang M, Goldenberg NA, et al (Univ of Colorado School of Medicine, Aurora; et al)
J Pediatr 161:682-688.e1, 2012

Objective.—To describe the course and management of thrombotic storm in 8 children.

Study Design.—Clinical data were collected and analyzed for consecutive children diagnosed with thrombotic storm, aged 6 months to 21 years inclusive, in the context of a single-institution prospective inception cohort study. Thrombotic storm was defined as newly diagnosed multisite venous thromboembolism (VTE) with acute thrombus progression despite conventional or higher than conventional dosing of heparin or low molecular weight heparin. All evaluations and therapies were ordered by the treating physicians in the context of clinical decision making.

Results.—Eight of the 178 children with VTE enrolled in the cohort between March 2006 and November 2009 were diagnosed with thrombotic storm. Antiphospholipid antibodies were acutely positive in 6 children, of whom heparin-induced thrombocytopenia was confirmed by serotonin release assay in 2 and atypical in 1. One child died. Five children received a direct thrombin inhibitor, titrated to achieve normalization of markedly elevated D-dimer levels. All children were transitioned to fondaparinux or enoxaparin before receiving extended anticoagulation with warfarin. Immunomodulatory therapy was instituted in all children. During follow-up (median duration, 3 years; range, 2-6 years), 3 of the 7 surviving children experienced recurrent VTE, and 4 children had clinically significant postthrombotic syndrome.

Conclusion.—Thrombotic storm is an infrequent but potentially fatal presentation of VTE in children. Administration of direct thrombin inhibitors and immune modulation can achieve quiescence, although long-term adverse outcomes are common.

▶ This report reminds us that venous thromboembolism (VTE) affects 5.8 children of every 100 000, at least based on data of discharges from pediatric hospitals. Most children seem to do very well, but there is a subset of youngsters who, despite conventional or even unconventional aggressive therapies with various forms of heparin, will exhibit rapid progression of thrombosis, known as *thrombotic storm*. The occurrence of rapid progression of thrombosis while on anticoagulant therapy raises concerns for catastrophic antiphospholipid antibody (APA) syndrome (CAPS) or (when accompanied by a rapid decline in platelet count) heparin induced thrombocytopenia and thrombosis syndrome or thrombotic thrombocytopenic purpura. In older age children and adults, Trousseau syndrome (cancer-associated migratory VTE) is also a diagnostic consideration. The overall inclusive term *thrombotic storm* is now currently used in the literature to describe a syndrome of VTE characterized by rapid development of multifocal thromboses of various etiologies outside of Trousseau syndrome with or without APA.

The authors of this report provide new information on thrombotic storm or CAPS in children. They examine the presentation, laboratory findings, complex management, survival, and thromboembolic outcomes in 8 consecutive children with thrombotic storm enrolled in an institutional-based prospective cohort study. In the children with thrombotic storm, antiphospholipid antibodies were observed in three-fourths of the patients. One in 4 experienced heparin-induced thrombocytopenia. One of the children died. Heparin alone and warfarin alone or both in combination were ineffective to treat the patients. Most patients received a direct thrombin inhibitor in an amount necessary to achieve normalization of markedly elevated D-dimer levels. All children were eventually able to be transitioned to fondaparinux or enoxaparin before receiving extended anticoagulation therapy with warfarin. Immunomodulatory therapy was instituted in all children. Over a 3-year follow-up, 3 of the children who survived did experience recurrent VTE.

The likelihood of VTE in families is dependent on the specific type of thrombophilia exhibited. The importance of identifying patients at risk for VTE cannot be overstated because of associated mortality, morbidity, and increased cost to society. However, mass screening for these inherited thrombophilias in the healthy population does not seem warranted at the current time, as the prevalence of a deficiency, for example, of protein C, protein S, and antithrombin, is less than 1%. In addition, thrombophilia testing is expensive and has ethical ramifications. Any child, however, with VTE as well as his or her relatives should be screened for inherited thrombophilia, including protein C and protein S and antithrombin deficiencies, along with factor V G1691A and factor II G20210A. For more on the topic of thrombophilia screening and tests, see the editorial by Bruce and Massicotte.[1]

J. A. Stockman III, MD

Reference

1. Bruce A, Massicotte MP. Thrombophilia screening: whom to test? *Blood.* 2012; 120:1353-1355.

Thrombosis from a Prothrombin Mutation Conveying Antithrombin Resistance

Miyawaki Y, Suzuki A, Fujita J, et al (Nagoya Univ Graduate School of Medicine, Japan; et al)

N Engl J Med 366:2390-2396, 2012

We identified a novel mechanism of hereditary thrombosis associated with antithrombin resistance, with a substitution of arginine for leucine at position 596 (p.Arg596Leu) in the gene encoding prothrombin (called prothrombin Yukuhashi). The mutant prothrombin had moderately lower activity than wild-type prothrombin in clotting assays, but the formation of thrombin—antithrombin complex was substantially impaired. A thrombin-generation assay revealed that the peak activity of the mutant prothrombin was fairly low, but its inactivation was extremely slow in reconstituted plasma. The Leu596 substitution caused a gain-of-function mutation in the prothrombin gene, resulting in resistance to antithrombin and susceptibility to thrombosis.

▶ There are many causes of an increased tendency to produce clots. Patients, however, with hereditary thrombophilia will frequently present with evidence of venous thrombosis at particularly young ages. Some of the genetic causes of thrombophilia include loss of function mutations in the natural anticoagulants antithrombin, protein C, and protein S along with gain-of-function mutations in procoagulant factors V (factor V Leiden) and II (prothrombin G20210A). It is believed that there are many undiscovered yet causative mutations as genetic etiologies of thrombophilia.

These authors describe a case of hereditary thrombosis caused by a novel mechanism of antithrombin resistance, a gain-of-function mutation in the gene encoding the clotting factor prothrombin, which they name prothrombin Yukuhashi.

The case that is described here is of a 17-year-old Japanese girl who experienced her first episode of deep vein thrombosis at age 11 years. Her family was from the town of Yukuhashi in the northern part of the Kyushu Islands. Her family history showed that 9 of her family members had one or more episodes of deep vein thrombosis, including 2 of the family members who had serious pulmonary embolism and 3 who had died from thrombosis. Five of the family members had onset of thrombosis at a very young age. Over the years, a number of the family members had routine studies to determine the etiology of their thrombophilia, but no disorder was identified, at least not until the investigators of this article did gene analysis on the prothrombin gene using specific gene primers by means of polymerase chain reaction. The authors found a novel missense mutation in the prothrombin gene that resulted in a variant prothrombin. The mutation occurred at a specific location at one of the antithrombin-binding sites where thrombin is inactivated by antithrombin with heparin.

Thus we now have one more cause of hereditary thrombophilia that should be looked for. It is likely that this new hereditary cause of thrombosis is quite rare in its occurrence, but worth looking for The mutation that results from the gene's effect results in slightly impaired but adequate procoagulant function of the mutant prothrombin, but considerably impaired inhibition of the mutant thrombin by antithrombin. Unfortunately, as of now, only fairly sophisticated gene testing will detect this disorder.

This commentary in the Blood chapter closes with a query having to do with a hematologic subject. For the 2012 Olympics, what was a predictable hematologic consequence? The prediction, which turned out to be correct, was that there would be a blood shortage as a result of individuals who might ordinarily donate blood staying home for days on end watching the Olympic Games on IV.[1] The prediction was forecasted based on the experience of very few blood donors arriving to Blood donor centers the day of a Royal wedding!

J. A. Stockman III, MD

Reference

1. Editorial Comment. Blood donors may stay home because of the Olympics. *BMJ.* 2012;344:4.

4   Child Development/ Behavior

Association Between Maternal Use of Folic acid Supplements and Risk of Autism Spectrum Disorders in Children
Surén P. Roth C. Bresnahan M. et al (Norwegian Inst of Public Health, Nydalen, Oslo; Columbia Univ, NY; et al)
JAMA 309.570-577, 2013

Importance.—Prenatal folic acid supplements reduce the risk of neural tube defects in children, but it has not been determined whether they protect against other neurodevelopmental disorders.

Objective.—To examine the association between maternal use of prenatal folic acid supplements and subsequent risk of autism spectrum disorders (ASDs) (autistic disorder, Asperger syndrome, pervasive developmental disorder—not otherwise specified [PDD-NOS]) in children.

Design, Setting, and Patients.—The study sample of 85 176 children was derived from the population-based, prospective Norwegian Mother and Child Cohort Study (MoBa). The children were born in 2002-2008; by the end of follow-up on March 31, 2012, the age range was 3.3 through 10.2 years (mean, 6.4 years). The exposure of primary interest was use of folic acid from 4 weeks before to 8 weeks after the start of pregnancy, defined as the first day of the last menstrual period before conception. Relative risks of ASDs were estimated by odds ratios (ORs) with 95% CIs in a logistic regression analysis. Analyses were adjusted for maternal education level, year of birth, and parity.

Main Outcome Measure.—Specialist-confirmed diagnosis of ASDs.

Results.—At the end of follow-up, 270 children in the study sample had been diagnosed with ASDs: 114 with autistic disorder, 56 with Asperger syndrome, and 100 with PDD-NOS. In children whose mothers took folic acid, 0.10% (64/61 042) had autistic disorder, compared with 0.21% (50/24 134) in those unexposed to folic acid. The adjusted OR for autistic disorder in children of folic acid users was 0.61 (95% CI, 0.41-0.90). No association was found with Asperger syndrome or PDD-NOS, but power was limited. Similar analyses for prenatal fish oil supplements showed no such association with autistic disorder, even though fish oil use was associated with the same maternal characteristics as folic acid use.

Conclusions and Relevance.—Use of prenatal folic acid supplements around the time of conception was associated with a lower risk of autistic disorder in the MoBa cohort. Although these findings cannot establish causality, they do support prenatal folic acid supplementation.

▶ Evidence suggests that autism spectrum disorders (ASDs) are associated with a combination of multiple genetic and environmental risk factors leading to variable clinical presentations. Given the interest in prenatal risk factors, some have theorized that nutritional exposures, such as folic acid intake, could increase the risk of autism. It is well known that folate and folic acid are sources of 1-carbon units essential for basic cellular processes, including DNA replication and DNA, RNA, and protein methylations. It is reasonable, therefore, to at least hypothesize that folic acid might affect numerous conditions either positively or negatively depending on timing and dose. We all know that randomized, controlled trials have documented that periconceptional folic acid supplementation does reduce the risk of neural tube defects and does so in up to 75% of cases. Now women of childbearing age routinely consume 400 μg/d of folic acid if they are following national recommendation standards. Studies have also found that periconceptional folic acid supplementation is associated with a reduced risk of severe language delay.[1]

Surén et al report results from a large study known as the *Norwegian Mother and Child Cohort Study*. This study looked at more than 85 000 children, including 114 who had an autism spectrum disorder. The authors reported an incidence of autistic disorder of 0.1% in offspring of mothers who took periconceptional folic acid supplements versus 0.21% in offspring who did not, for an adjusted odds ratio of 0.61. These findings clearly suggest that periconceptional folic acid supplementation is associated with a reduced risk of autistic disorders in the offspring of pregnant women. The findings actually make sense in light of several recent studies pointing to improved neurodevelopmental outcomes in children of mothers having higher folate concentrations or actually receiving folic acid supplements. Some have even talked about the possibility of preventing certain forms of autism in response to the discovery of inborn errors of metabolism associated with this disorder.

There is no question that the report of Surén et al needs to be followed by other population-based studies in other countries, including the United States. One of the conundrums is the fact that there seems to be a significant increase in ASD diagnoses over the last decade or 2 during a period in which folic acid supplementation in the periconceptional period has been the norm. This may be attributable to changes in diagnosis and surveillance or an actual real increase for other reasons in the prevalence of ASD attributable to as-yet unknown set of risk factors. The average daily consumption of folic acid in the United States is approximately 150 μg/d from food fortified with folic acid. This amount may, in fact, be too low to contribute measurably to a decline in prevalence such as seen in Norway. Future studies will be needed to sort this out.

This entry closes with an important comment about child development and the acquisition of language.[2] As infants start babbling at around age 6 months in preparation for talking, they shift from focusing on adults' eyes to paying special attention to speakers' mouths, a recent study finds. Babies start to lip read when they learn to babble. As tots become able to blurt out words and simple statements at age one, they go back to concentrating on adults' eyes. By two years of age, children with autism avoid eye contact and focus on speakers' mouths. It is suggested that with the new information on lip reading and babbling, perhaps disorders such as autism can be detected earlier.

J. A. Stockman III, MD

References

1. Roth C, Magnus P, Schjolberg S, et al. Folic acid supplements in pregnancy and severe language delay in children. *JAMA*. 2011;306:1566-1573.
2. Bower B. Babbling babies read adults' lips. *Science news*. 2012;181(3).

Age, Academic Performance, and Stimulant Prescribing for ADHD: A Nationwide Cohort Study

Zoëga H, Valdimarsdóttir UA, Hernández-Díaz S (Mount Sinai School of Medicine, NY; Univ of Iceland, Reykjavík; Harvard School of Public Health, Boston, MA)

Pediatrics 130:1012-1018, 2012

Background.—We evaluated whether younger age in class is associated with poorer academic performance and an increased risk of being prescribed stimulants for attention-deficit/hyperactivity disorder (ADHD).

Methods.—This was a nationwide population-based cohort study, linking data from national registries of prescribed drugs and standardized scholastic examinations. The study population comprised all children born in 1994—1996 who took standardized tests in Iceland at ages 9 and 12 ($n = 11\,785$). We estimated risks of receiving low test scores (0—10th percentile) and being prescribed stimulants for ADHD. Comparisons were made according to children's relative age in class.

Results.—Mean test scores in mathematics and language arts were lowest among the youngest children in the fourth grade, although the gap attenuated in the seventh grade. Compared with the oldest third, those in the youngest third of class had an increased relative risk of receiving a low test score at age 9 for mathematics (1.9; 95% confidence interval [CI] 1.6—2.2) and language arts (1.8; 95% CI 1.6—2.1), whereas at age 12, the relative risk was 1.6 in both subjects. Children in the youngest third of class were 50% more likely (1.5; 95% CI 1.3—1.8) than those in the oldest third to be prescribed stimulants between ages 7 and 14.

Conclusions.—Relative age among classmates affects children's academic performance into puberty, as well as their risk of being prescribed stimulants for ADHD. This should be taken into account when evaluating children's performance and behavior in school to prevent unnecessary stimulant treatment.

▶ How many times in practice have you been asked by a parent whether his or her youngster, who is due to start first grade, should be delayed for a year because the child is barely on the cusp of the minimal age to enter formal schooling? Obviously, birth cutoffs for school entry necessarily lead to an age span of at least 12 months within a classroom. A 5-year-old starting school at the earliest cutoff presents a significant difference in maturity and perhaps cognitive performance compared with a child essentially one year older who may also be in the same class, although most data suggest that being older relative to one's classmates has no long-term benefits.[1] All too often parents will hold back a youngster for a year before entering school so that they will be more mature and thus start off with an academic, social, and physical advantage. For the same reasons, some school districts have pushed back their birthday cutoffs to increase the average age of children entering, thus, improving their standardized test scores later.

Zoëga et al have designed a study to evaluate whether being young in a class is or is not associated with poor academic performance and an increased risk of being assigned a diagnosis of attention-deficit/hyperactivity disorder (ADHD). The investigators obtained nationwide data over a 7-year period on standardized test results and psychotropic drug prescription fills for national birth cohorts in the country of Iceland. They were able to link nationwide records from the database of National Scholastic Examinations, the Icelandic Population Registry, and the Icelandic Medicine's Registry. Fig 1 in the original article shows the performance on achievement tests mandatory for all children in the fourth (age 9) and seventh (age 12) grades in Iceland relative to age in the youngsters' classes.

The results of this population-based nationwide study indicate that being among the youngest students in a class is associated with academic underperformance during childhood. At age 9, the youngest third of children in their class had, compared with the oldest third, an 80% to 90% increased risk of scoring in the lowest centile on standardized tests. At age 12, the excess risk was 60% for both mathematics and language, indicating that the effect of relative age on academic achievement might ameliorate over time but is still at play into puberty. Furthermore, over 6 years of follow-up, the youngest third of children in the class were 50% more likely than the oldest third of their classmates to be prescribed stimulants for ADHD. It was also observed that the youngest children in class were less likely to enter high-end universities. Other studies have suggested that when compared with older peers, those younger have been shown to be less likely to excel in sports and to be at higher risk of emotional and behavioral problems.

Recently, Elder also showed that the youngest children in fifth and eighth grades are nearly twice as likely as their older classmates to use stimulants prescribed for ADHD. The latter authors argued that the diagnosis was largely driven by subjective comparisons across children in the same grade school.[2] In this same study of almost 12 000 US children followed from kindergarten to eighth grade, it was found that 8.4% of the youngest children in the class, born the month before their states' cutoff dates for kindergarten eligibility, were diagnosed with ADHD, compared with 5.1% of children born in the month immediately after the cutoff. These findings are consistent with those of one other report of Evans et al who found that children 7 years to 17 years old whose birth date fell in the 120 days before the school eligibility cutoff date, had, compared with those born in the 120 days after the cutoff, double the chance of being diagnosed or treated for ADHD.[3]

Zoëga et al suggest that the association of children's relative age to peers in a class with both academic performance and ADHD treatment may not be all that surprising. ADHD may affect academic performance, and academic performance may affect ADHD diagnosis. It is entirely possible that the increased risk observed of ADHD diagnosis in the youngest children in a class could partially be a mere consequence of their relative immaturity compared with older peers. If so, the consequence of a potential lifelong label of ADHD is a sorry price to pay for being the youngest in one's class.

This report should be read in detail by all pediatricians so that when the topic does come up in the office setting about whether to hold a child back is a wise decision, you have some information to assist in answering that question.

While on a topic having to do with child development, we close this commentary with mention of something having to so with memory and pigeons. It appears the expression "bird brain" has lost some if its meaning with new learnings about just how smart some birds are. Two investigators in Paris donned long white lab coats and spent several days feeding pigeons.[4] One investigator ignored the birds or chased them away while another fed the birds. Later the investigators swapped coats and also swapped roles. On returning to the area where the pigeons were fed, the pigeons flocked immediately to the individual who previously had fed them and ignored the individual who had been unfriendly. The investigators were of similar size and build. Since the lab coats covered more than 90% of the investigators bodies, it is assumed that pigeons could recognize and remember facial features. It should be noted that crows have already shown to be able to tell one person from another (http://scim.ag/_crows). An earlier experiment in the United States showed that the crows learned to distinguish between masks resembling a caveman and Vice President Dick Cheney!

J. A. Stockman III, MD

References

1. Stipek D. At what age should children enter kindergarten? A question for policy makers and parents. *SRCD Social Policy Report.* 2002;16:3-16.
2. Elder TE. The importance of relative standards in ADHD diagnoses: evidence based on exact birth dates. *J Health Econ.* 2010;29:641-656.
3. Evans WN, Morrill MS, Parente ST. Measuring inappropriate medical diagnosis and treatment in survey data: the case of ADHD among school-age children. *J Health Econ.* 2010;29:657-673.
4. Editorial comment. Pigeons don't forget a face. *Science.* 2011;333:274.

Prevalence and risk of violence against children with disabilities: a systematic review and meta-analysis of observational studies

Jones L, Bellis MA, Wood S, et al (Liverpool John Moores Univ, UK; et al)
Lancet 380:899-907, 2012

Background.—Globally, at least 93 million children have moderate or severe disability. Children with disabilities are thought to have a substantially greater risk of being victims of violence than are their non-disabled peers. Establishment of reliable estimates of the scale of the problem is an essential first step in the development of effective prevention programmes. We therefore undertook a systematic review and meta-analysis to synthesise evidence for the prevalence and risk of violence against children with disabilities.

Methods.—For this systematic review and meta-analysis, we searched 12 electronic databases to identify cross-sectional, case-control, or cohort studies reported between Jan 1, 1990, and Aug 17, 2010, with estimates of prevalence of violence against children (aged ≤ 18 years) with disabilities or their risk of being victims of violence compared with children without disabilities.

Findings.—17 studies were selected from 10 663 references. Reports of 16 studies provided data suitable for meta-analysis of prevalence and 11 for risk. Pooled prevalence estimates were 26·7% (95% CI 13·8—42·1) for combined violence measures, 20·4% (13·4—28·5) for physical violence, and 13·7% (9·2—18·9) for sexual violence. Odds ratios for pooled risk estimates were 3·68 (2·56—5·29) for combined violence measures, 3·56 (2·80—4·52) for physical violence, and 2·88 (2·24—3·69) for sexual violence. Huge heterogeneity was identified across most estimates ($I^2 > 75\%$). Variations were not consistently explained with meta-regression analysis of the characteristics of the studies.

Interpretation.—The results of this systematic review confirm that children with disabilities are more likely to be victims of violence than are their peers who are not disabled. However, the continued scarcity of robust evidence, due to a lack of well designed research studies, poor standards of measurement of disability and violence, and insufficient assessment of whether violence precedes the development of disability, leaves gaps in knowledge that need to be addressed.

▶ Before this article appeared, I was not familiar with the topic of violence against children with disabilities. Much is written, quite appropriately, about the estimated 53 000 children aged 0 to 17 who are murdered annually throughout the world.[1] Little, however, is written about violence against the estimated 5% of children (almost 93 million) birth through 14 years who have moderate or severe disability and a greater risk of violence taken out on them.[2] Children with disabilities are thought to be at greater risk of violence than those who are without, the reasons being related to social stigma and discrimination, negative traditional beliefs, ignorance within communities, lack of social support for care providers, types of impairment, and heightened vulnerability as a result of the need for increased care, including medical attention.

These authors undertook a systematic review and meta-analysis to identify the characteristics covering research into the prevalence and risk of violence perpetrated against children with disabilities who are 18 years of age and younger. The authors also assessed the quality of the research and undertook a quantitative synthesis of the evidence from the literature with a view toward identifying knowledge gaps and research priorities. They found 16 studies suitable for inclusion in a meta-analysis. The systematic review and meta-analysis did show that violence is an important problem for children with disabilities. The review itself is the first to provide estimates of the prevalence in risk of violence perpetrated against children with disabilities.

It seems fairly clear that children with mental or intellectual disability seem to have a higher prevalence and risk of violence than do children with other types of disabilities. This observation was most apparent for the prevalence of physical violence and emotional abuse and for the risk of sexual violence. Most of the data in this report, however, were from high-income countries such as the United States and European countries, leaving a huge gap in understanding the nature of the problem for most regions of the world, particularly for low-income and middle-income countries. Unfortunately, there was little information about school bullying of children with disabilities. When it comes to physical violence, it appears that 1 of 5 children with disabilities are subjected to this.

With data suggesting that up to a quarter of children with disabilities will experience violence within their lifetimes and that they are 3 to 4 times more likely to be victims of violence in comparison with their peers, there is a need to learn more about this problem and how to prevent it. Yes, there has been an increased awareness of violence against children in general as well as those with disabilities, but robust evidence continues to be scarce about what to do to eliminate this. The authors suggest what is needed: high-quality epidemiologic research that focuses on all types of disabilities using currently available standardized measures of disabilities and violence with a focus on low-income and middle-income families in particular where there is little evidence to provide directions in terms of prevention.

This commentary closes with an observation concerning IQ. It turns out that one's IQ in childhood is not immutable.[3] Back in 1994, investigators at the University College, London, tested the IQ of 33 14-year-olds. These same teens had MRI scans performed at that time. Four years later the teens were retested. The overall IQ score did not change from the prior testing (average IQ 112), but individual scores showed some significant variations. One teen's IQ dropped 18 points and another's rose 24 points. Some who scored high the first time scored even higher, and others who scored low the first time scored even lower. The IQ changes were accompanied by changes in brain grey matter. Boosts in verbal IQ came along with the development of denser gray matter in the left motor cortex, the area involved in speaking. Boosts in performance IQ, which measures abilities such as understanding images, were also associated with denser gray matter.

All of this suggests that the human brain is still "plastic" well into the teen years, something not observed in earlier studies.

J. A. Stockman III, MD

References

1. Pinherio PS. *World Report of Violence Against Children.* Geneva, Switzerland: ATAR Roto Presse SA; 2006.
2. World Health Organization. Global burden of disease. Disease and injury regional estimates. 2011. http://www.who.int/healthinfo/global_burden_disease/estimates_regional/en/index.html. Accessed December 26, 2012.
3. Sanders L. Teen years can warp the brain. *Science News.* 2011;11:12.

Does simultaneous bilingualism aggravate children's specific language problems?

Korkman M, Stenroos M, Mickos A, et al (Univ of Helsinki, Finland; Mental Care Ctr, City of Raseborg, Finland; Folkhälsan, Habiliteringen, Helsinki, Finland; et al)
Acta Paediatr 101:946-952, 2012

Aim.—There is little data on whether or not a bilingual upbringing may aggravate specific language problems in children. This study analysed whether there was an interaction of such problems and simultaneous bilingualism.

Methods.—Participants were 5- to 7-year-old children with specific language problems (LANG group, N = 56) or who were typically developing (CONTR group, N = 60). Seventy-three children were Swedish-Finnish bilingual and 43 were Swedish-speaking monolingual. Assessments (in Swedish) included tests of expressive language, comprehension, repetition and verbal memory.

Results.—Per definition, the LANG group had lower scores than the CONTR group on all language tests. The bilingual group had lower scores than the monolingual group only on a test of body part naming. Importantly, the interaction of group (LANG or CONTR) and bilingualism was not significant on any of the language scores.

Conclusions.—Simultaneous bilingualism does not aggravate specific language problems but may result in a slower development of vocabulary both in children with and without specific language problems. Considering also advantages, a bilingual upbringing is an option also for children with specific language problems. In assessment, tests of vocabulary may be sensitive to bilingualism, instead tests assessing comprehension, syntax and nonword repetition may provide less biased methods.

▶ There has been a fair amount written these days about bilingualism in a family and its effects on child development. In fact, growing up in a bilingual family could very well provide a youngster with the advantage of acquiring 2 languages simultaneously from the start of language development. This could, however, impose increased demands on the acquisition of vocabulary and linguistic structures in comparison with the demands of single language development. Data suggest that typically developing children do not suffer any major disadvantage from being simultaneously bilingual, with the exception of a distributed vocabulary and some cross-language influences. Little is known about the effects of a bilingual environment on children who have developmental delays, neurologic disorders, autism spectrum disorders, or significant hearing problems. Few studies have been undertaken to examine a possible risk of bilingual upbringing for children with specific language impairment or more generalized language impairment.

These authors have designed a study to determine whether simultaneous bilingualism could aggravate language problems. The study included 5-year-old to 7-year-old Finnish kindergarten or preschool students (in Finland, children start formal schooling when they reach 7 years of age). Studied were typically normally developing youngsters and those with specific language problems. The authors assessed monolingual and simultaneously bilingual children who either had specific language problems or were typically developing in their stronger language (Swedish). The authors found that bilingualism could result in slower development of vocabulary, but it does not seem to cause any specific language problems.

Because of the uncertainty concerning the effects of bilingualism, it is not uncommon that parents whose native languages are different are advised to choose only 1 language when communicating with a child who has language problems.[1] This study indicates that bilingualism does not overtax these children's language capacity. Still, the fact that simultaneously bilingual children from both groups did obtain slightly poorer scores on the body part naming subtests, the study could be seen as a reason to protect children from this negative effect by using only 1 language at home. However, this might restrict the interaction of a parent with a child, which would only make matters worse.

This commentary ends with the recognition that declines in intellect that come with age are actually occurring at earlier ages than one might think.[2] New research shows that cognitive decline can be detected as early as age 45 years. Investigators studied 5198 men and 2192 women aged 45-70 years during a 10-year period. The youngest participants in the study—45-49 years old at baseline—had a 3.6% decline in their reasoning abilities over 10 years. The decline in reasoning ability was 9.6% in the oldest men and 7.4% in the oldest women.

J. A. Stockman III, MD

References

1. Paradis J. Bilingual children with specific language impairment: theoretical and applied issues. *Appl Psycholinguist.* 2007;28:551-564.
2. Editorial comment. Early cognitive decline. *JAMA.* 2012;307:445.

Hypoxic and Hypercapnic Events in Young Infants During Bed-sharing

Baddock SA, Galland BC, Bolton DPG, et al (Univ of Otago, Dunedin, New Zealand)
Pediatrics 130:237-244, 2012

Objectives.—To identify desaturation events (arterial oxygen saturation [Sao_2] < 90%) and rebreathing events (inspired carbon dioxide (CO_2) > 3%), in bed-sharing (BS) versus cot-sleeping (CS) infants.

Methods.—Forty healthy, term infants, aged 0 to 6 months who regularly bed-shared with at least 1 parent > 5 hours per night and 40 age-matched CS infants were recruited. Overnight parent and infant behavior (via infrared video), Sao2, inspired CO_2 around the infant's face, and body temperature were recorded during sleep at home.

Results.—Desaturation events were more common in BS infants (risk ratio = 2.17 [95% confidence interval: 1.75 to 2.69]), associated partly with the warmer microenvironment during BS. More than 70% of desaturations in both groups were preceded by central apnea of 5 to 10 seconds with no accompanying bradycardia, usually in active sleep. Apnea > 15 seconds was rare (BS infants: 3 events; CS infants: 6 events), as was desaturation < 80% (BS infants: 3 events; CS infants: 4 events). Eighty episodes of rebreathing were identified from 22 BS infants and 1 CS infant, almost all preceded by head covering. During rebreathing, Sao_2 was maintained at the baseline of 97.6%.

Conclusions.—BS infants experienced more oxygen desaturations preceded by central apnea, partly related to the warmer microenvironment. Rebreathing occurred mainly during bed-sharing. Infants were at low risk of sudden infant death syndrome and maintained normal oxygenation. The effect of repeated exposure to oxygen desaturation in vulnerable infants is unknown as is the ability of vulnerable infants to respond effectively to rebreathing caused by head covering.

▶ This is a very important report. Most studies of infants sleep physiology are of solitary sleeping infants with few studies describing infants' responses to bed-sharing environments. Bed-sharing studies have reported decreased time in quiet sleep and increases in arousals, periodic breathing, increased inspired carbon dioxide, increased heart rates, and peripheral and axillary temperature increases. The study of Braddock et al was designed to investigate the usual sleep practices of infants in their own home to identify and compare desaturation events (arterial oxygen saturation < 90%) and rebreathing episodes (inspired carbon dioxide > 3%) between co-sleeping infants and infants left to sleep in their own independent environment (cribs/cots). Forty infants who regularly slept in a parent bed with 1 or both parents for a minimum of 5 hours a night and 40 matched independently sleeping infants who slept in a cot or bassinet for at least 5 hours a night were studied and compared.

This study found that infants who bed-share experience more episodes of mild oxygen desaturation associated with the warmer microenvironment and responded more frequently to rebreathing stimuli compared with infants who slept in a cot. More devastating events such as desaturations to < 80% and longer apneic episodes (> 15 seconds) were rare, but occurred in both groups of infants. Infants in this study were healthy and based on demographic characteristics were at low risk for sudden infant death syndrome. All responded appropriately to the potential stressors of cosleeping. It was clear, however, that bed-sharing infants were exposed to more rebreathe events than independently sleeping infants. This was associated with head covering by bedding or mother's clothing during supine or side positioning and less frequently from the infant's face positioned into a pillow during prone or side positioning. In response to this, it appears that infants may either increase ventilation effectively, remove themselves from the rebreathe situation, or have actions taken by the mother. Rebreathe events were identified in only 1 cot-sleeping infant swaddled in a muslin wrap who pulled the wrap over her face several times.

It is clear that desaturation events of < 90% is seen more often in bed-sharing infants than in those sleeping independently, although the importance of this event as a risk factor for sudden infant death syndrome is unclear. Episodic apnea and periodic breathing can occur in normal infants and are not observed more frequently in future sudden infant death victims. This study noted that almost all of the desaturation events were preceded by central apnea and were accompanied by a warmer microenvironment. The study also documented that warmer temperatures can trigger periodic breathing.

This report concluded that the presence of the mother and other bed partners and the physical environment of the adult bed lead to a different sleep environment for bed-sharing infants compared with those sleeping independently. This results in potentially compromising situations. Infant homeostatic responses and maternal interactions seem to keep these low-risk infants safe. However, the authors suggest that it is potentially hazardous for an infant to sleep in the same bed as their parent. The authors also acknowledge that bed sharing is a practice valued by many; thus, it is important to identify the specific dangers related to this practice. Keeping the environment smoke-free at all times, including during pregnancy, is perhaps the most important message one can pass on as well as avoiding the consumption of alcohol or sedating drugs on the bed-sharing night. The infant's face must be kept clear and the use of thick insulation as over-bedding must be avoided. There is no denying that bed sharing has special significance in many cultures and is widely practiced for perceived benefits in parent/infant bonding, encouraging breastfeeding, and reducing maternal sleep disruption and infant stress. These are all good influences. At the same time, the data from this report tell us that there are certain risk factors in bed sharing that should and can be avoided.

J. A. Stockman III, MD

Norms and Trends of Sleep Time Among US Children and Adolescents

Williams JA, Zimmerman FJ, Bell JF (UCLA (Univ of California, Los Angeles); Univ of Washington, Seattle)
JAMA Pediatr 167:55-60, 2013

Objectives.—To develop national sleep norms conditional on age and to examine stratification by sex, race/ethnicity, and changes over time.

Design.—Secondary analysis of a panel survey.

Setting.—The 3 waves (1997, 2002, and 2007) of the Child Development Supplement of the Panel Study of Income Dynamics, a nationally representative survey.

Participants.—Children from birth to 18 years with time-diary data were included: 2832 children in 1997, 2520 children in 2002, and 1424 children in 2007.

Main Exposure.—Age.

Main Outcome Measures.—Minutes of sleep for daytime and total sleep.

Results.—The 10th, 25th, 50th, 75th, and 90th percentiles of the distribution of children's minutes of sleep conditional on age were estimated using a double-kernel estimator that incorporates sample weights. Total average sleep was estimated at more than 13 hours a day for infants, decreasing steadily throughout childhood and early adolescence, reaching about 9 hours a day for 14- to 18-year-olds. The estimated conditional percentiles were higher on weekends than on weekdays for older children. The conditional percentiles for the weekend sleep minutes were flatter with respect to age than the weekday sleep minutes. The interquartile ranges were greater for children younger than 6 years and for teenagers. The medians stratified by race/ethnicity and sex were similar for most ages. For different survey years, the estimated medians were within a few minutes of each other.

Conclusions.—These estimates are consistent with the amount of sleep recommended for children, and no evidence was found of racial/ethnic differences.

▶ Great concern has been noted in the literature in recent years about the problem of sleep deprivation in children and, in particular, adolescents. Although sleep duration normal ranges have been obtained on random, representative samples of the population for some ages of children in Australia, Switzerland, and Italy, there are few comparative data on children in the United States.

These authors present the first large-scale nationally representative sleep duration norms for US children aged 0 to 18 years using sleep duration percentiles as the metric for reporting. Specifically, the investigators obtained data from parents who completed 24-hour time diaries on a random weekday and weekend day basis. The study confirms previous data from around the world showing that sleep duration steadily decreases with increasing age and very significantly from child to child. There is also a difference between weekdays and weekends.

In an editorial that accompanied this report, Jenni[1] noted that although these authors state that their estimates are in line with the guidelines for optimal sleep duration published by the Centers for Disease Control and Prevention suggesting that overall US children get an appropriate amount of sleep, it remains far from uncertain what a "normal," "ideal," or "adequate" sleep duration is for an individual child to promote optimal health and functioning. Jenni notes that relying on reports of sleep duration in children and adolescents at certain ages under normal, unconstrained conditions is not sufficient for determining optimal sleep time for individual children. The ideal would be to combine this information with studies of vigilance, sleepiness, and cognitive and emotional functioning under various circumstances such as sleep restriction or sleep extension. Therefore, a combination of these factors would be better to estimate true need for sleep. Unfortunately, studies that incorporate all these variables are scarce indeed. No optimal amount of sleep for the entire population of children can in fact be determined, but rather a range of hours should likely be considered. For instance, in this article some 4-year-old children seem to sleep only 9.5 hours a night, whereas others sleep for as long as 12.5 hours. Who is to say that 1 child is sleep deprived and the other is sacking in too much? These sleep durations do need to be correlated with the effects of too little sleep.

The authors of this article recommend that their percentiles be used as a clinical tool and suggest that if a child falls outside the median of the distribution, this could be a marker for further discussion with parents. Jenni, however, notes that this area is much more complex than simply trying to match up a certain number of hours with a child's sleep record. The data do not take into account frequent night awakenings. We all know individuals who do not sleep a lot yet seem perfectly fine, and others who get a good night's sleep and seem sleepy or unfocused during the day. One child who falls into the 10th percentile for sleep duration is not the same as another child who is in this same sleep percentile.

Despite all of the caveats noted by Jenni, the US sleep norms presented in this article are helpful for assisting in the interpretation of sleep duration. They simply cannot be used as an absolute benchmark. Fig 1 in the original article shows the ranges from this study and would be worthwhile copying for use in your practice with these understandings.

J. A. Stockman III, MD

Reference

1. Jenni OG. How much sleep is "normal" in children and adolescents? *JAMA Pediatr.* 2013;167:91-92.

Maternal Caffeine Consumption and Infant Nighttime Waking: Prospective Cohort Study

Santos IS, Matijasevich A, Domingues MR (Federal Univ of Pelotas, Brazil)
Pediatrics 129:860-868, 2012

Objective.—Coffee and other caffeinated beverages are commonly consumed in pregnancy. In adults, caffeine may interfere with sleep onset and have a dose-response effect similar to those seen during insomnia. In infancy, nighttime waking is a common event. With this study, we aimed to investigate if maternal caffeine consumption during pregnancy and lactation leads to frequent nocturnal awakening among infants at 3 months of age.

Methods.—All children born in the city of Pelotas, Brazil, during 2004 were enrolled on a cohort study. Mothers were interviewed at delivery and after 3 months to obtain information on caffeine drinking consumption, sociodemographic, reproductive, and behavioral characteristics. Infant sleeping pattern in the previous 15 days was obtained from a subsample. Night waking was defined as an episode of infant arousal that woke the parents during nighttime. Multivariable analysis was performed by using Poisson regression.

Results.—The subsample included 885 of the 4231 infants born in 2004. All but 1 mother consumed caffeine in pregnancy. Nearly 20% were heavy consumers ($\geq$300 mg/day) during pregnancy and 14.3% at 3 months postpartum. Prevalence of frequent nighttime awakeners (>3 episodes per night) was 13.8% (95% confidence interval: 11.5%−16.0%). The highest prevalence ratio was observed among breastfed infants from mothers consuming $\geq$300 mg/day during the whole pregnancy and in the postpartum period (1.65; 95% confidence interval: 0.86−3.17) but at a nonsignificant level.

Conclusions.—Caffeine consumption during pregnancy and by nursing mothers seems not to have consequences on sleep of infants at the age of 3 months.

▶ This interesting study was designed to assess the prevalence of heavy caffeine consumption by pregnant and working women and also to describe the nighttime sleep pattern of infants at 3 months of age to assess whether maternal caffeine consumption during pregnancy and periods of lactation would lead to more frequent nighttime awakening episodes in infants at 3 months of age. This is an important study in that coffee and other caffeinated beverages are commonly consumed during pregnancy. Maternal caffeine intake may affect the fetus for any number of reasons. Caffeine can readily cross the placenta. Its half-life is increased in late gestation in both the mother and the fetus. It is well known that the fetus has a very poor ability to metabolize caffeine and there is significant reuptake of caffeine from amniotic fluid through fetal swallowing. Caffeine is rapidly absorbed from the gastrointestinal tract and is distributed to saliva and the milk of lactating women, allowing newborns to be exposed to caffeine through breastfeeding. Physiologically, infants are unable to metabolize caffeine until three months of age. Prior to that, caffeine is excreted directly through the urine.

Santos et al studied a large number of women in Brazil who were heavy caffeine consumers during pregnancy and after childbirth. Study subjects took in 300 mg a day of caffeine. Caffeine sources included coffee and mate (a hot tea-like beverage highly consumed in portions of Brazil). Careful record was taken of nighttime awakenings in the infants during the 15 days prior to an average age of 3 months. The study revealed that prevalence of caffeine consumption is almost universal during pregnancy in the Brazilian population. The prevalence of heavy consumption ≥300 mg/day was 20% in pregnancy and 14.3% postpartum. It was observed that maternal caffeine consumption, even in large amounts during gestation and lactation, had no consequences on the sleep patterns of infants at 3 months of age. The authors had no explanation for this, but did suggest that infants of heavy caffeine-consuming mothers developed tolerance to caffeine. There also appeared to be no effect of caffeine on the infant's crying or of the prevalence of colic at 3 months of age.

The findings from this study confirm that the advised limit of caffeine consumption during pregnancy should be at a level of about 300 mg/day as documented by the fact that at least in this study, at such consumption levels there appears to be little effect on infant behavior. Whether we should regard the results of this study as good news or not is up to the reader, but at least we do not have to worry too terribly much about the behavioral consequences of caffeine consumption by mothers.

J. A. Stockman III, MD

Persistent Snoring in Preschool Children: Predictors and Behavioral and Developmental Correlates

Beebe DW, Rausch J, Byars KC, et al (Cincinnati Children s Hosp Med Ctr, OH; et al)
Pediatrics 130:382-389, 2012

Objective.—To clarify whether persistent snoring in 2- to 3-year-olds is associated with behavioral and cognitive development, and to identify predictors of transient and persistent snoring.

Methods.—Two hundred forty-nine mother/child pairs participated in a prospective birth cohort study. Based upon parental report of loud snoring ≥2 times weekly at 2 and 3 years of age, children were designated as non-snorers, transient snorers (snored at 2 or 3 years of age, but not both), or persistent snorers (snored at both ages). We compared groups by using validated measures of behavioral and cognitive functioning. Potential predictors of snoring included child race and gender, socioeconomic status (parent education and income), birth weight, prenatal tobacco exposure (maternal serum cotinine), childhood tobacco exposure (serum cotinine), history and duration of breast milk feeding, and body mass relative to norms.

Results.—In multivariable analyses, persistent snorers had significantly higher reported overall behavior problems, particularly hyperactivity, depression, and inattention. Nonsnorers had significantly stronger cognitive development than transient and persistent snorers in unadjusted analyses, but not after demographic adjustment. The strongest predictors of the presence and persistence of snoring were lower socioeconomic status and the absence or shorter duration of breast milk feeding. Secondary analyses suggested that race may modify the association of childhood tobacco smoke exposure and snoring.

Conclusions.—Persistent, loud snoring was associated with higher rates of problem behaviors. These results support routine screening and tracking of snoring, especially in children from low socioeconomic backgrounds; referral for follow-up care of persistent snoring in young children; and encouragement and facilitation of infant breastfeeding.

▶ It was in 2002 that the authors for the Section on Pediatric Pulmonology Subcommittee on Obstructive Sleep Apnea Syndrome study introduced a clinical practice guideline recommending that all physicians caring for children should routinely ask parents about snoring to screen for obstructive sleep apnea and milder forms of sleep-disordered breathing.[1] These recommendations were made because of the implications of obstructive sleep apnea, which is known to be associated with cognitive and behavioral problems in school-aged children even when formal polysomnography results have been negative or equivocal. Unfortunately, little is known about sleep-disordered breathing in very young children, although sleep-disordered breathing symptoms seem to have an upward infliction point between 2 and 3 years of age, a time in which snoring-related arousals from sleep correlate with early mental development. For these reasons, the impact of persistent snoring on preschool-aged children has remained largely unknown, although in older children persistent snoring does increase the chances of new or worsening behavioral problems.[2]

These authors designed a study to test whether children who persistently snore at 2 to 3 years of age will have more behavioral problems and poorer cognitive development by 3 years of age than children who did not snore at all. They also tested the hypothesis that demographic factors, infant feeding history, current body mass relative to norms, and prenatal and concurrent biomarkers for tobacco smoke exposure might also be associated with transient and persistent snoring. The investigators used data of mother—child pairs participating in the Health Outcomes and Measures of the Environment study, an ongoing prospective investigation in the Cincinnati, Ohio, metropolitan area. Snoring was assessed by using the validated Child Sleep Habits Questionnaire, a recognized instrument to detect the presence of sleep-disordered breathing problems.[3] Parents also completed the preschool form of the Behavior Assessment System for Children, also an extensively validated behavioral questionnaire. All children in the study also had an evaluation using the Bayley Scales of Infant Development. As predicted, children participating in this study who were persistent snorers had significantly higher behavior problem scores at 3 years of age than those who never snored or who were transient snorers. This article appears to be the first to examine the relationship between the persistence of snoring and behavioral functioning in preschool-aged children. These data are consistent with reports of older children. The authors were not able to provide definitive causal conclusions from their study. Nonetheless, findings are consistent with animal and observational human studies that suggest that sleep-disordered, breathing-mediated sleep disruption and intermittent hypoxia can result in elevated oxidative stress, generalized inflammation, and changes in neural and neurobehavioral functioning. Some of these findings in humans have been corrected by surgical treatment of childhood sleep-disordered breathing.

This article also found that children who were breastfed, particularly for long periods, were at markedly lower risk for persistent snoring. Whereas none of the children in the study who were breastfed for 12 months or more developed persistent snoring, one-fourth of those who were never breastfed or for only short periods of time, such as 1 month, became persistent snorers. One can only speculate as to why there is a negative association between lack of breast-feeding and snoring. The article also provides support for the belief that tobacco smoke is a risk factor for sleep-disordered breathing in youngsters in a family where there is a smoker. Birth weight, the child's sex, and age-corrected and gender-corrected body mass index were not consistently associated with either transient or persistent snoring.

The findings from this article clearly add to our body of knowledge about the cognitive, behavioral, and sociodemographic associations related to snoring. It is wise to follow the American Academy of Pediatrics' recommendations to screen for snoring. This should be done as early as 2 years of age to prevent the problems so well described in this study.

J. A. Stockman III, MD

References

1. Section on Pediatric Pulmonology, Subcommittee on Obstructive Sleep Apnea Syndrome, The American Academy of Pediatrics. Clinical practice guideline: diagnosis and management of childhood obstructive sleep apnea syndrome. *Pediatrics.* 2002;109:704-712.
2. Chervin RD, Ruzicka DL, Archbold KH, Dillon JE. Snoring predicts hyperactivity four years later. *Sleep.* 2005;28:885-890.
3. Byars KC, Yolton K, Rausch J, Lanphear B, Beebe DW. Prevalence, patterns, and persistence of sleep problems in the first 3 years of life. *Pediatrics.* 2012;129: e276-e284. www.pediatrics.org/cgi/content/full/129/2/e276.

Melatonin for sleep problems in children with neurodevelopmental disorders: randomised double masked placebo controlled trial

Gringras P, on behalf of the MENDS Study Group (St Thomas' Hosp, London, UK; et al)
BMJ 345:e6664, 2012

Objective.—To assess the effectiveness and safety of melatonin in treating severe sleep problems in children with neurodevelopmental disorders.

Design.—12 week double masked randomised placebo controlled phase III trial.

Setting.—19 hospitals across England and Wales.

Participants.—146 children aged 3 years to 15 years 8 months were randomised. They had a range of neurological and developmental disorders and a severe sleep problem that had not responded to a standardised sleep behaviour advice booklet provided to parents four to six weeks before randomisation. A sleep problem was defined as the child not falling asleep within one hour of lights out or having less than six hours' continuous sleep.

Interventions.—Immediate release melatonin or matching placebo capsules administered 45 minutes before the child's bedtime for a period of 12 weeks. All children started with a 0.5 mg capsule, which was increased through 2 mg, 6 mg, and 12 mg depending on their response to treatment.

Main Outcome Measures.—Total sleep time at night after 12 weeks adjusted for baseline recorded in sleep diaries completed by the parent. Secondary outcomes included sleep onset latency, assessments of child behaviour, family functioning, and adverse events. Sleep was measured with diaries and actigraphy.

Results.—Melatonin increased total sleep time by 22.4 minutes (95% confidence interval 0.5 to 44.3 minutes) measured by sleep diaries (n = 110) and 13.3 (−15.5 to 42.2) measured by actigraphy (n = 59). Melatonin reduced sleep onset latency measured by sleep diaries (−37.5 minutes, −55.3 to −19.7 minutes) and actigraphy (−45.3 minutes, −68.8 to −21.9 minutes) and was most effective for children with the longest sleep latency ($P = 0.009$). Melatonin was associated with earlier waking times than placebo (29.9 minutes, 13.6 to 46.3 minutes). Child behaviour and family functioning outcomes showed some improvement and favoured use of melatonin. Adverse events were mild and similar between the two groups.

Conclusions.—Children gained little additional sleep on melatonin; though they fell asleep significantly faster, waking times became earlier. Child behaviour and family functioning outcomes did not significantly improve. Melatonin was tolerable over this three month period. Comparisons with slow release melatonin preparations or melatonin analogues are required.

Trial Registration.—ISRCT No 05534585.

▶ This report from England represents a randomized, double-masked, multi-center, placebo-controlled phase III trial examining the potential benefits of melatonin for sleep disorders in children. Melatonin, produced by the pineal body, has clearly been documented to assist in the control of sleep. It can both initiate sleep and maintain sleep. Low concentrations of melatonin, as commonly seen in elderly people, are associated with insomnia. Studies have shown that treatment with melatonin can be effective in restoring normal sleep and improving quality of life in some people older than 55 years of age.[1] Melatonin has also been used to treat children with developmental disabilities and sleep difficulties and can be preferable to hypnotics, such as clonidine and benzodiazepines, which can have considerable side effects.

Gringras et al examined 146 children with neurodevelopmental delays and other disorders such as epilepsy, autism spectrum disorder, or both, that were associated with sleep disorders (delayed sleep onset or poor sleep maintenance, or both). In a double-blind manner, melatonin was compared with a placebo. The mean effect of melatonin was a shortened sleep latency, decreasing from 102 minutes at baseline to 55 minutes at week 12 of therapy. Melatonin prolonged total sleep time by approximately 40 minutes. Parent surveys indicated that parents did believe melatonin improved their children's quality of sleep and reduced their daytime sleepiness. Overall, treatment with melatonin resulted in better and longer sleep, which was a clinically important finding of this study.

One curious finding in this report was that children treated with melatonin woke up an average of 17 minutes earlier than before treatment and about 30 minutes earlier than those in the placebo group. Exogenous melatonin not only induces and maintains sleep, but it also affects the timing of its own synthesis and release by binding to receptors in the brain. Just as is true when people take melatonin for jet lag or to manage shift work, administering melatonin to children at a particular time will induce a time shift in the endogenous production of melatonin, resulting in earlier waking.

If a care provider decides to use melatonin to manage sleep disorders in children with neurodevelopmental disabilities, it should be recognized that in general, relatively small doses are needed. Although the parents in this study were instructed to give up to 12 mg of melatonin as deemed necessary, the average patient received only 0.5 mg to achieve the desirable effect. A little bit seems to go a long way.

J. A. Stockman III, MD

Reference

1. Lemoine P, Zisapel N. Prolonged-release formulation of melatonin (Circadin) for the treatment of insomnia. *Expert Opin Pharmacother.* 2012;13:895-905.

5 Dentistry and Otolaryngology (ENT)

Children's Dental Health, School Performance, and Psychosocial Well-Being

Guarnizo-Herreño CC, Wehby GL (Univ of Iowa)

J Pediatr 161:1153-1159.e2, 2012

Objective.—To assess the effects of dental health on school performance and psychosocial well-being in a nationally representative sample of children in the US.

Study Design.—We analyzed data from the 2007 National Survey of Children's Health for 40 752-41 988 children. The effects of dental problems and maternal-rated dental health on school performance and psychosocial well-being outcomes were evaluated using regression models adjusting for demographic, socioeconomic, and health characteristics.

Results.—Dental problems were significantly associated with reductions in school performance and psychosocial well-being. Children with dental problems were more likely to have problems at school (OR = 1.52; 95% CI: 1.37-1.72) and to miss school (OR = 1.42; 95% CI: 1.23-1.64) and were less likely to do all required homework (OR = 0.76; 95% CI: 0.68-0.85). Dental problems were associated with shyness, unhappiness, feeling of worthlessness, and reduced friendliness. The effects of dental problems on unhappiness and feeling of worthlessness were largest for adolescents between 15 and 17 years.

Conclusion.—Preventing and treating dental problems and improving dental health may benefit child academic achievement and cognitive and psychosocial development.

► Much has been written about dental health in children and adolescents; however, little has been documented about the link between the status of these youngsters' dental health and their psychological well-being. It seems intuitive that dental health may affect several domains of child development and growth as well as psychological well-being. After all, having good teeth does affect feeding, breathing, speaking, smiling, and social adaptation. Parents often will spend a lot of money on their offspring to show a good smile. On the other hand, consequences of dental diseases can include pain, discomfort, embarrassment, a challenge to cognitive development, reduced self-esteem, and impairments of daily life activities.[1] Dental caries in young children are known to be associated with being underweight, poor growth, irritability, and a high risk for hospitalization. Dental problems can also be associated with disturbed sleep and diminished learning capability.[2] Malocclusion has also been documented to be associated with a child's perceived attractiveness by others and social acceptance.[3]

To extend what is already known about the association between dental health and psychological well-being, the authors of this report evaluated the effects of child dental health status on school performance and psychosocial well-being in a large, nationally representative, US sample of children age 6 to 17 years. The authors controlled for several demographic, socioeconomic, and health confounding variables. It was found that poor child dental health is significantly associated with reduced school performance and psychosocial well-being even with adjustment for all the confounding factors. The evidence supports the Healthy People 2020 goals for reducing child dental problems and increasing children's access to preventative dental care through effective policies and public health interventions.[4] In this study, more than a quarter of children were shown to have at least one dental problem. About 30% of children experienced difficulties in school, and 80% missed at least one day of school per year for illness or injury. Children in this study with dental problems were more likely to have problems at school (odds ratio [OR] = 1.52) or missed school (OR = 1.42) and were less likely to do all of their homework. More specifically, children with dental problems were more likely to feel worthless/inferior and unhappy/sad/depressed, as well as being less likely to be friendly with other children. At the other end of the spectrum, very good/excellent dental health was associated with less shyness and more friendliness.

This report is not a perfect one. It is possible that psychosocial status has reverse effects on dental health and would bias the results. For example, less happy children with low self-esteem may have poorer dietary and teeth brushing habits. The authors could not completely exclude this potential bias, especially for the psychosocial outcomes results, but they re-estimated the dental health effects on schooling outcomes by adjusting for the psychosocial measures and found the same effects. For these reasons, it does seem reasonable that we should do the most possible to prevent and treat dental problems, not just because of the immediate consequences of the dental problems but because of the associated short- and long-term effects on psychosocial well-being.

J. A. Stockman III, MD

References

1. Jürgensen N, Petersen PE. Oral health and the impact of socio-behavioural factors in a cross sectional survey of 12-year old school children in Laos. *BMC Oral Health*. 2009;9:29.
2. Sheiham A. Dental caries affects body weight, growth and quality of life in pre-school children. *Br Dent J*. 2006;201:625-626.
3. Zhang M, McGrath C, Hägg U. The impact of malocclusion and its treatment on quality of life: a literature review. *Int J Paediatr Dent*. 2006;16:381-387.

4. *Healthy People 2020*. Washington, DC: Department of Health and Human Services; 2010. http://www.healthypeople.gov/2020. Accessed February 9, 2013.

Racial Disparity Trends in Children's Dental Visits: US National Health Interview Survey, 1964–2010

Isong IA, Soobader M-J, Fisher-Owens SA, et al (Harvard Med School, Boston, MA; StatWorks, Boston, MA; Univ of California, San Francisco; et al)
Pediatrics 130:306-314, 2012

Background and Objective.—Research that has repeatedly documented marked racial/ethnic disparities in US children's receipt of dental care at single time points or brief periods has lacked a historical policy perspective, which provides insight into how these disparities have evolved over time. Our objective was to examine the impact of national health policies on African American and white children's receipt of dental care from 1964 to 2010.

Methods.—We analyzed data on race and dental care utilization for children aged 2 to 17 years from the 1964, 1976, 1989, 1999, and 2010 National Health Interview Survey. Dependent variables were as follows: child's receipt of a dental visit in the previous 12 months and child's history of never having had a dental visit. Primary independent variable was race (African American/white). We calculated sample prevalences, and χ^2 tests compared African American/white prevalences by year. We age-standardized estimates to the 2000 US Census.

Results.—The percentage of African American and white children in the United States without a dental visit in the previous 12 months declined significantly from 52.4% in 1964 to 21.7% in 2010, whereas the percentage of children who had never had a dental visit declined significantly ($P < .01$) from 33.6% to 10.6%. Pronounced African American/white disparities in children's dental utilization rates, whereas large and statistically significant in 1964, attenuated and became nonsignificant by 2010.

Conclusions.—We demonstrate a dramatic narrowing of African American/white disparities in 2 measures of children's receipt of dental services from 1964 to 2010. Yet, much more needs to be done before persistent racial disparities in children's oral health status are eliminated (Fig 2).

▶ This report reminds us how far we have come or not come in providing dental care to minority children in the United States. It was back in the 1960s that America's War on Poverty and the Great Society initiated several health policies to increase access to care among low- and moderate-income groups in the United States. The Medicaid Expansion Act of 1965 took this a step further, as did the Early Periodic Screening, Diagnosis, and Treatment (EPSDT) Program under Medicaid in 1967. The next big step came with the Children's Health Insurance Program (CHIP) in 1997 that addressed several coverage gaps among low- and moderate-income children not poor enough to qualify

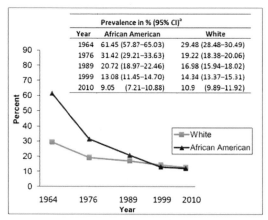

	Prevalence in % (95% CI)[a]	
Year	African American	White
1964	61.45 (57.87–65.03)	29.48 (28.48–30.49)
1976	31.42 (29.21–33.63)	19.22 (18.38–20.06)
1989	20.72 (18.97–22.46)	16.98 (15.94–18.02)
1999	13.08 (11.45–14.70)	14.34 (13.37–15.31)
2010	9.05 (7.21–10.88)	10.9 (9.89–11.92)

FIGURE 2.—Prevalence (weighted) with a history of never having had a dental visit for US children 2 to 17 years of age, by race, 1964–2010. [a]Estimates are age-standardized to the 2000 US Census. (Reprinted from Isong IA, Soobader M-J, Fisher-Owens SA, et al. Racial disparity trends in children's dental visits: US National Health Interview Survey, 1964–2010. *Pediatrics*. 2012;130:306-314, Copyright 2012, with permission from the American Academy of Pediatrics.)

for Medicaid. Most of the more recent legislative initiatives have played key roles in expanding access to dental care. Unlike for adults, Medicaid mandates that states provide dental care to children, and the EPSDT program requires that states do not limit medically necessary dental care. Dental care is now covered under the CHIP Reauthorization Act in all states, meaning that virtually all states cover at least basic dental services for children.

Isong et al have analyzed and compared trends in dental utilization rates among African-American children and white US children by using 1964 as the study baseline and 2010 as the study endpoint for determining the level of provision of dental care to children. The authors examined whether dental utilization rates among African-American and white US children had changed significantly from 1964 through 2010 and also determined whether historic African-American/ white disparities in children receiving dental care had changed at all during that period. They used data from the previously unavailable historic National Health Interview Survey (NHIS) database. The study was able to take nearly a half-century perspective on changes in children's use and disparities in dental care beginning before implementation of Medicaid and other Great Society programs of the 1960s.

The authors found that for the period spanning 1964 through 2010, one could demonstrate significant improvements in children's receipt of dental care overall as well as dramatic narrowing of African-American/white disparities. The study results indicated that utilization improvements were greater among publically insured children as well as poor and near-poor children. The programs disproportionately benefited African-American children largely because more were eligible for these programs. African-American children, although being only approximately half as likely as their white counterparts to have private health insurance in 2007, were almost 3 times as likely to have public coverage, primarily Medicaid or CHIP. The study documented achievement of near African-American/white equality in dental visits by 2010. Fig 2 shows the prevalence of those never having had a dental visit for US children 2 years to 17 years of age by race. One can see that by 2010 there was roughly parity between white children and children of African-American ancestry.

Recently reported was a study by Hakim et al that evaluated the prevalence of dental care visits in 2007 among Medicaid-enrolled children from birth through age 18 years.[1] The prevalence of having dental care visits ranges from 12% depending on age, to 49% with a median value of 33%, but did not exceed 50% in any one state. The mean percentage of change between 2000 and 2007 was 16%. Dental visits among toddlers and infants were low in all but 3 states, and in most states peaked at school entry at just more than 60%. In most states, there were few racial differences in the prevalence of dental visits in children enrolled in Medicaid programs. Overall, consistent with other reports, levels of dental care visits were low, but when the number of dental care visits was stratified by age and type of plan, striking patterns emerged, suggesting that a combination of school programs and having a medical home may have a very positive impact on dental care.

J. A. Stockman III, MD

Reference

1. Hakim RB, Babish JD, Davis AC. State of dental care among Medicaid-enrolled children in the United States. *Pediatrics*. 2012;130:5-14.

The role of antibiotics in the treatment of acute rhinosinusitis in children: a systematic review

Cronin MJ, Khan S, Saeed S (Betsi Cadwaladr Univ Health Board, Bangor, North Wales, UK)
Arch Dis Child 98:299-303, 2013

Objective.—A systematic review of randomised controlled trials reporting the efficacy of antibiotics compared with placebo in the treatment of acute rhinosinusitis in children.

Design.—Systematic review and meta-analysis.

Data Sources.—Cochrane Register of Controlled Trials, Medline, Embase and references obtained from retrieved articles.

Results.—Four studies fitted the selection criteria for inclusion. Risks for internal bias were thought to be small for each study, but external bias is potentially significant. The pooled OR for symptom improvement at 10−14 days favouring the use of antibiotics was 2.0 (95% CI 1.16 to 3.47; $I^2 = 14.8\%$).

Conclusions.—While the meta-analysis provides evidence to support the use of antibiotics for acute rhinosinusitis in children, it is the assessment of this review that such efficacy has not been adequately demonstrated. There remains a clear methodological challenge in the examination of this important clinical question; this challenge relates to difficulties in the application of appropriate diagnostic and inclusion criteria which are also consistent between studies.

▶ We all know that although most upper respiratory tract infections are caused by viral agents and generally are self-limiting, the use of antibiotics as a treatment remains high. The economic cost of such treatments is significant. A recent review of antibiotic prescribing trends here in the United States over a 10-year period has shown little change in the frequency of antibiotics prescribed for children with acute rhinosinusitis (about 75% of children diagnosed were prescribed antibiotics).[1] This is true in other developed countries as well. A Cochrane Review from 1995, and updated in 2002, has concluded that there is no good evidence for the routine use of prescribing antibiotics in children with acute rhinosinusitis.[2] Studies of antibiotic use in adults suggest a positive, albeit marginal, benefit of antibiotics.

The report by Cronin et al is a systematic review of the current evidence for the efficacy of antibiotics in the treatment of acute rhinosinusitis in children. As with all systematic reviews, a wide net was cast in the medical literature for relevant studies in this regard. After an initial 96 articles were screened that may have appeared initially relevant, ultimately 4 studies fit the selection criteria for inclusion.

The conclusion from this review is that the evidence to support the use of routine antibiotics remains unclear, despite the slightly positive findings on statistical analysis suggesting a small benefit over placebo effect in the use of antibiotics. The authors state that the evidence base is clearly inadequate and must be put into the context of the larger systematic reviews in the literature for adult patients, which shows only a small benefit from the use of antibiotics. The authors also note that future randomized and controlled trials on this subject are faced with the difficulty of bringing further uniformity and accuracy to the application of diagnosis. This has been a significant challenge all along.

This commentary closes with an observation. Were you aware that an enzyme on seaweed useful in cleaning the hulls of ships has the potential to be a treatment for chronic sinusitis? It appears that the enzyme, extracellular DNase produced by the marine-derived *Bacillus licheniformis*, can disperse bacterial biofilms. Studies performed in England show that seaweed extract is capable of breaking down biofilms that harbor bacterial organisms in the nasal passageways and sinuses.[3]

J. A. Stockman III, MD

References

1. Shapiro DJ, Gonzales R, Cabana MD, Hersh AL. National trends in visit rates and antibiotic prescribing for children with acute sinusitis. *Pediatrics.* 2011;127:28-34.
2. Morris P, Leach A. Antibiotics for persistent nasal discharge (rhinosinusitis) in children. *Cochrane Database Systemic Rev.* 2002;(4):CD001094.
3. Editorial comment. Seaweed enzyme for sinuses. *JAMA.* 2013;309:1336.

Age-Dependent Changes in the Size of Adenotonsillar Tissue in Childhood: Implications for Sleep-Disordered Breathing

Papaioannou G, Kambas I, Tsaoussoglou M, et al (Mitera Maternity and Children's Hosp, Athens, Greece; Univ of Athens School of Medicine and Aghia Sophia Children's Hosp, Greece)
J Pediatr 162:269 274.e4, 2013

Objective.—To analyze age-associated changes in linear and cross-sectional area (CSA) measurements of adenoid, tonsils, and pharyngeal lumen.

Study Design —Measurements were completed in head magnetic reso nance imaging examinations performed for diagnostic purposes. Linear and nonlinear regression models were applied to describe the effect of age on the size of soft tissues and upper airway

Results.—Magnetic resonance imaging data were analyzed in 149 children without snoring (aged 0-15.9 years) and in 33 children with snoring (aged 1.6-15 years). In the children without snoring, adenoid size increased during the first 7-8 years of life and then decreased gradually [% (adenoid oblique width/mental spine—clivus length) = 11.38 + 1.52 (age) − 0.11 (age)^2, $R^2 = 0.22$, $P < .01$; adenoid CSA = 90.75 + 41.93 (age) − 2.47 (age)^2; $R^2 = 0.50$; $P < .01$]. Nasopharyngeal airway CSA increased slowly up to age 8 years and rapidly thereafter. Similar patterns were noted for the tonsils and oropharyngeal airway. In contrast, in children with snoring, adenoid and tonsils were large irrespective of age, and nasopharyngeal airway size increased slowly with age.

Conclusions.—In children without snoring, growing adenotonsillar tissue narrows the upper airway lumen to variable degrees only during the first 8 years of life. In contrast, in children with snoring, appreciable

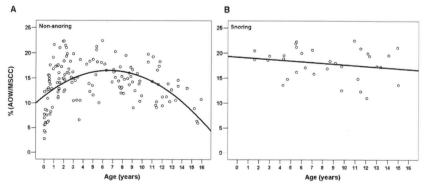

FIGURE 2.—**A,** Curve fitting (children without snoring) and **B,** line fitting (children with snoring) for the association of percentage AOW/MSCL with age. For children without snoring, $R^2 = 0.22$, $P < .01$; for children with snoring, $R^2 = 0.04$, $P = .27$. (Reprinted from Journal Pediatrics. Papaioannou G, Kambas I, Tsaoussoglou M, et al. Age-dependent changes in the size of adenotonsillar tissue in childhood: implications for sleep-disordered breathing. *J Pediatr* 2013;162:269-274.e4, Copyright 2013, with permission from Elsevier.)

pharyngeal lymphoid tissue enlargement is present during the preschool years and persists beyond the eighth birthday (Fig 2).

▶ This study is truly a first, as it uses a technology not heretofore used to assess the size of adenotonsillar tissue at varying ages. The technology, of course, is magnetic resonance imaging (MRI), a safe and highly accurate way to measure tissue volume. The trick in this particular study was to find a group of otherwise generally well children who were undergoing an MRI of the head for unrelated purposes. Children excluded from this study were those with symptoms of acute or lower respiratory tract infection; a history of adenoidectomy or tonsillectomy; a history of craniofacial, neuromuscular, or genetic disorder; and brain tumors. Before this study was published, the general thought, based on plain cranial radiographs, was that during preschool years, the adenoids grow progressively in children without obstructive sleep-disordered breathing, restricting the upper airway lumen to variable degrees such that even small increases beyond this normal growth would potentially cause some obstructive symptomatology.

This study was performed in Greece. Subjects younger than 4 years and older uncooperative children were sedated with intravenous propofol. A total of 185 children underwent MRI of the head for unrelated clinical purposes. Comparisons were made between these normal children and those who had evidence of obstructive airway disease resulting in symptoms such as snoring.

The results of this study show that during the first 8 years of life, pharyngeal lymphoid tissue does restrict the upper airway lumen to varying degrees in most children. After that age, however, overgrowth of adenotonsillar tissue resolves in children without snoring but persists in children with snoring. To say this differently, the size of the oropharyngeal airway in children with snoring does not change significantly as these youngsters age. Although the nasopharyngeal airway lumen of children with snoring does become progressively wider, it tends to be narrower relative to that of children without sleep-disordered breathing. Given that there is some narrowing of the airway in most children until age 8, virtually anything that stimulates lymphoid cellular proliferation can be a cause of some obstructive symptoms. For most children, however, they are scot-free in this regard after the age of 8 years.

This commentary in the Dentistry and Otolaryngology chapter closes with an interesting tidbit about the nose. Researchers in Germany have determined that over many thousands of years the human nose adapts to its environment.[1] They examined the nasal cavities of 100 human skulls using computer-aided instruments and found that the nasal cavities of cold, dry populations are relatively high and show a more abrupt change in diameter in the upper part of the cavity than those of hot, humid climate populations. This narrowing of the long passage-way is presumed to enhance contact between the air and the mucosal tissue, which would better warm and humidify the air. The longer passage-way also would allow more time for the air to warm.

What's in your nose?

J. A. Stockman III, MD

Reference

1. Raymond J. The shape of a nose. *Scientific American.* 2012;8:27.

Relationships among Obstructive Sleep Apnea, Anthropometric Measures, and Neurocognitive Functioning in Adolescents with Severe Obesity

Hannon TS, Rofey DL, Ryan CM. et al (Indiana Univ School of Medicine, Indianapolis; Univ of Pittsburgh School of Medicine, PA; et al)
J Pediatr 160:732-735, 2012

Objective.—To explore associations between measures of obstructive sleep apnea (OSA) and sleep quality, anthropometrics, and neurocognitive functioning in severely obese adolescents.

Study Design.—This was a cross-sectional pilot study performed at an academic medical center in 37 severely obese (body mass index [BMI] > 97th percentile) adolescents. Study evaluations included polysomnography, BMI, waist circumference, and standardized neurocognitive tests to assess memory, executive functioning, psychomotor efficiency, academic achievement, and an approximation of full-scale IQ. Outcome data were evaluated categorically, based on clinical criteria for the diagnosis of OSA, and continuously to quantify associations between sleep parameters, anthropometrics, and neurocognitive test results.

Results.—Sleep fragmentation and poorer sleep quality were associated with reduced psychomotor efficiency, poorer memory recall, and lower scores on standardized academic tests. Having evidence of OSA was associated with lower math scores, but not with other neurocognitive measures. BMI and waist circumference were negatively associated with oxygen saturation.

Conclusion.—Our pilot study findings suggest that sleep fragmentation and poorer sleep quality have implications for neurocognitive functioning in obese adolescents. The epidemic of childhood obesity has dire implications, not only for increasing cardiometabolic pathology, but also for possibly promoting less readily apparent neurologic alterations associated with poor sleep quality.

▶ There seems to be much written these days about the relationship of obesity and sleep apnea. Hannon et al examined the potential associations between sleep-disordered breathing and obesity by doing a battery of cognitive tests in slightly more than 3 dozen severely overweight children. Youngsters with evidence of sleep fragmentation and poor quality of sleep were more likely to manifest reduced psychomotor efficiency, memory recall, and had lower scores on standardized academic tests. This population of obese children was without evidence of sleep apnea, but they did by and large (90%) have obvious snoring and some degree of sleep-disordered breathing. The findings from this report indicate that even small subclinical alterations in sleep can impose deleterious effects on thought processing in susceptible individuals—specifically, overweight children.

If you add to the information from this study the body of evidence now linking sleep-disordered breathing with inflammatory mediator increases, sleepiness, and endothelial dysfunction that have also been associated with cognitive defects, and you can see the magnitude of what many of us otherwise would have thought was a very innocuous problem.

Recently a linkage between obesity and asthma was observed in a report of Rastogi et al.[1] The latter study showed that obesity appears to shift T-cell lymphocytes to enhance Th1 responses and the inflammatory effects exhibit a U-shaped relationship with asthma. However, an even more recent report by Ross et al did not identify such relationships between asthma and obesity in a small cohort of 108 children attending an asthma clinic.[2] In the latter report, there was an association between asthma and sleep-disordered breathing. This association has been observed in adults and more recently confirmed in African-American children with a history of poorly controlled asthma associated with more severe sleep-disordered breathing.[3] Needless to say, we are beginning to see a common thread between the existence of a potential asthma severity independent overlap with sleep-disordered breathing and possibly also with obesity. It is possible now to speculate that obesity, a cause of chronic systemic low-grade inflammatory processes, can amplify the intrinsic susceptibility to sleep-disordered breathing, this leading to poorer cognitive outcomes, and now an added risk of reactive airway disease manifesting as classical asthma. Thus, if you are obese, be prepared to snore a lot and to have a higher risk of heart disease and reactive airway disease. The long-term outcome for obese children in this regard is not looking rosy.

J. A. Stockman III, MD

References

1. Rastogi D, Canfield SM, Andrade A, et al. Obesity-associated asthma in children: a distinct entity. *Chest.* 2012;141:895-905.
2. Ross KR, Storfer-Isser A, Hart MA, et al. Sleep-disordered breathing is associated with asthma severity in children. *J Pediatr.* 2012;160:736-742.
3. Ramagopal M, Mehta A, Roberts DW, et al. Asthma as a predictor of obstructive sleep apnea in urban African-American children. *J Asthma.* 2009;46:895-899.

Association Between Treated and Untreated Obstructive Sleep Apnea and Risk of Hypertension

Marin JM, Agusti A, Villar I, et al (Hospital Universitario Miguel Servet, Zaragoza, Spain; Hosp Clinic, Barcelona, Spain; Aragon Inst of Health Sciences, Zaragoza, Spain; et al)
JAMA 307:2169-2176, 2012

Context.—Systemic hypertension is prevalent among patients with obstructive sleep apnea (OSA). Short-term studies indicate that continuous positive airway pressure (CPAP) therapy reduces blood pressure in patients with hypertension and OSA.

Objective.—To determine whether CPAP therapy is associated with a lower risk of incident hypertension.

Design, Setting, and Participants.—A prospective cohort study of 1889 participants without hypertension who were referred to a sleep center in Zaragoza, Spain, for nocturnal polysomnography between January 1, 1994, and December 31, 2000. Incident hypertension was documented at annual follow-up visits up to January 1, 2011. Multivariable models adjusted for confounding factors, including change in body mass index from baseline to censored time, were used to calculate hazard ratios (HRs) of incident hypertension in participants without OSA (controls), with untreated OSA, and in those treated with CPAP therapy according to national guidelines.

Main Outcome Measure.—Incidence of new-onset hypertension.

Results.—During 21 003 person-years of follow-up (median, 12.2 years), 705 cases (37.3%) of incident hypertension were observed. The crude incidence of hypertension per 100 person-years was 2.19 (95% CI, 1.71-2.67) in controls, 3.34 (95% CI, 2.85-3.82) in patients with OSA ineligible for CPAP therapy, 5.84 (95% CI, 4.82-6.86) in patients with OSA who declined CPAP therapy, 5.12 (95% CI, 3.76-6.47) in patients with OSA nonadherent to CPAP therapy, and 3.06 (95% CI, 2.70-3.41) in patients with OSA and treated with CPAP therapy. Compared with controls, the adjusted HRs for incident hypertension were greater among patients with OSA ineligible for CPAP therapy (1.33; 95% CI, 1.01-1.75), among those who declined CPAP therapy (1.96; 95% CI, 1.44-2.66), and among those nonadherent to CPAP therapy (1.78; 95% CI, 1.23-2.58), whereas the HR was lower in patients with OSA who were treated with CPAP therapy (0.71; 95% CI, 0.53-0.94).

Conclusion.—Compared with participants without OSA, the presence of OSA was associated with increased adjusted risk of incident hypertension; however, treatment with CPAP therapy was associated with a lower risk of hypertension.

▶ Obstructive sleep apnea is a common problem in both adults and children. As noted elsewhere, obstructive sleep apnea can be associated in children with a higher risk of cognitive deficits and asthma. This report from Spain, which includes a number of young adults as well as older individuals, suggests a causal link between obstructive sleep apnea and hypertension, a finding previously suggested in the literature. The Wisconsin Sleep Cohort Study of middle-aged adults did find a strong dose-response relationship between baseline obstructive sleep apnea severity and hypertension 4 years later.[1] These findings are consistent with an association between obstructive sleep apnea, hypertension, and obesity. In adults, at least, blood pressure elevations in those with obstructive sleep apnea can be reduced with the use of continuous positive airway pressure (CPAP) therapy.

The report by Marin et al tells us about the association between obstructive sleep apnea and hypertension, testing the hypothesis that those who strictly adhere to CPAP use will have a reduction in their risk of hypertension. With a median of 12.2 years of follow-up, the study found a strong dose-response relationship between obstructive sleep apnea and hypertension and a strong association between adhering to CPAP therapy and a lower incidence of hypertension, after adjustment for important known confounders. This study significantly advances our understanding of the relationship between obstructive sleep apnea, hypertension, and the benefit of CPAP therapy, at least in an adult population including young adults. Unfortunately, many questions remain regarding obstructive sleep apnea, hypertension, and the management of both. In children, we tend not to use CPAP therapy but rather attempt to address the underlying cause of the disturbed sleep patterns so frequently seen as a result of obesity. Obesity, alone, however, is not the sole cause of obstructive sleep apnea, and it may be worthwhile to consider using CPAP, at least in the older teen population with evidence of sleep apnea, if we truly believe that the latter increases one's risk of inflammation, hypertension, cognitive defects, and potentially reactive airway disease. In adults, evidence does support the treatment of obstructive sleep apnea to improve symptoms, quality of life, and cardiovascular endpoints. Treatment of obstructive sleep apnea may not only reduce blood pressure but may in fact prevent long-term hypertension in those who are at highest risk. Clearly, there needs to be much more in the way of investigation of these associations in children because studies of adults can only give us clues as to what might be going on in the young population.

J. A. Stockman III, MD

Reference

1. Young T, Finn L, Peppard PE, et al. Sleep disordered breathing and mortality: 18-year follow-up of the Wisconsin sleep cohort. *Sleep.* 2008;31:1071-1078.

Outpatient Tonsillectomy in Children: Demographic and Geographic Variation in the United States, 2006

Boss EF, Marsteller JA, Simon AE (Johns Hopkins Univ School of Medicine, Baltimore, MD; Johns Hopkins Bloomberg School of Public Health, Baltimore, MD; Natl Ctr for Health Statistics, Hyattsville, MD)
J Pediatr 160:814-819, 2012

Objectives.—To examine geographic and demographic variation for outpatient tonsillectomy in children nationally.

Study Design.—The 2006 National Survey of Ambulatory Surgery was analyzed to describe outpatient tonsillectomy in children. Rates by age, sex, region, urban/rural residence, and payment source were calculated with 2006 population estimates from the Census Bureau and the National Health Interview Survey as denominators. Rates were compared with Z tests.

Results.—In 2006, approximately 583 000 (95% CI, 370 000-796 000) outpatient tonsillectomy procedures were performed in children in the United States. Rates per 10 000 children were lower in children 13 to 17 years old (33.8 per 10 000) than in both children 7 to 12 years old (91.3; $P < .05$) and children 0 to 6 years old (102.9; $P < .001$). Compared with the South, tonsillectomy rates were lower in the West (29 per 10 000 versus 125 per 10 000; $P < .01$) and not significantly different in other regions. Compared with large central metropolitan areas, tonsillectomy rates were higher in small/medium metropolitan areas (118 per 10 000 versus 42 per 10 000; $P < .05$), and not significantly different in large fringe or non-metropolitan areas. Tonsillectomy rates were similar for children insured by Medicaid compared with those insured by private sources. Compared with older children (13-17 years), children in the younger age groups (0-6 years, 7-12 years) underwent tonsillectomy more commonly for airway obstruction (69.5% and 59.2% versus 34.3%, $P < .05$ for both). Compared with older children, younger children (0-6 years) underwent tonsillectomy less commonly for infection (40.4% versus 61.0% [7-12 years] and 72.2% [13-17 years], $P < .001$ for both).

Conclusions.—Use of tonsillectomy in the ambulatory setting varies across age groups, geographic regions, levels of urbanization, and indication. Further research is warranted to examine these differences.

▶ Tonsillectomy rates have waxed and waned over the years. Goodman et al note that peak rates of tonsillectomy probably occurred in the 1930s and 1940s. For example, among 1000 typical 11-year-old children in New York City in 1932–1933, 61% had their tonsils removed.[1] During the same period, some 93.5% of all children had either had a tonsillectomy or had received at least 1 recommendation for the procedure. Uncertainty about the value of the procedure began to appear in the literature half a century ago. Tonsillectomy rates declined precipitously and reached their nadir during the 1980s. Rates of tonsillectomy have recently increased fairly dramatically. Between 1996 and 2006, the ambulatory tonsillectomy rate for US children younger than age 15 years approximately doubled from 4.97 to 8.7 per 1000 children. Converted to numbers, this represents an additional quarter of a million procedures per year.[2] It seems likely that the pickup in tonsillectomies in recent years is the result of the belief on the part of some that the procedure may alleviate obstructive sleep apnea.

Given that little is actually known about the national epidemiology of tonsillectomy, Boss et al attempted to look at why tonsillectomies are being performed in such high numbers using data from the National Survey of Ambulatory Surgery. The study demonstrated significant demographic and geographic variation in tonsillectomy rates for children. In 2006, there were an estimated 583 000 ambulatory tonsillectomy procedures performed in the United States. It is well known that fewer than 10% of tonsillectomies now are done in hospital; thus these numbers do provide a basis to look at the epidemiology of tonsillectomy. The data from this report show that in youngsters up to 6 years of age undergoing tonsillectomy, the primary indication for tonsillectomy was airway obstruction or sleep disturbance (69.5%). At 7 to 12 years of age, 59.2% of the procedures related to airway obstruction or sleep disturbances. Tonsillectomies for children in the oldest age group (13 to 17 years), however, were performed more commonly for infection than for airway obstruction because 65.7% of children had an indication of infection, compared with 27.8% of children who had an indication for airway obstruction only. It should be noted that tonsillectomy was performed concurrently with adenoidectomy in 90.1% of children. About 1 in 5 children who underwent a tonsillectomy also underwent tympanic membrane procedures or sinonasal procedures. There were higher rates of tonsillectomy in the southern states in comparison to the western United States. There were also higher rates of tonsillectomy in urban settings even when corrected for population densities.

The literature has suggested that variation in tonsillectomy rates may also be explained by physician-to-population ratio for pediatric otolaryngologists. Currently, the average distance to a pediatric otolaryngologist in the United States is 48.5 miles, suggesting that geographic barriers may exist for some patients. It has also been suggested that insurance status may affect a child's propensity to undergo tonsillectomy. For example, a survey of otolaryngologists in southern California recently indicated that only 19% of otolaryngologists would perform a tonsillectomy on a child on Medicaid, largely because of poor reimbursement and high administrative demands.[3]

Despite the increase in numbers of tonsillectomies, largely the result of management of obstructive sleep apnea, current practices are poorly supported by research. Indeed, an accurate diagnosis of obstructive sleep apnea can only be made with polysomnography and there are no real studies that have been properly designed to tell whether tonsillectomy is effective for accurately diagnosed obstructive sleep apnea. It is doubtful that most children will have undergone sleep studies prior to tonsillectomy. For those with well-documented apnea, tonsillectomy often provides immediate improvement, but not resolution of the problem.[4] We are still waiting for a randomized clinical trial of tonsillectomy in the management of obstructive sleep apnea. In the absence of such a trial, it appears that twice as many tonsillectomies are being performed these days in comparison to when there was no fad surrounding obstructive sleep apnea and its role in the health of children.

J. A. Stockman III, MD

References

1. American Child Health Association. *Physical Defects: the Pathway to Correction.* New York: American Child Health Association; 1934.
2. Owings MF, Kozak LJ. Ambulatory and inpatient procedures in the United States, 1996. *Vital Health Statistic Med 13.* 1998:1-119.
3. Wang EC, Choe MC, Meara JG, Koempel JA. Inequality of access to surgical specialty health care: why children with government-funded insurance have less access than those with private insurance in Southern California. *Pediatrics.* 2004;114:e584-e590.
4. Bhattacharjee R, Kheirandish-Gozal L, Spruyt K, et al. Adenotonsillectomy outcomes in treatment of obstructive sleep apnea in children: a multicenter retrospective study. *Am J Respir Crit Care Med.* 2010;182:676-683.

Perioperative Dexamethasone Administration and Risk of Bleeding Following Tonsillectomy in Children: A Randomized Controlled Trial

Gallagher TQ, Hill C, Ojha S, et al (Naval Med Ctr Portsmouth, VA; Dartmouth Hitchcock Med Ctr, Lebanon, NH; Massachusetts Eye and Ear Infirmary, Boston; et al)

JAMA 308:1221-1226, 2012

Context.—Corticosteroids are commonly given to children undergoing tonsillectomy to reduce postoperative nausea and vomiting; however, they might increase the risk of perioperative and postoperative hemorrhage.

Objective.—To determine the effect of dexamethasone on bleeding following tonsillectomy in children.

Design, Setting, and Patients.—A multicenter, prospective, randomized, double-blind, placebo-controlled study at 2 tertiary medical centers of 314 children aged 3 to 18 years undergoing tonsillectomy without a history of bleeding disorder or recent corticosteroid medication use and conducted between July 15, 2010, and December 20, 2011, with 14-day follow-up. We tested the hypothesis that dexamethasone would not result in 5% more bleeding events than placebo using a noninferiority statistical design.

Intervention.—A single perioperative dose of dexamethasone (0.5 mg/kg; maximum dose, 20 mg), with an equivalent volume of 0.9% saline administered to the placebo group.

Main Outcome Measures.—Rate and severity of posttonsillectomy hemorrhage in the 14-day postoperative period using a bleeding severity scale (level I, self-reported or parent-reported postoperative bleeding; level II, required inpatient admission for postoperative bleeding; or level III, required reoperation to control postoperative bleeding).

Results.—One hundred fifty-seven children (median [interquartile range] age, 6 [4-8] years) were randomized into each study group, with 17 patients (10.8%) in the dexamethasone group and 13 patients (8.2%) in the placebo group reporting bleeding events. In an intention-to-treat analysis, the rates of level I bleeding were 7.0% (n = 11) in the dexamethasone group and 4.5% (n = 7) in the placebo group (difference, 2.6%; upper limit 97.5% CI, 7.7%; P for noninferiority = .17); rates of level II bleeding were 1.9% (n = 3) and 3.2% (n = 5), respectively (difference, −1.3%; upper limit 97.5% CI, 2.2%; P for noninferiority < .001); and rates of level III bleeding were 1.9% (n = 3) and 0.6% (n = 1), respectively (difference, 1.3%; upper limit 97.5% CI, 3.8%; P for noninferiority = .002).

Conclusions.—Perioperative dexamethasone administered during pediatric tonsillectomy was not associated with excessive, clinically significant level II or III bleeding events based on not having crossed the noninferior threshold of 5%. Increased subjective (level I) bleeding events caused by dexamethasone could not be excluded because the noninferiority threshold was crossed.

Trial Registration.—clinicaltrials.gov Identifier: NCT01415583.

▶ Systemic steroids are frequently used to reduce postoperative nausea and vomiting in patients who have undergone a tonsillectomy. These symptoms and signs are a major source of morbidity in youngsters who have this surgical procedure performed. There are adequate data to show that perioperative administration of corticosteroids effectively manages postoperative nausea and vomiting. This modality of therapy also allows a more rapid resumption of a normal diet, improved pain control, and decreased airway swelling. These benefits have been known for many years. In fact, 2 meta-analyses have demonstrated the benefits of a single dose of dexamethasone in controlling postoperative nausea and vomiting following tonsillectomy.[1,2] The American Academy of Otolaryngology's Head and Neck Surgery Clinical Practice Guidelines on Pediatric Tonsillectomy strongly recommend the use of perioperative corticosteroids.

Although corticosteroids seem to work for certain purposes, there has been some concern that they may increase the risk of postoperative bleeding. A randomized controlled trial has suggested that a single dose of intraoperative dexamethasone significantly increases the probability of posttonsillectomy hemorrhage events.[3]

The authors of this article undertook a clinical trial to address the concerns about bleeding events in children associated with dexamethasone use during tonsillectomy. The study itself was a multicenter, prospective, randomized, double-blind, placebo-controlled study at 2 tertiary medical centers and involved hundreds of children undergoing splenectomy. Those children who received dexamethasone received a single perioperative dose (0.5 mg/kg). Control patients received saline. The patients ranged in age from 3 to 18 years and mostly underwent tonsillectomy for either management of sleep-disordered breathing or infectious tonsillitis. Seventeen patients in the dexamethasone group reported bleeding events, while 13 patients in the placebo group reported bleeding events.

The authors hypothesized that there would not be more bleeding events in the dexamethasone group compared with the saline placebo group. In fact, the conclusion of this article, which represented a prospective randomized study of 314 children undergoing tonsillectomy, was that perioperative dexamethasone administration was not associated with more level II or III bleeding events than placebo. Increased subjective (level I) bleeding events noted with dexamethasone could not be excluded. The data from this report are consistent with another recent meta-analysis of randomized controlled trials undertaken recently in Canada.[4] The latter employed data from Medline, Embase, the Cochrane Central Register of Controlled Trials, Scopus, Web of Science, Intute, Biosis, OpenSINGLE, the National Technical Information Services, and Google Scholar. In this meta-analysis, it was clear that perioperative administration of systemic steroids in patients undergoing tonsillectomy did not increase the risk of perioperative bleeding.

J. A. Stockman III, MD

References

1. Goldman AC, Govindaraj S, Rosenfeld RM. A meta-analysis of dexamethasone use with tonsillectomy. *Otolaryngol Head Neck Surg.* 2000;123:682-686.
2. Steward DL, Welge JA, Myer CM. Do steroids reduce morbidity of tonsillectomy? Meta-analysis of randomized trials. *Laryngoscope.* 2001;111:1712-1718.
3. Czarnetzki C, Elia N, Lysakowski C, et al. Dexamethasone and risk of nausea and vomiting and postoperative bleeding after tonsillectomy in children: a randomized trial. *JAMA.* 2008;300:2621-2630.
4. Plante J, Turgeon AF, Zarychanski R, et al. Effect of systemic steroids on post-tonsillectomy bleeding and re-interventions: meta-analysis of randomized controlled trials. *BMJ.* 2012;345:14.

Congenital Cytomegalovirus Is the Second Most Frequent Cause of Bilateral Hearing Loss in Young French Children

Avettand-Fenoë V, Marlin S, Vauloup-Fellous C, et al (Hosp Necker-Enfants-Malades, Paris, France; Hosp Trousseau, Paris, France; Univ Paris-Sud, France; et al)
J Pediatr 162:593-599, 2013

Objective.—To estimate the prevalence of congenital cytomegalovirus (cCMV) among causes of bilateral hearing loss in young French children.

Study Design.—Children < 3 years old with hearing loss were prospectively included at their first visit to a referral center. Cytomegalovirus polymerase chain reaction was performed on dried blood spots from Guthrie cards. Medical records were reviewed.

Results.—One hundred children with bilateral hearing loss were included at a median age of 15 months; the prevalence of cCMV was 8% (8/100) (95% CI, 2.7%-13.3%) in this population and 15.4% (8/52) in the subpopulation of children with profound bilateral hearing loss. Delayed neurodevelopment and brain abnormalities on computed tomography scan were found more often in children with cCMV than in children with hearing loss without cCMV ($P = .027$, $P = .005$). In 6 of 8 cCMV cases, cCMV infection had not been diagnosed before the study.

Conclusions.—In a comprehensive study of the causes of bilateral hearing loss in young French children, cCMV is the second most frequent cause of hearing loss after connexin mutations. It underlines that a majority of French children with hearing loss and cCMV are not diagnosed early and therefore may not benefit from early intervention including the possibility of neonatal antiviral treatment. These results make the case for promoting systematic cytomegalovirus screening in neonates with confirmed hearing loss identified through neonatal hearing screening.

▶ We know that congenital cytomegalovirus (cCMV) is a major cause of hearing loss. The hearing loss can be present at birth or can be delayed in onset, in which case the etiology can be often difficult to determine. These investigators from France have tackled the issue of the true prevalence of cCMV as a cause of hearing loss by examining the Guthrie cards of children evaluated for hearing loss to apply polymerase chain reaction (PCR) assays on the dried blood spot to detect CMV. In the absence of universal neonatal screening for cCMV infection, CMV PCR on neonatal Guthrie cards has been proposed as a way of obtaining a retrospective diagnosis of cCMV in children with hearing loss.

Using the strategy described to estimate the prevalence of cCMV in a population of young French children with bilateral hearing loss, the investigators found a prevalence of cCMV of 8%. It should be noted that the prevalence of cCMV reported in this study reflects only the proportion of cCMV among French children with bilateral hearing loss and not the prevalence of cCMV in the total population of children with hearing loss. It should be noted that, because in France Guthrie cards are discarded after 2 to 3 years depending on the regional laboratory, older children could not be enrolled in this study. An important observation in this study was that 75% of the CMV-infected children with bilateral hearing loss did not have a diagnosis of cCMV before participating in this study.

By the way, as noted in the title of this report, cCMV is the second most frequent cause of bilateral hearing loss. The most common cause of hearing loss remains connexin mutations.

J. A. Stockman III, MD

Tympanometry in Discrimination of Otoscopic Diagnoses in Young Ambulatory Children

Helenius KK, Laine MK, Tähtinen PA, et al (Turku Univ Hosp, Finland)
Pediatr Infect Dis J 31:1003-1006, 2012

Background.—Tympanometry can indicate middle ear effusion in children referred for tympanostomy tube placement. In outpatient setting, objective adjunctive tools are needed to diagnose the otitis media spectrum.

Methods.—We enrolled and followed 515 children aged 6–35 months at primary care level. We compared tympanometry with pneumatic otoscopy and evaluated the proportions of type A, C1, C2, Cs and B tympanograms in relation to specific otoscopic diagnoses in 2206 and 1006 examinations at symptomatic and asymptomatic visits, respectively.

Results.—At symptomatic visits, different peaked tympanograms were associated with a healthy middle ear as follows: type A in 78%, type C1 in 62%, type C2 in 54% and type Cs in 18% of examinations. In contrast, any peaked tympanogram was related to healthy middle ear in 67% of examinations. Flat (type B) tympanogram was related to otitis media with effusion in 44% and to acute otitis media in 56% of examinations, respectively. At asymptomatic visits, the peaked tympanograms together were associated with a healthy middle ear in 87% of otoscopic examinations. Flat tympanogram indicated otitis media with effusion as well in 87% of examinations.

Conclusions.—Tympanometry is not a useful tool in detecting specific otoscopic diagnoses because it cannot distinguish between otitis media with effusion and acute otitis media. However, among outpatients all peaked tympanograms suggest a healthy middle ear and a flat tympanogram is useful in detecting any middle ear effusion. Thus, tympanometry can be used as an adjunctive tool, but accurate diagnosis requires careful pneumatic otoscopy.

▶ Tympanometry has been available for a number of decades as an adjunctive diagnostic tool to detect the presence of middle ear fluid and otitis media. The primary diagnosis generally lies on the use of pneumatic otoscopy, but the latter is a subjective assessment of otoscopic findings. That is why tympanometry has seemed so attractive as an adjunctive technique for diagnosis.

Helenius et al have collected a large database that includes young patients with a wide range of otoscopic findings from the healthy middle ear with or without middle ear effusion to full-blown acute otitis media with bullae on the tympanic membrane. The database allowed the investigators to assess the relationship between tympanograms and otoscopic diagnoses. The study was undertaken to evaluate the usefulness of tympanometry in detecting specific otoscopic diagnoses of otitis media in children in a primary care setting; 515 children were evaluated. Some children were symptomatic and others asymptomatic. The investigators performed spectral gradient acoustic reflectometry, tympanometry, and pneumatic otoscopy. Pneumatic otoscopy served as the diagnostic standard. Patients were classified into 5 categories: healthy ear (no pathologic otoscopic findings), air-interface otitis media with effusion, complete otitis media with effusion, air-interface acute otitis media, and complete acute otitis media. The diagnosis of acute otitis media required middle ear effusion, acute inflammatory signs in the tympanic membrane, and the presence of acute symptoms.

This study found that tympanometry is not useful in detecting specific otoscopic diagnoses of otitis media, although it is able to differentiate middle ears with effusion from those without effusion. To say this differently, tympanometry is able to tell the clinician that a child's ears are normal if the findings on tympanometry are normal. If the findings on tympanometry are abnormal, all that tympanometry tells you is that there is fluid in the middle ear, not whether the patient has acute otitis media. Although a flat tympanogram indicates middle ear effusions, it is not verification of acute otitis media even when a child is symptomatic. Consequently, the diagnosis of acute otitis media and otitis media with effusion should always be verified by pneumatic otoscopy. As of now, the eyes are the best technology for the diagnosis of acute otitis media.

J. A. Stockman III, MD

Development and Validation of a New Grading Scale for Otitis Media
Lundberg T, Hellström S, Sandström H (Umeå Univ, Sweden; Karolinska Univ Hosp, Stockholm, Sweden)
Pediatr Infect Dis J 32:341-345, 2013

Background.—Grading of acute otitis media (AOM) is important in clinical situations as well as in research. Current grading scales for AOM have used a 6 to 9 point scoring system primarily based on variation

TABLE 1.—Description of Items

Item	Description
Effusion	Fluid level visible or notable effusion in middle ear. Effusion can be transparent, opaque or hemorrhagic
Position	1. Retracted TM with protruding lateral process of malleus; the reflex may be divided and the annulus fibrosus may be protruding. 2. Normal position. 3. Bulging TM with loss of normal anatomical structure, shattered or absent reflex.
Vascularization	Visible vascularization with radiant arteries in pars flaccida, over handle of malleus, over entire TM and/or on the outside the margins of the TM.
Bullae	One or more bullous formation on TM.
Hemorrhagic (later described as chagrinated)	Visible hemorrhage spread diffusely over TM, most often with keratin patches (highly deformed TM with keratin patches).
Perforation	Visible perforation of TM or the finding of purulent fluid in the ear canal.

TABLE 2.—Development of the Scale. Version 3 is the Final Scale

Grade	Version 1	Version 2	Version 3
0	0: Normal	0: Normal	0: Normal
1	1: Transparent, retracted	1R: Transparent, retracted	1R: Transparent, retracted
		1F: Transparent, clear fluid level	1F: Transparent, clear fluid level
2	2: Transparent, fluid level	2RF: Transparent, retracted with clear fluid level	2RF: Transparent, retracted with clear fluid level
		2OF: Transparent, opaque fluid level	2OF: Transparent, opaque fluid level
3	3: Opaque, normal position	3: Opaque, normal position	3: Opaque, normal position
4	4: Opaque and bulging	4: Opaque and bulging	4: Opaque and bulging
	4B: Bullous formation	4B: Bullous formation	
	4H: Hemorrhagic	4C: Chagrinated	
5		5: Perforation	5B: Bullous formation
			5C: Chagrinated or perforation

of redness and bulging of the tympanic membrane (TM). This study aimed to develop and validate a new scale for grading AOM.

Method.—The scale was developed in 3 stages based on 32 patients with images taken of the TM when a child attended healthcare centre with othalgia and at follow-up visits. Content validity was used as the method for the first 2 stages. An expert panel reviewed the scale and repeated the process on a revised scale. Reliability was tested with a different expert panel that used the final scale on a sample of TM images in a test—retest and inter-rater and intra-rater agreements were calculated.

Results.—The scale was developed in 3 steps using expert committees. During the process the description of vascularization was judged to be of insufficient importance for our scale. Inter-rater agreement was moderate ($\kappa = 0.52$) and intra-rater agreement was good ($\kappa = 0.66$ to 0.89) in the test—retest of the final scale.

Conclusions.—The developed AOM image-based grading scale demonstrates substantial inter- and intra-rater reliability with potential use in clinical research and telemedicine applications. Furthermore, the parameter "redness of TM" is of less importance in our scale as compared with other available grading systems (Tables 1 and 2).

▶ One wonders why this report has been such a long time coming. The literature has only one image-based grading scale for acute otitis media (AOM) that has been developed for clinical use.[1] Lundberg et al have addressed this by developing a consensus of a grading system for AOM based on digital images, a consensus of 2 general practitioners, and 2 ear-nose-throat (ENT) specialists. Table 1 describes the characteristics that the evaluators were asked to examine in the digital images. The development of the image scale went through several iterations (version 1, version 2, and version 3). Table 2 shows the evolution. Version 3 is the final scale that is recommended. As others have used this scale, the interrater agreement was found to be very high, meaning that the scale could be used by multiple other care providers with a fair degree of accuracy.

The authors of this report believe that the new scale could contribute to an important move toward improving the grading of AOM by creating a common lexicon based on hardcore images that can be archived in a patient's record.

While on the topic of AOM, investigators recently examined the temporal association between circulating respiratory viruses and the occurrence of pediatric cases of AOM. Seasonal respiratory syncytial virus, human metapneumovirus, and influenza activity were found to be temporally associated with increased numbers of diagnoses of AOM among children. These findings support the role of individual respiratory viruses in the development of AOM and underscore the potential for respiratory viral vaccines to remarkably reduce the burden of AOM.[2]

J. A. Stockman III, MD

References

1. Friedman NR, McCormick DP, Pittman C, et al. Development of a practical tool for assessing the severity of acute otitis media. *Pediatr Infect Dis J*. 2006;25:101-107.
2. Stockmann C, Ampofo K, Hersh AL, et al. Seasonality of acute otitis media and the role of respiratory viral activity in children. *Pediatr Infect Dis J*. 2013;32:314-319.

Tympanostomy With and Without Adenoidectomy for the Prevention of Recurrences of Acute Otitis Media: A Randomized Controlled Trial

Kujala T, Alho O-P, Luotonen J, et al (Univ of Oulu, Finland)
Pediatr Infect Dis J 31:565-569, 2012

Background.—The prevention of otitis media, particularly among infants, remains a controversial issue. We evaluated the efficacy of insertion of tympanostomy tubes with and without adenoidectomy for preventing recurrent acute otitis media (AOM) in young children.

Methods.—We randomly assigned 300 children aged 10 months to 2 years who had recurrent AOM to groups receiving tympanostomy tubes (Tymp) (n = 100), tympanostomy tubes with adenoidectomy (TympAde) (n = 100) or neither (Contr) (n = 100). All the children were followed up for 12 months.

Results.—The primary outcome was intervention failure (2 AOM episodes in 2 months, 3 in 6 months or persistent effusion lasting for 2 months). Intervention failed in 21% of cases (21/100) in the Tymp group, 16% (16/100) in the TympAde group and 34% (34/100) in the Contr group. The absolute differences were −13% [95% confidence interval (CI) −25% to −1%, $P = 0.04$] between the Tymp and Contr groups and −18% (95% CI −30 to −6%, $P = 0.004$) between the TympAde and Contr groups.

Conclusions.—Insertion of tympanostomy tubes alone or with adenoidectomy was effective in preventing recurrent AOM episodes in children younger than 2 years of age.

▶ The insertion of tympanostomy tubes is the second most frequently performed pediatric surgical procedure, after circumcision, in the United States. It is generally used to prevent recurrent acute otitis media (AOM). This, if associated with hearing loss, has been suspected to lead to long-term impairment of speech and cognitive abilities. It is for this reason that over several decades investigators have attempted to determine the best way to prevent episodes of recurrent AOM. A recent Cochrane review included only 2 randomized trials looking at the evidence for tympanostomy as a method of reducing episodes of recurrent AOM in children younger than 3 years of age.[1] Evidence to date suggests that adenoidectomy alone is ineffective in preventing recurrent AOM in children younger than 2 years of age.[2] Most of the evidence to date suggests that tympanostomy tubes do have a significant role in maintaining time without recurrent AOM at least in the first 6 months after insertion, but research has been limited to suggest a benefit beyond 6 months after insertion.

These authors have designed a randomized controlled study to clarify the efficacy of tympanostomy tube placement versus tympanostomy tube placement with adenoidectomy versus a control group that received neither therapy. Three hundred eligible children were randomized to these 3 management arms. Intervention failed during the 1-year follow-up in 21% of cases in the tympanostomy group, 16% in the tympanostomy/adenoidectomy group, and 34% in the control group. Insertion of tympanostomy tubes and tympanostomy tubes with adenoidectomy reduced the risk of failure by 38% and 53%, respectively, compared with the group of children who received no treatment. To avoid 1 failure, the investigators noted that they would have to place tympanostomy tubes in 8 children or place and perform tympanostomy tubes adenoidectomy on 6 with a 95% confidence interval to significantly lower the rate of recurrent AOM. The differences in time to failure between the tympanostomy and control groups and tympanostomy/adenoidectomy and control groups were significant as well. Altogether, 48% of children in the tympanostomy group, 49% in the tympanostomy/adenoidectomy group, and 34% in the control group had no episodes of AOM during the follow-up period. There was no significant difference in the long term between tympanostomy and tympanostomy/adenoidectomy managements in the time to failure or in the proportion of children with no AOM episodes. It should be noted that there were no serious complications (hemorrhage or anesthetic) recorded in any of the children who participated in the trial.

The results of this study should be given attention, particularly because of how commonly these procedures are performed. In Pittsburgh, for example, 6% of all children had received tympanostomy tubes before their second birthday.[3] Over 600 000 tympanostomy tubes were placed in children younger than 15 years of age in the United States in 2006.[4] It is likely that the data emanating from this study in Finland will be used to support the continuing use of tympanostomy tubes. Tympanostomy tubes are usually inserted under general anesthesia. The procedure is simple, but performing adenoidectomy at the same time makes the procedure significantly more invasive, with additional surgical and anesthetic risks. Given the marginal benefits described in this article and elsewhere of the role of adenoidectomy, clinicians should remember the possibilities of complications and weigh them against the possible benefits. The authors conclude that tympanostomy tube insertion is reasonably efficient in preventing AOM episodes in children younger than 2 years of age, the group at highest risk for developing recurrent AOM.

J. A. Stockman III, MD

References

1. McDonald S, Langton Hewer CD, Nunez DA. Grommets (ventilation tubes) for recurrent acute otitis media in children. *Cochrane Database Syst Rev.* 2008;(4). CD004741.
2. Koivunen P, Uhari M, Luotonen J, et al. Adenoidectomy versus chemoprophylaxis and placebo for recurrent acute otitis media in children under 2 years of age: randomised controlled trial. *BMJ.* 2004;328:487.
3. Paradise JL, Rockett HE, Colborn DK, et al. Otitis media in 2253 Pittsburgh-area infants: prevalence and risk factors during the first two years of life. *Pediatrics.* 1997;99:318-333.
4. Cullen KA, Hall MJ, Golosinski YA. *Ambulatory surgery in the United States, 2006.* Hyattsville, MD: National Center for Health Statistics. http://www.cdc.gov/nchs/data/nhsr/nhsr011.pdf. 2009. Accessed April 13, 2012.

Specialised treatment based on cognitive behaviour therapy versus usual care for tinnitus: a randomised controlled trial

Cima RFF, Maes IH, Joore MA, et al (Maastricht Univ, Netherlands; Univ Hosp Maastricht, Netherlands; et al)
Lancet 379:1951-1959, 2012

Background.—Up to 21% of adults will develop tinnitus, which is one of the most distressing and debilitating audiological problems. The absence of medical cures and standardised practice can lead to costly and prolonged treatment. We aimed to assess effectiveness of a stepped-care approach, based on cognitive behaviour therapy, compared with usual care in patients with varying tinnitus severity.

Methods.—In this randomised controlled trial, undertaken at the Adelante Department of Audiology and Communication (Hoensbroek, Netherlands), we enrolled previously untreated Dutch speakers (aged >18 years) who had a primary complaint of tinnitus but no health issues precluding participation. An independent research assistant randomly allocated patients by use of a computer-generated allocation sequence in a 1:1 ratio, stratified by tinnitus severity and hearing ability, in block sizes of four to receive specialised care of cognitive behaviour therapy with sound-focused tinnitus retraining therapy or usual care. Patients and assessors were masked to treatment assignment. Primary outcomes were health-related quality of life (assessed by the health utilities index score), tinnitus severity (tinnitus questionnaire score), and tinnitus impairment (tinnitus handicap inventory score), which were assessed before treatment and at 3 months, 8 months, and 12 months after randomisation. We used multilevel mixed regression analyses to assess outcomes in the intention-to-treat population. This study is registered with ClinicalTrials. gov, number NCT00733044.

Findings.—Between September, 2007 and January, 2011, we enrolled and treated 492 (66%) of 741 screened patients. Compared with 247 patients assigned to usual care, 245 patients assigned to specialised care improved in health-related quality of life during a period of 12 months (between-group difference 0·059, 95% CI 0·025 to 0·094; effect size of Cohen's $d = 0·24$; $p = 0·0009$), and had decreased tinnitus severity ($-8·062$, $-10·829$ to $-5·295$; $d = 0·43$; $p < 0·0001$) and tinnitus impairment ($-7·506$, $-10·661$ to $-4·352$; $d = 0·45$; $p < 0·0001$). Treatment seemed effective irrespective of initial tinnitus severity, and we noted no adverse events in this trial.

Interpretation.—Specialised treatment of tinnitus based on cognitive behaviour therapy could be suitable for widespread implementation for patients with tinnitus of varying severity.

▶ Tinnitus is a fairly common problem in adults. It can also present itself in the pediatric age population, mostly in teenagers. As many as 1 in 5 adults will at some point in their lives have tinnitus, manifesting as the perception of a noxious disabling internal sound without an external source. Tinnitus can be one of the most distressing and debilitating audiological disorders, affecting many aspects of daily life. Cognitive impairments and negative emotions associated with tinnitus are especially bothersome for both patients and their families. Because tinnitus cannot be easily objectively quantified, various therapies for its treatment have been largely difficult to find and usually are unsuccessful. It is fair to say that there is no standardized practice in this regard, although there are 2 main treatment approaches that many use. One is based on retraining designed to mask tinnitus at the sound perception level in combination with structured counseling. This neuro-physiological model aims to ameliorate tinnitus distress through education and exposure to neutral external sound. Through habituation to this neutral sound, patients are expected to have diminished annoyance from tinnitus. Supporting evidence for this retraining therapy is fairly scanty. The second main approach is cognitive behavior therapy. This includes psychoeducation, relaxation, exposure techniques, and behavioral reactivation, often in combination with mindfulness-based training. Once again, although treatment of tinnitus with such therapy can reduce distress and improve quality of life, large-scale and well-controlled trials are still needed.

These authors have developed a new multidisciplinary protocol for treatment of tinnitus including a stepped-care cognitive behavior therapy approach with elements from tinnitus retraining therapy. They performed a randomized controlled study to assess the effectiveness of this specialized treatment protocol. Two hundred forty-seven patients were allocated to usual care and 245 patients were allocated to specialized care, consisting of cognitive behavior therapy enriched with elements of tinnitus retraining therapy. The therapy was aggressive and designed to overcome the general thinking in the medical community that nothing can be done to treat tinnitus. After 12 months, the stepped specialized care program was superior to usual care both in health-related quality-of-life measurements and tinnitus-specific questionnaires. The fact that the outcomes were so positive argues against another common belief, that nonpharmacologic interventions cannot be investigated with the same methodological rigor as pharmacologic interventions in double-blind, randomized, controlled trials. This article clearly shows this is not the case.

The essential feature of the study carried out by these authors is that specialized care for tinnitus must be carried out in a multidisciplinary fashion. The study design was carried out by audiologists, psychologists, speech therapists, movement therapists, physical therapists, and social workers. The actual implementation approaches were not entirely new since they combined components of cognitive behavioral therapy and tinnitus retraining therapy, the most widely used treatment strategies used. The difference is that the techniques used were implemented by a multidisciplinary team and studied very carefully.

It goes without saying that future advances in the management of tinnitus must be based on a better understanding of the pathophysiology of the problem. There are well-known causes of tinnitus, some of which can either be prevented or managed if the cause is identified. For example, exposure to loud noise from portable music devices can induce noise-related hearing loss associated with tinnitus. Ear wax irritating the eardrum can cause tinnitus. Otosclerosis (stiffening of the bones of the middle ear) can also cause hearing loss and tinnitus, albeit not in the pediatric age group. Curiously, stress and depression frequently are associated with tinnitus and seem to aggravate it. Last, acoustic neuromas, also called vestibular schwannoma, can cause tinnitus, but the tinnitus in these cases tends to be only in one ear. A rare cause of tinnitus in children is arterial venous malformations in and about the middle ear. Other causes in children include chemotherapeutic agents such as vincristine, certain diuretics, and when taken in high doses, aspirin.

J. A. Stockman III, MD

6 Endocrinology

Congenital Hypothyroidism Caused by Excess Prenatal Maternal Iodine Ingestion

Connelly KJ, Boston BA, Pearce EN, et al (Oregon Health & Science Univ Doernbecher Children's Hosp, Portland; Boston Univ School of Medicine, MA; et al)
J Pediatr 161:760-762, 2012

We report the cases of 3 infants with congenital hypothyroidism detected with the use of our newborn screening program, with evidence supporting excess maternal iodine ingestion (12.5 mg/d) as the etiology. Levels of whole blood iodine extracted from their newborn screening specimens were 10 times above mean control levels. Excess iodine ingestion from nutritional supplements is often unrecognized.

▶ Most of us learn during residency training that exposure of the fetus in utero or shortly after birth to large amounts of iodine can cause neonatal hypothyroidism. This occurs either through placental transfer of iodine or via breast milk feedings. The authors of this report present 3 cases of infants with congenital hypothyroidism detected by newborn screening. The mothers of 3 of these infants were ingesting a nutritional supplement whose iodine content far exceeded the normal daily recommended intake. The mothers had elevated iodine levels in their urine and breast milk samples. It is known that iodine freely crosses the placenta and that such transfer is essential for normal neonatal thyroid function and neurocognitive development. If there is excess iodine delivered to the fetal thyroid or the neonatal thyroid, it can cause a transient decrease in thyroid hormone production. This is a physiologic response that protects against overproduction of thyroid hormone due to iodine excess. This mechanism also is capitalized upon to shut down thyroid function at the time of radiation exposure in older children and adults. Eventually in older children and adults, this effect of excess iodine, known as the Wolff-Chaikoff effect, burns itself out after a few days of exposure to protect against the development of hypothyroidism. Unfortunately for the neonate, the thyroid gland is unable to escape the effects of the acute Wolff-Chaikoff effect, making the infant and fetus much more susceptible to iodine-induced hypothyroidism. This is a well-described problem in certain parts of the world such as Japan, where diets are high in iodine from the eating of iodine-rich seaweed, resulting in elevated iodine levels in maternal urine, serum, and breast milk and abnormal thyroid function in infants.

The infants described in the report of Connelly et al were detected with newborn screening as having hypothyroidism. A quick maternal history pinpointed the cause of the problem. The infants all demonstrated elevated iodine content in their urine. All recovered normal thyroid function after the maternal exposure ceased.

So what is the lesson to be learned here? With the increasing use of nutritional supplements these days, one must be wary during pregnancy about women unknowingly taking excess amounts of iodine. In the 3 cases reported, all the infants' mothers reported taking a supplement known as Iodoral (Optimox Corporation, Torrance, CA). Iodoral tablets contain 12.5 mg iodine. These tablets are taken usually once daily. The 3 cases demonstrate the potential hazard of the use of nutritional supplements containing iodine amounts far in excess of the 1100 ug/d total intake considered by the US Institute of Medicine to be the safe upper limit for iodine ingestion.[1]

J. A. Stockman III, MD

Reference

1. Otten J, Hellwig J, Meyers L. *Dietary reference intakes: essential guide to nutrient requirements.* Washington, DC: The National Academies Press, 2006.

β-Cell Dysfunction in Adolescents and Adults with Newly Diagnosed Type 2 Diabetes Mellitus

Elder DA, Herbers PM, Weis T, et al (Cincinnati Children's Hosp Med Ctr, OH; et al)
J Pediatr 160:904-910, 2012

Objective.—To compare β-cell function in adolescents and adults with newly diagnosed type 2 diabetes (T2DM).

Study Design.—Thirty-nine adolescents with T2DM, 38 age- and weight-matched control subjects, and 19 adults with T2DM were studied. The adolescent subjects with diabetes were divided on the basis of whether they needed insulin to control their initial hyperglycemia. The primary outcome variable was the disposition index, computed from the acute insulin response to glucose corrected for insulin sensitivity (1/Homeostatic model assessment of insulin resistance).

Results.—The disposition index was significantly reduced in all 3 diabetic groups (control $n = 3360$, adolescents with T2DM without insulin $n = 630$, adolescents with T2DM with insulin $n = 120$, adults with T2DM $n = 200$; $P < .001$), and the adolescents with more severe hyperglycemia at diagnosis had lower disposition index than those with a more modest presentation ($P < .05$).

Conclusion.—At the time of diagnosis, adolescents with T2DM have significant β-cell dysfunction, comparable with adults newly diagnosed with T2DM. Thus, severe β-cell impairment can develop within the first two decades of life and is likely to play a central role in the pathogenesis of T2DM in adolescents.

▶ It has been known for some years that the pathophysiology of type 2 diabetes mellitus relates to 2 problems: insulin resistance and β-cell dysfunction. Most of the data in this regard have been derived from studies of adults. Which of these abnormalities is primary has also been a source of some debate. Both loss of insulin secretion and insulin resistance seem to play a role in childhood onset of type 2 diabetes. Although insulin resistance has been shown to be familial in origin, with exacerbation by a number of environmental factors, the triggers for loss of insulin secretion have remained less well understood. It is thought that β-cell dysfunction may occur some years before the initiation of a need for management of type 2 diabetes mellitus. These authors demonstrate that β-cell function is measured by the disposition index (representing the product of insulin secretion and insulin sensitivity), and it is decreased in adolescence with new-onset diabetes compared with controls but similar to adults with new-onset type 2 diabetes.

The findings in this article also demonstrate that adolescents with type 2 diabetes mellitus have marked impairment of insulin secretion at the time of diagnosis, even after a short course of treatment to correct hyperglycemia. A wide range of insulin secretory capacity was observed in subjects with the most severe hyperglycemia at presentation, prompting insulin treatment at diagnosis. These findings do not support the hypothesis that adolescents with new onset type 2 diabetes mellitus have relatively greater preservation of β-cell function than adults with newly diagnosed type 2 diabetes mellitus. The findings also indicate that severe β-cell impairment is comparable with that of adults who have recently been diagnosed with type 2 diabetes mellitus and is a central feature of the presence of type 2 diabetes mellitus in adolescents.

In summary, adolescents with new onset type 2 diabetes mellitus do have impaired insulin secretion and response to glucose and other agents such as arginine. The situation is comparable to or worse than that for adults in whom diabetes was recently diagnosed. The authors could not determine from their studies whether abnormalities of insulin secretion in adolescents with diabetes are long-standing, with slow progression similar to the model for adult type 2 diabetes, or whether they develop more rapidly shortly before clinical presentation. Thus, adolescents with type 2 diabetes seem to share some key defects of insulin secretion with adults who have diabetes, but we need to learn more about the pathogenesis and natural history across the age spectrum of these disorders in disparate age groups.

J. A. Stockman III, MD

Nocturnal Glucose Control with an Artificial Pancreas at a Diabetes Camp

Phillip M, Battelino T, Atlas E, et al (Natl Ctr for Childhood Diabetes, Petah Tikva, Israel; Univ of Ljubljana, Slovenia; et al)
N Engl J Med 368:824-833, 2013

Background.—Recent studies have shown that an artificial-pancreas system can improve glucose control and reduce nocturnal hypoglycemia. However, it is not known whether such results can be replicated in settings outside the hospital.

Methods.—In this multicenter, multinational, randomized, crossover trial, we assessed the short-term safety and efficacy of an artificial pancreas system for control of nocturnal glucose levels in patients (10 to 18 years of age) with type 1 diabetes at a diabetes camp. In two consecutive overnight sessions, we randomly assigned 56 patients to receive treatment with an artificial pancreas on the first night and a sensor-augmented insulin pump (control) on the second night or to the reverse order of therapies on the first and second nights. Thus, all the patients received each treatment in a randomly assigned order. The primary end points were the number of hypoglycemic events (defined as a sensor glucose value of <63 mg per deciliter [3.5 mmol per liter] for at least 10 consecutive minutes), the time spent with glucose levels below 60 mg per deciliter (3.3 mmol per liter), and the mean overnight glucose level for individual patients.

Results.—On nights when the artificial pancreas was used, versus nights when the sensor-augmented insulin pump was used, there were significantly fewer episodes of nighttime glucose levels below 63 mg per deciliter (7 vs. 22) and significantly shorter periods when glucose levels were below 60 mg per deciliter ($P = 0.003$ and $P = 0.02$, respectively, after adjustment for multiplicity). Median values for the individual mean overnight glucose levels were 126.4 mg per deciliter (interquartile range, 115.7 to 139.1 [7.0 mmol per liter; interquartile range, 6.4 to 7.7]) with the artificial pancreas and 140.4 mg per deciliter (interquartile range, 105.7 to 167.4 [7.8 mmol per liter; interquartile range, 5.9 to 9.3]) with the sensor-augmented pump. No serious adverse events were reported.

Conclusions.—Patients at a diabetes camp who were treated with an artificial-pancreas system had less nocturnal hypoglycemia and tighter glucose control than when they were treated with a sensor-augmented insulin pump. (Funded by Sanofi and others; ClinicalTrials.gov number, NCT01238406.)

▶ This is an interesting and important report dealing with a fairly common problem. Increasingly, we are hearing about a fully automated artificial pancreas system as a means to control nocturnal glucose levels. Such systems link glucose sensors with insulin pumps through computerized control algorithms. These control insulin delivery in response to real-time sensor data. Studies have been carried out in inpatient settings that show such systems improve glucose control and reduce the risk of nocturnal hypoglycemia in children, adolescents, and adults. The report of Phillip et al adds to our current understandings by taking what we have learned from the hospital setting into the ultimate outpatient setting, youth camps, one each in Israel, Slovenia, and Germany. The diabetes Wireless Artificial Pancreas Consortium (DREAM) undertook this study on patients who were 10 to 18 years of age and who were already receiving insulin pump therapy for at least 3 months.

In 2 consecutive overnight sessions, subjects were assigned to receive treatment with an artificial pancreas on the first night and a sensor-augmented insulin pump (the control) on the second night or the reverse on the first and second nights. The artificial pancreas model was one using MD-Logic. This is a wireless, fully automated, closed-loop system using an algorithm based on fuzzy logic theory, a learning algorithm, and an alerts module and personal system setting. The alerts model includes real-time alarms such as impending hypoglycemia and long-standing hyperglycemia. The algorithm for alerts integrates information derived from past glucose levels, insulin delivery (time and dose), and models of insulin pharmacodynamics. The hypoglycemia alarms are designed to operate in instances in which impending hypoglycemia cannot be avoided by only withholding the dose of insulin. The primary endpoints in this study were the number of hypoglycemic events (defined according to the European Guidelines for Hypoglycemia as a sensor value of < 63 mL/dL for at least 10 consecutive minutes), the time during which glucose levels were less than 60 mg/dL, and mean overnight glucose levels for individual patients.

It was clear that when the artificial pancreas was used at night, there were fewer episodes of nighttime glucose levels less than 63 mg/dL and shorter periods when glucose levels were less than 60 mg/dL. Being that glucose values for individual mean glucose levels were approximately 15 mg/dL lower with the use of the artificial pancreas compared with the sensor augmented pump, the improved results seem to be related to a combined effect of better control of the amount of insulin provided and better control of the timing of insulin delivery, together with the presence of an alarm module, in the artificial pancreas.

The camp was chosen as a location of the study because it represents a transitional phase between a hospital clinical research center setting and a child's home. Nonetheless, the camp itself provides the elements of a real-life setting in a place in which health care needs still can be met by the research team. It will be interesting to see how the data from this report ultimately translate into clinical practice, but the results from this study do demonstrate the utility and success of the artificial pancreas model.

J. A. Stockman III, MD

Clinical Presentation of Children With Premature Adrenarche

von Oettingen J, Sola Pou J, Levitsky LL, et al (Massachusetts General Hosp for Children and Harvard Med School, Boston; Hospital Universitari de Girona, Girona, Spain)
Clin Pediatr 51:1140-1149, 2012

Objectives.—To describe the phenotype of premature adrenarche (PA) patients, elucidate historical and physical correlates, and distinguish PA from late-onset congenital adrenal hyperplasia (LOCAH).

Study Design.—Retrospective chart review of 122 patients (91 female and 31 male) with PA and 11 with LOCAH.

Results.—In PA patients, birth weight was <2 standard deviation scores (SDSs) in 6%, and 14% were premature. Body mass index SDSs were high (2.00 ± 1.84). Bone age (BA) SDS was >2 in 31% and was greater in boys than in girls; PA subjects were taller, and the predicted height was at or above genetic potential. Dehydroepiandrosterone sulfate (DHEAS) was higher in boys. LOCAH patients had earlier pubic hair, more advanced BA, lower height SDSs, lower adult height prediction, and higher adrenal androgen levels.

Conclusion.—Patients with PA tend to be overweight with BA acceleration but normal height prediction. LOCAH is distinguished by earlier presentation and higher 17-hydrocyprogesterone and adrenal androgens.

▶ This article from the United States and Spain provides valuable new information about the clinical presentation of youngsters with premature adrenarche. Premature adrenarche refers to the onset of increased adrenal androgen production shortly before the onset of gonadarche (the earliest detectable changes of puberty) and is associated with the appearance of apocrine, body odor, and acne or oily skin as well as pubic and axillary hair growth. Premature adrenarche refers to the onset of such symptoms before age 8 years in girls and 9 years in boys and is usually associated with increasing levels of adrenal androgens in the pubertal range. Premature pubarche more specifically refers to the early onset of pubic or axillary hair growth in those age groups. Premature adrenarche has been seen in youngsters with increased body mass index and with premature pubarche, and in some populations, low birth weight and smallness for gestational age may be risk factors. At one time, premature adrenarche was thought to be a benign variant of normal adrenarche, but more and more reports have appeared linking premature adrenarche to functional hyperadrenalism, polycystic ovary syndrome, hyperinsulinism, and metabolic syndrome. Premature adrenarche also must be distinguished from pathologic conditions that may present with similar symptoms and require treatment, including late onset congenital adrenal hyperplasia and virilizing adrenal or gonadal tumors. Premature adrenarche is more common in black and non-Hispanic white children and is up to 10 times more common in girls than boys.

These authors now describe the phenotypic characteristics in some detail for boys and girls with premature adrenarche. Their study represented a retrospective chart review of patients seen on a pediatric endocrine service. The data from this report represent the largest study to date of premature adrenarche, which importantly contains information on boys with the disorder. It is the first study to specifically describe differences in presentation between sexes. The data show that girls are symptomatic about 14 to 17 months earlier than boys, consistent with previous descriptions from the literature. Almost two-thirds of boys and girls in this study with premature adrenarche were either overweight or obese. Height and bone age were both advanced in affected individuals. Despite the advanced bone age, youngsters with premature adrenarche ultimately had normal height predictions. Patients with late onset congenital adrenal hyperplasia generally presented earlier and had significantly higher levels of adrenal hormones when assayed.

J. A. Stockman III, MD

Incidence and Characteristics of Pseudoprecocious Puberty Because of Severe Primary Hypothyroidism

Cabrera SM, Dimeglio LA, Eugster EA (Indiana Univ School of Medicine, Indianapolis)
J Pediatr 162:637-639, 2013

Severe primary hypothyroidism is a presumed rare cause of pseudoprecocious puberty (PsPP). Here, we report a 24% incidence of PsPP among 33 children with profound hypothyroidism. Those with PsPP were older and trended toward a higher thyroid stimulating hormone. Increased awareness of PsPP can hasten diagnosis and appropriate treatment.

▶ This article reminds us that profound primary hypothyroidism can be a cause of early secondary sexual development. This is a variety of pseudoprecocious puberty, also known as Van Wyk-Grumbach syndrome. Those affected have the usual classical features of hypothyroidism, including delayed linear growth and skeletal maturation, but affected girls have breast development, galactorrhea, and/or vaginal bleeding, while boys have testicular enlargement without virilization. Girls demonstrate large multicystic ovaries and an enlarged uterus on pelvic ultrasound. Affected individuals have low thyroxine levels in association with markedly elevated thyroid-stimulating hormone (TSH). They also show elevated prolactin, normal to high estradiol, and follicle-stimulating hormone (FSH). In addition, there are suppressed luteinizing hormone levels consistent with profound hypothyroidism and FSH-predominant gonadotropin-independent puberty. FSH predominance is believed to be caused by prolactin-induced reduction and the frequency of gonadotropin-releasing hormone pulsatility, a condition that increases FSH expression while inhibiting luteinizing hormone expression.

Before this article appeared, there was little information about how frequently pseudoprecocious puberty occurs as a result of severe primary hypothyroidism. The investigators examined the records of all children diagnosed with Hashimoto thyroiditis diagnosed over a 10-year period at Riley Hospital for Children in Indianapolis. They were able to find more than 5 dozen children with this diagnosis who had markedly elevated TSH levels of 100 or more. Thirty-four percent of this group had goiters. More than half had final heights that were in excess of 2 standard deviations below their target height. Thirty-three of the 62 children were of prepubertal age and were thus able to be evaluated for the presence of pseudoprecocious puberty. The incidence of pseudoprecocious puberty in these profoundly hypothyroid children was 24% with a predominance of girls (75% of the total).

It is not exactly known what the precise cause of pseudoprecocious puberty is in relationship to profound hypothyroidism. Nonetheless, if you see a child who is profoundly hypothyroid, examine that youngster closely if he or she is in an age group where pseudoprecocious puberty might be evolving. Contrarily, if you see a child with what looks like precocious puberty, plan to rule out hypothyroidism as a potential etiology. Obviously, this is an unusual and perhaps even rare association, but at least think of it.

J. A. Stockman III, MD

Random Luteinizing Hormone Often Remains Pubertal in Children Treated with the Histrelin Implant for Central Precocious Puberty
Lewis KA, Eugster EA (Indiana Univ School of Medicine, Indianapolis)
J Pediatr 162:562-565, 2013

Objective.—To investigate the use of random ultrasensitive (US) luteinizing hormone (LH) levels to monitor children being treated with a histrelin implant for central precocious puberty (CPP).

Study Design.—This was a prospective, uncontrolled, observational study at a pediatric endocrinology tertiary center. Thirty-three children (26 girls; mean age 7.2 ± 2.5 years) treated with a histrelin implant for CPP were enrolled. A random US LH measurement was obtained at 6 months, and a gonadotropin-releasing hormone analog stimulation test was performed at 12 months. Clinic visits occurred at baseline and at 6-month intervals.

Results.—In 59% of the patients (17 of 29), the 6-month random US LH exceeded the prepubertal range of ≤ 0.3 IU/L. In contrast, gonadotropin-releasinghormone analog stimulation tests revealed complete hypothalamic-pituitary-gonadal axis suppression (peak LH < 4 IU/L) in all 31 patients who underwent testing. US LH levels were highly correlated with peak stimulated LH levels. The mean peak stimulated LH level was higher in patients with a pubertal random LH than in those with a prepubertal random LH (1.2 ± 0.5 IU/L vs 0.5 ± 0.1 IU/L; $P < .01$). No patient had clinical evidence of pubertal progression.

Conclusion.—The random US LH level does not revert to a prepubertal range in more than one-half of patients with a histrelin implant and documented hypothalamic-pituitary-gonadal axis suppression. Long-term studies are needed to elucidate the optimal strategy for monitoring treatment in children with CPP.

▶ Histrelin is a nonapeptide analog of gonadotropin-releasing hormone (GnRH) with added potency. It acts on particular cells of the pituitary glands called *gonadotropes*. It stimulates gonadotropes to release luteinizing hormone (LH) and follicle-stimulating hormone. Thus, it is considered a GnRH agonist. Histrelin is marketed by Endo pharmaceuticals under the brand names Vandas and Supprelin LA. Its standard use is to treat hormone-sensitive cancers of the prostate in men and uterine fibroids in women. In addition, histrelin has been proven to be highly effective in treating central precocious puberty in children. It is available as a daily intramuscular injection or as a 12-month subcutaneous implant (Vandas), usually used for the palliative treatment of advanced prostate cancer. A 12-month subcutaneous implant (Supprelin LA) for central precocious puberty (CPP) was approved in 2007 by the US Food and Drug Administration.

The report of Lewis et al reminds us that currently there is no consensus regarding routine biochemical monitoring of GnRH agonist therapy during treatment. It has been suggested, however, that a random ultrasensitive (US) LH level greater than the prepubertal range may indicate inadequate suppression from GnRH agonist therapy. To determine whether this is so, Lewis et al designed a prospective study to look at boys and girls treated with histrelin implant for CPP. All these youngsters had precocious puberty and were being treated with a histrelin implant. The data from this report showed that a random US LH level does not return to the prepubertal range in at least half of patients with histrelin implants. Although these data do not necessarily indicate treatment failure, they are very worrisome. The authors of this report do say that whether US LH levels should be measured at all as part of routine clinical care in patients being treated for CPP remains open to debate given that growth velocity, pubertal progression, and bone age advancement are likely the most important indicators of therapeutic efficacy. It is entirely possible that prepubertal random US LH levels on histrelin may simply reflect that the child is further along in pubertal development when GnRH agonist therapy was initiated, as suggested by the pubertal LH values in the girls who were postmenarchal and the boys with larger testicular volumes in this report. The authors conclude that further study is needed to determine the optimal approach to the monitoring of CPP in patients with histrelin implants or other modes of delivery of GnRH agonist therapy.

Please do not think that the safety and efficacy of GnRH agonist therapy for CPP is disputed. It is not. It is simply that the optimal strategy for monitoring the effectiveness of this therapy has not yet been established.

J. A. Stockman III, MD

Growth during Infancy and Childhood, and Adiposity at Age 16 Years: Ages 2 to 7 Years Are Pivotal

Liem ET, van Buuren S, Sauer PJJ, et al (Univ of Groningen, The Netherlands; Netherlands Organization for Applied Scientific Research TNO, Leiden)
J Pediatr 162:287-292.e2, 2013

Objective.—To assess the period during infancy and childhood in which growth is most associated with adolescent adiposity and the metabolic syndrome (MS) and whether this differs depending on maternal smoking during pregnancy.

Study Design.—A longitudinal population-based cohort study among 772 girls and 708 boys.

Results.—Weight gains between ages 2-4 years and ages 4-7 years were most strongly associated with higher body mass index (BMI), sum of skinfold measurements, body fat percentage, and waist circumference at age 16. A one SD increase in weight between ages 2-4 and 4-7 years was associated with increases in outcome measures of +0.82 to +1.47 SDs (all $P < .001$), and with a less favorable MS score. In children whose mothers smoked during pregnancy, the association of relative weight gain during ages 2-4 years with adolescent BMI was stronger than in children whose mothers did not smoke. For adolescent BMI, the increase was 0.42 SD higher ($P = .01$). This was similar for the other adiposity measures.

Conclusions.—Large relative increases in weight from ages 2 to 7 years are associated with adolescent adiposity and MS. This is more pronounced in adolescents whose mothers smoked during pregnancy.

▶ This report from the Netherlands assesses the period during infancy and childhood in which growth is most associated with adolescent adiposity and corresponding metabolic traits. It has been thought for some time that critical time periods exist in which accelerated growth constitutes a risk factor for subsequent adiposity and its associated metabolic complications. Specifically, these critical time periods have been thought to include gestation, early infancy, the period of adiposity rebound, and adolescence. Several reviews have shown positive correlations between rapid growth and early childhood (from birth to age 2 years and from age 2 to 7 years) and adolescent and adult overweight. Early adiposity rebound has been found to be associated with adult overweight, independent of the body mass index when the adiposity rebound began. Unfortunately, strong evidence on the relative importance of these critical periods is lacking, thus, the value of the report of Liem et al.

Liem et al undertook a cohort study among 772 girls and 708 boys and showed that weight gains between 2 and 4 years and 4 to 7 years were most strongly associated with higher body mass index, percentage of body fat, and waist circumference by age 16. Such factors were also associated with less favorable metabolic syndrome scores. These findings were much more exaggerated in children of mothers who smoked during pregnancy.

Findings from these reports support an early start of preventative strategies, perhaps as early as 2 years of age. Such interventions should target children whose mothers have smoked during pregnancy.

More data are appearing in the literature suggesting that the cardiovascular complications of obesity are appearing earlier in life. A study, for example, among 3832 US service personnel who died in combat operations between 2000 and 2011 showed that 12.1% already had evidence of coronary or aortic atherosclerosis at autopsy. Some 8.5% had coronary atherosclerosis, which was severe in 2.3%. The mean age was just 26 years. This and other autopsy studies going back more than half a century remind us that atherosclerosis begins early and is the result of the usual combination of risk factors.[1]

J. A. Stockman III, MD

Reference

1. Webber BJ, Seguin PG, Burnett DG, Clark LL, Otto JL. Prevalence of and risk factors for autopsy determined atherosclerosis among US service members, 2001–2011. *JAMA*. 2012;308:2577-2583.

Effect of Inhaled Glucocorticoids in Childhood on Adult Height

Kelly HW, for the CAMP Research Group (Univ of New Mexico, Albuquerque; et al)
N Engl J Med 367:904-912, 2012

Background.—The use of inhaled glucocorticoids for persistent asthma causes a temporary reduction in growth velocity in prepubertal children. The resulting decrease in attained height 1 to 4 years after the initiation of inhaled glucocorticoids is thought not to decrease attained adult height.

Methods.—We measured adult height in 943 of 1041 participants (90.6%) in the Childhood Asthma Management Program; adult height was determined at a mean ($\pm$SD) age of 24.9 $\pm$ 2.7 years. Starting at the age of 5 to 13 years, the participants had been randomly assigned to receive 400 μg of budesonide, 16 mg of nedocromil, or placebo daily for 4 to 6 years. We calculated differences in adult height for each active treatment group, as compared with placebo, using multiple linear regression with adjustment for demographic characteristics, asthma features, and height at trial entry.

Results.—Mean adult height was 1.2 cm lower (95% confidence interval [CI], -1.9 to -0.5) in the budesonide group than in the placebo group ($P = 0.001$) and was 0.2 cm lower (95% CI, -0.9 to 0.5) in the nedocromil group than in the placebo group ($P = 0.61$). A larger daily dose of inhaled glucocorticoid in the first 2 years was associated with a lower adult height (-0.1 cm for each microgram per kilogram of body weight) ($P = 0.007$). The reduction in adult height in the budesonide group as compared with the placebo group was similar to that seen after 2 years of treatment (-1.3 cm; 95% CI, -1.7 to -0.9). During the first 2 years, decreased growth velocity in the budesonide group occurred primarily in prepubertal participants.

Conclusions.—The initial decrease in attained height associated with the use of inhaled glucocorticoids in prepubertal children persisted as a reduction in adult height, although the decrease was not progressive or cumulative. (Funded by the National Heart, Lung, and Blood Institute and the National Center for Research Resources; CAMP ClinicalTrials. gov number, NCT00000575.)

▶ There has been a lot of controversy over the potential side effects of corticosteroids on the growth of children with asthma. Inhaled corticosteroids are the recommended therapy for persistent asthma in youngsters and there are good data to indicate that the use of inhaled corticosteroids may reduce growth velocity by an average of 1 cm on average during the first few years of therapy. This reduction has been reported for low-to-medium doses. The general belief, however, has been that although the use of steroids may slow growth, youngsters with asthma so treated tend to grow for a longer period before reaching adult height and thus are more likely than not to achieve a normal height. The authors of this report previously examined data from the Childhood Asthma Management Program (CAMP) clinical trial suggesting that participants in a trial receiving budesonide had not caught up with the heights of participants in the placebo group after 4.8 years of follow-up. The purpose of the current study was to continue the height follow-up of the CAMP participants to assess the effects of budesonide (Pulmicort Turbuhaler, AstraZeneca) and nedocromil (Tilade, Rhone-Poulenc Rorer).

The CAMP clinical trial had children entered into it from December 1993 through September 1995. More than 1000 children between the ages of 5 and 13 years with mild-to-moderate asthma entered the double-blind, placebo-controlled CAMP trial, which compared the efficacy and safety of inhaled budesonide with nedocromil administered by means of a metered-dose inhaler and placebo. Albuterol was used for asthma symptoms in all 3 groups. Height and weight were measured in these youngsters every 6 months during the initial 4.5 years of observational follow-up and 1 to 2 times a year during the next 8 years. Adult height was determined at a mean age of 24.9 ± 2.7 years. Tanner staging was performed annually until the participants were 18 years of age or had attained sexual maturity.

The results of the current study indicated that the adjusted mean adult height was 1.2 cm lower in the budesonide group than in the placebo group (171.1 cm vs 172.3 cm, $P = .001$); the mean adult height in the nedocromil group (172.1 cm) was similar to that in the placebo group ($P = .61$). This deficit in adult height in the budesonide group compared with the placebo group was greater for women (-1.8 cm) than for men (-0.8). Although the deficit was greater for participants who were younger at trial entry than for those who were older and greater for whites than for other races or ethnic groups, the effect of budesonide on adult height did not vary significantly according to the age at trial entry, race or ethnic group, or duration of asthma at trial entry. The deficit in the adjusted mean height in the budesonide group as compared with the placebo group was 1.3 cm after 2 years of treatment and 1.2 cm at the end of the CAMP trial and persisted into adulthood without progressing further.

The authors of this report concluded that the reduction in growth seen in the first few years of administration of inhaled corticosteroids in prepubertal children persists as lowered adult height. This very modest difference in height has to be weighed against the benefits of the use of corticosteroids in controlling persistent asthma and the effects of uncontrolled asthma itself on overall well-being. It was also concluded that the most appropriate dose of steroids is the lowest dose that can effectively control one's asthma. No surprise with the latter conclusion.

J. A. Stockman III, MD

The world's tallest nation has stopped growing taller: the height of Dutch children from 1955 to 2009

Schönbeck Y, Talma H, van Dommelen P, et al (Netherlands Organisation for Applied Scientific Res (TNO), Leiden; Free Univ Med Ctr (VUmc), Amsterdam, The Netherlands; et al)
Pediatr Res 73:371-377, 2013

Background.—Records show that mean height in The Netherlands has increased since 1858. This study looks at whether this trend in the world's tallest nation is continuing. We consider the influence of the geographical region, and of the child and parental education, on changes in height.

Methods.—We compared the height of young Dutch people aged 0–21 y as determined on the basis of the growth study of 2009, with the height data from growth studies conducted in 1955, 1965, 1980, and 1997.

Results.—The analysis sample included 5,811 boys and 6,194 girls. Height by age was the same as in 1997. Mean final height was 183.8 cm (SD = 7.1 cm) in boys and 170.7 cm (SD = 6.3 cm) in girls. The educational levels of both children and their parents are positively correlated with mean height. Since 1997, differences between geographical regions have decreased but not vanished, with the northern population being the tallest.

Conclusion.—The world's tallest population has stopped growing taller after a period of 150 y, the cause of which is unclear. The Dutch may have reached the optimal height distribution. Alternatively, growth-promoting environmental factors may have stabilized in the past decade, preventing the population from attaining its full growth potential.

▶ I think everyone knows the human race has been gradually getting taller, at least in developing countries. This trend was thought to be the result of improvements in the nutritional, hygienic, economic, and health status of the populations of the better-off nations. The authors of this report from the Netherlands actually pose the question: "Do we believe that we could all be giants if living conditions for humans were to improve further, or is there some maximum (and presumably optimal) population average beyond which our species will not grow, no matter how favorable the circumstances?"

If you are not aware, the Dutch population is the tallest in the world, and this population has been well studied. Before 1955, the population height in the Netherlands was estimated on the basis of data for those inducted into the military, that is, men and then nonrandom samples from the general population. Between 1955 and 1997, there were a number of cross-sectional nationwide growth studies in the Netherlands showing that Dutch adults are among the tallest people in the world with women measuring almost 171 cm (5 feet, 7.25 inches) and men 184 cm (6 feet, 1.5 inches). Data going back in time show that people in the Netherlands have been growing taller since 1858. At that time, those entering the military were of an average height of just 163 cm. Thus, there has been a gain of height of 21 cm over just 140 years. Nonetheless, in the Netherlands, as in most northern European countries, the upward trend is slowing down significantly. There is some suggestion here in the United States that the continuing growth observed here in the United States has flattened out and may be even reversing slightly.[1]

The report of Schönbeck et al tells us about new data related to height from the Fifth Dutch Growth Study carried out in 2009. The report addresses several questions. Is the 140-year trend of increasing height in the world's tallest nation still continuing? If not, has there been a compression of height variation? Do regional/geographic/educational levels affect the development of mean height? The study sample consisted of more than 10 000 children of Dutch origin who were followed up over a number of years. The data show that over a 12-year interval between 1997 and 2009, there was a very slight increase in mean height in early puberty in boys and girls, indicating that they were taller at a younger age than in 1997. However, this did not affect the final height of either gender, as no significant differences in final height were seen compared with 1997. There was also no compression of height variation observed. Thus, the standard deviations within each age group remained similar over a 12-year period. Thus, the secular height trend toward increasing heights spanning 150 years appears to have come to an end, at least temporarily. The cause is not clear. Economic factors are not likely to be involved because gross domestic product in the Netherlands has not fallen off. Indeed, it increased exponentially between 1920 and 2008. Various measures of social and psychoemotional status also have shown no significant changes over the interval.

Given that the Dutch are the tallest people in the world and that they are no longer growing taller, the authors of this report hypothesize that the mean height of the population has reached the maximum possible. It is entirely possible that the height achieved in this population is the best it ever will be, meaning that the ideal average height achieved by boys is 184 cm and 171 cm for girls.

If you want to learn more about the opposite end of this scale, short stature in children and what to do about it, see the superb review of this topic by Allen and Cuttler.[2]

J. A. Stockman III, MD

References

1. Komlos J. The recent decline in the height of African-American women. *Econ Hum Biol*. 2010;8:58-66.
2. Allen DB, Cuttler L. Clinical practice. Short stature in childhood—challenges and choices. *N Engl J Med*. 2013;368:1220-1228.

7 Gastroenterology

Management of Ingested Magnets in Children

Hussain SZ, Bousvaros A, Gilger M, et al (WK Pediatric Gastroenterology & Res, Shreveport, LA; Children's Hosp, Boston, MA; Texas Children's Hosp, Houston; et al)
J Pediatr Gastroenterol Nutr 55:239-242, 2012

We describe a comprehensive algorithm for the management of ingested rare-earth magnets in children. These newer and smaller neodymium magnets sold as adult toys are much stronger than the traditional magnets, and can attract each other with formidable forces. If >1 magnet is swallowed at the same time, or a magnet is co-ingested with another metallic object, the loops of intestine can be squeezed between them resulting in bowel damage including perforations. An algorithm that uses the number of magnets ingested, location of magnets, and the timing of ingestion before intervention helps to delineate the roles of the pediatric gastroenterologists and surgeons in the management of these cases (Figs 1 and 3).

▶ This report tells us that neodymiums, rare-earth magnets, are not our grandfathers' magnets. They are composed of iron, boron, and neodymium. They are at least 5 to 10 times more powerful than traditional magnets. They were invented by General Motors and Sumitomo Special Metals in 1982 and are now used in many toys and modern household products, including cordless tools, hard drives, magnetic resonance imaging instruments, and hybrid electric engines. Ingested neodymium magnets are a serious health hazard for children with an extremely high risk of intestinal obstruction.

In 2006 the US Consumer Product Safety Commission raised the recommended age for magnetic children's toys from 3 to 6 years to ensure children's safety. Nonetheless, increasing reports of the swallowing of rare-earth neodymium magnets have surfaced. Many of these reports have appeared since 2008 and involve small neodymium magnets sold as a part of a cube of magnets marketed as desk toys and stress relievers for adults. The Consumer Product Safety Commission has received reports of toddlers finding loose magnets left within their reach. Adolescents and teenagers use these high-powered magnets to mimic body piercings by placing two or more on their earlobe, tongue, or nose, which has resulted in magnets being unintentionally inhaled and swallowed.

In 2008 the first magnet ball cube toy, the NeoCube, was developed, followed by the Bucky Ball in 2009. These adult desk toys rapidly became popular and increased exposure to neodymium magnets to children. Each unit of a neodymium magnet has approximately 125 to greater than 1000 magnetic balls (Fig 1) and

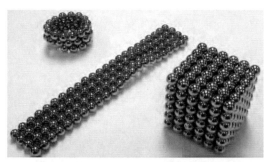

FIGURE 1.—High-powered ball bearing neodymium magnets in adult toys sold on the Internet as "New Magnetic Magnet Balls Beads Sphere Puzzle Cube." (From *www.cpsc.gov*, November 10, 2011, press release.) (Reprinted from Hussain SZ, Bousvaros A, Gilger M, et al. Management of ingested magnets in children. *J Pediatr Gastroenterol Nutr.* 2012;55:239-242. © 2012 with permission by the AAP.)

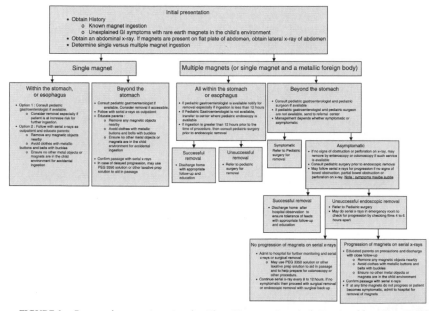

FIGURE 3.—Rare-earth magnet ingestion algorithm. GI = gastrointestinal. (Reprinted from Hussain SZ, Bousvaros A, Gilger M, et al. Management of ingested magnets in children. *J Pediatr Gastroenterol Nutr.* 2012;55:239-242. © 2012 with permission by the AAP.)

can be purchased on the Internet and other retail outlets. In 2009 the Consumer Product Safety Commission issued a ban on the sale of rare earth magnets to children younger than 14 years of age. If ingested, the swallowing of more than one magnet will cause one bowel wall to be attracted to another bowel wall containing magnets and does so with extreme magnetic force, resulting in ischemia and pressure injuries that can result in bowel perforation, volvulus, fistula, and severe infection. These problems can occur within 8 hours.

The report of Hussain et al describes a comprehensive algorithm for the management of ingested rare-earth magnets in children. The algorithm (Fig 3) allows a clinician to more quickly evaluate the seriousness of the problem created by the ingestion of magnets. The initial step in the evaluation is to confirm the diagnosis of magnet ingestion in a child presenting with gastrointestinal symptoms such as vomiting and abdominal pain. This is done by x-ray. The next step is to determine whether only a single magnet was ingested versus multiple magnets or a single magnet with a co-ingestion of another metallic object. To determine whether only a single magnet was ingested, multiple radiologic views are necessary because it is possible for magnets to stack on one another, overlap on a single view, and be misdiagnosed as a single magnet. A single magnet swallowed can be managed conservatively with appropriate education of the parents and child. It is the child with multiple magnets that will get into potential problems. Multiple magnet ingestions or co-ingestion of a single magnet and another metallic object should be treated with increased urgency because of the risk of perforation. The time interval between ingestion and presentation along with the location of the magnets determines the next step in the algorithm. Children with delayed presentation of more than 12 hours after ingestion seem to sustain more complications such as perforation and fistulae. If there is any concern, the magnets need to get out. There has been debate about the use of laxative agents to expedite the progression of a magnetic object through the intestine. There are no established data to support this approach and therefore endoscopic removal should be performed under general anesthesia with a protected airway. These objects can be very difficult to remove even with endoscopy.

The authors of this report do us all a service by reminding us of the many problems caused by magnets that are ingested by children. They also tell us that pediatric surgeons should be involved early in complicated cases, especially those with multiple magnet ingestions that are determined to be located distal to the stomach as well as with those that have had a significant period of time elapse between magnet ingestion and clinical intervention.

J. A. Stockman III, MD

Esophageal Sphincter Device for Gastroesophageal Reflux Disease

Ganz RA, Peters JH, Horgan S, et al (Minnesota Gastroenterology, Plymouth, MN; Univ of Rochester School of Medicine and Dentistry, NY; Univ of California, San Diego, La Jolla; et al)
N Engl J Med 368:719-727, 2013

Background.—Patients with gastroesophageal reflux disease who have a partial response to proton-pump inhibitors often seek alternative therapy. We evaluated the safety and effectiveness of a new magnetic device to augment the lower esophageal sphincter.

Methods.—We prospectively assessed 100 patients with gastroesophageal reflux disease before and after sphincter augmentation. The study did not include a concurrent control group. The primary outcome measure was normalization of esophageal acid exposure or a 50% or greater reduction in exposure at 1 year. Secondary outcomes were 50% or greater improvement in quality of life related to gastroesophageal reflux disease and a 50% or greater reduction in the use of proton-pump inhibitors at 1 year. For each outcome, the prespecified definition of successful treatment was achievement of the outcome in at least 60% of the patients. The 3-year results of a 5-year study are reported.

Results.—The primary outcome was achieved in 64% of patients (95% confidence interval [CI], 54 to 73). For the secondary outcomes, a reduction of 50% or more in the use of proton-pump inhibitors occurred in 93% of patients, and there was improvement of 50% or more in quality-of-life scores in 92%, as compared with scores for patients assessed at baseline while they were not taking proton-pump inhibitors. The most frequent adverse event was dysphagia (in 68% of patients postoperatively, in 11% at 1 year, and in 4% at 3 years). Serious adverse events occurred in six patients, and in six patients the device was removed.

Conclusions.—In this single-group evaluation of 100 patients before and after sphincter augmentation with a magnetic device, exposure to esophageal acid decreased, reflux symptoms improved, and use of proton-pump inhibitors decreased. Follow-up studies are needed to assess long-term safety. (Funded by Torax Medical; ClinicalTrials.gov number, NCT00776997.)

▶ Some pediatric patients were included in the study of a new esophageal sphincter device used in the management of gastroesophageal reflux disease. Thus, this report should be of interest to those providing care to pediatric patients, at least at the older age spectrum of pediatrics. We all know that the fundamental pathogenic abnormality in gastroesophageal reflux disease is an incompetent lower esophageal sphincter. Medical management usually involves methods to suppress acid formation, most commonly with proton-pump inhibitors. These are hardly perfect agents, however, and a fair percentage of patients are not treatable in this way. These agents, of course, do not deal with the structural underlying problem of an incompetent sphincter, and, therefore, do not necessarily have an effect on reflux itself. Currently, the only established option for patients who do not respond to aggressive medical management is antireflux surgery, typically with the Nissen fundoplication. Even when needed, one will find potential side effects with this type of approach, including abdominal bloating, increased flatulence, inability to belch or vomit, and persistent dysphasia.

Ganz et al tell us about augmentation of the role of the esophageal sphincter with a magnetic device that may provide an alternative treatment for patients who have incomplete symptom relief with proton-pump inhibitors or who are reluctant to undergo formal surgical fundoplication. The device in question is designed to augment sphincter function with a magnetic ring that improves the barrier function of the sphincter without altering the hiatal and gastric anatomy or interfering with swelling, belching, or vomiting. Ganz et al report on a 3-year study showing outcomes of a clinical trial assessing the efficacy and safety of a magnetic device for sphincter augmentation. The esophageal sphincter device is implanted with the use of a standard laparoscopic technique commonly used by surgeons who otherwise might have performed a fundoplication. The device itself uses magnetic attraction through adjacent magnetic beads, which augments the resistance of the esophageal sphincter to the abnormal opening associated with reflux. Each bead contains a sealed core of magnetic neodymium iron boride that produces a precise and permanent force of attraction. The beads are connected to adjacent beads by small wires that allow the device to expand. The device is sized to fit around the external diameter of the esophagus without compressing the underlying muscle. The beads separate with the transport of food or increased intragastric pressure associated with belching or vomiting. No dietary restrictions are needed after implantation (Fig 1 in the original article). In a way, one can think of this as a not-too-tight rubberband that can expand and contract as needed based on internal luminal pressure within the lower end of the esophagus. Others have tried a similar approach by placing a loose ligature around the lower esophageal sphincter, but, unfortunately, this approach does not allow yielding of the esophagus when challenged by gastric distention or by swallowing. The expandable medical device for augmentation of the sphincter provides greater control of resistance to sphincter effacement and opening that is provided by previous devices, because it allows for expansion of the passage of food and also permits belching and vomiting. In this report, persistent dysphasia that led to the removal of the device developed in just 3% of patients. When necessary, the device was readily and easily removed.

The most worrisome complication, theoretically, is that the placement of a foreign body around a mobile muscular tube such as the esophagus might cause erosion of tissue. At the time of the publication of this report, there had been almost 500 magnetic implants with a median implant duration of almost 3 years. No erosions or migrations have been reported. The risk over a longer period, however, is unknown. That said, this single-group trial did show that a magnetic device designed to augment the lower esophageal sphincter can be implanted safely with the use of standard laparoscopic techniques. The device decreases exposure to esophageal acid, improves reflux symptoms, and allows sensation of proton-pump inhibitors in most patients. This Star Wars approach seems reasonable in patients who are not responding to medical therapy who are at the older age spectrum of pediatrics.

J. A. Stockman III, MD

Health Status of Children Alive 10 Years after Pediatric Liver Transplantation Performed in the US and Canada: Report of the Studies of Pediatric Liver Transplantation Experience

Ng VL, for the Studies of Pediatric Liver Transplantation (SPLIT) Research Group (The Hosp for Sick Children and Univ of Toronto, Ontario, Canada; et al)
J Pediatr 160:820-826.e3, 2012

Objectives.—To determine clinical and health-related quality of life outcomes, and to derive an "ideal" composite profile of children alive 10 years after pediatric liver transplantation (LT) performed in the US and Canada.

Study Design.—This was a multicenter cross-sectional analysis characterizing patients enrolled in the Studies of Pediatric Liver Transplantation database registry who have survived > 10 years from LT.

Results.—A total of 167 10-year survivors were identified, all of whom received daily immunosuppression therapy. Comorbidities associated with the post-LT course included post-transplantation lymphoproliferative disease (in 5% of patients), renal dysfunction (9%), and impaired linear growth (23%). Health-related quality of life, as assessed by the PedsQL 4.0 Generic Core Scales, revealed lower patient self-reported total scale scores for 10-year survivors compared with matched healthy children (77.2 ± 12.9 vs 84.9 ± 11.7; $P < .001$). At 10 years post-LT, only 32% of patients achieved an ideal profile of a first allograft stable on immunosuppression monotherapy, normal growth, and absence of common immunosuppression-induced sequelae.

Conclusion.—Success after pediatric LT has moved beyond patient survival. Availability of an ideal composite profile at follow-up provides opportunities for patients, families, and healthcare providers to identify broader sets of outcomes at earlier stages, ultimately contributing to improved outcomes after pediatric LT.

▶ There are good data telling us about long-term outcomes in adults who have undergone liver transplant. One can expect an overall life expectancy in excess of 20 years in adults posttransplant. Unfortunately, patient survival and longevity in children who have undergone liver transplantation remains unknown, although it is thought to be likely greater than that noted in adults. Ng et al have undertaken a multicenter analysis to look at data from the Studies of Pediatric Liver Transplantation Database Registry. This registry was established in 1995 as a prospective data repository for children undergoing liver transplantation in the United States and Canada. This database is the largest detailed database of pediatric liver transplant recipients internationally.

The report of Ng et al was designed to look at the characteristics of children who survived a minimum of 10 years after liver transplantation. The study showed that in this population, survival rates for the first liver transplant were 94% at 1 year and 88% at 10 years. It is clear that effective immunosuppression is the key to the success of pediatric liver transplantation. The study confirms that daily immunosuppression with calcineurin inhibitor agents and newer options such as sirolimus remains the present clinical practice for long-term survivors of pediatric liver transplantation in the United States and Canada. Unfortunately, 1 in 5 children after liver transplantation are still on steroids at their 10th anniversary posttransplant. Longer duration of steroid exposure was associated with both growth impairment and limited catch-up growth. This study also confirmed the relatively low prevalence of specific immune and nonimmune complications associated with long-term immunosuppression use. Nonetheless, surprisingly, 10% of long-term survivors had missed more than 20 days of school in the preceding year with resultant significant impact on health-related quality of life issues. This finding suggests that chronic medication exposure may adversely impact health status by increasing the risk of community-acquired infections that cause lost school days.

The bottom line from this report is that survivorship is no longer the major issue posttransplant for liver disease. Quality of life issues must be looked at because only 32% of patients surviving 10 years after transplant achieved an ideal profile with respect to normal growth and overall absence of common immunosuppression-induced sequelae.

J. A. Stockman III, MD

Increasing Prevalence of Nonalcoholic Fatty Liver Disease Among United States Adolescents, 1988-1994 to 2007-2010

Welsh JA, Karpen S, Vos MB (Emory Univ School of Medicine, Atlanta, GA)
J Pediatr 162:496-500.e1 2013

Objective.—To assess recent trends in nonalcoholic fatty liver disease (NAFLD) prevalence among US adolescents.

Study Design.—Cross-sectional data from 12 714 12-19 year olds (exclusions: chronic hepatitis, hepatotoxic medications) in the National Health and Examination Survey between 1988-1994 and 2007-2010 were used to estimate trends in suspected NAFLD, defined as overweight (body mass index ≥ 85th percentile) plus elevated alanine aminotransferase levels (boys > 25.8 U/L; girls > 22.1 U/L). Linear trends in prevalence and the independent effect of demographic indicators and adiposity on NAFLD risk were tested using regression models. Complex sampling methods and P values of <.05 were used to assess statistical significance.

Results.—Suspected NAFLD prevalence (SE) rose from 3.9% (0.5) in 1988-1994 to 10.7% (0.9) in 2007-2010 ($P < .0001$), with increases among all race/ethnic subgroups, males and females, and those obese (P trend ≤ .0006 for all). Among those obese, the multivariate adjusted odds of suspected NAFLD were higher with increased age, body mass index, Mexican American race, and male sex; the adjusted odds in 2007-2010 were 2.0 times those in 1988-1994. In 2007-2010, 48.1% (3.7) of all obese males and 56.0% (3.5) of obese Mexican American males had suspected NAFLD.

Conclusion.—Prevalence of suspected NAFLD has more than doubled over the past 20 years and currently affects nearly 11% of adolescents and one-half of obese males. The rapid increase among those obese, independent of body mass index, suggests that other modifiable risk factors have influenced this trend.

▶ As most of us now know, nonalcoholic fatty liver disease has become the most common form of liver disease in children. It is associated with obesity and is known to lead to cirrhosis and liver failure over time. Separate from that, it is a risk factor for cardiovascular disease and hepatic cancer. The ability to estimate the prevalence of nonalcoholic fatty liver disease in adolescents has been difficult because of the lack of a solid database in this regard. Clinicians looking for the disorder usually screen for it with serum transaminase levels. The 95th percentile for alanine aminotransferase (ALT) levels now runs 25.8 U/L for boys and 22.1 U/L for girls.[1]

Welsh et al used national data collected using the same or similar methods over the past 3 decades to estimate what the current nonalcoholic fatty liver disease prevalence is among US adolescents and also examined trend lines in that regard. The comparative information was collected on 12- to 19-year-olds enrolled in the National Health and Nutrition Examination Survey 1988 to 1994 (NHANES III) and also the most recent version of the same survey. ALT levels were part of the information gathering, and nonalcoholic fatty liver disease was defined using the cutoffs already mentioned in otherwise obese adolescents whose body mass index for age and sex was greater than the 85th percentile.

It was clear from the findings of this study that the prevalence of suspected nonalcoholic fatty liver disease has increased substantially, doubling among US adolescents over a 30-year period. Both boys and girls experienced an increased incidence of this disorder. The prevalence of nonalcoholic fatty liver disease ran 3.9% during the 1988 to 1994 period and 10.7% by 2007 to 2008. Mathematically, this represents approximately 2 million current teens affected by nonalcoholic fatty liver disease. The greatest increase was seen in the US teen population among Mexican-American youngsters. In 2007 to 2010, 48% of obese boys and 56% of obese Mexican-American boys had suspected nonalcoholic fatty liver disease.

The information from this study will turn out to be a major determinant of the number of nonpediatric hepatologists that will be needed in the next 20 to 30 years. Nonalcoholic fatty liver disease is a problem that is not going away any time soon.

J. A. Stockman III, MD

Reference

1. Schwimmer JB, Dunn W, Norman GJ, et al. SAFETY study: alanine aminotransferase cutoff values are set too high for reliable detection of pediatric chronic liver disease. *Gastroenterology.* 2010;138:1357-1364.

Pediatric Obesity and Gallstone Disease
Koebnick C, Smith N, Black MH, et al (Kaiser Permanente Southern California, Pasadena, CA; et al)
J Pediatr Gastroenterol Nutr 55:328-333, 2012

Objectives.—The aim of the present study was to investigate the association between childhood and adolescent obesity, the risk of gallstones, and the potential effect modification by oral contraceptive use in girls.

Methods.—For this population-based cross-sectional study, measured weight and height, oral contraceptive use, and diagnosis of cholelithiasis or choledocholithiasis were extracted from the electronic medical records of 510,816 patients ages 10 to 19 years enrolled in an integrated health plan, 2007—2009.

Results.—We identified 766 patients with gallstones. The adjusted odds ratios (95% CI) of gallstones for under-/normal-weight (reference), overweight, moderate obesity, and extreme obesity in boys were 1.00, 1.46 (0.94%—2.27%), 1.83 (1.17%—2.85%), and 3.10 (1.99%—4.83%) and in girls were 1.00, 2.73 (2.18%—3.42%), 5.75 (4.62%—7.17%), and 7.71 (6.13%—9.71%), respectively (P for interaction sex × weight class < 0.001). Among girls, oral contraceptive use was associated with higher odds for gallstones (odds ratio 2.00, 95% CI 1.66%—2.40%). Girls who used oral contraceptives were at higher odds for gallstones than their counterparts in the same weight class who did not use oral contraceptives (P for interaction weight class × oral contraceptive use 0.023).

Conclusions.—Due to the shift toward extreme childhood obesity, especially in minority children, pediatricians can expect to face increasing numbers of children and adolescents affected by gallstone disease.

► A great deal is known about the causes of gallstones in adults. For example, several risk factors for gallstones in adults have been well established, including age, female sex, Hispanic ethnicity, obesity, the use of female sex hormones, pregnancy, sedentary lifestyle, and a family history of gallstones. There is relatively little, information, however, available regarding these same risk factors in children. Generally speaking, when one encounters a child with gallstones, one tends to think of hemolytic diseases as a high probability diagnosis. Some clinical reports, however, suggest that hemolytic diseases are no longer the most frequent cause of pediatric gallbladder disease.[1] In fact, obesity may be replacing hemolytic disease as the most frequent cause of gallstones and cholecystitis in the younger age group. As the prevalence of obesity has increased in children, so have the surgical rates for cholecystectomy.

Koebnick et al undertook a study to evaluate the relationship between gallstones and body mass index using a set of data for children enrolled in a large population-based cohort study, the Kaiser Permanente Southern California Children's Health Study. Kaiser Permanente Southern California is the largest health care provider in Southern California and provides health care service to more than 3.4 million members, about 16% of the total population in its service areas. Given the large amount of data collected as part of the ongoing studies in Southern California, there was access to databases showing the prevalence of gallstone formation and correlations were possible with body weight, body mass index, race/ethnicity/socioeconomic status, and the use of oral contraceptives.

Data from this report show that the prevalence of overweight, obesity, and extreme obesity in children in Southern California enrolled in the Kaiser programs was 19.6%, 13.7%, and 7.7%, respectively. Almost 800 children were gleaned from the Kaiser databases to have an established diagnosis of gallstones in the gallbladder or biliary ducts. The adjusted odds ratios for gallstones were higher in girls (OR 4.42), older children (OR 5.50), Hispanics (OR 1.55), and individuals living in areas with low neighborhood education (OR 1.23). Oral contraceptive use was associated with higher odds for gallstones (OR 2.00).

Thus, excessive body weight, being Hispanic, and being on oral contraceptives are the most significant risk factors for the development of gallstones in children. In this study, Hispanic youth have 55% higher odds for the development of gallstone disease than their non-Hispanic white counterparts, even after adjusting for sex, body weight, age, and low neighborhood education level. This suggests that racial and ethnic disparities as described extensively in adults also exist in children. The data are clear that the obesity epidemic seen in the United States is putting more children at risk for the development of gallbladder disease and gallstone formation. It is best for anyone in a primary care practice to keep an eye out for this problem because it is occurring with increasing frequency these days.

J. A. Stockman III, MD

Reference

1. Miltenburg DM, Schaffer R 3rd, Breslin T, Brandt ML. Changing indications for pediatric cholecystectomy. *Pediatrics.* 2000;105:1250-1253.

Definitions of Pediatric Pancreatitis and Survey of Present Clinical Practices
Morinville VD, on Behalf of the INSPPIRE Group (McGill Univ, Montreal, Canada; et al)
J Pediatr Gastroenterol Nutr 55:261-265, 2012

Objectives.—There is limited literature on acute pancreatitis (AP), acute recurrent pancreatitis (ARP), and chronic pancreatitis (CP) in children. The International Study Group of Pediatric Pancreatitis: In Search for a Cure (INSPPIRE) consortium was formed to standardize definitions, develop diagnostic algorithms, investigate disease pathophysiology, and design prospective multicenter studies in pediatric pancreatitis.

Methods.—Subcommittees were formed to delineate definitions of pancreatitis, and a survey was conducted to analyze present practice.

Results.—AP was defined as requiring 2 of the following: abdominal pain compatible with AP, serum amylase and/or lipase values ≥3 times upper limits of normal, and imaging findings of AP. ARP was defined as ≥2 distinct episodes of AP with intervening return to baseline. CP was diagnosed in the presence of typical abdominal pain plus characteristic imaging findings, or exocrine insufficiency plus imaging findings, or endocrine insufficiency plus imaging findings. We found that children with pancreatitis were primarily managed by pediatric gastroenterologists. Unless the etiology was known, initial investigations included serum liver enzymes, triglycerides, calcium, and abdominal ultrasound. Further investigations (usually for ARP and CP) included magnetic resonance or other imaging, sweat chloride, and genetic testing. Respondents' future goals for INSPPIRE included determining natural history of pancreatitis, developing algorithms to evaluate and manage pancreatitis, and validating diagnostic criteria.

Conclusions.—INSPPIRE represents the first initiative to create a multicenter approach to systematically characterize pancreatitis in children.

TABLE 1.—Definitions of Pancreatitis in Children

Entity	Clinical Definition
AP	Requires at least 2 of 3 criteria: 1. Abdominal pain suggestive of, or compatible with AP (ie, abdominal pain of acute onset, especially in the epigastric region) 2. Serum amylase and/or lipase activity at least 3 times greater than the upper limit of normal (IU/L) 3. Imaging findings characteristic of, or compatible with AP (eg, using U/S, CECT, EUS, MRI/MRCP)
Pediatric onset	First episode of AP occurring before the patient's 19th birthday
ARP	Requires at least 2 distinct episodes of AP (each as defined above), along with: • Complete resolution of pain (≥1-month pain free interval between the diagnoses of AP) OR • Complete normalization of serum pancreatic enzyme levels (amylase and lipase), before the subsequent episode of AP is diagnosed, along with complete resolution of pain symptoms, irrespective of a specific time interval between AP episodes
CP	Requires at least 1 of the following[‡]: 1. Abdominal pain consistent with pancreatic origin and imaging findings suggestive of chronic pancreatic damage* 2. Evidence of exocrine pancreatic insufficiency[†] and suggestive pancreatic imaging findings* 3. Evidence of endocrine pancreatic insufficiency[‡] and suggestive pancreatic imaging findings* OR • Surgical or pancreatic biopsy specimen demonstrating histopathologic features compatible with CP

AP = acute pancreatitis; ARP = acute recurrent pancreatitis; CECT = contrast-enhanced computerized tomography; CP = chronic pancreatitis; EUS = endoscopic ultrasonography; MRI/MRCP = magnetic resonance imaging/magnetic resonance cholangiopancreatography; U/S = transabdominal ultrasonography.

*Suggestive imaging findings of chronic pancreatitis/chronic pancreatic damage including: ductal changes (irregular contour of the main pancreatic duct or its radicles, intraductal filling defects; calculi, stricture or dilation) and parenchymal changes (generalized or focal enlargement, irregular contour [accentuated lobular architecture], cavities, calcifications, heterogeneous echotexture). Imaging modalities may include CT, MRI/MRCP, ERCP; U/S; EUS (in which at least 5 EUS features [as defined by the Rosemont classification (19)] must be fulfilled).

[†]Exocrine pancreatic insufficiency to be diagnosed via fecal elastase-1 monoclonal assay <100 μg/g stool (2 separate samples done ≥1 month apart); or coefficient of dietary fat absorption <90% on a 72-hour fecal fat collection. Neither test should be performed during an acute pancreatitis episode because the results may be temporarily low. Children with classic cystic fibrosis, exhibiting early-onset pancreatic insufficiency without earlier evidence of any meaningful pancreas sufficiency, typically should not be diagnosed as having CP. They do not have chronic abdominal pain and pancreatic imaging findings described in the CP criteria.

[‡]Endocrine pancreatic insufficiency to be diagnosed via 2006 World Health Organization criteria for the diagnosis of diabetes mellitus (fasting glucose ≥7.0 mmol/L (126 mg/dL) or plasma glucose ≥11.1 mmol/L (200 mg/dL) 2 hours after glucose load 1.75 g/kg children (to maximum 75-g glucose load) (20).

Future aims include creation of patient database and biologic sample repository (Table 1).

▶ This report emanates from a research consortium known as the International Study Group of Pediatric Pancreatitis: In Search for a Cure (INSPPIRE). INSPPIRE was created to provide information on acute and chronic pancreatitis in children. Heretofore, there has been limited literature regarding acute recurrent pancreatitis and chronic pancreatitis in children, and little is known about the epidemiology and natural history of either. There is no evidence-based diagnostic, prognostic, and treatment guidelines for either of these disorders, leaving pediatricians to rely on diagnostic, prognostic and treatment guidelines that have been handed down from adult medicine. In fact, the etiologies of pancreatitis in children are markedly different from those of adults, and all the prognostic algorithms and therapeutic guidelines largely are inconsiderate of the unique age-related requirements of childhood.

The report of Morinville et al represents a study undertaken by INSPPIRE to develop a consensus statement on the definitions of childhood-onset acute pancreatitis, acute recurrent pancreatitis, and chronic pancreatitis; the delineation of estimates of the prevalence of these disorders; and the defining characteristics of diagnosis, evaluation, and management. The study group reviewed available literature for consensus on definitions of the disorders and surveyed pediatric gastroenterologists to ascertain data on the number of children with acute pancreatitis, acute recurrent pancreatitis, and chronic pancreatitis seen throughout the United States.

Table 1 illustrates the consensus of INSPPIRE regarding all types of pancreatitis in children (younger than 19 years). It is noted that lipase elevations may be more sensitive than amylase elevations in finding younger children with pancreatitis. Also, pediatric care providers are more selective in the types of imaging studies they perform to limit radiation exposure. Imaging features compatible with acute pancreatitis include pancreatic edema, pancreatic or peripancreatic necrosis, peripancreatic inflammation, acute fluid collections, pancreatic hemorrhage, pancreatic abscess, and pancreatic pseudocyst. Transabdominal ultrasound scan is most frequently used to rule out obstructive etiologies, such as a choledochal cyst, traumatic injury, tumor, or stones.

The clinical survey information obtained from pediatric gastroenterologists yielded a great amount of data, as there was a 91% response rate. The majority of respondents felt that the number of admissions for acute pancreatitis to children's facilities had significantly increased in the previous 3 years. Among the survey findings was the observation that resolution of abdominal pain was the most important factor in a pediatric gastroenterologist's decision concerning when to begin oral feedings (50% of respondents). Forty-four percent of participants would often use enteral tube feedings in the course of management of acute pancreatitis. Morphine or related opioids drugs were the medications of choice for control of pain in acute pancreatitis (94%). Ninety-four percent of respondents would order genetic testing to rule out cystic fibrosis in any child with acute recurrent pancreatitis or chronic pancreatitis, regardless of age. All of the participants also measured fetal elastase levels to diagnose or monitor for pancreatic exocrine insufficiency, whereas only 44% also performed a 3-day stool collection for fecal fat analysis.

INSPPIRE represents the first initiative to create a multicenter approach to systematically characterizing pancreatitis in children. This group is now formalizing standard definitions of acute pancreatitis, acute recurrent pancreatitis, and chronic pancreatitis in children that can be used in future research efforts. It is clear that pediatric pancreatitis differs in practice from that of adults. There are infrequent uses of invasive workups (eg, endoscopic retrograde cholangiopancreatography, endoscopic ultrasound) as first-line testing. By contrast, ultrasound scan is used in the initial presentation much more commonly than computed tomography scanning to limit radiation exposure, and magnetic resonance imaging is frequently performed in cases of acute recurrent pancreatitis, acute pancreatitis, and chronic pancreatitis, emphasizing the importance of detecting anatomic abnormalities in children. It appears that pediatric subspecialists are relatively conservative with the workup of a single episode of acute pancreatitis, but detailed investigation is implemented once a child presents with acute recurrent pancreatitis or chronic pancreatitis. In the latter situations, it is imperative to rule out variants of cystic fibrosis.

J. A. Stockman III, MD

Severe Abdominal Trauma Involving Bicycle Handlebars in Children

Alkan M, Iskit SH, Soyupak S, et al (Cukurova Univ Faculty of Medicine, Adana, Turkey)
Pediatr Emerg Care 28:357-360, 2012

Objectives.—To emphasize the severity of the underlying injury which may not be realized during the initial patient admission to the emergency department.

Methods.—A retrospective case note review of children admitted to our institution with the severe abdominal injury.

Results.—Eight children were identified with the severe abdominal injury secondary to the trauma from a bicycle handlebar that needed special care in the intensive care unit. All injuries were due to blunt trauma. The mean delay from the time of the accident to the time of presentation was 34.5 hours. All patients had an imprint of the handlebar edge on the hypochondrium. There were 3 pancreatic lacerations, 1 duodenal laceration, 1 jejunal laceration, 1 liver laceration, 1 abdominoinguinal laceration that all required open surgery, and 1 duodenal hematoma that resolved in 4 weeks follow-up period. The patients who required open surgery were evaluated with computed tomographic scans before surgery.

Conclusions.—Children with an imprint made by the handlebar edge on the abdominal wall or give a clear history of injuries by a bicycle handlebar should be treated with great care. Early computed tomography evaluation may help to reduce the morbidity resulting from the delay in diagnosis of injuries to the internal organs (Table 1).

▶ There is not one among us who is not familiar with bicycle handlebar injuries. It is estimated that bicycle accidents account for somewhere between 5% and 14% of blunt abdominal trauma in children.[1] These injuries can be fatal. The reason why is that a fair percentage of the injuries are initially missed, as is true of other forms of blunt abdominal trauma.

These authors designed a study whose conclusion was that physicians who manage pediatric trauma need to have a high index of suspicion of serious intra-abdominal organ injury when first assessing children who have sustained trauma from bicycle handles. The investigators reviewed data on patients with bicycle handlebar injuries from September 2007 through September 2008 who were in the intensive care unit in the pediatric surgery department at the University of Cukurova, Adana, Turkey. This hospital is a referral hospital for a

TABLE 1.—Types of Internal Organ Injury, Management and Admission Time

Sex	Age, y	Organ Injury	Operation	Admission Time, hours
Male	10	Duodenal laceration	Laparotomy, resection with anastomosis	4
Male	13	Liver laceration	Laparotomy, liver laceration oversewed	6
Female	8	Pancreas tail transection	Laparotomy, necrotic tissue debrided and distal pancreatectomy	48
Male	8	Pancreas laceration	Laparotomy, necrotic tissue debrided	72
Male	8	Pancreas laceration	Laparotomy, necrotic tissue debrided	48
Female	14	Jejunal laceration	Laparotomy, jejunal resection with anastomosis	48
Male	7	Abdomino-inguinal laceration	Laparotomy, exploration, necrotic tissue debrided	2
Male	7	Duodenal hematoma	Non-operative treatment	48

city and surrounding area of approximately 1.9 million inhabitants. Reported on were 8 patients who ended up in the intensive care unit as a result of blunt abdominal trauma from a bicycle handlebar injury. Boys were affected more often than girls (3.3:1) and the mean age of trauma was 9.6 years. The mechanism of the accident was similar in all patients and involved loss of control of a bicycle, the wheel of their bikes turning 90 degrees, and the abdomen being impacted by the end of a handlebar. The children initially showed no signs of severe injury when examined by their local medical practitioners and were initially sent home. They presented to an emergency room 34.5 hours (on average) after the accident with complaint of abdominal pain and vomiting. The types of internal organ injury are shown in Table 1.

The morbidity of handlebar injuries is often underappreciated as evidenced by the delayed diagnosis in this series. Physicians are often placed in the dilemma when examining children who have had handlebar injury as to whether or not a CT scan is indicated. It is unfortunate that severe intra-abdominal damage may take more than a day to manifest its actual severity. During this period, the seriousness of the underlying injury may very well not be realized. Needless to say, all children presenting to an emergency room or office setting after bicycle accidents should be treated with a high index of suspicion regarding the potential for an underlying intra-abdominal injury. The approach should be one of repeated regular clinical examination and the use of CT examination based on judicious judgment.

J. A. Stockman III, MD

Reference

1. Acton CH, Thomas S, Clark R, Pitt WR, Nixon JW, Leditschke JF. Bicycle incidents in children—abdominal trauma and handlebars. *Med J Aust.* 1994;160: 344-346.

Spectrum of Gastroparesis in Children

Waseem S, Islam S, Kahn G, et al (Indiana Univ School of Medicine, Indianapolis; Univ of Florida, Gainesville; et al)
J Pediatr Gastroenterol Nutr 55:166-172, 2012

Background.—Gastroparesis (GP) is characterized by delayed gastric emptying in the absence of mechanical outlet obstruction. Symptoms may include nausea, vomiting, bloating, early satiety, abdominal pain, and weight loss. Delayed gastric emptying of a solid-phase meal assessed by radionuclear scintigraphy is the criterion standard for diagnosis. The prevalence of GP is difficult to estimate due to the lack of a validated, widely available diagnostic test that can be applied in primary care. The extent of this problem in children is unknown.

Methods.—We studied a cohort of children with GP diagnosed by radionuclear scintigraphy to identify demographics, symptoms, comorbidities, treatment, and outcomes. A retrospective analysis of 239 patients between ages 0 and 21 years was performed.

Results.—The mean age of presentation was 7.9 years, and boys and girls were almost equally affected, that is, 48.5% and 51.5%, respectively. Vomiting was the most frequent presenting symptom (68%), followed by abdominal pain (51%), nausea (28%), weight loss (27%), early satiety (25%), and bloating (7%). Almost 75% of patients responded to intravenous erythromycin administered provocatively during gastric scintigraphy. In a majority of the patients, no cause was identified, that is, idiopathic GP (70%), followed by drugs (18%) and postsurgical (12.5%) causes. Only 4% patients had diabetic GP, and our population was essentially narcotic naïve (2%). After an average of 24 months' follow-up, the most common complication was esophageal reflux (67%). Despite different therapeutic modalities, by the end of the follow-up period, a significant improvement in symptoms was reported by an average of 60%, regardless of sex, age, or degree of emptying delay.

Conclusions.—GP has a good prognosis in childhood despite different etiologies, symptom presentation, and therapy.

▶ Pediatricians do not tend to think a whole lot about the entity known as gastroparesis. Nausea, vomiting, and abdominal pain are among the most common complaints in children. When these symptoms are persistent, one needs to consider functional causes, including gastroesophageal reflux, peptic ulcer disease, functional dyspepsia, and gastroparesis. Gastroparesis is a motor and sensory disorder of the stomach characterized by delayed gastric emptying in the absence of mechanical obstruction. Symptoms related to gastroparesis classically include nausea, vomiting, early satiety, bloating, postprandial fullness, abdominal pain, and weight loss. Although the etiology and management of gastroparesis has been well studied in the adult population, in the pediatric population the literature on the subject is quite limited, leaving many children untreated.

Waseem et al provide us with a great deal of information by examining a cohort of children with gastroparesis diagnosed by radionuclide scintography.

They examined the demographics, symptoms, comorbidities, treatment, and outcomes in a retrospective analysis of 239 patients between the ages of infancy and 21 years.

This study revealed important findings. Girls seem to be slightly more affected than boys with a gender difference increasing more significantly as children get older. By 17 years of age, two-thirds of affected individuals are girls, for example. Most cases of gastroparesis appear to be idiopathic (70%). Diabetes is a common cause when a cause can be found. Still, diabetes as a cause of gastroparesis runs just 4% in comparison to data from the adult literature showing that about one-third of adults with gastroparesis have diabetes mellitus. In this report, almost 40% of patients had comorbidities that may have contributed to gastroparesis. In the pediatric population, abdominal pain is the most common presenting feature. In adults, nausea and vomiting predominate. This study also demonstrated that most treat gastroparesis with erythromycin administered orally.

This report represents the first large hospital-based study to describe the demographics, etiologies, and outcomes of gastroparesis in the pediatric age population. It is an uncommon condition, but still represents a major cause of disease burden and is often overlooked. Most patients with gastroparesis need continuous medical care and there are limited therapeutic choices available to clinicians to manage this problem. This study does provide the basis for future studies that can focus on risk stratification of children with gastroparesis as well as establishing a baseline for treatment protocols.

Remember, all that is abdominal pain, nausea, and vomiting need not reflect a simple diagnosis. At least think about gastroparesis as 1 etiologic possibility for such symptoms.

J. A. Stockman III, MD

Total and Abdominal Obesity Are Risk Factors for Gastroesophageal Reflux Symptoms in Children
Quitadamo P, Buonavolontà R, Miele E, et al (Univ "Federico II," Naples, Italy)
J Pediatr Gastroenterol Nutr 55:72-75, 2012

Objectives.—The association between GERD and obesity has been frequently reported in adults. Data in children are scarce and inconclusive, evaluating only general obesity. Central adiposity has never been investigated in children as a possible risk factor for GERD. The aims of the present study were to evaluate the prevalence of gastroesophageal reflux disease (GERD) symptoms in overweight and obese children in comparison with a general normal-weight population and whether the GERD symptoms are associated with waist circumference (WC).

Methods.—The study population consisted of 153 healthy children. A detailed clinical history and a physical examination were obtained from each patient. A questionnaire on reflux symptoms was completed by caregivers.

Results.—The reflux symptomatic score resulted significantly higher in obese than in normal-weight children and in children with WC > 90th percentile compared with those with WC < 75th percentile.

Conclusions.—These preliminary data show that both total and abdominal obesity are risk factors for the development of GERD symptoms in children. The risk of GERD symptoms rises progressively with the increase in both body mass index and waist circumference, even in normal-weight children.

▶ For those who are well into adulthood, the relationship between obesity and gastroesophageal reflux disease (GERD) is well established. The relationship, however, in the pediatric age group has been somewhat more controversial. If one looks at the literature of the relationship between obesity and GERD, the relationship between the 2 conditions has yet to provide clear answers. Patel et al have reviewed esophageal histology from 230 pediatric patients undergoing upper endoscopy and compared objective signs of reflux esophagitis with body mass index.[1] The investigators could not find a significantly greater prevalence of esophagitis in overweight children, but in this report the majority of patients were taking antireflux medication and only 1 histological criterion was used. Thus the true prevalence of reflux symptoms in this 1 particular study was potentially underestimated. On the other hand, Hancox et al did observe positive associations between symptoms of GERD (heartburn and regurgitation) and asthma in young adults, findings independent of body mass index and smoking.[2] Other studies have noted though a positive association between obesity and reflux.[3]

Quitadamo et al have studied the relationship between weight and reflux by examining the relationship between waist circumference and the presence of GERD symptoms. The intent was to evaluate the possible role of visceral adiposity on the occurrence of reflux. They found a positive relationship between waist circumference and GERD symptoms, noting that even moderate increases of waist circumference within the range of normal may be associated with increased risks of GERD. This study was conducted in a well-child clinic in children without obvious complaints of GERD.

It may be that total and abdominal obesity are risk factors for reflux symptoms in children and are independent risk factors. The risk of GERD symptoms as noted in this report seems to rise progressively with increasing body mass index and waist circumference, even among normal-weight children. For those with GERD, in addition to the routine use of antireflux medications, one should consider weight reduction, even for some whose weight is within the normal range.

J. A. Stockman III, MD

References

1. Patel NR, Ward MJ, Beneck D, Cunningham-Rundles S, Moon A. The association between childhood overweight and reflux esophagitis. *J Obes.* 2010;2010:136909.
2. Hancox RJ, Pouton R, Taylor DR, et al. Associations between respiratory symptoms, lung function and gastro-oesophageal reflux symptoms in a population-based birth cohort. *Respir Res.* 2006;7:142.
3. Teitelbaum JE, Sinha P, Micale M, Yeung S, Jaeger J. Obesity is related to multiple functional abdominal diseases. *J Pediatr.* 2009;154:444-446.

Clinical Presentation, Response to Therapy, and Outcome of Gastroparesis in Children

Rodriguez L, Irani K, Jiang H, et al (Children's Hosp, Boston, MA; Massachusetts General Hosp, Boston; Children's Hosp Boston, MA)

J Pediatr Gastroenterol Nutr 55:185-190, 2012

Objectives.—The aims of the present study was to define the clinical features, response to therapy, and outcome of pediatric gastroparesis.

Methods.—Retrospective review of 230 children with gastroparesis. Demographics, gastric emptying times, symptoms, response to medications, and outcome were determined for each of 3 groups (infants, children, and adolescents).

Results.—Mean age was 9 years, with boys predominating among infants and girls among adolescents. Postviral gastroparesis occurred in 18% and mitochondrial dysfunction (MD) in 8%. Symptoms varied with age, with children experiencing more vomiting and adolescents reporting more nausea and abdominal pain. The addition of promotility drugs was an effective therapy. Overall rates of symptom resolution were 22% at 6 months, 53% at 18 months, and 61% at 36 months, with median time to resolution of 14 months. Factors associated with symptom resolution included younger age, male sex, postviral gastroparesis, shorter duration of symptoms, response to addition of promotility therapy, and absence of MD. In multivariate analysis, longer duration of symptoms and MD both predicted lower rates of resolution, whereas younger age and response to addition of promotility therapy predicted a higher rate.

Conclusions.—Pediatric gastroparesis is a complex condition with variable symptomatology and outcome depending on multiple parameters. Understanding the clinical features and response to therapy will improve our diagnosis and treatment of this disorder.

▶ This is another report having to do with gastroparesis. The report expands our understanding of the clinical presentation of the disorder, its natural history, and response to therapy. One of the most important factors to patients with gastroparesis as well as to their families is knowing whether and when to expect resolution of this chronic and often debilitating condition. In the study of Rodriguez et al, the overall rate of symptom resolution was 52%, which was achieved at a median of 14 months from the time of diagnosis. In those patients in whom symptoms ultimately resolved, 84% did so by 12 months and the rest by 36 months. Several factors appear to be predictive of the likelihood of symptom resolution. These include younger age, shorter duration of symptoms, absence of mitochondrial dysfunction, and response to promotility drugs.

Postviral gastroparesis appears to be a common cause, accounting for 18% of all cases in the present study. Of 41 patients with postviral gastroparesis, three-quarters responded positively to promotility agents and 63% ultimately reported symptom resolution. The addition of promotility medications was associated with a favorable symptomatic response in just over half of subjects, independent of age. Again, erythromycin was the drug most often used for this purpose.

Metoclopramide resulted in low resolution rates. The authors reported a significant response rate to domperidone.

The authors of this report suggest that prospective studies are needed to define standardized protocols for gastric-emptying studies in children and also to define the role of promotility drugs and other therapies in treating pediatric gastroparesis. The disorder is an orphan disease that requires collaborative study intervention.

J. A. Stockman III, MD

Incidence of Peptic Ulcer Bleeding in the US Pediatric Population
Brown K, Lundborg P, Levinson J, et al (AstraZeneca R&D, Wilmington, DE AstraZeneca R&D, Mölndal, Sweden)
J Pediatr Gastroenterol Nutr 54:733-736, 2012

Objectives —The aim of the present study was to determine the incidence of peptic ulcer bleeding (PUB) in pediatric patients.

Methods.—A hospital inpatient database, Premier Perspective, and an insurance claims database, MarketScan, were analyzed to estimate upper and lower limits for the annual incidence of PUB in the US pediatric population.

Results.—Using data from the Premier Perspective database and database-specific projection methodology, the total number of cases of hospitalization of pediatric patients for PUB in the United States in 2008 was estimated to be between 378 and 652. This translated to an incidence of 0.5 to 0.9/100,000 individuals in the pediatric population. Using data from the MarketScan database, the incidence of PUB in the insured pediatric population was estimated to be 4.4/100,000 individuals. Overall, 17.4% of insured pediatric patients diagnosed as having any upper gastrointestinal ulcer in 2008 were reported to have developed PUB.

Conclusions.—The estimated incidence of PUB in the US pediatric population in 2008 ranged from 0.5 to 4.4/100,000 individuals. The total number of cases of PUB in pediatric patients in the United States each year was thus estimated to be between 378 and 3250. Such estimates provide a likely lower and upper limit for the total number of cases of the condition annually.

▶ Peptic ulcer bleeding (PUB) is a well-characterized disorder in the adult population. In adults, the most common risk factors for PUB are infection with *Helicobacter pylori*, increasing age, treatment with nonsteroidal anti-inflammatory drugs, smoking, and previous gastrointestinal complications. The clinical course and presentation of peptic ulcer disease and its complications including PUB have been thought to be similar in both adults and children. Those caring for youngsters who have PUB generally use therapies that have been put on the market only for adults. Unfortunately, risk factors for PUB have not been studied extensively in children, although they are thought to be much lower in incidence than in adults. Brown et al have designed a retrospective study to estimate the annual incidence of PUB in pediatric patients 1 year to 17 years of age in the United States.

According to 2008 data, the authors found that the incidence of PUB was 0.5 to 0.9/100 000 and 4.4/100 000 individuals, using inpatient pediatric database information and an insurance claims database, respectively. These numbers can be translated into somewhere between an occurrence of 378 and 3250 pediatric PUB cases per year. The authors indicate that to their knowledge, their study is the first to offer an estimate of the overall incidence of PUB in the general US pediatric population.

The authors of this report do acknowledge that it is unknown whether the incidence of pediatric PUB is the same in insured and uninsured patients. This may lead to inaccuracy in the estimate of the total number of cases in the overall population extrapolated from the databases used. It is also possible that the hospitals included in the database may not be fully representative of the overall US population. Nonetheless, one can conclude that PUB is rare in the pediatric population, at least in this country. This does not mean, however, that when it does occur, PUB is not serious, as we see in the report that follows.

J. A. Stockman III, MD

Predictors of Clinically Significant Upper Gastrointestinal Hemorrhage Among Children With Hematemesis

Freedman SB, Stewart C, Rumantir M, et al (The Hosp for Sick Children, Toronto, Ontario, Canada; Univ Hosp of Wales, Cardiff, UK)
J Pediatr Gastroenterol Nutr 54:737-743, 2012

Objectives.—The aim of the study was to determine the proportion of children with hematemesis who experience a clinically significant upper gastrointestinal hemorrhage (UGIH) and to identify variables predicting their occurrence.

Methods.—A retrospective cohort study was conducted. All of the emergency department visits by children ages 0 to 18 years who presented with hematemesis between 2000 and 2007 were reviewed. The primary aim of the study was to determine the proportion of children who developed a clinically significant UGIH; the secondary aim was to identify risk factors predictive of a clinically significant UGIH. A significant UGIH was defined by any of the following: hemoglobin drop >20 g/L, blood transfusion, or emergent endoscopy or surgical procedure.

Results.—Twenty-seven of 613 eligible children (4%; 95% confidence interval 3%–6%) had a clinically significant UGIH. Clinically significant hemorrhages were associated with older age (9.7 vs 2.9 years; $P < 0.001$), vomiting moderate to large amounts of fresh blood (58% vs 20%; $P < 0.001$), melena (37% vs 5%; $P < 0.001$), significant medical history (63% vs 24%; $P < 0.001$), unwell appearance (44% vs 6%; $P < 0.001$), and tachycardia (41% vs 10%; $P < 0.001$). The frequency of laboratory investigations increased with age ($P < 0.001$). The hemoglobin level was the only laboratory investigation whose results differed between those with and without significant bleeds. The presence of any one of the following characteristics identified all of the children with a clinically significant hemorrhage: melena, hematochezia, unwell appearance, or a moderate to large volume of fresh blood in the vomitus, sensitivity 100% (95% confidence interval 85%–100%).

Conclusions.—The occurrence of a clinically significant UGIH was uncommon among children with hematemesis, especially in well-appearing children without melena, hematochezia, or who had not vomited a moderate to large amount of fresh blood.

▶ As noted in the report by Brown et al[1] dealing with the incidence of pediatric peptic ulcer bleeding in the United States, it is a relatively rare problem. Likewise, as we see in this article, hematemesis is also an uncommon pediatric emergency department chief complaint. These authors conducted a retrospective cohort study looking at all children up to 18 years of age who presented to the emergency department between May 1, 2000, and April 30, 2007, with a chief complaint or diagnosis consistent with hematemesis. This single-center study was conducted at the Hospital for Sick Children, a tertiary referral children's hospital in downtown Toronto. The study attempted to identify variables predicting the occurrence of hematemesis.

In noting that hematemesis is an uncommon pediatric emergency department chief complaint, the authors also observed that only 4% of children with hematemesis once evaluated were determined to have clinically significant upper gastrointestinal tract hemorrhage. To the authors' knowledge, there have been no studies that specifically examined clinically significant upper gastrointestinal tract hemorrhage in this pediatric age population. The authors did find that older children were at increased risk and that all significant cases associated with hemorrhage could be identified by the presence of 1 of 4 factors: an unwell appearance, a history of melena, a history of hematochezia, or a large volume of fresh blood in the vomitus. These factors therefore can help guide clinical decision making when evaluating a child for hematemesis. These findings of significant upper intestinal tract hemorrhage being an infrequent occurrence are supported by pediatric intensive care unit data reporting only 2% of critically ill patients experiencing such hemorrhage.[2] It should be noted that most children with clinically significant upper gastrointestinal hemorrhage did have notable medical histories, including portal hypertension, upper gastrointestinal bleeding, gastric or duodenal ulcer, gastroesophageal reflux, and coagulation disorders.

Although these authors found the presence of a large volume of blood in the vomitus to be a predictor of a clinically significant upper gastrointestinal hemorrhage, previous reports have found the visual estimation of blood loss to be highly inaccurate, either by laypeople or by health care professionals. Parents, for example, overestimate blood volumes nearly three-quarters of the time by a factor of 1.5 to 5 depending on the volume and mode of presentation, while physicians tend to underestimate blood loss with nurses being somewhat more accurate than either parents or physicians.[3] Both physicians and nurses tend to overestimate small volumes and underestimate larger ones, and these inaccuracies do not decrease with increasing experience. Despite such inaccuracies and the potential discrepancies that are inherent in chart reviews, the authors of this report did find a correlation between the perception of large volume and clinically significant upper gastrointestinal hemorrhage. With these factors in mind, history and physical examination can play a role in identifying children who appear to be at greatest risk for clinically significant upper gastrointestinal hemorrhage. A child who is unwell, has a history of melena, a history of hematochezia, and a moderate to large volume of fresh blood in the vomitus should set off serious alarms. Add to that older age, a significant medical history, and the presence of tachycardia and you know you have a problem on your hands. All these factors should be taken into consideration when evaluating children with upper gastrointestinal tract hemorrhage.

J. A. Stockman III, MD

References

1. Brown K, Lundborg P, Levinson J, Yang H. Incidence of peptic ulcer bleeding in the US pediatric population. *J Pediatr Gastroenterol Nutr.* 2012;54:733-736.
2. Chaïbou M, Tucci M, Dugas MA, Farrell CA, Proulx F, Lacroix J. Clinically significant upper gastrointestinal bleeding acquired in a pediatric intensive care unit: a prospective study. *Pediatrics.* 1998;102:933-938.
3. Tebruegge M, Misra I, Pantazidou A, et al. Estimating blood loss: comparative study of the accuracy of parents and health care professionals. *Pediatrics.* 2009; 124:e729-e736.

Helicobacter pylori and Infantile Colic

Ali AM (Al-Azhar Univ, Cairo, Egypt)
Arch Pediatr Adolesc Med 166:648-650, 2012

Objective.—To determine whether *Helicobacter pylori* is associated with infantile colic.

Design.—Case-control study.

Settings.—Local tertiary hospital in rural Gizan, Saudi Arabia.

Participants.—A total of 55 patients with infantile colic who were 2 weeks to 4 months of age and who fulfilled modified Wessel criteria (ie, crying and fussy behavior) and a total of 30 healthy controls with no history of colic who were matched by country of origin, age, sex, and ethnicity to the 55 colicky infants.

Main Outcome Measure.—*Helicobacter pylori* infection determined by *H pylori* stool antigen testing.

Results.—Of the 55 patients presenting with infantile colic, 45 (81.8%) tested positive for *H pylori*; of the 30 healthy controls, 7 (23.3%) tested positive for *H pylori* (odds ratio, 15.3 [95% CI, 17.9-29.8]).

Conclusion.—*H pylori* infection is associated with infantile colic and may be a causative factor.

▶ This past year marked the 30th anniversary of the discovery of *Helicobacter pylori*. In the interval of 30 years, we have come to recognize that this organism is the most prevalent gastric microbial pathogen. It is a cause of asymptomatic gastritis at one end of a spectrum and, at the other end, peptic ulcerations and gastric malignancies. It is estimated that more than half of the world's population are infected with this pathogen. The prevalence, however, varies widely by age, country of origin, ethnic background, and socioeconomic conditions in early childhood.

Ali has designed a study to examine the potential association between *H pylori* and a common occurrence, infant colic. The etiology of the latter has remained a puzzle, despite the fact that as common as colic is, no investigator to date has been able to find an etiologic link that is readily correctable. This author looked at 55 infants with colic and compared them with healthy controls matched for age, sex, and other variables. A strong association was found between *H pylori* infection and infantile colic in this particular group of infants. The logical question, however, is whether the association is one of cause and effect. Other studies have suggested that the association could be causal. It has even been suggested that dosing with probiotics may help improve colic symptoms.[1] It has also been suggested that *H pylori* stimulates the release of interleukin-8 from gastric epithelia, initiating inflammatory damage to the gastric mucosa and predisposing to colic.

Whether the information provided by this article in any way might change how colic is managed is hard to say. If the author of this article is correct, perhaps a short course of treatment would be in order. It is likely that such a trial will appear in the literature fairly soon. Fortunately, such treatment is relatively innocuous.

J. A. Stockman III, MD

Reference

1. Zhou C, Ma FZ, Deng XJ, Yuan H, Ma HS. Lactobacilli inhibit interleukin-8 production induced by Helicobacter pylori lipopolysaccharide-activated Toll-like receptor 4. *World J Gastroenterol*. 2008;14:5090-5095.

Lactobacillus reuteri DSM 17938 for the Management of Infantile Colic in Breastfed Infants: A Randomized, Double-Blind, Placebo-Controlled Trial
Szajewska H, Gyrczuk E, Horvath A (The Med Univ of Warsaw, Poland)
J Pediatr 162:257-262, 2013

Objective.—To determine whether administration of *Lactobacillus reuteri* (*L reuteri*) DSM 17938 is beneficial in breastfed infants with infantile colic.

Study Design.—Eighty infants aged <5 months with infantile colic (defined as crying episodes lasting 3 or more hours per day and occurring at least 3 days per week within 7 days prior to enrollment), who were exclusively or predominantly (>50%) breastfed were randomly assigned to receive *L reuteri* DSM 17938 (10^8 colony-forming units) (n = 40) or an identically appearing and tasting placebo (n = 40), both orally, in 5 drops, 1 time daily, for 21 days. The primary outcome measures were the treatment success, defined as the percentage of children achieving a reduction in the daily average crying time $\geq 50\%$, and the duration of crying (minutes per day) at 7, 14, 21, and 28 days after randomization.

Results.—The rate of responders to treatment was significantly higher in the probiotic group compared with the placebo group at day 7 ($P = .026$), at day 14 (relative risk (RR) 4.3, 95% CI 2.3-8.7), at day 21 (RR 2.7, 95% CI 1.85-4.1), and at day 28 (RR 2.5, 95% CI 1.8-3.75). In addition, throughout the study period, the median crying time was significantly reduced in the probiotic group compared with the control group.

Conclusion.—Exclusively or predominantly breastfed infants with infantile colic benefit from the administration of *L reuteri* DSM 17938 compared with placebo.

▶ There actually is a standardized definition for what constitutes infantile colic.[1] The criteria for infantile colic include all the following in infants from birth through 4 months of age: paroxysms of irritability, fussing, or crying that start and stop without obvious cause; episodes lasting 3 or more hours per day and occurring at least 3 days per week for at least 1 week; and failure to thrive. Colic usually is at its worst at age 6 weeks and almost invariably resolves by around 4 months of age. The etiology of infantile colic has remained an enigma. Some have theorized that it is the result of painful intestinal contractions, lactose intolerance, food hypersensitivity, altered gastrointestinal tract microbiota, gas, parent misinterpretation of what otherwise is a normal crying baby, or an assorted combination of these. The list of therapies to manage colic is almost too long to summarize, but it usually includes the use of various formulas, sucrose, herbal teas, soy formula, lactose-reduced formula, and fiber-enriched formulas. Parents will often try walking around with the infant or employing music, vibration, or massage. Despite all the purported therapies, none have proven effective.

In recent times, investigators have begun to look at the use of probiotics as part of the management of colic. In 2007, a randomized, controlled trial in breastfed infants showed that the administration of *Lactobacillus reuteri* ATCC 5573, when compared with simethicone, did in fact reduce crying time, although there were a number of methodological concerns about the design of this study.[2] A subsequent study by the same investigators found similar results using a different strain of organism given the fact that the original trial used a strain of *Lactobacillus* that had been found to potentially carry transferable resistance traits for tetracycline and lincomycin.

These authors undertook a clinical study to compare the effectiveness of *L reuteri* DSM 17938 in comparison with a placebo in the treatment of breastfed infants with infantile colic in a double-blind, randomized, controlled trial to see again whether this particular strain of *Lactobacillus* would be effective in the management of infantile colic. The study was carried out in a family primary care practice in Warsaw, Poland. Participants in the study had to be full-term infants aged 5 months or less with the standard definition of infantile colic. The infants either were exclusively or predominantly (> 50%) breastfed. None of the infants exhibited chronic disease, gastrointestinal disorders, or had use of antibiotics or probiotic pharmaceutical products within a week of the study. The treatment outcomes looked for included a reduction in daily average crying time of 50% or more. Data from this study showed that the use of *L. reuteri* was associated with treatment success and reduced crying times at 1, 2, 3, and 4 weeks after randomization. These findings are consistent with findings from a prior study. Treatment success, defined as a 50% reduction in crying time compared with baseline, was more likely in the probiotic group compared with a placebo group. The results were quite impressive.

It is not precisely known how *L reuteri* might exert its beneficial effects as part of the management of infantile colic. It has been suggested that the result is caused by the effect of *L reuteri* on gut motility and function, colonic sensory nerves, colon contractile activity, and pain perception. The authors feel that exclusively or predominantly breastfed infants with infantile colic could benefit from treatment with *L reuteri* DSM 17938. The issue is whether the self-limiting condition is worthy of such treatment. Given the fact that there seems to be no other effective therapy for infantile colic and the fact that probiotics are known to be quite safe, it may be time to think about their use as part of the management of this very common infant disorder, at least in the restricted population (breastfed infants) that has been studied.

J. A. Sturkman III, MD

References

1. Hyman PE, Milla PJ, Benninga MA, Davidson GP, Fleisher DF, Taminiau J. Childhood functional gastrointestinal disorders: neonate/toddler. *Gastroenterology.* 2006;130:1519-1526.
2. Savino F, Pelle E, Palumeri E, Oggero R, Miniero R. Lactobacillus reuteri (American Type Culture Collection Strain 55730) versus simethicone in the treatment of infantile colic: a prospective randomized study. *Pediatrics.* 2007;119:e124-e130.

Gut-directed hypnotherapy for functional abdominal pain or irritable bowel syndrome in children: a systematic review

Rutten JMTM, Reitsma JB, Vlieger AM, et al (Emma Children's Hosp AMC, Amsterdam, The Netherlands; Univ Med Ctr Utrecht, The Netherlands; St Antonius Hosp Nieuwegein, The Netherlands)
Arch Dis Child 98:252-257, 2013

Objectives.—Gut directed hypnotherapy (HT) is shown to be effective in adult functional abdominal pain (FAP) and irritable bowel syndrome (IBS) patients. We performed a systematic review to assess efficacy of HT in paediatric FAP/IBS patients.

Methods.—We searched Medline, Embase, PsychINFO, Cumulative Index to Nursing and Allied Health Literature databases and Cochrane Central Register of Controlled Trials for randomised controlled trials (RCT) in children with FAP or IBS, investigating efficacy of HT on the following outcomes: abdominal pain scores, quality of life, costs and school absenteeism.

Results.—Three RCT comparing HT to a control treatment were included with sample sizes ranging from 22 to 52 children. We refrained from statistical pooling because of low number of studies and many differences in design and outcomes. Two studies examined HT performed by a therapist, one examined HT through self-exercises on audio CD. All trials showed statistically significantly greater improvement in abdominal pain scores among children receiving HT. One trial reported beneficial effects sustained after 1 year of follow-up. One trial reported statistically significant improvement in quality of life in the HT group. Two trials reported significant reductions in school absenteeism after HT.

Conclusions.—Therapeutic effects of HT seem superior to standard medical care in children with FAP or IBS. It remains difficult to quantify exact benefits. The need for more high quality research is evident.

▶ It is now clear that behavioral approaches, including cognitive behavioral therapy (CBT) and hypnosis, are among the very most effective treatments for irritable bowel disease and functional abdominal pain. The success of these treatments has been confirmed in both randomized, controlled trials and large case series. CBT has demonstrated efficacy with an average of 78% improvement in bowel habits, and treatment lasts up to 4 years.[1]

While less rigorously studied until recently, gut-directed hypnotherapy has been shown to target many of the underlying psychophysiologic processes of irritable bowel syndrome (IBS), including visceral hypersensitivity, pain, somatization, and catastrophizing, as well as improving colonic motility and altering gut secretions.[2] Response rates to hypnotherapy in refractory cases approach 85%, which is slightly better than those of CBT, but there have been no comparative effectiveness trials to confirm this.

Hypnotherapy for IBS has been studied more extensively in adults than in children,[3] and because children are known to be better at doing self-hypnosis, it is reasonable to assume that results in children would probably be even better than those in adults.[4] In a randomized, controlled trial from 2007 using hypnotherapy in pediatric patients with IBS and functional abdominal pain (FAP), significant improvement took place in as early as one week, revealing long-term improvement in 85% of the hypnosis patients compared with 25% of the standard medical treatment group, at 1-year follow-up.[5] Five years later, the same group of patients continued to show maintenance of their improvement in 68% of the hypnosis group, whereas this remained true in only 20% of the standard treatment group.[6] In addition, hypnosis can help comorbid features of both IBS and inflammatory bowel disease (IBD), including positively influencing coping behaviors, reducing stress, facilitating sleep, modulating depression or anxiety, and contributing positively to overall wellness.[7]

In patients with ulcerative colitis, medical hypnosis has been found to decrease inflammation when measured systemically as well as locally in rectal mucosa. Results from Keefer et al[8] showed a 57% decrease in relapse over 12 months, in patients with ulcerative colitis and IBD, compared with 18% of control patients, as measured by hospitalizations, outpatient visits, and emergency room visits. Although hypnosis has been shown to be effective in treating IBS and FAP, both of which are considered to be functional diseases, what is exciting about the Keefer et al study is that it shows the efficacy of behavioral therapy in the treatment of biopsy-proven organic disease.

Looking more broadly at the applications of medical hypnosis, it has also been shown to be efficacious either as a primary therapy or as an adjunctive treatment for pain,[9] migraine, recurrent, and daily headache,[10] tics,[11] and nocturnal enuresis.[12] Often, hypnosis can allow medication to be decreased and even discontinued. Hypnosis can also be helpful for performance anxieties of all types,[13] habit disorders, and even hyperhidrosis.[14]

Hypnosis is an effective therapy for FAP and IBS...and that's not BS! Even patients with hyperhidrosis can be helped when they learn self-hypnosis. And children with motivation can cure their night-time urination. Too bad it can't cure halitosis!

J. E. Lazarus, MD, FAAP

References

1. Ford AC, Talley NJ, Schoenfeld PS, Quigley EM, Moayyedi P. Efficacy of antidepressants and psychological therapies in irritable bowel syndrome: systematic review and meta-analysis. *Gut.* 2009;58:367-378.
2. Palsson O. Hypnosis treatment for gut problems. *Eur Gastroenterol Hepatol Rev.* 2010;6:42-46.
3. Brent M, Lobato D, LeLeiko N. Psychological treatments for pediatric functional gastrointestinal disorders. *J Pediatr Gastroenterol Nutr.* 2009;48:13-21.
4. Palsson OS, Whitehead WE. The growing case for hypnosis as adjunctive therapy for functional gastrointestinal disorders. *Gastroenterology.* 2002;123:2132-2135.
5. Vlieger AM, Menko-Frankenhuis C, Wolfkamp SC, Tromp E, Benninga MA. Hypnotherapy for children with functional abdominal pain or irritable bowel syndrome: a randomized controlled trial. *Gastroenterology.* 2007;133:1430-1436.
6. Vlieger AM, Rutten JM, Govers AM, Frankenhuis C, Benninga MA. Long-term follow-up of gut-directed hypnotherapy vs. standard care in children with functional abdominal pain or irritable bowel syndrome. *Am J Gastroenterol.* 2012;107:627-631.
7. Keefer L. Presentation at American Society of Clinical Hypnosis Annual Scientific Meeting. March 18, 2013; Louisville, KY.
8. Keefer L, Kiebles JL, Martinovich Z, Cohen E, Van Denburg A, Barrett TA. Behavioral interventions may prolong remission in patients with inflammatory bowel disease. *Behav Res Ther.* 2011;49:145-150.
9. Kuttner L. Favorite stories: a hypnotic pain-reduction technique for children in acute pain. *Am J Clin Hypn.* 1988;30:289-295.
10. Olness K, MacDonald JT, Uden DL. Comparison of self-hypnosis and propranolol in the treatment of juvenile classic migraine. *Pediatrics.* 1987;79:593-597.
11. Lazarus JE, Klein SK. Nonpharmacological treatment of tics in Tourette syndrome adding videotape training to self-hypnosis. *J Dev Behav Pediatr.* 2010;31:498-504.
12. Olness K. The use of self-hypnosis in the treatment of childhood nocturnal enuresis. A report on forty patients. *Clin Pediatr (Phila).* 1975;14:273-275, 278-279.
13. Pates J, Maynard I. Effects of hypnosis on flow states and golf performance. *Percept Mot Skills.* 2000;91:1057-1075.
14. Kohen D, Olness K. *Hypnosis and Hypnotherapy with Children.* 3rd ed. New York, NY: Guilford Publications, Inc, 1996, 2011.

Diagnostic Imaging and Negative Appendectomy Rates in Children: Effects of Age and Gender

Bachur RG, Hennelly K, Callahan MJ, et al (Children's Hosp and Harvard Med School, Boston, MA)
Pediatrics 129:877-884, 2012

Background and Objectives.—Diagnostic imaging is often used in the evaluation of children with possible appendicitis. The utility of imaging may vary according to a patient's age and gender. The objectives of this study were (1) to examine the use of computed tomography (CT) and ultrasound for age and gender subgroups of children undergoing an appendectomy; and (2) to study the association between imaging and negative appendectomy rates (NARs) among these subgroups.

Methods.—Retrospective review of children presenting to 40 US pediatric emergency departments from 2005 to 2009 (Pediatric Health Information Systems database). Children undergoing an appendectomy were stratified by age and gender for measuring the association between ultrasound and CT use and the outcome of negative appendectomy.

Results.—A total of 8 959 155 visits at 40 pediatric emergency departments were investigated; 55 227 children had appendicitis. The NAR was 3.6%. NARs were highest for children younger than 5 years (boys 16.8%, girls 14.6%) and girls older than 10 years (4.8%). At the institutional level, increased rates of diagnostic imaging (ultrasound and/or CT) were associated with lower NARs for all age and gender subgroups other than children younger than 5 years, The NAR was 1.2% for boys older than 5 years without any diagnostic imaging.

Conclusions.—The impact of diagnostic imaging on negative appendectomy rate varies by age and gender. Diagnostic imaging for boys older than 5 years with suspected appendicitis has no meaningful impact on NAR. Diagnostic strategies for possible appendicitis should incorporate the risk of negative appendectomy by age and gender.

▶ Elsewhere a report is summarized describing low-dose computed tomography (CT) to be as adequate as standard dose CT for diagnosing appendicitis in older children and young adults.[1] Although adults treated with low-dose CT scans as part of the evaluation of appendicitis were slightly more likely to need at least 1 additional test, the difference in outcome otherwise was not significant. The authors suggested that low-dose radiation protocols are reasonable alternatives to regular CT in hospitals with experienced radiologists. The report of Bachur et al tells us about a retrospective review of children presenting to emergency rooms in the United States over a recent 5-year period detailing the role of ultrasound and CT scan on the outcome of surgeries showing negative appendectomies. With appendicitis being the most common surgical emergency in children, this report is important for all of us. Without question, advanced imaging with CT and ultrasound has become routine in many children undergoing diagnostic evaluation for pediatric appendicitis because of the relatively limited performance of clinical intuition and clinical decision rules. CT scans have been shown to have superior diagnostic performance as compared with ultrasound, but exposes the patient to ionizing radiation. When CT was introduced as a diagnostic tool for pediatric appendicitis, the diagnostic sensitivity reduced the need for routine admission of patients with equivocal findings for serial examination. In addition, CT was expected to identify early appendicitis and thereby reduce perforation rates. The actual improvement in perforation rates has been quite variable in a number of reports. The report of Bachur et al tells us that negative appendectomy rates are highest for children younger than 5 years and girls older than 10 years and are reduced through the use of advanced diagnostic imaging. The authors suggest that routine use of CT and ultrasound should be limited, however, in boys older than 5 years with suspected appendicitis and no other clinical concerns, given the relatively low negative appendectomy rate independent of any imaging technique.

The concern still exists that CT scans performed for any reason in children carry an increased subsequent risk of malignancy. The publication of a scientific study reporting the potential risk of brain cancer and leukemia from CT scans in children was reported in the popular press.[2] As a result, parents and other caregivers have expressed increasing concern about CT scans and many are afraid to allow their children to undergo a CT scan, even though the benefit of the test may very well outweigh risks depending on the clinical situation. June 12, 2012, saw the press release from the American Board of Radiology indicating that all American Board of Radiology—certified radiologists and medical physicists are tested as part of their validation to ensure that they have the skills to perform pediatric CTs of the highest quality with the least radiation dose. That same board convened a large consensus development conference in August 2012 as the first of a series of national summits aimed to address safety issues in our current system of medical imaging. For more on this topic, see www.abr.org.

J. A. Stockman III, MD

References

1. Kim K, Kim YH, Kim SY, et al. Low-dose abdominal CT for evaluating suspected appendicitis. *N Engl J Med.* 2012;366:1596-1605.
2. Pearce MS, Salotti JA, Little MP, et al. Radiation exposure from CT scans in childhood and subsequent risk of leukaemia and brain tumours: a retrospective cohort study. *Lancet.* 2012;380:499-505.

Advanced Radiologic Imaging for Pediatric Appendicitis, 2005-2009: Trends and Outcomes

Bachur RG, Hennelly K, Callahan MJ, et al (Children's Hosp and Harvard Med School, Boston, MA)
J Pediatr 160:1034-1038, 2012

Objectives.—To examine the variability in the use of computed tomography (CT) and ultrasound (US) for children with appendicitis and identify associations with clinical outcomes, and to demonstrate any trends in diagnostic imaging between 2005 and 2009.

Study Design.—This was a retrospective review of children evaluated for appendicitis in an emergency department between 2005 and 2009 using an administrative database of 40 pediatric institutions in the United States. Imaging utilization by institutions was studied for association with 3 clinical outcomes.

Results.—A total of 55 238 children with appendicitis were studied. Utilization of CT and US varied widely across institutions, with medians of 34% (IQR, 21%-49%) for CT and 6% (IQR, 2%-26%) for US. Increased use of US or a combination of CT and US (but not of CT use alone) was associated with a lower negative appendectomy rate. Imaging was not associated with other clinical outcomes. In children with appendicitis, the use of US has increased since 2007, whereas that of CT has decreased.

Conclusion.—There is considerable variation in the use of CT and US for children with appendicitis at major pediatric institutions. At the institutional level, increased use of US or combined US and CT is associated with a lower negative appendectomy rate. Despite the better diagnostic accuracy of CT compared with US, the use of CT is decreasing.

▶ This article emanates from the Division of Emergency Medicine and the Department of Radiology at the Children's Hospital, Boston. It adds to our body of knowledge regarding the use of computed tomography (CT) scanning and ultrasound for the diagnosis of appendicitis in children. Elsewhere the emerging role of low-dose CT has been discussed, but this article gives us a much broader understanding about the utilization of either CT scans or ultrasound by examining the administrative databases of more than 40 pediatric institutions here in the United States. These institutions represent major pediatric centers and often serve as national models for pediatric care. Almost 9 million emergency department visits were analyzed from which a total of 55 238 cases of appendicitis were identified. These records represented a 5-year period spanning January 1, 2005, through December 31, 2009. The trends during this 5-year period showed an increasing rate of ultrasound and a decreasing use of CT scanning. Presumably this finding is the result of an increased awareness of the risk of ionizing radiation and numerous scientific publications with thoughtful commentaries that likely have had a significant influence on clinical practice.

Use of CT and ultrasound varies quite widely across institutions. This institution-based variability was not linked to outcomes of perforation rate or rate of return for "missed" appendicitis. It was fairly clear that when CT was introduced as a diagnostic tool for appendicitis in children, its great diagnostic sensitivity obviated the need for routine admission of patients with equivocal findings for serial clinical examination. It had been thought that CT would identify early cases of appendicitis and thereby reduced the rate of perforation; this decreased rate was inconsistently appreciated in previous investigations and was not associated with CT rates at all in the present study. Nonetheless, the data from this article continue to support the inverse association between diagnostic imaging and lower negative appendectomy rates. Of note, institutions that use ultrasound infrequently have the greatest negative appendectomy rates, supporting the need for experienced ultrasonographers.

Overall, the median institutional rate of using either CT or ultrasound was 48%. It will be interesting to see if there is a rebound rise in the use of CT now that we have learned low-dose imaging CT is almost as good as standard CT, presumably with a much lower risk of the development of secondary malignancy.

J. A. Stockman III, MD

Low-Dose Abdominal CT for Evaluating Suspected Appendicitis

Kim K, Kim YH, Kim SY, et al (Seoul Natl Univ Bundang Hosp, Gyeonggi-do, South Korea; et al)

N Engl J Med 366:1596-1606, 2012

Background.—Computed tomography (CT) has become the predominant test for diagnosing acute appendicitis in adults. In children and young adults, exposure to CT radiation is of particular concern. We evaluated the rate of negative (unnecessary) appendectomy after low-dose versus standard-dose abdominal CT in young adults with suspected appendicitis.

Methods.—In this single-institution, single-blind, noninferiority trial, we randomly assigned 891 patients with suspected appendicitis to either low-dose CT (444 patients) or standard-dose CT (447 patients). The median radiation dose in terms of dose—length product was 116 mGy·cm in the low-dose group and 521 mGy·cm in the standard-dose group. The primary end point was the percentage of negative appendectomies among all nonincidental appendectomies, with a noninferiority margin of 5.5 percentage points. Secondary end points included the appendiceal perforation rate and the proportion of patients with suspected appendicitis who required additional imaging.

Results.—The negative appendectomy rate was 3.5% (6 of 172 patients) in the low-dose CT group and 3.2% (6 of 186 patients) in the standard-dose CT group (difference, 0.3 percentage points; 95% confidence interval, −3.8 to 4.6). The two groups did not differ significantly in terms of the appendiceal perforation rate (26.5% with low-dose CT and 23.3% with standard-dose CT, $P = 0.46$) or the proportion of patients who needed additional imaging tests (3.2% and 1.6%, respectively; $P = 0.09$).

Conclusions.—Low-dose CT was noninferior to standard-dose CT with respect to negative appendectomy rates in young adults with suspected appendicitis. (Funded by GE Healthcare Medical Diagnostics and others; ClinicalTrials.gov number, NCT00913380.)

► There is no question that the use of computed tomography (CT) has a definitive role in the diagnosis of appendicitis. When compared with ultrasonography, increased use of CT has been consistently found to coincide with a reduction in the rate of negative (unnecessary) appendectomies without an increase in the rate of appendiceal perforations. The routine use of CT in patients suspected of having appendicitis has also been reported to be cost-effective because it prevents delayed or inaccurate diagnoses. The rub, however, with CT scans is the radiation dose required. Many patients in whom appendicitis is suspected are children or young adults and radiation exposure from CT is of particular concern in this age population. Although the issue continues to be debated, concern that even a single typical abdominal CT examination might confer a small but real risk of carcinogenesis is increasing. Thus it would be terrific if one could figure out a way of lowering the dose of radiation when performing a CT scan in young people.

Several exploratory studies have shown that reducing radiation dose by 50% to 80% does not significantly hinder the diagnosis of appendicitis, although low-dose CT techniques have not gained wide acceptance as yet because of concern that increased image noise will degrade image quality, resulting in misdiagnosis or overdiagnosis. To address this, Kim et al have designed a randomized, controlled trial establishing the role of low-dose CT in diagnosing appendicitis. Patients as young as 15 years of age were included in this study, making the results appropriate for at least the adolescent age group in terms of its conclusions. Outcomes were looked at with 2 doses of radiation. The low-dose radiation CT scan involved approximately one-fifth the radiation dosage as the standard CT.

In this study, the low-dose CT group was noninferior to the standard-dose CT group with regard to negative appendectomy rates. Neither the appendiceal perforation rate nor the diagnostic performance of CT for appendicitis differed significantly between the 2 groups.

There has been a huge increase in the use of CT for diagnostic imaging for patients with suspected appendicitis over the past 10 to 15 years in the United States. It is estimated that more than a quarter million appendectomies are performed each year and the majority of these involve a patient undergoing preoperative CT scan. There are many more patients for whom the results on CT scan are negative. Although the individual risk for cancer induced by a single CT examination is likely to be extremely low, when one looks at the magnitude of the number of scans performed simply to make or rule out a diagnosis of appendicitis, the effect on the incidence of cancer can be quite dramatic. The findings from this report support those of previous exploratory studies supporting a reduction in radiation dose when CT is used in the diagnosis of appendicitis. The excellent findings from this report can be attributed to improved imaging capabilities of modern CT scanners and the intrinsic simplicity of CT image interpretation in diagnosing appendicitis, which may offset the loss in image quality resulting from low-dose CT techniques. There is little reason to use standard dose radiation in young patients with appendicitis.

This commentary closes with an observation having to do with radiation and one that may cause you to never want to eat a certain fruit again. There was no worse comparative than that made by US presidential advisor John Holdren describing a communication strategy (which was never implemented) after the March 2011 Fukushima nuclear accident, comparing the nuclear fallout radiation from Japan to the natural radiation from ingesting potassium-40 in a banana.[1] He later said: *"We called it the banana standard. We thought this was a great idea, to show people that any radiation doses experienced by Americans would be small compared, essentially to eating a banana, but apparently some people in the banana industry took offense."* ... DUH.

J. A. Stockman III, MD

Reference

1. Editorial comment. They said that! *Science.* 2012;336:1083.

Association between Early Childhood Otitis Media and Pediatric Inflammatory Bowel Disease: An Exploratory Population-Based Analysis
Shaw SY, Blanchard JF, Bernstein CN (Univ of Manitoba, Winnipeg, Canada)
J Pediatr 162:510-514, 2013

Objective.—To determine whether a diagnosis of otitis media in the first 5 years of childhood is associated with the development of pediatric inflammatory bowel disease (IBD).

Study Design.—This was a nested case control analysis of a population-based IBD database in Manitoba, Canada. A total of 294 children with IBD diagnosed between 1989 and 2008 were matched to 2377 controls, based on age, sex, and geographic region. The diagnosis of otitis media was based on physician claims. IBD status was determined based on a validated administrative database definition. Multivariate conditional logistic regression models were used to model the association between otitis media and IBD, adjusted for annual physician visits.

Results.—Approximately 5% of the IBD cases and 12% of the controls did not have an otitis media diagnosis before that IBD case date. By age 5 years, 89% of the IBD cases had at least one diagnosis of otitis media, compared with 82% of the controls. In multivariate analyses, compared with cases and controls without an otitis media diagnosis, individuals with an otitis media diagnosis by age 5 years were 2.8-fold more likely to be an IBD case (95% CI, 1.5-5.2; $P = .001$). This association was detected in stratified models examining Crohn's disease and ulcerative colitis separately.

Conclusion.—Compared with controls, subjects diagnosed with IBD were more likely to have had at least one early childhood episode of otitis media before their diagnosis. We suspect that otitis media serves as a proxy measure of antibiotic use.

▶ More evidence is being uncovered that suggests antibiotic use in early infancy may be strongly linked to the development of inflammatory bowel disease (IBD) in children. Several years ago, investigators began to suggest that such a linkage would exist. More specifically, those infants who received at least one antibiotic prescription had at least a 2.5 times greater risk for development of IBD than matched counterparts who had not received antibiotics. Researchers also found that otitis media was by far the most common diagnosis associated with antibiotic prescriptions with other respiratory infections trailing far behind. The 2 most common classes of antibiotics used were penicillin-type drugs and sulfonamide.[1]

In the report abstracted, Shaw et al from Manitoba, Winnipeg, Canada, uncovered additional information in this regard after examining the university's IBD Epidemiology Database. This population-based database has information on all IBD cases in Manitoba, including patient prescription data, from 1995 onward. Data from 36 children with IBD diagnosed between 1996 and 2008 were identified in the database. The investigators pulled information from the database on 10 matched controls for each case. The mean age at diagnosis for the patients and controls was 8.4 years. Fifty-eight percent of patients and 39% of controls had received at least one antibiotic prescription. When the investigators matched controls with patients by age, sex, and region of residence, they calculated an odds ratio 2.9 for development of IBD with at least one antibiotic prescription using a conditional logistic regression analysis. When they separated the genders, they uncovered an odds ratio of 6.68 among boys and 1.44 among girls. Overwhelmingly, the most common indication for antibiotic treatment had been management of otitis media. Upper respiratory tract infections accounted for just 12% of antibiotic prescriptions, lower respiratory tract infections for 9%, and other indications for 19%.

It was not clear from this report why there was such a strong association between antibiotic use and the development of IBD in boys or whether otitis media itself is somehow directly associated with the development of IBD and antibiotic use is merely a proxy.

This report is merely one of a spate of recently published studies that strongly suggest that patients with IBD in childhood are more likely to have been prescribed antibiotics early in life. It cannot be disputed that the incidence of IBD has recently increased in pediatric populations, particularly in high-resource countries. A 5% to 7% annual increase in IBD has been reported over a recent 10-year period in Canada, and another study has found that the incidence of IBD has increased 6% to 8% per year in Finland.[2]

The authors of this report conclude their discussion of this topic by indicating that their study provides an impetus for further exploration of the gut microbiome in young children who have IBD, as well as an investigation of how the gut microbiome may be altered for extended periods, perhaps even permanently by antibiotic use early in life.[3]

J. A. Stockman III, MD

References

1. Shaw SY, Blanchard JF, Bernstein CN. Association between the use of antibiotics in the first year of life and pediatric inflammatory bowel disease. *Am J Gastroenterol.* 2010;105:2687-2692.
2. Benchimol EI, Guttmann A, Griffiths AM, et al. Increasing incidence of paediatric inflammatory bowel disease in Ontario, Canada: evidence from health administrative data. *Gut.* 2009;58:1490-1497.
3. Lehtinen P, Ashorn M, Iltanen S, et al. Incidence trends of pediatric inflammatory bowel disease in Finland, 1987–2003, a nationwide study. *Inflamm Bowel Dis.* 2011;17:1778-1783.

Familial Diarrhea Syndrome Caused by an Activating *GUCY2C* Mutation

Fiskerstrand T, Arshad N, Haukanes BI, et al (Haukeland Univ Hosp, Bergen, Norway; Indian Inst of Science, Bangalore; et al)
N Engl J Med 366:1586-1595, 2012

Background.—Familial diarrhea disorders are, in most cases, severe and caused by recessive mutations. We describe the cause of a novel dominant disease in 32 members of a Norwegian family. The affected members have chronic diarrhea that is of early onset, is relatively mild, and is associated with increased susceptibility to inflammatory bowel disease, small-bowel obstruction, and esophagitis.

Methods.—We used linkage analysis, based on arrays with single-nucleotide polymorphisms, to identify a candidate region on chromosome 12 and then sequenced *GUCY2C*, encoding guanylate cyclase C (GC-C), an intestinal receptor for bacterial heat-stable enterotoxins. We performed exome sequencing of the entire candidate region from three affected family members, to exclude the possibility that mutations in genes other than *GUCY2C* could cause or contribute to susceptibility to the disease. We carried out functional studies of mutant GC-C using HEK293T cells.

Results.—We identified a heterozygous missense mutation (c.2519G→T) in *GUCY2C* in all affected family members and observed no other rare variants in the exons of genes in the candidate region. Exposure of the mutant receptor to its ligands resulted in markedly increased production of cyclic guanosine monophosphate (cGMP). This may cause hyperactivation of the cystic fibrosis transmembrane regulator (CFTR), leading to increased chloride and water secretion from the enterocytes, and may thus explain the chronic diarrhea in the affected family members.

Conclusions.—Increased GC-C signaling disturbs normal bowel function and appears to have a proinflammatory effect, either through increased chloride secretion or additional effects of elevated cellular cGMP. Further investigation of the relevance of genetic variants affecting the GC-C—CFTR pathway to conditions such as Crohn's disease is warranted. (Funded by Helse Vest [Western Norway Regional Health Authority] and the Department of Science and Technology, Government of India.)

▶ I have to confess some degree of ignorance in not knowing much, if anything, about familial diarrhea, a not-so-pleasant diagnosis for those who have it. All of us know about the common causes of chronic diarrhea. These include, in part, irritable bowel syndrome, inflammatory bowel disease, infectious diarrhea, paraneoplastic syndrome presenting with diarrhea, celiac disease, malabsorption syndrome, and disorders resulting in bacterial overgrowth in the small intestine. More recently, studies have focused on the importance of genetic factors in the development of many cases of chronic diarrhea. These genetic factors can provide insight into the pathophysiology of intestinal diseases and also suggest new forms of therapy. For example, irritable bowel syndrome does aggregate strongly within families. There is a genetic predisposition to Crohn disease, particularly that associated with ileitis. To date, however, no major genes causing these disorders have been found. There are rare inherited forms of chronic diarrhea that have been reported. Nearly all of these are severe, autosomal recessive, single-gene diseases that usually manifest as early as the newborn period.

Investigators from Norway have studied a single large family with a dominantly inherited, fully penetrant syndrome of chronic diarrhea and dysmotility. Gastrointestinal (GI) disorders running within this family include Crohn disease, small bowel obstruction, and esophagitis with or without esophageal hernia. They studied more than 32 affected individuals from 3 branches of the same family, as well as 14 unaffected family members. All had DNA studies in addition to very detailed histories and physical examinations. Colonoscopies were done in affected family members with the chronic diarrhea syndrome. These were unremarkable. The affected family members had on average 3.6 stools per day that typically were watery or very loose and were accompanied by abdominal pain and meteorism. Ten of the family members had previously undergone laparotomy for suspected small bowel obstruction, confirmed in 8 family members. The obstruction resulted from volvulus, adhesions, or ileal inflammation. Eight family members had also been hospitalized for dehydration, metabolic acidosis, and electrolyte disturbances in the newborn period. All the common causes of chronic diarrhea had been excluded with prior studies. Specific DNA studies documented an inheritance pattern consistent with a dominant mutation in an autosomal gene, the result of a specific missense mutation. The genetic mutation appeared to cause excess activation of guanylate cyclase C receptors, resulting in elevated levels of cellular cyclic guanosine monophosphate. This ultimately causes increased GI tract chloride secretion via the cystic fibrosis transmembrane conductance regulator. This creates an osmotic drive that results in the secretion of sodium ions and hence water into the intestinal lumen. This effect is particularly prominent in the ileum, which may be the reason why so many family members affected with this disorder have had intestinal obstructions.

As rare as this syndrome may well be, it serves as a model for any one of a number of GI disorders that result from increased GI motility secondary to electrolyte and fluid excretion excesses. It could be that the pathways affected will ultimately serve as a target for further search of mechanisms of disease and the development of unique therapies for some of the more common disorders presenting in similar ways.

This commentary on the GI tract closes with a little-known fact about a large percentage of folks in India who are without bathroom facilities. Open defecation still occurs. Recently, the Development Ministry called for an end to open defecation by 2022 as part of the country's Total Sanitation Campaign. Fifty-four percent of India's population practices open defecation, representing 58% of the total world's population who have few alternatives to this practice.[1]

J. A. Stockman III, MD

Reference

1. Editorial Comment. No more open defecation. *Lancet.* 2012;379:1.

Probiotics for the Prevention and Treatment of Antibiotic-Associated Diarrhea: A Systematic Review and Meta-analysis

Hempel S, Newberry SJ, Maher AR, et al (Southern California Evidence-Based Practice Ctr, Santa Monica, CA; RAND, Santa Monica, CA)
JAMA 307:1959-1969, 2012

Context.—Probiotics are live microorganisms intended to confer a health benefit when consumed. One condition for which probiotics have been advocated is the diarrhea that is a common adverse effect of antibiotic use.

Objective.—To evaluate the evidence for probiotic use in the prevention and treatment of antibiotic-associated diarrhea (AAD).

Data Sources.—Twelve electronic databases were searched (DARE, Cochrane Library of Systematic Reviews, CENTRAL, PubMed, EMBASE, CINAHL, AMED, MANTIS, TOXLINE, ToxFILE, NTIS, and AGRICOLA) and references of included studies and reviews were screened from database inception to February 2012, without language restriction.

Study Selection.—Two independent reviewers identified parallel randomized controlled trials (RCTs) of probiotics (*Lactobacillus, Bifidobacterium, Saccharomyces, Streptococcus, Enterococcus, and/or Bacillus*) for the prevention or treatment of AAD.

Data Extraction.—Two independent reviewers extracted the data and assessed trial quality.

Results.—A total of 82 RCTs met inclusion criteria. The majority used *Lactobacillus*-based interventions alone or in combination with other genera; strains were poorly documented. The pooled relative risk in a DerSimonian-Laird random-effects metaanalysis of 63 RCTs, which included 11 811 participants, indicated a statistically significant association of probiotic administration with reduction in AAD (relative risk, 0.58; 95% CI, 0.50 to 0.68; $P < .001$; I^2, 54%; [risk difference, -0.07; 95% CI, -0.10 to -0.05], [number needed to treat, 13; 95% CI, 10.3 to 19.1]) in trials reporting on the number of patients with AAD. This result was relatively insensitive to numerous subgroup analyses. However, there exists significant heterogeneity in pooled results and the evidence is insufficient to determine whether this association varies systematically by population, antibiotic characteristic, or probiotic preparation.

Conclusions.—The pooled evidence suggests that probiotics are associated with a reduction in AAD. More research is needed to determine which probiotics are associated with the greatest efficacy and for which patients receiving which specific antibiotics.

▶ Everyone knows that antibiotics may disturb the flora of the gastrointestinal tract. When this occurs, clinical symptoms including diarrhea may develop in as many as 30% of patients. Symptoms can range from mild and self-limiting to severe, particular in *Clostridium difficile* infections. Antibiotic-associated diarrhea is an important reason for nonadherence with antibiotic treatment.

Some have proposed probiotics as a partial solution to antibiotic-associated diarrhea. Recall that probiotics are micro-organisms intended to have a health benefit when consumed. Symbiotics refer to preparations in which probiotic organisms and prebiotics (nondigestible food ingredients that may benefit the host by selectively stimulating bacteria in the colon) are combined. Theoretically, probiotics maintain or can restore gut microecology during or after antibiotic treatment through receptor competition, competition for nutrients, inhibition of epithelial and mucosal adherence pathogens, introduction of lower colonic pH favoring the growth of nonpathogenic species, stimulation of immunity, or production of antimicrobial substances.

A recent Cochrane review[1] on pediatric antibiotic-associated diarrhea has suggested a protective association of probiotic use in preventing this problem in children. Most prior reviews have been nonsystematic, have focused on specific patient populations or probiotic genera, and have not included the latest clinical trials.

These authors revisited the topic of the benefits of probiotics for management of antibiotic-associated diarrhea by undertaking a systematic review and meta-analysis of the literature to evaluate the available evidence on probiotics and symbiotic interventions, including the genera *Lactobacillus*, *Bifidobacterium*, *Saccharomyces*, *Streptococcus*, *Enterococcus*, and *Bacillus*, alone or in combination for the prevention and treatment of antibiotic-associated diarrhea. A total of 82 randomized controlled trials were of sufficient quality to include in this meta-analysis.

The primary finding of the review of these authors was that using probiotics as an adjunct therapy reduces the risk of antibiotic-associated diarrhea by approximately 58%. The existing evidence for the prevention or treatment consists primarily of *Lactobacillus* interventions, either alone or in combination with other probiotics. The trials predominantly use the lactic acid—producing bacteria *L casei*. The relative efficacy of probiotic interventions may be strain specific. This article did not provide information about which population of patients would benefit most from adjunctive probiotic therapy.

It should be noted that in rare cases, probiotics have been linked to serious adverse outcomes such as fungemia and bacterial sepsis. Hence, the potential adverse effects of probiotics must be reviewed with the efficacy data, especially because little research has focused on the adverse effects of probiotics used in clinical practice. Although none of the included clinical trials in this systematic review reported such adverse events, it is noteworthy that few trials have addressed these outcomes, especially since cases of such infections suspected to be associated with the administered organisms were reported decades ago.

In summary, this review found sufficient evidence to conclude that using probiotics as an adjunctive therapy is associated with a reduced risk of antibiotic-associated diarrhea. Future studies will be necessary to assess which patients might benefit most from this form of therapy, and studies should be designed to explicitly determine the possibility of adverse outcomes in order to better refine our understandings of the use of probiotics in the prevention of antibiotic-associated diarrhea.

J. A. Stockman III, MD

Reference

1. Johnston BC, Goldenberg JZ, Vandvik PO, Sun X, Guyatt GH. Probiotics for the prevention of pediatric antibiotic-associated diarrhea. *Cochrane Database Syst Rev.* 2011;(11):CD004827.

Probiotics for the Prevention of *Clostridium difficile*—Associated Diarrhea: A Systematic Review and Meta-analysis

Johnston BC, Ma SSY, Goldenberg JZ, et al (The Hosp for Sick Children Res Inst, Toronto, Ontario, Canada; Bastyr Univ, Kenmore, WA; McMaster Univ, Hamilton, Ontario, Canada; et al)
Ann Intern Med 157:878-888, 2012

Background.—Antibiotic treatment may disturb the resistance of gastrointestinal flora to colonization. This may result in complications, the most serious of which is *Clostridium difficile*—associated diarrhea (CDAD).

Purpose.—To assess the efficacy and safety of probiotics for the prevention of CDAD in adults and children receiving antibiotics.

Data Sources.—Cochrane Central Register of Controlled Trials, MEDLINE, EMBASE, CINAHL, Allied and Complementary Medicine Database, Web of Science, and 12 gray-literature sources.

Study Selection.—Randomized, controlled trials including adult or pediatric patients receiving antibiotics that compared any strain or dose of a specified probiotic with placebo or with no treatment control and reported the incidence of CDAD.

Data Extraction.—Two reviewers independently screened potentially eligible articles; extracted data on populations, interventions, and outcomes; and assessed risk of bias. The Grading of Recommendations Assessment, Development and Evaluation guidelines were used to independently rate overall confidence in effect estimates for each outcome.

Data Synthesis.—Twenty trials including 3818 participants met the eligibility criteria. Probiotics reduced the incidence of CDAD by 66% (pooled relative risk, 0.34 [95% CI, 0.24 to 0.49]; $I^2 = 0\%$). In a population with a 5% incidence of antibiotic-associated CDAD (median control group risk), probiotic prophylaxis would prevent 33 episodes (CI, 25 to 38 episodes) per 1000 persons. Of probiotic-treated patients, 9.3% experienced adverse events, compared with 12.6% of control patients (relative risk, 0.82 [CI, 0.65 to 1.05]; $I^2 = 17\%$).

Limitations.—In 13 trials, data on CDAD were missing for 5% to 45% of patients. The results were robust to worst-plausible assumptions regarding event rates in studies with missing outcome data.

Conclusion.—Moderate-quality evidence suggests that probiotic prophylaxis results in a large reduction in CDAD without an increase in clinically important adverse events.

▶ Both children and adults who are exposed to broad-spectrum antibiotics for long periods of time, particularly those who are hospitalized, are at significantly increased risk for the development of antibiotic-associated diarrhea attributable to *Clostridium difficile*. *C difficile* is the pathogen most often associated with opportunistic proliferation after breakdown of colonization resistance caused by antibiotic administration. The spectrum of *C difficile*—related disease ranges from asymptomatic intestinal colonization to diarrhea, colitis and pseudomembranous colitis, and death. About 10 years ago, hospitals in several high-income countries began to experience a dramatic rise in both the incidence and severity of *C difficile*—associated diarrhea. Reports from the United States also demonstrated an almost 2-fold increase in the fatality rate related to *C difficile*—associated diarrhea. In adults at least, 1 of 10 patients who acquire *C difficile* will die.

So what does this have to do with the topic in this article? Probiotics are microorganisms that are believed to counteract disturbances in intestinal flora and thereby reduce the risk for colonization by various pathogenic bacteria. The rationale for probiotic administration includes reinoculation of disturbed indigenous microflora secondary to antibiotic use and the inhibition of pathogen adhesion, colonization, and invasion of the gastrointestinal mucosa. Probiotics are increasingly used in capsule form and as dietary-based supplements, often sold in health food stores and supermarkets. If probiotics are effective in the management of gastrointestinal tract disorders related to antibiotic overuse, their low cost and the low incidence of adverse side effects would make them a very attractive choice to help diminish the prevalence of *C difficile*—associated diarrhea.

These authors conducted a systematic review to determine the efficacy and safety of probiotics for the prevention of *C difficile*—associated diarrhea in both adults and children who are taking antibiotics. The authors undertook a full data review using the Cochrane Central Register of Controlled Trials, MEDLINE, Embase, the Cumulative Index to Nursing and Allied Health Literature, Allied and Contemporary Medicine Database, Web of Science, and 12 other literature review sources. Twenty acceptable trials were found that included almost 4000 participants. The gist of this meta-analysis was that probiotics reduce the incidence of *C difficile*—associated diarrhea by as much as 66%. Few side effects were observed related to the use of probiotics.

These authors suggest that there is a moderate level of quality evidence supporting the use of probiotics in preventing *C difficile*—associated diarrhea. Given the low cost of probiotics and the moderate-quality evidence suggesting the absence of important side effects, there seems to be no reason not to encourage the use of probiotics in patients who are taking antibiotics who are at any kind of appreciable risk for the development of *C difficile*—associated diarrhea.

J. A. Stockman III, MD

Duodenal Infusion of Donor Feces for Recurrent *Clostridium difficile*

van Nood E, Vrieze A, Nieuwdorp M, et al (Univ of Amsterdam, The Netherlands; et al)

N Engl J Med 368:407-415, 2013

Background.—Recurrent *Clostridium difficile* infection is difficult to treat, and failure rates for antibiotic therapy are high. We studied the effect of duodenal infusion of donor feces in patients with recurrent *C. difficile* infection.

Methods.—We randomly assigned patients to receive one of three therapies: an initial vancomycin regimen (500 mg orally four times per day for 4 days), followed by bowel lavage and subsequent infusion of a solution of donor feces through a nasoduodenal tube; a standard vancomycin regimen (500 mg orally four times per day for 14 days); or a standard vancomycin regimen with bowel lavage. The primary end point was the resolution of diarrhea associated with *C. difficile* infection without relapse after 10 weeks.

Results.—The study was stopped after an interim analysis. Of 16 patients in the infusion group, 13 (81%) had resolution of *C. difficile*—associated diarrhea after the first infusion. The 3 remaining patients received a second infusion with feces from a different donor, with resolution in 2 patients. Resolution of *C. difficile* infection occurred in 4 of 13 patients (31%) receiving vancomycin alone and in 3 of 13 patients (23%) receiving vancomycin with bowel lavage ($P < 0.001$ for both comparisons with the infusion group). No significant differences in adverse events among the three study groups were observed except for mild diarrhea and abdominal cramping in the infusion group on the infusion day. After donor-feces infusion, patients showed increased fecal bacterial diversity, similar to that in healthy donors, with an increase in Bacteroidetes species and clostridium clusters IV and XIVa and a decrease in Proteobacteria species.

Conclusions.—The infusion of donor feces was significantly more effective for the treatment of recurrent *C. difficile* infection than the use of vancomycin. (Funded by the Netherlands Organization for Health Research and Development and the Netherlands Organization for Scientific Research; Netherlands Trial Register number, NTR1177.)

▶ The management of patients with recurrent *Clostridium difficile* infection is most problematic. *C difficile* has become the most commonly identified cause of nosocomial infectious diarrhea in the United States. In fact, the incidence of such infections and its severity have been on the increase and are associated with significant mortality in both children and adults. In both populations, antibiotic therapy more often than not will resolve the problem, but at least 1 of 4 infected individuals will have a recurrence of *C difficile*—related diarrhea, and in some patients, this results in disastrous consequences. The rub with this problem is that once the disorder manifests itself again, the recurrence risk for third attacks increases very significantly. For patients who have multiple recurrences, the likelihood of a subsequent recurrence is well over 50%.

Most are not aware of this, but it was well over 50 years ago that in the United States we saw the first administration of feces by enema to matched patients with fulminant, life-threatening pseudomembranous enterocolitis, an infection we now know is caused by *C difficile*.[1] In the ensuing half decade, in addition to *C difficile* being identified as the causative organism of pseudomembranous enterocolitis, effective antibiotic treatments were identified, but failure of antibiotics to eliminate recurrence in some patients became obvious. In the same interim period of time, only patients with the most recalcitrant cases of *C difficile* infection have been likely to undergo fecal microbiota transplantation (FMT). FMT has been the management of last resort, yet systematic review reveals that the reported efficacy of FMT in treating recurrent *C difficile* infection is greater than 90%.[2]

Needless to say, the procedure is esthetically quite unappealing and somewhat logistically challenging in terms of harvesting stool and processing suitable donor material. These facts and the lack of efficacy data from randomized, controlled trials have led to the use of FMT on an exceptional rather than regular basis.

That is where this article becomes important. In this study, investigators compared the duodenal infusion of donor feces after vancomycin therapy and bowel lavage with vancomycin therapy either alone or with bowel lavage absent FMT. The outcome data indicated an 81% response rate with FMT, a response rate greater than vancomycin therapy either alone (31%) or with bowel lavage (23%). The study was conducted in patients with relapse *C difficile* infection in whom standard therapy with vancomycin had failed. The results were so positive that the study was closed to new patients well before the planned time period. The data from this report are quite consistent with earlier systematic reviews of uncontrolled case series in which FMT administered through the stomach or via small intestine showed an overall response rate of about 80%.

In an editorial that accompanied this report by Kelly,[3] the issue of the residual antipathy toward fecal therapy was addressed. It was suggested that resistance to FMT could be reduced by banking suitable material from anonymous screened donors because this would more distance the recipient from the stool donation and provide physicians with quite readily accessible, quality-controlled treatment materials. Needless to say, even better would be the use of precultured bacteria to colonize the bowel. The latter theoretically would diminish the potential for inadvertent transmission of disease-carrying pathogens in stool. The editorial that accompanied this article also suggested that this current article might encourage and facilitate the design of similar trials of intestinal microbiota therapy for various other common conditions, such as inflammatory bowel disease, irritable bowel syndrome, the prevention of colorectal cancer, and certain metabolic disorders. There is an interesting summary of the use of cut microbiota that is worth reading.[4]

This commentary closes with a question. Who holds the record for having the greatest infestation with the whipworm Trichuris trichiura? In modern man, having an estimated 200 whipworms in one's gut would be considered a very heavy infestation. The record, however, in this regard appears to now be held by a 200-year-old mummy from Piraino, Italy.[5] This particular whipworm buries its tail into the gut wall and excretes eggs into the infected individual's feces.

Investigators examined a fecal sample from the body of a clergyman buried in a crypt in the Cathedral of Piraino. Conditions in the crypt are so dry, bodies there naturally mummify. One gram of this man's feces was determined to contain 34 529 whipworm eggs, reflecting a total whipworm burden estimated to be as high as 7430 worms. This is the highest worm infestation recorded in archaeological history!

J. A. Stockman III, MD

References

1. Eiseman B, Silen W, Bascom GS, Kauvar AJ. Fecal enema as an adjunct in the treatment of pseudomembranous enterocolitis. *Surgery.* 1958;44:854-859.
2. Gough E, Shaikh H, Manges AR. Systematic review of intestinal microbiota transplantation (fecal bacteriotherapy) for recurrent *Clostridium difficile* infection. *Clin Infect Dis.* 2011;53:994-1002.
3. Kelly CP. Fecal microbiota transplantation—an old therapy comes of age. *N Engl J Med.* 2013;368:474-475.
4. Shanahan F. The gut microbiota in 2011: translating the microbiota to medicine. *Nat Rev Gastroenterol Hepatol.* 2011;9:72-74.
5. Editorial comment. One sick mummy gets a double diagnosis. *Science.* 2011;333:403.

8 Genitourinary Tract

Costs and Effectiveness of Neonatal Male Circumcision
Kacker S, Frick KD, Gaydos CA, et al (Johns Hopkins Univ, Baltimore, MD)
Arch Pediatr Adolesc Med 166:910-918, 2012

Objective.—To evaluate the expected change in the prevalence of male circumcision (MC)—reduced infections and resulting health care costs associated with continued decreases in MC rates. During the past 20 years, MC rates have declined from 79% to 55%, alongside reduced insurance coverage.

Design.—We used Markov-based Monte Carlo simulations to track men and women throughout their lifetimes as they experienced MC procedure-related events and MC-reduced infections and accumulated associated costs. One-way and probabilistic sensitivity analyses were used to evaluate the impact of uncertainty.

Setting.—United States.

Participants.—Birth cohort of men and women.

Intervention.—Decreased MC rates (10% reflects the MC rate in Europe, where insurance coverage is limited).

Outcomes Measured.—Lifetime direct medical cost (2011 US$) and prevalence of MC-reduced infections.

Results.—Reducing the MC rate to 10% will increase lifetime health care costs by $407 per male and $43 per female. Net expenditure per annual birth cohort (including procedure and complication costs) is expected to increase by $505 million, reflecting an increase of $313 per forgone MC. Over 10 annual cohorts, net present value of additional costs would exceed $4.4 billion. Lifetime prevalence of human immunodeficiency virus infection among males is expected to increase by 12.2% (4843 cases), high- and low-risk human papillomavirus by 29.1% (57124 cases), herpes simplex virus type 2 by 19.8% (124767 cases), and infant urinary tract infections by 211.8% (26876 cases). Among females, lifetime prevalence of bacterial vaginosis is expected to increase by 51.2% (538865 cases), trichomoniasis by 51.2% (64585 cases), high-risk human papillomavirus by 18.3% (33148 cases), and low-risk human papillomavirus by 12.9% (25837 cases). Increased prevalence of human immunodeficiency virus infection among males represents 78.9% of increased expenses.

187

Conclusion.—Continued decreases in MC rates are associated with increased infection prevalence, thereby increasing medical expenditures for men and women.

▶ This is an interesting report that does some theoretical modeling to suggest what the consequences would be in the United States if there is a further decline in male circumcision rates from an already low percentage (55%) down to just 10%. The authors used a Monte Carlo simulation to track men and women throughout their lifetimes as they experienced male circumcision procedure—related events and male circumcision—reduced infections along with the accumulated associated cost. The data indicate that should there be a reduction in male circumcision rates to 10% of all boys born, there would be an increase in lifetime health care cost of approximately $407 per male and $43 per female. Over 10 annual birth cohorts, the net present value of these additional costs would exceed $4.4 billion. Lifetime prevalence rates of human immunodeficiency virus (HIV) infection among males would increase by 12.2%, high- and low-risk human papillomavirus infection by 29.1%, herpes simplex virus type 2 infection by 19.8% and infant urinary tract infections by 211.8%. Among females, lifetime prevalence of bacterial vaginosis would increase by 51.2%, trichomoniasis by 51.2%, high-risk human papillomavirus by 18.3%, and low-risk human papillomavirus by 12.8%. Of the overall increased cost associated with a reduction in male circumcision, more than three-quarters of the added cost is related to the increase in the potential prevalence of HIV infection among males.

There is no question that male circumcision does lower HIV rates. For example, an increase in male circumcision in a South African community was documented to coincide with lower overall HIV rates among adult men.[1] Researchers in South Africa devised a program starting in 2008 that provided free circumcision for men plus condoms and counseling. Within 3 years, the adult male circumcision rate jumped from 17% to 54%, and the prevalence of HIV infection decreased from 15.4% to 12.3% when adjusted for condom usage. Presumably, these decreases in HIV prevalence in men would lead to a decrease in HIV rates for their female partners. The goal in South Africa is to achieve circumcision rates of approximately 80%, which seems doable according to health officials there.

Circumcision of newborn boys has been medically documented since ancient times. It is primarily elective, is sometimes done by religious scholars, and is considered sacred to the Jewish and Muslim faiths. Yet many today consider it to be a human-rights violation. The global debate over religious circumcision erupted anew in June 2012, when the German city of Cologne banned the procedure and charged a rabbi with inflicting physical harm on an infant after he did the operation.[2] Other countries have imposed similar bans at a time when recently the American Academy of Pediatrics (AAP) released its circumcision policy statement on August 27, 2012, indicating that the benefits of circumcision for newborn boys outweighed the risks, especially with regard to a decrease in the risk of acquiring a sexually transmitted infection. This policy statement may be found at the *www. aap.org* website. The statement supports circumcision for those who choose it for religious reasons but does not recommend the procedure to be done on all newborn boys. The position of the AAP is that the operation should be available to all US families who request it and for it to be covered by Medicaid. Readers will recall that back in 1999 the AAP declared that despite the potential health benefits of circumcision in newborn boys, they felt unable to recommend the practice, and as a result, circumcision rates decreased from 67% to 55% in the United States.

The AAP's current position on circumcision is likely to cause a resurgence of requests for nonmedically indicated circumcision in newborn boys. Commentaries that have appeared in Europe have suggested that there should be a respectful dialogue between clinicians and religious leaders and effective training schemes for both to ensure that all circumcisions are done in a safe and sterile environment with adequate pain control. Needless to say the debate over the pros and cons of circumcision will not end anytime soon.

J. A. Stockman III, MD

References

1. Seppa N. Male circumcision lowers HIV rate. Community programs changing public opinion of procedure. *Science News*. August 25, 2012:11.
2. Editorial comment. Safeguarding male circumcision *Lancet*. 2012;380:860

Association of Malodorous Urine With Urinary Tract Infection in Children Aged 1 to 36 Months

Gauthier M, Gouin S, Phan V, et al (Univ of Montreal, Quebec, Canada)
Pediatrics 129:885-890, 2012

Objective.—To determine whether parental reporting of malodorous urine is associated with urinary tract infection (UTI) in children.

Methods.—We conducted a prospective consecutive cohort study in the emergency department of a pediatric hospital from July 31, 2009 to April 30, 2011. All children aged between 1 and 36 months for whom a urine culture was prescribed for suspected UTI (ie, unexplained fever, irritability, or vomiting) were assessed for eligibility. A standardized questionnaire was administered to the parents by a research assistant. The primary outcome measure was a UTI.

Results.—Three hundred ninety-six children were initially enrolled, but 65 were excluded a posteriori either because a urine culture, although prescribed, was not done (11), was collected by bag (39), and/or showed gross contamination (25). Therefore, 331 children were included in the final analysis. Their median age was 12 months (range, 1—36). Criteria for UTI were fulfilled in 51 (15%). A malodorous urine was reported by parents in 57% of children with UTI and in 32% of children without UTI. On logistic regression, malodorous urine was associated with UTI (odds ratio 2.83, 95% confidence interval: 1.54—5.20). This association remained statistically significant when adjusted for gender and the presence of vesicoureteral reflux (odds ratio 2.73, 95% confidence interval: 1.46—5.08).

Conclusions.—Parental reporting of malodorous urine increases the probability of UTI among young children being evaluated for suspected UTI. However, this association is not strong enough to definitely rule in or out a diagnosis of UTI.

▶ The authors of this report tell us something that parents have known for a long time, and that is that stinky urine portends a urinary tract infection. Or does it? This is the subject of this report. Given the debate as to how far one should go to evaluate the presence of a urinary tract infection, any additional clinical clue to the diagnosis that has sufficient predictive ability would help practitioners decide when to evaluate a young child for a possible urinary tract infection. So far, few investigators have actually looked at the value of malodorous urine as a predictor of urinary tract infection, and the results of prior reports have been quite contradictory.

The objective of the study of Gauthier et al was to determine whether parent reporting of malodorous urine is associated with the probability of a urinary tract infection in young children. The investigators designed a prospective emergency department study in a pediatric university-affiliated tertiary care center in Montreal, Canada. All children between 1 and 36 months of age for whom a urine culture was requested entered the study. A number of variables were looked at, and parents were asked 2 questions: Have you noticed that your child's urine smelled stronger than usual, and have you noticed that your child's urine smelled offensive? Urinary tract infection criteria were fulfilled in 15% of the children for whom a urinary culture was obtained. In these patients, the infection was suspected because of fever without a source. No urinary tract infection was found in afebrile children suspected of having this infection because of unexplained vomiting or irritability. Urine cultures were positive for *Escherichia coli* in 82% of cases. Malodorous urine was reported by parents in 57% of children with a urinary tract infection and in 32% of children without a urinary tract infection. This symptom standing by itself was associated with a risk of urinary tract infection with an odds ratio of 2.83. On multiple logistic regression, the association between malodorous urine remained statistically significant when adjusting for other known risk factors, such as gender and the presence of urinary tract reflux (odds ratio 2.73). Malodorous urine showed a sensitivity of 0.57 and a specificity of 0.68 for urinary tract infection, leading to a positive likelihood ratio of 1.79 and a negative likely ratio of 0.63.

This study concluded that there is an association between parent reporting of malodorous urine and urinary tract infection in young children. This association between smelly urine and urinary tract infection was at least as significant as the association with female gender, past medical history of urinary tract infection, and urinary tract reflux. At the same time, however, 40% of children with urinary tract infection did not have malodorous urine, and slightly more than 30% of parents reported malodorous urine in children without a urinary tract infection. Needless to say, parent reporting of malodorous urine does not have a sufficiently high sensitivity or specificity to definitely rule in or rule out a urinary tract infection. This really is not any different than other symptoms used to define "classical" urinary tract infection.

If there is a message to take home from this report, it is that smelly urine should make the clinician somewhat more suspicious of a urinary tract infection when one gets this history in a young child who has a fever without a source. What would be most useful, however, would be to design a study in which multiple factors were put together, including smelly urine, to derive a multi-source predictive determination. While waiting for such a report, we should at least put some modest value on the presence or absence of smelly urine.

J. A. Stockman III, MD

Urinary Incontinence in Young Nulligravid Women: A Cross-sectional Analysis
O'Halloran T, Bell RJ, Robinson PJ, et al (Monash Univ, Melbourne, Victoria, Australia)
Ann Intern Med 157:87-93, 2012

Background.—Although pregnancy is a risk factor for urinary incontinence (UI), the extent of UI in nulligravid women has not been reported.
Objective.—To investigate the rate of UI in a sample of young nulligravid women and its potential risk factors and effect on quality of life.
Design.—Cross-sectional, self-administered questionnaire-based study.
Setting.—University campuses and medical and allied health clinics.
Participants.—Nulligravid Australian women aged 16 to 30 years.
Measurements.—The Questionnaire for Urinary Incontinence Diagnosis, the Psychological General Well Being Index (PGWBI), the King's Health Questionnaire, and the International Physical Activity Questionnaire-Short Form. Demographic variables and potential risk factors were also documented.
Results.—1018 of 1620 questionnaires (63%) were returned, and 1002 provided analyzable data. The mean age of participants was 22.5 years (SD, 3.2). The rate of any UI was 12.6% (95% CI, 10.5% to 14.7%). Incontinence was slightly more common in students than in nonstudents (13.2% [CI, 11.0% to 15.8%] vs. 10.6% [CI, 6.7% to 14.6%]). Rates of UI varied according to sexual activity and use of combined oral contraceptives (COCs), with highest rates reported by students who were ever sexually active and not using COCs (21.5% [CI, 16.7% to 27.3%]). Women with UI reported significantly lower overall well-being than women without UI and had worse PGWBI scores related to anxiety, depression, positive well-being, and self-control.
Limitation.—A convenience sample of healthy, well-educated women was recruited, and response rates and participant characteristics varied by setting.
Conclusion.—In a sample of young nulligravid women, UI was associated with ever being sexually active and no COC use, as well as lower

psychological well-being. Further research is needed to assess the prevalence and risk factors for UI in nulligravid women.

▶ This report tells us about urinary incontinence in young women who have never been pregnant. The study does include teenagers and therefore the information should be valuable to those who provide care to older-aged teens.

It is well known that pregnancy contributes to the development of urinary incontinence, and data do seem to indicate that incontinence before one becomes pregnant predisposes a woman to pregnancy-related urinary incontinence. Although substantial literature exists on the prevalence of urinary incontinence in women at midlife or later, few studies have investigated this problem in young nulliparous women. For women who have been pregnant at least once, the reported prevalence of urinary tract incontinence ranges from 10% to 12% in women at 30 years of age and 20% in women 31 to 40 years of age. Data from the literature suggest that young, unmarried, nulliparous students report that as many as 50% are affected by stress urinary incontinence. Symptoms that have been associated with urinary incontinence in young women include physical activity, nocturnal bed-wetting before 18 years of age, and urinary tract infections.

O'Halloran et al designed a study aimed at investigating the rate of urinary incontinence in a sample of nulligravid women age 16 to 30 years of age. The study was entirely questionnaire-based. The survey instrument began with an explanatory statement that indicated the aim of the survey was "to determine how many young women experience a problem with bladder control in the form of urine leakage either in routine activities or when undertaking sporting activities." Women were instructed not to complete the survey if they believed they had symptoms of a urinary tract infection or had been treated for a urinary tract infection in the preceding 3 months. Also excluded were women who had chronic severe medical conditions, including diabetes or renal, liver, or respiratory disease. Women who were pregnant or who had ever been pregnant were also excluded. The survey was carried out on college campuses and in medical clinics. A total of 1018 questionnaires was returned and analyzed. The mean age of the respondents was 22.5 years (SD 3.2); 76.4% of the women were college students.

The rate of any urinary incontinence in the returned questionnaires was 12.6%. Incontinence was slightly more common in students than in nonstudents (13.2% vs 10.6%). For the subtypes of urinary incontinence, the estimates were 6.2% for stress-only urinary incontinence, 4.5% for urge-only urinary incontinence, and 1.9% for mixed urinary incontinence. Rates of urinary incontinence varied by reported sexual activity (ever or never) and oral contraceptive use. Students who were sexually active and not using an oral contraceptive reported higher rates of urinary incontinence (21.5%) than those who were never sexually active and not using an oral contraceptive (10.1%) or those who were sexually active and using an oral contraceptive (9.7%). Women with urinary incontinence had significantly lower psychological well-being as exemplified by certain questions on the survey than women without urinary incontinence. More than half of women with urinary incontinence reported worrying about odor and almost half were careful about fluid intake or needed to change their underclothes at least sometimes. More than one-third of the women with urinary incontinence reported wearing pads to keep dry.

This report suggests that urinary incontinence may be more of a problem than one might have suspected among never-pregnant women, including teens. This report appears to be the first study of its type to examine urinary incontinence in women who had never been pregnant. It should be noted that the study found no association between urinary incontinence and age, body mass index, physical activity, or history of urinary tract infection. This may have been a consequence of the study cohort being relatively young, physically active, and predominantly of normal body weight.

The finding of a lower psychological well-being among women with urinary incontinence should not be surprising. Urinary incontinence has been associated with a sense of shame and fear of humiliation in prior studies. Younger women have been shown to be subject to greater distress and restriction of activities than older women. One-half of women with urinary incontinence in this report did restrict their fluid intake to prevent leakage and were worried about odor. These findings highlight that the consequences of urinary incontinence in young women are not limited to bothersome symptoms, but include adverse effects on behavior and psychological well-being.

J. A. Stockman III, MD

Comparison of Risk Prediction Using the CKD-EPI Equation and the MDRD Study Equation for Estimated Glomerular Filtration Rate

Matsushita K, for the Chronic Kidney Disease Prognosis Consortium (Johns Hopkins Univ, Baltimore, MD; et al)
JAMA 307:1941-1951, 2012

Context.—The Chronic Kidney Disease Epidemiology Collaboration (CKD-EPI) equation more accurately estimates glomerular filtration rate (GFR) than the Modification of Diet in Renal Disease (MDRD) Study equation using the same variables, especially at higher GFR, but definitive evidence of its risk implications in diverse settings is lacking.

Objective.—To evaluate risk implications of estimated GFR using the CKD-EPI equation compared with the MDRD Study equation in populations with a broad range of demographic and clinical characteristics.

Design, Setting, and Participants.—A meta-analysis of data from 1.1 million adults (aged ≥ 18 years) from 25 general population cohorts, 7 high-risk cohorts (of vascular disease), and 13 CKD cohorts. Data transfer and analyses were conducted between March 2011 and March 2012.

Main Outcome Measures.—All-cause mortality (84 482 deaths from 40 cohorts), cardiovascular mortality (22 176 events from 28 cohorts), and end-stage renal disease (ESRD) (7644 events from 21 cohorts) during 9.4 million person-years of follow-up; the median of mean follow-up time across cohorts was 7.4 years (interquartile range, 4.2-10.5 years).

Results.—Estimated GFR was classified into 6 categories (≥ 90, 60-89, 45-59, 30-44, 15-29, and <15 mL/min/1.73 m^2) by both equations.

Compared with the MDRD Study equation, 24.4% and 0.6% of participants from general population cohorts were reclassified to a higher and lower estimated GFR category, respectively, by the CKD-EPI equation, and the prevalence of CKD stages 3 to 5 (estimated GFR <60 mL/min/1.73 m^2) was reduced from 8.7% to 6.3%. In estimated GFR of 45 to 59 mL/min/1.73 m^2 by the MDRD Study equation, 34.7% of participants were reclassified to estimated GFR of 60 to 89 mL/min/1.73 m^2 by the CKD-EPI equation and had lower incidence rates (per 1000 person-years) for the outcomes of interest (9.9 vs 34.5 for all-cause mortality, 2.7 vs 13.0 for cardiovascular mortality, and 0.5 vs 0.8 for ESRD) compared with those not reclassified. The corresponding adjusted hazard ratios were 0.80 (95% CI, 0.74-0.86) for all-cause mortality, 0.73 (95% CI, 0.65-0.82) for cardiovascular mortality, and 0.49 (95% CI, 0.27-0.88) for ESRD. Similar findings were observed in other estimated GFR categories by the MDRD Study equation. Net reclassification improvement based on estimated GFR categories was significantly positive for all outcomes (range, 0.06-0.13; all $P < .001$). Net reclassification improvement was similarly positive in most subgroups defined by age (<65 years and ≥65 years), sex, race/ethnicity (white, Asian, and black), and presence or absence of diabetes and hypertension. The results in the high-risk and CKD cohorts were largely consistent with the general population cohorts.

Conclusion.—The CKD-EPI equation classified fewer individuals as having CKD and more accurately categorized the risk for mortality and ESRD than did the MDRD Study equation across a broad range of populations.

▶ This article is mostly based on data from adults, but the study did include some teenagers as well. The conclusions from the report are likely accurate for use by pediatricians and pediatric nephrologists.

Glomerular filtration rate (GFR) is used in the diagnosis of chronic kidney disease. Most laboratories no longer report just serum creatinine levels. Rather, they calculate from the serum creatinine an estimated GFR based on characteristics that additionally include height and weight. Indeed, clinical guidelines now recommend reporting estimated GFR when serum creatinine level is measured. Currently, about 85% of laboratories report an estimated GFR. This percentage is probably less in laboratories providing only pediatric services. More recently, however, it has been proposed that an alternative be used to estimate GFR. This alternative applies different coefficients to the same 4 variables used to calculate the estimated GFR (age, sex, race, and serum creatinine level). It is thought that the new equation (known as the Chronic Kidney Disease Epidemiology Collaboration [CKD-EPI] equation) estimates measured GFR more accurately.

These authors have looked at the comparability of 2 methods of calculating estimated GFR to determine the risk implications of estimated GFR using CKD-EPI equations compared with the standard methodology for calculating GFR. They found that 1 in 4 individuals using the new methodology were reclassified as having lesser degrees of chronic renal failure in comparison with the existing methodology used to calculate GFR. The findings from this article largely apply to adults but can be extrapolated to children. With respect to the adult population, tens of thousands of individuals thought to have significant chronic renal failure could be reclassified to have lesser degrees of the problem.

It will be interesting to see how these data are looked at in our pediatric-age populations. All too often we have to use "hand-me-down" studies from adult populations.

J. A. Stockman III, MD

Estimating Glomerular Filtration Rate from Serum Creatinine and Cystatin C
Inker LA, for the CKD EPI Investigators (Tufts Med Ctr, Boston, MA, et al)
N Engl J Med 367:20-29, 2012

Background.—Estimates of glomerular filtration rate (GFR) that are based on serum creatinine are routinely used; however, they are imprecise, potentially leading to the overdiagnosis of chronic kidney disease. Cystatin C is an alternative filtration marker for estimating GFR.

Methods.—Using cross-sectional analyses, we developed estimating equations based on cystatin C alone and in combination with creatinine in diverse populations totaling 5352 participants from 13 studies. These equations were then validated in 1119 participants from 5 different studies in which GFR had been measured. Cystatin and creatinine assays were traceable to primary reference materials.

Results.—Mean measured GFRs were 68 and 70 ml per minute per 1.73 m^2 of body-surface area in the development and validation data sets, respectively. In the validation data set, the creatinine−cystatin C equation performed better than equations that used creatinine or cystatin C alone. Bias was similar among the three equations, with a median difference between measured and estimated GFR of 3.9 ml per minute per 1.73 m^2 with the combined equation, as compared with 3.7 and 3.4 ml per minute per 1.73 m^2 with the creatinine equation and the cystatin C equation ($P = 0.07$ and $P = 0.05$), respectively. Precision was improved with the combined equation (interquartile range of the difference, 13.4 vs. 15.4 and 16.4 ml per minute per 1.73 m^2, respectively [$P = 0.001$ and $P < 0.001$]), and the results were more accurate (percentage of estimates that were >30% of measured GFR, 8.5 vs. 12.8 and 14.1, respectively [$P < 0.001$ for both comparisons]). In participants whose estimated GFR based on creatinine was 45 to 74 ml per minute per 1.73 m^2, the combined equation improved the classification of measured GFR as either less than 60 ml per minute per 1.73 m^2 or greater than or equal to 60 ml per minute per 1.73 m^2 (net reclassification index, 19.4% [$P < 0.001$]) and correctly reclassified 16.9% of those with an estimated GFR of 45 to 59 ml per minute per 1.73 m^2 as having a GFR of 60 ml or higher per minute per 1.73 m^2.

Conclusions.—The combined creatinine−cystatin C equation performed better than equations based on either of these markers alone and may be useful as a confirmatory test for chronic kidney disease. (Funded by the National Institute of Diabetes and Digestive and Kidney Diseases.)

▶ There is a fair amount being written today about better ways to improve estimating glomerular filtration rates (GFR). This article describes a new combined creatinine–cystatin-C estimating equation that provides greater precision and accuracy for classification of the GFR. Most clinicians are familiar with the fact that clinical laboratories now routinely report an estimated GFR when a serum creatinine is measured. Unfortunately, such GFR estimates are relatively imprecise because of the variation in non-GFR determinants of serum creatinine, which may be affected in both acute and chronic illnesses. Such imprecision can either over-estimate or underestimate the likelihood of chronic renal failure, particularly in teenagers and adults.

For those who are not familiar with cystatin-C, it is considered to be an alternative to serum creatinine for estimating GFR. In recent years, it has been consistently shown to be a better marker than creatinine. Estimated GFR based on cystatin-C in fact could be used as a confirmatory test for an adverse prognosis in patients suspected of having chronic kidney disease. That is exactly what this article shows, specifically that combined creatinine–cystatin-C determined together appears to produce a very accurate assessment of GFR.

In an editorial that accompanied this article, Weir[1] tells us how important this particular report is. It reminds us that automated reporting of GFR has generally resulted in earlier recognition of chronic kidney disease in all age groups, but misdiagnosis remains an important concern. This is a particularly important issue for the elderly population in whom gradual onset of chronic kidney disease is common, but it still applies to pediatrics as well. Weir[1] suggests that this new improved estimating formula using creatinine and cystatin-C could be used as a confirmatory test for kidney disease in patients whose estimated GFR, derived from a creatinine-based formula, is right on the cusp of a number suggesting chronic renal failure (60 mL/min/1.73 m^2).

All clinicians should stay tuned to the story regarding GFR determination based on both creatinine and cystatin-C. There is probably a lot more we will learn in the next few years about this.

J. A. Stockman III, MD

Reference

1. Weir MR. Improving the estimating equation for GFR—A clinical perspective. *N Engl J Med*. 2012;367:75-76.

Peginesatide for Anemia in Patients with Chronic Kidney Disease Not Receiving Dialysis

Macdougall IC, for the PEARL Study Groups (King's College Hosp, London, UK; et al)
N Engl J Med 368:320-332, 2013

Background.—Peginesatide is a peptide-based erythropoiesis-stimulating agent (ESA) that may have therapeutic potential for anemia in patients with advanced chronic kidney disease. We evaluated the safety and efficacy of peginesatide, as compared with another ESA, darbepoetin, in 983 such patients who were not undergoing dialysis.

Methods.—In two randomized, controlled, open-label studies (PEARL 1 and 2), patients received peginesatide once a month, at a starting dose of 0.025 mg or 0.04 mg per kilogram of body weight, or darbepoetin once every 2 weeks, at a starting dose of 0.75 µg per kilogram. Doses of both drugs were adjusted to achieve and maintain hemoglobin levels between 11.0 and 12.0 g per deciliter for 52 weeks or more. The primary efficacy end point was the mean change from the baseline hemoglobin level to the mean level during the evaluation period; noninferiority was established if the lower limit of the two-sided 97.5% confidence interval was -1.0 g per deciliter or higher. Cardiovascular safety was evaluated on the basis of an adjudicated composite end point.

Results.—In both studies and at both starting doses, peginesatide was noninferior to darbepoetin in increasing and maintaining hemoglobin levels. The mean differences in the hemoglobin level with peginesatide as compared with darbepoetin in PEARL 1 were 0.03 g per deciliter (97.5% confidence interval [CI], -0.19 to 0.26) for the lower starting dose of peginesatide and 0.26 g per deciliter (97.5% CI, 0.04 to 0.48) for the higher starting dose, and in PEARL 2 they were 0.14 g per deciliter (97.5% CI, -0.09 to 0.36) and 0.31 g per deciliter (97.5% CI, 0.08 to 0.54), respectively. The hazard ratio for the cardiovascular safety end point was 1.32 (95% CI, 0.97 to 1.81) for peginesatide relative to darbepoetin, with higher incidences of death, unstable angina, and arrhythmia with peginesatide.

Conclusions.—The efficacy of peginesatide (administered monthly) was similar to that of darbepoetin (administered every 2 weeks) in increasing and maintaining hemoglobin levels. However, cardiovascular events and mortality were increased with peginesatide in patients with chronic kidney disease who were not undergoing dialysis. (Funded by Affymax and Takeda Pharmaceutical; ClinicalTrials.gov numbers, NCT00598273 [PEARL 1], NCT00598442 [PEARL 2], NCT00597753 [EMERALD 1], and NCT00597584 [EMERALD 2].)

▶ This study did include older teenage patients, and, therefore, the information provided is of significant relevance to the care of children, at least in the older age set of children with chronic renal failure.

We all know that a major problem associated with chronic renal failure is the development of anemia, with all of its signs and symptoms. When it becomes severe enough, both children and adults with chronic renal failure are given erythropoiesis-stimulating agents to help correct their anemia instead of what was done years ago, treatment with transfusional therapy. The introduction of erythropoiesis-stimulating agents has markedly improved the lives of many patients with chronic renal disease who in the past would have been transfusion dependent. The most commonly used erythropoiesis-stimulating agents have been varieties of recombinant human erythropoietin. Recombinant human erythropoietin is highly effective but short acting. More recently, second-generation products have become available with an extended duration of action, in particular darbepoetin-α, which has an altered glycosylation pattern and a continuous erythropoietin-receptor activator called methoxy polyethylene glycol-epoetin-β. This is the first product approved for dosing every 2 weeks and the second for dosing once a month.

Although many are using variations of these agents to correct anemia, we have learned, at least in older patients, that it is best to leave the anemia only partially corrected in order to avoid now well-known cardiovascular complications of normal or slightly high hemoglobin levels. Unfortunately, it is not known whether these negative effects of the complete correction of anemia are caused primarily by high hemoglobin levels, from excessive use of erythropoiesis-stimulating agents, or both.

These authors report the results of several randomized, controlled, open-label trials that have compared the efficacy of peginesatide with standard erythropoiesis-stimulating agents. The former is a peptide-based erythropoietic agent, a dimeric pegylated peptide. Peptide-based erythropoietic agents such as peginesatide are not homologous with erythropoietin and therefore exhibit no antibody cross-activity. This means that patients with transfusion-dependent chronic kidney disease without antibody-mediated pure red cell aplasia may be "rescued" after treatment with drugs of this class. Peginesatide has been recently approved in the United States for patients undergoing hemodialysis but not for patients who are not receiving hemodialysis. One of the advantages of this drug is that it requires less-frequent dosing and does not induce pure red cell aplasia, but antibody development against this compound, although infrequent, may reduce its efficacy.

The authors show that peginesatide can be administered monthly and its effect is similar to that of other erythropoiesis-stimulating agents in increasing and maintaining hemoglobin levels. Unfortunately, cardiovascular events and mortality were shown to be slightly increased in patients with chronic renal disease who were not undergoing dialysis. As with any new class of drugs, prolonged exposure and monitoring will be necessary to know what the benefit–risk ratio is of this new class of erythropoiesis-stimulating agents. Another issue is cost. Expensive new drugs like peginesatide will need to be proven to be significantly better than older erythropoiesis-stimulating agents if they are to be a substitute for the latter. Only time will tell whether this is true.

J. A. Stockman III, MD

Tolvaptan in Patients with Autosomal Dominant Polycystic Kidney Disease

Torres VE, for the TEMPO 3:4 Trial Investigators (Mayo Clinic, Rochester, MN; et al)

N Engl J Med 367:2407-2418, 2012

Background.—The course of autosomal dominant polycystic kidney disease (ADPKD) is often associated with pain, hypertension, and kidney failure. Preclinical studies indicated that vasopressin V_2-receptor antagonists inhibit cyst growth and slow the decline of kidney function.

Methods.—In this phase 3, multicenter, double-blind, placebo-controlled, 3-year trial, we randomly assigned 1445 patients, 18 to 50 years of age, who had ADPKD with a total kidney volume of 750 ml or more and an estimated creatinine clearance of 60 ml per minute or more, in a 2:1 ratio to receive tolvaptan, a V_2-receptor antagonist, at the highest of three twice daily dose regimens that the patient found tolerable, or placebo. The primary outcome was the annual rate of change in the total kidney volume. Sequential secondary end points included a composite of time to clinical progression (defined as worsening kidney function, kidney pain, hypertension, and albuminuria) and rate of kidney-function decline.

Results.—Over a 3-year period, the increase in total kidney volume in the tolvaptan group was 2.8% per year (95% confidence interval [CI], 2.5 to 3.1), versus 5.5% per year in the placebo group (95% CI, 5.1 to 6.0; $P < 0.001$). The composite end point favored tolvaptan over placebo (44 vs. 50 events per 100 follow-up-years, $P = 0.01$), with lower rates of worsening kidney function (2 vs. 5 events per 100 person-years of followup, $P < 0.001$) and kidney pain (5 vs. 7 events per 100 person-years of followup, $P = 0.007$). Tolvaptan was associated with a slower decline in kidney function (reciprocal of the serum creatinine level, -2.61 [mg per milliliter]$^{-1}$ per year vs. -3.81 [mg per milliliter]$^{-1}$ per year; $P < 0.001$). There were fewer ADPKD-related adverse events in the tolvaptan group but more events related to aquaresis (excretion of electrolyte-free water) and hepatic adverse events unrelated to ADPKD, contributing to a higher discontinuation rate (23%, vs. 14% in the placebo group).

Conclusions.—Tolvaptan, as compared with placebo, slowed the increase in total kidney volume and the decline in kidney function over a 3-year period in patients with ADPKD but was associated with a higher discontinuation rate, owing to adverse events. (Funded by Otsuka Pharmaceuticals and Otsuka Pharmaceutical Development and Commercialization; TEMPO 3:4 ClinicalTrials.gov number, NCT00428948.)

▶ Autosomal dominant polycystic kidney disease (ADPKD) remains the most common kidney disease of genetic origins and is among a handful of leading causes of end-stage renal disease. The disorder generally results in death by the sixth decade of life in about half of affected individuals. It results in the ongoing development of renal cysts, kidney pain, hypertension, and renal failure. Thus far, there have been no effective therapies to halt the progression of the disorder. It has been suggested from animal studies that the antidiuretic hormone arginine vasopressin and its messenger adenosine-3-, 5-cyclic monophosphate (cAMP) promote kidney cyst formation. In animal studies, the suppression of vasopressin release by pharmacologic or other means slows the progression of cyst formation. One such agent appears to be tolvaptan, a vasopressin V_2-receptor antagonist. This is a drug that is approved for the treatment of dilutional hyponatremia or volume overload in heart failure in various parts of the world.

The Tolvaptan Efficacy and Safety in Management of Autosomal Dominant Polycystic Kidney Disease and Its Outcomes (TEMPO) 3:4 trial, a large, phase II study, reported by these authors, evaluated the efficacy of tolvaptan in more than 1400 patients with ADPKD. At baseline, the mean age of participating patients was 39 years. Kidney function was preserved, but nearly 80% of the patients had hypertension. Kidney size was increased by a factor of 5, and half the patients who were enrolled in this study reported kidney pain. The study met its primary and secondary endpoints: Tolvaptan, when given at an average dose of 95 mg per day over a 3-year period, slowed the usual increase in kidney volume by 50% and reduced the decline in glomerular filtration rate (GFR). Part of the reduction in kidney volume was likely a result of early reduction in the secretion of cysts fluid. The effect on GFR became apparent only after the first year of treatment. Unfortunately, a number of patients treated with this drug discontinued tolvaptan because of its aquaretic side effects, namely, thirst, polydipsia, polyuria, and nocturia. Tolvaptan treatment was also associated with elevated liver enzymes, hypernatremia, and increased levels of uric acid and gout. Nonetheless, compared with patients who were in the placebo control group, significantly fewer patients who received tolvaptan had adverse events related to their kidney disease, such as kidney and back pain, hematuria, and urinary tract infection.

Obviously, the study, although undertaken in adults, has clear implications for insights into what might turn out to be the long-term best types of therapy for management of children with polycystic kidney disease. We do not know if tolvaptan might be a useful treatment for the majority of patients with the disorder or whether it is best prescribed for those at greatest risk for progression to end-stage renal disease. The side effects of an aquaretic drug will affect the quality of life in a very substantial number of patients treated with it. This needs to be weighed against the possible effects of delayed dialysis and transplantation, decreased kidney pain, and fewer urinary tract infections. Some patients may opt out of such treatments by receiving preemptive kidney transplantation before the initiation of dialysis rather than undergo treatment with a drug that has such bothersome side effects. Those patients who for whatever reason begin to rapidly progress might choose a short-term therapy with drugs that do have side effects. In any event, we now have at least 1 class of drugs that does show some effectiveness in the management of a disease for which no therapy previously was available.

J. A. Stockman III, MD

9 Heart and Blood Vessels

Azithromycin and the Risk of Cardiovascular Death
Ray WA, Murray KT, Hall K, et al (Vanderbilt Univ School of Medicine, Nashville, TN)
N Engl J Med 366:1881-1890, 2012

Background.—Although several macrolide antibiotics are proarrhythmic and associated with an increased risk of sudden cardiac death, azithromycin is thought to have minimal cardiotoxicity. However, published reports of arrhythmias suggest that azithromycin may increase the risk of cardiovascular death.

Methods.—We studied a Tennessee Medicaid cohort designed to detect an increased risk of death related to short-term cardiac effects of medication, excluding patients with serious noncardiovascular illness and person-time during and shortly after hospitalization. The cohort included patients who took azithromycin (347,795 prescriptions), propensity-score—matched persons who took no antibiotics (1,391,180 control periods), and patients who took amoxicillin (1,348,672 prescriptions), ciprofloxacin (264,626 prescriptions), or levofloxacin (193,906 prescriptions).

Results.—During 5 days of therapy, patients taking azithromycin, as compared with those who took no antibiotics, had an increased risk of cardiovascular death (hazard ratio, 2.88; 95% confidence interval [CI], 1.79 to 4.63; $P < 0.001$) and death from any cause (hazard ratio, 1.85; 95% CI, 1.25 to 2.75; $P = 0.002$). Patients who took amoxicillin had no increase in the risk of death during this period. Relative to amoxicillin, azithromycin was associated with an increased risk of cardiovascular death (hazard ratio, 2.49; 95% CI, 1.38 to 4.50; $P = 0.002$) and death from any cause (hazard ratio, 2.02; 95% CI, 1.24 to 3.30; $P = 0.005$), with an estimated 47 additional cardiovascular deaths per 1 million courses; patients in the highest decile of risk for cardiovascular disease had an estimated 245 additional cardiovascular deaths per 1 million courses. The risk of cardiovascular death was significantly greater with azithromycin than with ciprofloxacin but did not differ significantly from that with levofloxacin.

Conclusions.—During 5 days of azithromycin therapy, there was a small absolute increase in cardiovascular deaths, which was most pronounced among patients with a high baseline risk of cardiovascular disease. (Funded by the National Heart, Lung, and Blood Institute and the Agency for Healthcare Quality and Research Centers for Education and Research on Therapeutics.)

▶ Although this article deals with a side effect of azithromycin in adults, this broad spectrum macrolide antibiotic could theoretically have exactly the same set of consequences in children if they were so predisposed in terms of existing heart disease. It is well known that 2 related drugs, erythromycin and clarithromycin, can increase the risk of ventricular arrhythmias and are associated with an increased risk of sudden death. Accumulating evidence has begun to indicate that azithromycin may also have proarrhythmic effects. There are more than half a dozen published reports of patients with normal baseline QT intervals in whom azithromycin had arrhythmia-related adverse cardiac effects, including pronounced QT-interval prolongation, torsades de pointes, and polymorphic ventricular tachycardia, the latter in the absence of QT-interval prolongation. The US Food and Drug Administration's Adverse Event Reporting System includes at least 20 reports of torsades de pointes associated with azithromycin.[1] Many pediatric websites have picked up on this relationship between azithromycin and arrhythmias in adults and have suggested that this antibiotic should be used very cautiously in children who have underlying cardiac problems, including arrhythmias that might predispose them to the development of ventricular tachycardia or ventricular fibrillation.

These authors studied the Tennessee Medicaid Database that included over one-third of a million prescriptions for azithromycin and were able to compare reported side effects in over a million individuals prescribed common antibiotics. Among patients who took azithromycin, there were 29 cardiovascular deaths during a typical 5-day course of treatment. Of these, 22 were sudden cardiac deaths. Compared with other commonly used antibiotics such as amoxicillin, azithromycin was associated with almost a 3-fold increased risk for sudden cardiac death and other cardiovascular deaths. This increase in the risk of cardiovascular death was most pronounced in patients who were among the upper 10% of risk factors for cardiovascular disease. There was no increased risk of death from non-cardiovascular causes among patients who took azithromycin.

It should be noted that the increased risk of cardiovascular death during a usual 5-day course of azithromycin does not persist after a course of the antibiotic has ended. Although concentrations of azithromycin remain elevated in tissues for several days after cessation of oral therapy, serum concentrations decline more rapidly. As with many other drugs with proarrhythmic effects, an elevated serum concentration is a key determinant of increased risk, which is an important reason why rapid infusion of erythromycin is not recommended at any age. Again, the mean age of the patients evaluated as part of this study from Tennessee data was that of a young, middle-aged adult population (mean age 48.6 years). This does not mean that children are off scot-free, however. It would be wise to be cautious about the use of this antibiotic in children who have underlying structural or rhythm cardiac abnormalities.

J. A. Stockman III, MD

Reference

1. Poluzzi E, Raschi E, Moretti U, De Ponti F. Drug-induced torsades de pointes: data mining of the public version of the FDA Adverse Event Reporting System (AERS). *Pharmacoepidemiol Drug Saf.* 2009;18:512-518.

Tracking of clustered cardiovascular disease risk factors from childhood to adolescence

Bugge A, El-Naaman B, McMurray RG, et al (Univ of Southern Denmark, Odense, Denmark; Univ of North Carolina, Chapel Hill)
Pediatr Res 73:245-249, 2013

Background.—Clustering of cardiovascular disease (CVD) risk factors has been found in children as young as 9 y of age. However, the stability of this clustering over the course of childhood has yet to be determined. The purpose of this study was to determine the tracking of clustered CVD risk from young school age through adolescence and to examine differences in tracking between levels of overweight/obesity and cardiorespiratory fitness (VO_{2peak}).

Methods.—Beginning at 6 y, children ($n − 434$) were measured three times in 7 y. Anthropometrics, blood pressure, and VO_{2peak} were measured. Fasting blood samples were analyzed for CVD risk factors. A clustered risk score (z-score) was constructed by adding sex-specific z-scores for blood pressure, homeostatic model assessment (HOMA-IR), triglyceride (TG), skinfolds, and negative values of high-density lipoprotein cholesterol (HDLc) and VO_{2peak}.

Results.—Significant tracking coefficients were found between clustered z-score at all time intervals ($r = 0.514$, 0.559, and 0.381 between ages 6−9, 9−13, and 6−13 y, respectively, all $P < 0.0001$). Tracking was higher for low-fit children, whereas no clear pattern was found for different levels of body fat.

Conclusion.—We found that clustered z-score is a fairly stable characteristic through childhood. Implementation of preventive strategies could therefore start at early school age.

▶ This report makes some interesting and important observations. The report notes that 3 or more cardiovascular disease risk factors have been found in more than 3 times as many participants than expected based on data from one of their earlier studies. This corresponds to 13.8% of the population in young children.[1] It is generally accepted that despite differences seen in many study designs, the literature has consistently documented the finding of the tracking of cardiometabolic risk factors clustering from childhood and adolescence into adulthood.[2] These clusterings are largely related to lifestyle factors, including obesity and cardiorespiratory fitness.

The authors of this report designed a study to evaluate the tracking of cardiovascular risk factors in young children using 3 time points from 6 to 13 years of age and also examined how different levels of overweight/obesity and cardiorespiratory fitness influence these risk factors. Only one study before this one in children has examined the effect of obesity on tracking of clustered factors, and no prior studies have looked at the effect of cardiorespiratory status in detail. Needless to say, the study was examining only the short-term tracking of a clustering of such risk factors in an otherwise normal youth population from early school age to the beginning of adolescence. This report observed moderate to high levels of tracking between all of the measured time points. Depending on the risk factor examined, when compared with baseline, children who had a risk factor at the first time point studied were 2.3 times to 30.8 times more likely to have the same cardiovascular risk factor in later childhood.

The authors of this report concluded that moderate to strong tracking can be observed between the ages of 6 years and 13 years when it comes to cardiovascular risk factors. The bottom line is if you have cardiometabolic risk factors in young childhood, chances are overwhelming that these will track through your entire school-age grouping of children. These results have important implications for instituting preventative strategy in early childhood.

While on the topic of the impact of things that can shorten one's life, it is interesting to observe new information about how long we can expect to live. Data from Great Britain suggest that around 13% of girls born in 1951 are expected to be alive in 2051. For girls born in 2013, nearly 40% are estimated to be alive in 2113. It is further estimated that around 60% of girls born in 2016 might expect to live long enough to receive a message from the reigning British monarch that they had reached the 100-year mark in life. Changes in the global burden of disease have shown that part of this is because of a significant decrease in the number of deaths in children less than 5 years, which has declined by some 60% when compared with 1970.[3]

J. A. Stockman III, MD

References

1. Andersen LB, Bugge A, Dencker M, Eiberg S, El-Naaman B. The association between physical activity, physical fitness and development of metabolic disorders. *Int J Pediatr Obes.* 2011;1:29-34.
2. Camhi SM, Katzmarzyk PT. Tracking of cardiometabolic risk factor clustering from childhood to adulthood. *Int J Pediatr Obes.* 2010;5:122-129.
3. Appleby J. How long can we expect to live. *BMJ.* 2013;346:f331.

Effect of physical inactivity on major non-communicable diseases worldwide: an analysis of burden of disease and life expectancy
Lee I-M, for the Lancet Physical Activity Series Working Group (Harvard Med School, Boston, MA; et al)
Lancet 379:219-229, 2012

Background.—Strong evidence shows that physical inactivity increases the risk of many adverse health conditions, including major non-communicable diseases such as coronary heart disease, type 2 diabetes, and breast and colon cancers, and shortens life expectancy. Because much of the world's population is inactive, this link presents a major public health issue. We aimed to quantify the effect of physical inactivity on these major non-communicable diseases by estimating how much disease could be averted if inactive people were to become active and to estimate gain in life expectancy at the population level.

Methods.—For our analysis of burden of disease, we calculated population attributable fractions (PAFs) associated with physical inactivity using conservative assumptions for each of the major non-communicable diseases, by country, to estimate how much disease could be averted if physical inactivity were eliminated. We used life-table analysis to estimate gains in life expectancy of the population.

Findings.—Worldwide, we estimate that physical inactivity causes 6% (ranging from 3·2% in southeast Asia to 7·8% in the eastern Mediterranean region) of the burden of disease from coronary heart disease, 7% (3·9–9·6) of type 2 diabetes, 10% (5·6–14·1) of breast cancer, and 10% (5·7–13·8) of colon cancer. Inactivity causes 9% (range 5·1–12·5) of premature mortality, or more than 5·3 million of the 57 million deaths that occurred worldwide in 2008. If inactivity were not eliminated, but decreased instead by 10% or 25%, more than 533 000 and more than 1·3 million deaths, respectively, could be averted every year. We estimated that elimination of physical inactivity would increase the life expectancy of the world's population by 0·68 (range 0·41–0·95) years.

Interpretation.—Physical inactivity has a major health effect worldwide. Decrease in or removal of this unhealthy behaviour could improve health substantially.

▶ Readers of my work most likely know that I abhor exercise as much as I do getting a flat tire, but ancient physicians, including those from China in 2600 BC and Hippocrates as early as 400 BC, believed in the value of physical activity for health. Plato is also said to have remarked "lack of activity destroys the good condition of every human being while movement and methodical physical exercise save it and preserve it."[1] We now know that physical activity is a significant predictor of cardiovascular disease, type 2 diabetes mellitus, obesity, some cancers, poor skeletal health, some aspects of mental health, and overall mortality as well as poor quality of life. Men and women of all ages, socioeconomic groups, and ethnicities are healthier if they achieve the public health recommendation of at least 150 minutes per week of moderate-intensity aerobic physical activity, such as brisk walking. Immediate and future health benefits are also clearly described for children and adolescents for whom at least 60 minutes per day of vigorous or moderate physical activity is recommended. Data from 2008 show that 63% of deaths worldwide were due to noncommunicable diseases, mainly diseases of the heart and vascular system, diabetes mellitus, cancers, and obstructive pulmonary disease. Compared with inactive individuals, those who are active, but at levels less than recommended (about 1.5 hours per week), have been shown to live about 3 years longer.

Lee et al calculated population-attributable fractions associated with physical inactivity by country to estimate how much disease could be averted if physical inactivity were eliminated. The authors estimated that physical inactivity causes 6% to 10% of the major noncommunicable diseases of coronary artery disease, type 2 diabetes, and breast and colon cancers. They also calculated that unhealthy behavior in this regard causes 9% of premature mortality or more than 5.3 million of the 57 million deaths occurring annually. With elimination of physical inactivity, it is projected that life expectancy of the world's population could be expected to increase by 0.68 years. These findings make physical inactivity similar to the established risk factors of smoking and obesity. Needless to say, these are only averages. For individuals who move from inactive to active, one might expect a greater increase in life expectancy. Studies done here in the United States have estimated that inactive people would gain 1.3 to 3.7 years from age 50 by becoming active.

I guess it is time to get moving.

J. A. Stockman III, MD

Reference

1. Das P, Horton R. Rethinking our approach to physical activity. *Lancet*. 2012;380: 189-190.

Serum uric acid in US adolescents: distribution and relationship to demographic characteristics and cardiovascular risk factors
Shatat IF, Abdallah RT, Sas DJ, et al (Med Univ of South Carolina Children's Hosp, Charleston; et al)
Pediatr Res 72:95-100, 2012

Introduction.—Despite being associated with multiple disease processes and cardiovascular outcomes, uric acid (UA) reference ranges for adolescents are lacking. We sought to describe the distribution of UA and its relationship to demographic, clinical, socioeconomic, and dietary factors in US adolescents.

Methods.—A nationally representative subsample of 1,912 adolescents 13—18 y of age, from the National Health and Nutrition Examination Survey (NHANES) for the years 2005—2008 representing 19,888,299 adolescents, was used for this study. Percentiles of the distribution of UA were estimated using quantile regression. Linear regression models examined the association of UA with demographic, socioeconomic, and dietary factors.

Results.—The mean UA level was 5.14 ± 1.45 mg/dl. It increased with increasing age and was higher in non-Hispanic whites, male sex, those with higher BMI z-scores, and those with higher systolic blood pressure (BP). In fully adjusted linear regression models, sex, age, race, and BMI were independent determinants of higher UA.

TABLE 1.—Nationally Representative Percentiles of Uric Acid Distribution in 13—18-y-Old Persons, NHANES 2005—2008

| | Uric Acid (mg/l)[a] Weighted Percentiles | | | | | | | |
	1st	5th	25th	50th	75th	95th	99th	*n*
Overall	2.80	3.40	4.20	5.00	5.00	7.40	8.70	1,912
13—14 y	2.80	3.40	4.20	4.80	5.60	6.90	8.30	607
15—16 y	2.80	3.40	4.10	5.00	5.80	7.60	8.50	666
17—18 y	2.80	3.50	4.40	5.30	6.00	7.90	9.50	639
Male	3.30	4.10	5.10	5.70	6.40	8.00	9.50	939
Female	2.50	3.20	3.90	4.40	5.00	5.90	6.60	973
Non-Hispanic white	2.80	3.50	4.30	5.10	5.90	7.60	8.70	579
Male	3.40	4.20	5.10	5.80	6.40	8.10	9.70	287
Female	2.50	3.20	4.00	4.50	5.20	6.10	6.60	292
Non-Hispanic black	2.50	3.30	4.00	4.80	5.60	6.80	8.40	567
Male	3.10	4.00	4.80	5.40	6.10	7.30	8.50	280
Female	2.20	2.90	3.70	4.20	4.80	5.80	6.90	287
Mexican American	2.90	3.20	4.00	4.90	5.80	7.30	7.90	541
Male	3.30	4.20	5.00	5.60	6.60	7.70	8.50	262
Female	2.70	3.00	3.70	4.10	4.90	5.90	6.20	279

NHANES, National Health and Nutrition Examination Survey.
[a]Uric acid conversion from conventional units to SI units: 1 mg/dl = 59.48 μmol/l.

Discussion.—This study defines serum UA reference ranges for adolescents. It also reveals some intriguing relationships between UA and demographic and clinical characteristics that warrant further studies to examine the pathophysiological role of UA in various disease processes (Table 1).

▶ More information has appeared in the literature in recent years linking elevated uric acid levels to a variety of problems in both adults and children. In humans and higher primates, uric acid is the final oxidation product of purine metabolism and is excreted in the urine. Elevated serum uric acid levels result either exogenously from increased intake of purine-rich foods, or endogenously from increased production as seen in certain malignancies and inborn errors of metabolism. Increased uric acid levels can also result from decreased renal clearance.

The literature shows a relationship between uric acid homeostasis and health and disease. For example, elevated uric acid levels are associated with hypertension as well as with diabetes, cardiovascular disease, endothelial dysfunction, obesity, metabolic syndrome, nephrolithiasis, intellectual disability, and all-cause mortality. Unfortunately, despite multiple investigations into the relationship between uric acid and hypertension in children, little is known about the normal range of serum uric acid levels in children and adolescents. Shatat et al add to our knowledge by examining serum uric acid distributions in a large, nationally representative group of adolescents in the United States as well as examining the relationship between uric acid values and dietary and demographic variables including a potential relationship with hypertension. Almost 2000 adolescents, 13 to 18 years of age, were reviewed using data from the National Health and Nutrition Examination Survey for the years 2005 to 2008.

Table 1 shows the percentiles of uric acid distribution in the teenage cohort examined in this study.

The study showed that the mean uric acid in teenagers is 5.14 to 1.45 mg/dL (range 1st 99th percentile, 2.8–8.7 mg/dL). Uric acid levels were found to be higher in boys than in girls. Levels increase with body mass index in a linear fashion. The study also found a relationship between socioeconomic status and obesity in both children and adults with the highest uric acid levels associated with the highest percentage of children living in poverty, whereas uric acid levels in the range 4.3 to 5.1 mg/dL were associated with the lowest percentage of poverty. A strong association was found between uric acid levels and the presence of hypertension.

As we learn more about the relationship between uric acid and certain cardiovascular risk factors, it is likely that guidelines will be developed for both detecting and managing uric acid levels in children and adolescents. It is far too early to tell exactly where data from the report of Shatat et al will lead us, but the report is an important one as it is the first to clearly define serum uric acid levels in adolescents.

J. A. Stockman III, MD

Trends in Serum Lipids Among US Youths Aged 6 to 19 Years, 1988-2010
Kit BK, Carroll MD, Lacher DA, et al (Natl Ctr for Health Statistics, Hyattsville, MD; et al)
JAMA 308:591-600, 2012

Context.—For more than 20 years, primary prevention of coronary heart disease has included strategies intended to improve overall serum lipid concentrations among youths.

Objective.—To examine trends in lipid concentrations among youths from 1988-1994 through 2007-2010.

Design, Setting, and Participants.—Cross-sectional analysis of serum lipid concentrations among 16 116 youths aged 6 to 19 years who participated in the nationally representative National Health and Nutrition Examination Survey during 3 time periods: 1988-1994, 1999-2002, and 2007-2010.

Main Outcome Measures.—Among all youths, mean serum total cholesterol (TC), non–high-density lipoprotein cholesterol (non–HDL-C), high-density lipoprotein cholesterol (HDL-C); and among adolescents only, low-density lipoprotein cholesterol (LDL-C) and geometric mean triglyceride levels. Trends in adverse lipid concentrations are reported for TC levels of 200 mg/dL and greater, non–HDL-C levels of 145 mg/dL and greater, HDL-C levels of less than 40 mg/dL, LDL-C levels of 130 mg/dL and greater, and triglyceride levels of 130 mg/dL and greater.

Results.—Among youths aged 6 to 19 years between 1988-1994 and 2007-2010, there was a decrease in mean TC (from 165 mg/dL [95% CI, 164-167] to 160 mg/dL [95% CI, 158-161]; $P < .001$) and a decrease in the prevalence of elevated TC (from 11.3% [95% CI, 9.8%-12.7%] to 8.1% [95% CI, 6.7%-9.5%]; $P = .002$). Mean HDL-C significantly increased between 1988-1994 and 2007-2010, but the prevalence of low HDL-C did not change. Mean non–HDL-C and prevalence of elevated non–HDL-C both significantly decreased over the study period. In 2007-2010, 22% (95% CI, 20.3%-23.6%) of youths had either a low HDL-C level or high non–HDL-C, which was lower than the 27.2% (95% CI, 24.6%-29.7%) in 1988-1994 (P —.001). Among adolescents (aged 12-19 years) between 1988-1994 and 2007-2010, there was a decrease in mean LDL-C (from 95 mg/dL [95% CI, 92-98] to 90 mg/dL [95% CI, 88-91]; P =.003) and a decrease in geometric mean triglycerides (from 82 mg/dL [95% CI, 78-86] to 73 mg/dL [95% CI, 70-76]; P < .001). Prevalence of elevated LDL-C and triglycerides between 1988-1994 and 2007-2010 also significantly decreased.

Conclusions.—Between 1988-1994 and 2007-2010, a favorable trend in serum lipid concentrations was observed among youths in the United States but almost 1 in 10 had elevated TC in 2007-2010.

▶ It is not clear why, but youngsters in the United States finally are seeing improvements in their overall cholesterol levels.[1] Improvement in lipid values in children and adolescents as reported by Kit et al provides remarkable reason for optimism. In this study based on cross-sectional National Health and Nutrition Examination Survey (NHANES) data involving more than 16 000 participants from 1988 through 1994 and 2007 through 2010 were reviewed. The authors report that total cholesterol levels declined a mean of 5 mg/dL in children 16 to 19 years of age over the past 2 decades. Non-high-density lipoprotein (non-HDL) decreased a mean of 8 mg/dL across all ages. Low-density lipoprotein (LDL) and triglyceride levels both declined (5 mg/dL and 9 mg/dL, respectively). Furthermore, HDL increased by 2 mg/dL.

An editorial that accompanied this report by de Ferranti discusses the potential reasons why childhood cholesterol levels seem to have improved.[2] With increasing pediatric obesity, a decrease in physical activity, and an increase in screen time, along with poor overall diet, one would think that lipid levels would be moving in the wrong direction rather than the opposite. Several possibilities, however, might explain the results found by Kit et al. It is conceivable that the data reported are inaccurate. That is highly unlikely given the careful nature with which the NHANES studies have been conducted. Another possible explanation is that the changes in pediatric lipid levels reported by Kit et al merely represent a temporary decline that will worsen in the coming years. However, cholesterol levels also declined in adults between 1960 and 2006, according to the NHANES data, suggesting a population-wide trend that may be at play during childhood. A plausible explanation for improved childhood lipid values could be individual interventions to improve cardiovascular disease risk factors, either lifestyle modification or pharmacologic treatments. For a number of years now, lipid-lowering interventions have been recommended by the American Academy of Pediatrics and the American Heart Association, including the use of statins for select high-risk children. Although there has not been a wholesale stampede to the use of statins in children, clearly a number of high-risk children are now being treated who were not being treated before.

Is it possible that improvements in serum lipids are the result of healthier life-styles? All the data to date suggest that US children are unlikely to be following heart-healthy habits. Overall, Kit et al found improved HDL and lower triglycer-ides suggesting that changes in childhood obesity rates are not the cause of the lipid values reported. A more plausible explanation for the cholesterol improve-ment is dietary shifts at a population level. Indeed, dietary intake of fat has declined over the past several decades and some studies suggest that substitu-tion of carbohydrates for dietary fat, particularly poor-quality high carbohydrates, might promote obesity yet explain some of the lipid changes reported by Kit et al. The wholesale decline in the use of trans fats as a food preservative may also play a role.

It will be interesting to see if the improvements in childhood and adolescent lipid levels over the past 2 decades are sustained. If so and if the trends continue, they should have important impact on outcomes related to cardiovas-cular disease.

J. A. Stockman III, MD

References

1. Roger VL, Go AS, Lloyd-Jones DM, et al; American Heart Association Statistics Committee and Stroke Statistics Subcommittee. Heart disease and stroke statistics — 2012 update: a report from the American Heart Association. *Circulation.* 2012;125: e2-e220.
2. de Ferranti SD. Declining cholesterol levels in US youths: a reason for optimism. *JAMA.* 2012;308:621-622.

Lipid-Related Markers and Cardiovascular Disease Prediction

The Emerging Risk Factors Collaboration (Univ of Cambridge, England; et al)
JAMA 307:2499-2506, 2012

Context.—The value of assessing various emerging lipid-related markers for prediction of first cardiovascular events is debated.

Objective.—To determine whether adding information on apolipopro-tein B and apolipoprotein A-I, lipoprotein(a), or lipoprotein-associated phospholipase A_2 to total cholesterol and high-density lipoprotein choles-terol (HDL-C) improves cardiovascular disease (CVD) risk prediction.

Design, Setting, and Participants.—Individual records were available for 165 544 participants without baseline CVD in 37 prospective cohorts (calendar years of recruitment: 1968-2007) with up to 15 126 incident fatal or nonfatal CVD outcomes (10 132 CHD and 4994 stroke outcomes) during a median follow-up of 10.4 years (interquartile range, 7.6-14 years).

Main Outcome Measures.—Discrimination of CVD outcomes and reclassification of participants across predicted 10-year risk categories of low (<10%), intermediate (10%-<20%), and high (≥20%) risk.

Results.—The addition of information on various lipid-related markers to total cholesterol, HDL-C, and other conventional risk factors yielded improvement in the model's discrimination: C-index change, 0.0006

(95% CI, 0.0002-0.0009) for the combination of apolipoprotein B and A-I; 0.0016 (95% CI, 0.0009-0.0023) for lipoprotein(a); and 0.0018 (95% CI, 0.0010-0.0026) for lipoprotein-associated phospholipase A_2 mass. Net reclassification improvements were less than 1% with the addition of each of these markers to risk scores containing conventional risk factors. We estimated that for 100 000 adults aged 40 years or older, 15 436 would be initially classified at intermediate risk using conventional risk factors alone. Additional testing with a combination of apolipoprotein B and A-I would reclassify 1.1%; lipoprotein(a), 4.1%; and lipoprotein-associated phospholipase A_2 mass, 2.7% of people to a 20% or higher predicted CVD risk category and, therefore, in need of statin treatment under Adult Treatment Panel III guidelines.

Conclusion.—In a study of individuals without known CVD, the addition of information on the combination of apolipoprotein B and A-I, lipoprotein(a), or lipoprotein-associated phospholipase A_2 mass to risk scores containing total cholesterol and HDL-C led to slight improvement in CVD prediction.

▶ This report from the Emerging Risk Factors Collaboration was designed to determine whether adding apolipoproteins and lipoproteins to routine measurement of total cholesterol and high-density lipoprotein (HDL) cholesterol is associated with improved risk prediction for cardiovascular disease. This study was performed in adults but presumably has some relevance to the lipid profile recommendations that will be handed down to the pediatric age group. In this large, multicenter study that included 165 544 patients without baseline known cardiovascular disease, there were 15 126 new fatal or nonfatal cardiovascular disease outcomes over a median follow-up of 10.4 years. Overall, replacement of the total cholesterol and HDL cholesterol with apolipoproteins or their ratios was not associated with improved cardiovascular disease risk prediction, whereas adding lipoprotein factors and HDL cholesterol was associated with slight improvement in cardiovascular disease risk prediction.

Given that there is only a slight increase in the predictive value of adding additional cardiovascular risk factor indicators to the usual lipid profile one most frequently orders, the added cost seems hardly worth the effort. As of now, total cholesterol and HDL cholesterol seem to be the way to go.

J. A. Stockman III, MD

Surrogate Lipid Markers for Small Dense Low-Density lipoprotein Particles in Overweight Youth
Burns SF, Lee SJ, Arslanian SA (Univ of Pittsburgh Med Ctr, PA)
J Pediatr 161:991-996, 2012

Objectives.—To determine if the ratio of triglycerides to high-density lipoprotein cholesterol (TG/HDL) and non-HDL cholesterol concentration could identify youth with small dense low-density lipoprotein (LDL).

Study Design.—One hundred forty-one (75 black and 66 white) over-weight adolescents (9 to <18 years) had a fasting measurement of plasma lipids and LDL particle concentrations and size. Receiver operating characteristic curves were used to indicate the ability of different TG/HDL ratios and non–HDL cholesterol concentrations to identify overweight youth with atherogenic LDL concentration and size.

Results.—Youth with a TG/HDL ratio of ≥3 vs <3 had higher concentrations of small dense LDL (1279.5 ± 60.1 vs 841.8 ± 24.2 nmol/L, $P < .001$) and smaller LDL particle size (20.3 ± 0.1 vs 21.2 ± 0.1 nm, $P < .001$). In receiver operating characteristic analyses a TG/HDL cut-point of 3 best predicted LDL concentration in white youth, and 2.5 in black youth. Non-HDL cholesterol cut-point of 120 mg/dL and 145 mg/dL predicted LDL particle concentration in white and in black youth, respectively. TG/HDL ratio with body mass index or waist circumference explained 71% and 79% of the variance, respectively, in total small LDL.

Conclusions.—TG/HDL ratio and non–HDL cholesterol can identify overweight youth with atherogenic LDL particles. These easily obtained clinical lipid markers, in combination with body mass index and waist circumference, could be cost effective, in observational or interventional studies, for screening and follow-up of youth at heightened risk for atherogenic LDL.

▶ A great deal has been written over several decades about the role of fats in our blood and the development of vascular disease, specifically fat related to atherogenesis. Previously, Burns et al studied the ratio of fasting triglycerides to high-density lipoprotein (TG/HDL) cholesterol and showed that this ratio can predict insulin resistance in young people.[1] In obese 13- to 16-year-old teenagers, TG/HDL cholesterol levels were found to explain 32% and 16% of the individual variation in low-density lipoprotein (LDL) particle size, respectively. Previously, the TG/HDL marker had been suspected to identify the presence of small dense LDL in obese youth. More recently, TG/HDL ratio has been shown to be negatively related to LDL particle size and large LDL concentration in youth and is positively related to small LDL concentration in adults.[2] On the basis of these studies, the current report by Burns et al evaluated whether TG/HDL ratio could predict a method of early identification of youth at risk for atherogenic LDL particles in later life.

There is no argument that a critical risk factor for early onset of cardiovascular disease is the level of LDL cholesterol, and lowering LDL cholesterol has been and remains a primary focus of reducing the risk of coronary heart disease and stroke. Unfortunately, a substantial number of patients in whom cardiovascular disease develops have normal or minimally elevated LDL cholesterol levels. In fact, the most prevalent lipid pattern in individuals presenting with a cardiovascular event is a combined dyslipidemia characterized on a standard lipid profile by elevated triglycerides, decreased HDL cholesterol, and normal or minimally elevated LDL cholesterol. This is the profile seen in insulin resistance and the metabolic syndrome, usually in the context of obesity. What Burns et al have done is extend our knowledge of these lipids, showing why dyslipidemia with

LDL cholesterol levels less than their traditional cutoff for risk is still an LDL problem.

Burns et al show that teenagers with a TG/HDL ratio ≥3 versus less than 3 had higher concentrations of small dense LDL and smaller LDL particle size. Amazingly, TG/HDL ratio for body mass index or waist circumference explained most of the variance in small LDL. They also found that the thresholds for lipid and lipoprotein levels predictive of LDL particles vary by race.

In the study of Burns et al, the presence of small dense LDL concentration and smaller LDL particle size was found to be related to both TG/HDL ratio and adiposity. The data also support previous findings that abdominal adiposity along with whole-body adiposity play an important role in determining lipid profiles in both black and white children. The authors also found that the inclusion of waist circumference to body mass index significantly improves the prediction of the lipid component of the metabolic syndrome in overweight children. Moreover, it was found that LDL particle size and concentrations differed significantly between children above and below the 90th percentile for waist circumference.

TG/HDL ratios and non-HDL cholesterol are easily obtained as part of lipid profiles, and have been shown to identify overweight youth with atherogenic LDL particles. If you order these studies and combine them with information provided by body mass index and waist circumference, you will have a good handle on which overweight children are at greatest risk for long-term problems with atherogenesis. The authors of this report say that such an approach is very cost effective for screening purposes. To read more about the new thinking in terms of LDL particles and their size, see the superb review by Rae-Ellen Kavey and Michele Mietus Snyder.[3]

J. A. Stockman III, MD

References

1. Hannon TS, Bacha F, Lee SJ, Janosky J, Arslanian SA. Use of markers of dyslipidemia to identify overweight youth with insulin resistance. *Pediatr Diabetes.* 2006;7:260-266.
2. Weiss R, Otvos JD, Sinnreich R, Miserez AR, Kark JD. The triglyceride to high-density lipoprotein-cholesterol ratio in adolescence and subsequent weight gain predict nuclear magnetic resonance-measured lipoprotein subclasses in adulthood. *J Pediatr.* 2011;158:44-50.
3. Kavey RE, Mietus-Snyder M. Beyond cholesterol: the atherogenic consequences of combined dyslipidemia. *J Pediatr.* 2012;161:977-999.

Lipoprotein Subfractions by Ion Mobility in Lean and Obese Children

Benson M, Hossain J, Caulfield MP, et al (Nemours Children's Clinic, Jacksonville, FL; Alfred I. Dupont Hosp for Children, Wilmington, DE; Quest Diagnostics Nichols Inst, San Juan Capistrano, CA)
J Pediatr 161:997-1003.e6, 2012

Objective.—To establish normative data for lipoprotein subfractions using a novel ion mobility assay in healthy lean children and to compare their data with those of obese children preselected with normal glucose, blood pressure, and relatively normal lipids.

Study Design.—Fasting blood samples in 162 children aged 7.0-18.9 years (75 lean [body mass index: 18.6 ± 6.6 kg/m^2] and 87 obese [body mass index: 31.7 ± 5.4 kg/m^2]) were analyzed. Correlation of lipoprotein subfractions with anthropometric and laboratory markers was performed. Principal component analysis was used to avoid using correlated variables.

Results.—Normative data for lipid subfractions were obtained in healthy children. Lean children had higher high-density lipoprotein (HDL)-large (76%), HDL-small (13%), and HDL-total (27%) compared with obese ($P < .01$), and lower low-density lipoprotein (LDL)-medium (-30%, $P < .01$) and medium + small (-21%, $P = .02$) as well as LDL-total (-13%, $P = .035$). In both groups, the LDL component was higher in males and pubertal children ($P < .01$). Prepubertal children had a higher HDL component than pubertal ones ($P < .004$). Adjusting for sex and pubertal status LDL component was positively, and HDL component negatively, correlated with obesity ($P < .004$).

Conclusions.—Despite relatively normal triglycerides and cholesterol measured with standard assays at screening, ion mobility analysis showed significant differences in lipid and apolipoprotein subfractions between lean and obese children, even those prepubertal. Long-term, prospective follow-up may better characterize the predictability of lipid subfractions for future cardiovascular disease risk in children (Fig).

▶ This is another article showing how far we have come in understanding which specific lipid profiles are most predictive of atherogenesis in later life and how to detect these different lipid components. Lipoproteins comprise a very heterogeneous group of particles. This includes different size, density, and apolipoprotein concentrations.

One way to sort out various lipid components is to use a methodology known as ion mobility analysis, a novel assay designed to more accurately characterize circulating lipid and lipoprotein subfractions. It has been postulated that measurement of smaller, more atherogenic lipid subfractions may in theory provide additional biomarkers to predict the risk of cardiovascular disease in adults.

These authors designed a study to establish the normal range of data for these lipid subfractions in a cohort of healthy lean children and then compared them with a group of obese children who had no associated medical conditions. The authors also attempted to correlate these lipid measures with known inflammatory markers, sex, pubertal status, and markers of adiposity. This was done in an obese population of prepubertal and adolescent children.

In this study, large numbers of obese children had their blood samples analyzed. The children all displayed normal blood pressure, fasting glucose, total cholesterol levels (< 200 mg/dL), and triglycerides levels (< 130 mg/dL) and normal or mildly decreased high-density lipoprotein (HDL). Obesity was defined as a body mass index (BMI) greater than 95% for children in North

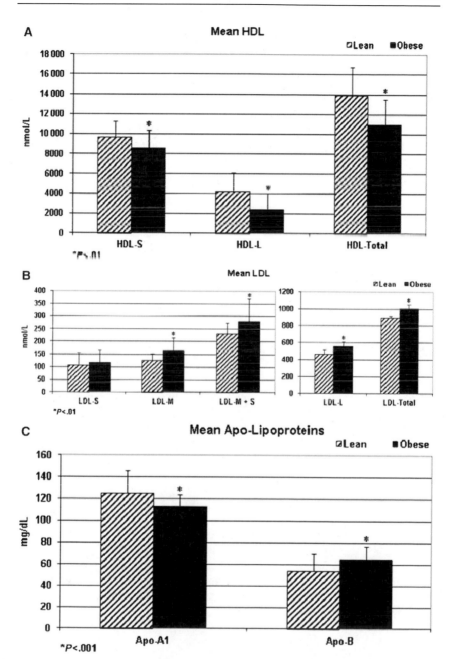

FIGURE.—A, Mean HDL, B, LDL, and C, Apo-B subfractions in lean and obese children. Differences in LDL-VS disappeared after correction for triglyceride and HDL concentrations. M, medium; S, small; L, large. (Reprinted from Journal Pediatrics from Benson M, Hossain J, Caulfield MP, et al. Lipoprotein subfractions by ion mobility in lean and obese children. *J Pediatr.* 2012;161:997-1003.e6, Copyright 2013, with permission from Elsevier.)

America. An ion mobility assay was used to measure lipoprotein subfractions in plasma. In brief, this technology is capable of measuring and quantifying lipoprotein particles from small dense HDL to large buoyant very low density lipoprotein. The ion mobility assay works on the principle that particles of a given size and charge behave in a predictable manner when carried in a laminar airflow and subjected to an electric field. It takes just 2 minutes to do such an analysis.

The results from this study showed differences in many lipoprotein subfractions between obese and lean children, despite relatively normal cholesterol and triglyceride concentrations and normal to minimally decreased HDL as measured by conventional assays. These differences were already apparent even before the onset of puberty, underscoring the fact that cardiovascular risk factors can be picked up early in life with such sophisticated studies. The article extends the hypothesis that HDL in childhood is an important risk factor, but there are striking differences evident in subfractions of lipids even in prepubertal children, not just in total HDL, but also in small and large HDL subfractions. The data showed the most significant variations are seen in HDL subfractions. These lipoprotein subfractions correlate significantly with other markers of insulin sensitivity, including inflammatory and thrombosis markers such as fibrinogen. The data also show the compounding effects of obesity as measured by BMI (waist circumference and percentage of fat mass), sex, and pubertal status.

The authors could not say whether lipoprotein subfractions, if measured, could actually provide additional risk stratification, but other studies as reported in this year's YEAR BOOK OF PEDIATRICS suggest that these may be powerful markers to identify children at risk for cardiovascular disease.[1]

It is a whole new world now in predicting the risk of atherogenesis. Soon it will be routine for us to go beyond measuring cholesterol levels and triglyceride levels. These lipid subfractions are likely to turn out to be something that will be part of our lipid profiles in the very near future. If you want to follow the progress of information into the future, the tables in the original article present the normative lipid and lipoprotein subfraction levels reported in this study.

J. A. Stockman III, MD

Reference

1. Burns SF, Lee SJ, Arslanian SA. Surrogate lipid markers for small dense low-density lipoprotein particles in overweight youth. *J Pediatr.* 2012;161:991-996.

Efficacy and safety of a microsomal triglyceride transfer protein inhibitor in patients with homozygous familial hypercholesterolaemia: a single-arm, open-label, phase 3 study
Cuchel M, for the Phase 3 HoFH Lomitapide Study investigators (Univ of Pennsylvania, Philadelphia; et al)
Lancet 381:40-46, 2013

Background.—Patients with homozygous familial hypercholesterolaemia respond inadequately to existing drugs. We aimed to assess the efficacy and safety of the microsomal triglyceride transfer protein inhibitor lomitapide in adults with this disease.

Methods.—We did a single-arm, open-label, phase 3 study of lomitapide for treatment of patients with homozygous familial hypercholesterolemia. Current lipid lowering therapy was maintained from 6 weeks before baseline through to at least week 26. Lomitapide dose was escalated on the basis of safety and tolerability from 5 mg to a maximum of 60 mg a day. The primary endpoint was mean percent change in levels of LDL cholesterol from baseline to week 26, after which patients remained on lomitapide through to week 78 for safety assessment. Percent change from baseline to week 26 was assessed with a mixed linear model.

Findings.—29 men and women with homozygous familial hypercholesterolaemia, aged 18 years or older, were recruited from 11 centres in four countries (USA, Canada, South Africa, and Italy). 23 of 29 enrolled patients completed both the efficacy phase (26 weeks) and the full study (78 weeks). The median dose of lomitapide was 40 mg a day. LDL cholesterol was reduced by 50% (95% CI −62 to −39) from baseline (mean 8·7 mmol/L [SD 2·9]) to week 26 (4·3 mmol/L [2·5]; $p < 0.0001$). Levels of LDL cholesterol were lower than 2·6 mmol/L in eight patients at 26 weeks. Concentrations of LDL cholesterol remained reduced by 44% (95% CI −57 to −31; $p < 0.0001$) at week 56 and 38% (−52 to −24; $p < 0.0001$) at week 78. Gastrointestinal symptoms were the most common adverse event. Four patients had aminotransaminase levels of more than five times the upper limit of normal, which resolved after dose reduction or temporary interruption of lomitapide. No patient permanently discontinued treatment because of liver abnormalities.

Interpretation.—Our study suggests that treatment with lomitapide could be a valuable drug in the management of homozygous familial hypercholesterolaemia.

▶ This article tells us about the efficacy of a new agent that is being explored as part of the treatment of patients with homozygous familial hypercholesterolemia. This study includes some teenagers and therefore is of value for those engaged in the care of children with this hereditary disorder.

Homozygous familial hypercholesterolemia is an inherited disorder caused mainly by mutations in both low-density lipoprotein (LDL) receptor alleles. The disorder is difficult to treat. Currently available lipid-lowering therapies, even if combined with LDL apheresis, rarely achieve optimal LDL cholesterol concentrations in patients with homozygous familial hypercholesterolemia, leaving these patients at extremely high risk for early onset cardiovascular disease and reduced life expectancy. Statin therapy will delay the onset of cardiovascular events to some extent and can prolong survival, but only modestly reduces LDL cholesterol levels. Even with statin therapy, the average age of death for a child diagnosed with familial hypercholesterolemia is very young, with few patients surviving into their 40s.

This article reports on the efficacy and safety of lomitapide, an oral inhibitor of microsomal transfer protein (MTP), in 29 older teenagers and young adults with homozygous familial hypercholesterolemia. MTP is a key protein involved in the assembly and secretion of ApoB-containing lipoproteins in the liver and intestines. The complete absence of MTP causes abetalipoproteinemia, a rare disorder characterized by failure to thrive, steatorrhea, deficiency of the fat-soluble vitamins, and extremely low or undetectable concentrations of ApoB-containing lipoproteins. Inhibition of MTP, therefore, is potentially a powerful therapeutic method to reduce the production of very low-density lipoproteins, the precursors of LDL. These authors, using a median dose of 40 mg lomitapide per day, showed a reduction in LDL cholesterols of 50% in patients with familial hypercholesterolemia. Unfortunately, as was expected based on the drug's mechanism of action, gastrointestinal side effects were common in 80% of patients, and 30% of patients had a 3-fold elevation in liver enzymes sometime during treatment therapy.

Despite the limitations of this nonrandomized study, the results are impressive and suggest that a new agent is now available to patients with homozygous familial hypercholesterolemia. What we do not know is the long-term potential risk of such therapy. Also, the drug is somewhat difficult to use since its dosing has to be titrated in individual patients according to gastrointestinal side effects, liver enzyme elevations, and the amount of hepatic fat accumulation that occurs as the result of the use of this drug.

There are other ways that are being examined to manage patients with familial hypercholesterolemia. For example, in patients with heterozygous familial hypercholesterolemia, monoclonal antibodies directed against protein convertase subtilisin/kexin type 9 (PCSK9) have been shown to reduce LDL cholesterol by as much as 50% to 60% on top of high-dose statins.[1]

None of the agents studied so far have produced the kind of LDL cholesterol reduction levels that we would like to see, and therefore the ultimate test of any lipid-modifying therapy remains a reduction in cardiovascular events and improved survival. Hopefully, the addition of drugs such as described in this article will improve long-term survival if the side effects of such agents can be reduced.

J. A. Stockman III, MD

Reference

1. Stein EA, Gipe D, Bergeron J, et al. Effect of a monoclonal antibody to PCSK9, REGN727/SAR236553, to reduce low-density lipoprotein cholesterol in patients with heterozygous familial hypercholesterolaemia on stable statin dose with or without ezetimibe therapy: a phase 2 randomised controlled trial. *Lancet.* 2012; 380:29-36.

Efficacy, safety, and tolerability of a monoclonal antibody to proprotein convertase subtilisin/kexin type 9 as monotherapy in patients with hypercholesterolaemia (MENDEL): a randomised, double-blind, placebo-controlled, phase 2 study

Koren MJ, Scott R, Kim JB, et al (Jacksonville Ctr for Clinical Res, FL; Amgen, Thousand Oaks, CA; et al)
Lancet 380:1995-2006, 2012

Background.—Proprotein convertase subtilisin/kexin type 9 (PCSK9) increases serum LDL-cholesterol (LDL-C) concentrations. We assessed the effects of AMG 145, a human monoclonal antibody against PCSK9, in patients with hypercholesterolaemia in the absence of concurrent lipid-lowering treatment.

Methods.—In a phase 2 trial done at 52 centres in Europe, the USA, Canada, and Australia, patients (aged 18−75 years) with serum LDL-C concentrations of 2·6 mmol/L or greater but less than 4·9 mmol/L were randomly assigned equally through an interactive voice response system to subcutaneous injections of AMG 145 70 mg, 105 mg, or 140 mg, or placebo every 2 weeks; subcutaneous AMG 145 280 mg, 350 mg, or 420 mg or placebo every 4 weeks; or oral ezetimibe 10 mg/day. The primary endpoint was percentage change from baseline in LDL-C concentration at week 12. Analysis was by modified intention to treat. Study personnel and patients were masked to treatment assignment of AMG 145 or placebo. Ezetimibe assignment was open label. This trial is registered with ClinicalTrials.gov, number NCT01375777.

Findings.—406 patients were assigned to AMG 145 70 mg (n = 45), 105 mg (n = 46), or 140 mg (n = 45) every 2 weeks; AMG 145 280 mg (n = 45), 350 mg (n = 45), or 420 mg (n = 45) every 4 weeks; placebo every 2 weeks (n = 45) or every 4 weeks (n = 45); or ezetimibe (n = 45). AMG 145 significantly reduced LDL-C concentrations in all dose groups (mean baseline LDL-C concentration 3·7 mmol/L [SD 0·6]; changes from baseline with every 2 weeks AMG 145 70 mg −41·0% [95% CI −46·2 to −35·8]; 105 mg −43·9% [−49·0 to −38·7]; 140 mg −50·9% [−56·2 to −45·7]; every 4 weeks AMG 145 280 mg −39·0% [−44·1 to −34·0]; 350 mg −43·2% [−48·3 to −38·1]; 420 mg −48·0% [−53·1 to −42·9]; placebo every 2 weeks −3·7% [−9·0 to 1·6]; placebo every 4 weeks 4·5% [−0·7 to 9·8]; and ezetimibe −14·7% [−18·6 to −10·8]; $p < 0.0001$ for all doses *vs* placebo or ezetimibe). Treatment-emergent adverse events occurred in 136 (50%) of 271 patients in the AMG 145 groups, 41 (46%) of 90 patients in the placebo groups, and 26 (58%) of 45 patients in the ezetimibe group; no deaths or serious treatment-related adverse events were reported.

Interpretation.—The results of our study support the further assessment of AMG 145 in long-term studies with larger and more diverse populations including patients with documented statin intolerance.

▶ For both children and adults at risk for vascular disease resulting from hyperlipidemia, the lowering of low-density lipoprotein cholesterol (LDL-C) with statins has broadly proven benefits for both primary and secondary prevention of complications of heart disease. Current consensus statements recommend consideration of an aggressive treatment goal of an LDL-C of less than 1.8 mmol/L for high-risk or very high-risk adults. It is not clear what the ideal ranges are in children in terms of lowering of LDL-C, but aggressive treatment is clearly needed in some patients. Unfortunately, there are some adults and children who cannot tolerate any statin or a dose high enough to achieve desired targeted LDL-C reductions.

Proprotein convertase subtilisin/kexin type 9 (PCSK9) is a serine protease that binds to the LDL receptor. PCSK9 has emerged as a target for lowering LDL-C in the management of hyperlipidemia. By way of background, serum LDL-C is regulated by LDL receptors on hepatocytes. These receptors bind LDL-C and clear it from plasma. After clearance of LDL-C through endocytosis, LDL receptors with attached PCSK9 are directed to lysosomes for degradation, whereas LDL receptors free of bound PCSK9 recycle to the plasma membrane. By this mechanism, extracellular PCSK9 reduces the available number of LDL receptors on the hepatocyte surface, increasing serum LDL-C concentrations. Knowledge of this has stimulated interest in treatments that block the effects of PCSK9, particularly in patients with high lipid levels who remain inadequately treated on high doses of statins or who cannot tolerate the complications related to statin therapy.

This article tells us about a human monoclonal immunoglobulin-G2 antibody against PCSK9 in patients with hypercholesterolemia who have been on statins. The antibody used is called AMG 145. In adults randomly assigned to AMG or placebo, marked reductions in lipid levels were seen. AMG 145 significantly reduced the LDL-C concentration from baseline values compared with placebo by up to 66%. AMG 145 was well tolerated with no dose-related or dose-frequency-related increase in reported adverse effects.

It appears that statins in and of themselves are not the perfect treatment for reducing LDL-C levels. Statins, particularly at high doses, lead to increases in liver enzymes in as many as 3% of patients. Intolerable muscle pain can also occur in both adults and youngsters treated with statins. It may be that in such circumstances and in patients who do not get good effects from statins the agent described in this article could be helpful. Although AMG 145 and similar agents are still in the testing period, the results of treatment with these agents are quite phenomenal. The related agent RN-316, made by Pfizer Pharmaceutical, reduces LDL levels by up to 75% during a 12-week trial.[1]

J. A. Stockman III, MD

Reference

1. Statin substitute shows promise. *Science News.* December 15, 2012:9.

Prevalence of Persistent Prehypertension in Adolescents

Acosta AA, Samuels JA, Portman RJ, et al (Texas A&M Univ College of Medicine, Temple; Univ of Texas Med School at Houston; Bristol-Myers Squibb, Princeton, NJ; et al)
J Pediatr 160:757-761, 2012

Objective.—To measure the prevalence of persistent prehypertension in adolescents.

Study Design.—We collected demographic and anthropometric data and 4 oscillometric blood pressure (BP) measurements on 1020 students. The mean of the second, third, and fourth BP measurements determined each student's BP status per visit, with up to 3 total visits. Final BP status was classified as normal (BP < 90th percentile and 120/80 mm Hg at the first visit), variable (BP > 90th percentile or 120/80 mm Hg at the first visit and subsequently normal), abnormal (BP ≥ 90th percentile or 120/80 mm Hg at 3 visits but not hypertensive), or hypertensive (BP ≥ 95th percentile at 3 visits). The abnormal group included those with persistent prehypertension (BP ≥ 90th percentile or 120/80 mm Hg and < 95th percentile on 3 visits). Statistical analysis allowed for comparison of groups and identification of characteristics associated with final BP classification.

Results.—Of 1010 students analyzed, 71.1% were classified as normal, 15.0% as variable, 11.5% as abnormal, and 2.5% as hypertensive. The prevalence of persistent prehypertension was 4.0%. Obesity similarly affected the odds for variable BP (OR, 3.9; 95% CI, 2.5-6.0) and abnormal BP (OR, 3.4; 95% CI, 2.0-5.9), and dramatically increased the odds for hypertension (OR, 38.4; 95% CI, 9.4-156.6).

Conclusion.—Almost 30% of the students had at least one elevated BP measurement significantly influenced by obesity. Treating obesity may be essential to preventing prehypertension and/or hypertension.

▶ The term *prehypertension* has crept into the pediatric literature in the past decade or so. In 2003, the Seventh Report of the Joint National Committee on Prevention, Detection, Evaluation, and Treatment of High Blood Pressure recommended that adults having systolic blood pressure between 120 and 139 and/or diastolic blood pressure between 80 mm Hg and 89 mm Hg be defined as having prehypertension. This term prehypertension was developed to alert clinicians that there are patients who may have a risk for progression to hypertension and cardiovascular disease who have modest aberrations in blood pressure. The report from 2003 suggested that such individuals undergo lifestyle changes to reduce their risk of cardiovascular disease and the development of hypertension. It was not long after this seventh report of the Joint National Committee on Prevention, Detection, Evaluation, and Treatment of High Blood Pressure that the National High Blood Pressure Education Program Working Group updated the classification system of blood pressure in children and adolescents to parallel the adult classification system, changing the terminology from high normal to prehypertension for blood pressures between the 90th percentile and the 95th percentile based on age. Again, the classification prehypertension was developed to alert pediatricians to the risk of these blood pressure levels and to encourage lifestyle modifications in this cohort of children and adolescents. This is especially true because it is known that children with hypertension are more likely to become adults with hypertension. It is also known that nonhypertensive children in the upper centiles of blood pressure are at increased risk for developing adult hypertension.

One of the problems defining either hypertension or prehypertension in adolescents is the variability in blood pressure measurement to measurement. Acosta et al looked at more than 1000 Houston area high school students, determining blood pressure levels on at least 3 visits. In this cohort, almost 20% of the population had a mean blood pressure in the prehypertensive range at the first visit. Similar to other well-documented observations for hypertension, a large percent of these children subsequently normalized. After repeated measures, only 4% had persistent prehypertension. Thus the prevalence of hypertension in this study is consistent with that reported in other studies of hypertension ranging from 2.2% to 4.5% on repeated measures. Those at greatest risk for prehypertension and hypertension were boys, those with an increased body mass index, and those with an elevated heart rate.

There are a lot of lessons to be learned from this report. Many in practice will do a follow-up blood pressure only for those whose mean blood pressure on a single visit is ≥95th percentile. Clearly this is not the best screen in the world. Be aware that a single normal blood pressure measurement does not rule out the child at greatest risk. At the same time, almost half of students in this report with prehypertension at the first visit do in fact normalize on subsequent visits, whereas 4% have a blood pressure persistently in the prehypertensive range. Perhaps those who are overweight might be the ones to more carefully follow-up as overweight in this report as noted was significantly associated with the abnormal blood pressures found.

Although the association between hypertension and obesity has been well studied, the exact mechanism of this relationship is still not understood. Also, we do know from past studies that there is an association between elevated heart rate and obesity and higher urinary catecholamine levels have been documented in hypertensive children. The findings from the report of Acosta et al are consistent with these prior studies. There is also evidence suggesting that an elevated blood pressure may in fact precede future weight gain. Thus the relationship between body mass index and blood pressure is a very complex affair, to say the least.

It will be interesting to see what the follow-up is of this report over time. Is it possible that those youngsters who have prehypertension on their first visit who normalize on subsequent visits in fact do turn out to be at higher risk of later hypertension? Only time will tell. Perhaps we are headed into a new category of hypertension preprehypertension for those who sporadically have elevated blood pressures. We do know that "white-coat hypertension" is in fact a risk for the development of persistent hypertension, and it may be that children who have sporadic elevations of blood pressure will have a similar fate.

J. A. Stockman III, MD

Efficacy of immunoglobulin plus prednisolone for prevention of coronary artery abnormalities in severe Kawasaki disease (RAISE study): a randomised, open-label, blinded-endpoints trial
Kobayashi T, on behalf of the RAISE study group investigators (Gunma Univ Graduate School of Medicine, Japan; et al)
Lancet 379:1613-1620, 2012

Background.—Evidence indicates that corticosteroid therapy might be beneficial for the primary treatment of severe Kawasaki disease. We assessed whether addition of prednisolone to intravenous immunoglobulin with aspirin would reduce the incidence of coronary artery abnormalities in patients with severe Kawasaki disease.

Methods.—We did a multicentre, prospective, randomised, open-label, blinded-endpoints trial at 74 hospitals in Japan between Sept 29, 2008, and Dec 2, 2010. Patients with severe Kawasaki disease were randomly assigned by a minimisation method to receive either intravenous immunoglobulin (2 g/kg for 24 h and aspirin 30 mg/kg per day) or intravenous immunoglobulin plus prednisolone (the same intravenous immunoglobulin regimen as the intravenous immunoglobulin group plus prednisolone 2 mg/kg per day given over 15 days after concentrations of C-reactive protein normalised). Patients and treating physicians were unmasked to group allocation. The primary endpoint was incidence of coronary artery abnormalities during the study period. Analysis was by intention to treat. This trial is registered with the University Hospital Medical Information Network clinical trials registry, number UMIN000000940.

Findings.—We randomly assigned 125 patients to the intravenous immunoglobulin plus prednisolone group and 123 to the intravenous immunoglobulin group. Incidence of coronary artery abnormalities was significantly lower in the intravenous immunoglobulin plus prednisolone group than in the intravenous immunoglobulin group during the study period (four patients [3%] *vs* 28 patients [23%]; risk difference 0·20, 95% CI 0 12-0·28, $p < 0·0001$). Serious adverse events were similar between both groups: two patients had high total cholesterol and one neutropenia in the intravenous immunoglobulin plus prednisolone group, and one had high total cholesterol and another non-occlusive thrombus in the intravenous immunoglobulin group.

Interpretation.—Addition of prednisolone to the standard regimen of intravenous immunoglobulin improves coronary artery outcomes in patients with severe Kawasaki disease in Japan. Further study of intensified primary treatment for this disease in a mixed ethnic population is warranted.

▶ The saga of the use of corticosteroids as part of the management of Kawasaki disease is a sorted one. Ever since the disorder was first described in Japan in 1969, investigators have been trying to determine the best way to treat it and, more importantly, to prevent the long-term complications of the disorder, particularly the formation of vascular aneurysms. From everything we know, it is clear that high-dose intravenous immunoglobulin is the treatment of choice and should be given as soon as possible and certainly within the first 10 days of illness to decrease the prevalence of coronary artery aneurysms. When given in this manner, the reduction in the prevalence of the latter is from 20% to less than 5%.

The steroid treatment of Kawasaki disease has a checkered history. Other vasculitides respond to corticosteroids, and thus we would expect that Kawasaki disease would as well. Steroid trials have had mixed results. A randomized study undertaken by the Pediatric Heart Network assessed the use of intravenous methylprednisolone in a single pulsed dose before treatment with intravenous immunoglobulin. This study did not show any benefit in terms of reduction of coronary outcomes.[1] A meta-analysis concluded that an addition of steroids to conventional treatment, while reducing the need for retreatment with intravenous immunoglobulin, had no effect on the incidence of coronary artery aneurysms.[2]

These authors conducted a controlled trial to assess the role of immunoglobulin plus steroid therapy as part of the management of Kawasaki disease. The article provides compelling evidence for intensified primary treatment with corticosteroids plus intravenous immunoglobulin, showing benefit to high-risk patients. The authors randomly assigned 125 patients with severe Kawasaki disease to an intravenous immunoglobulin plus prednisolone group and 123 patients to an intravenous immunoglobulin alone group. All patients also received aspirin. High-risk patients had characteristics such as a low serum sodium, very short history of fever prior to onset of clinical disease, liver enzyme elevations, elevations of white blood cell neutrophil counts, and a low platelet count. In addition a high C-reactive protein concentration and young age (less than 12 months) were also high-risk factors. The differences in this article from that of the Pediatric Heart Network Trial most likely represent findings based on patient selection and treatment duration.

An editorial by Son and Newburger[3] accompanied this article. The editorial comments that although the findings of the study of these authors conclusively show the efficacy of the addition of prednisolone to conventional treatment for Kawasaki disease in high-risk Japanese children, several obstacles prevent the generalization of this steroid regimen to a wider population with the disease. The translation of the data from this article into clinical practice is very much dependent on the identification of patients at risk for intravenous immunoglobulin resistance. Unfortunately, risk scores that have been developed in Asia do not adequately identify patients in other racial and ethnic groups that may be at risk for such resistance.[4] A second challenge relates to differences in health care systems in Japan and other developed countries. In the United States, patients with Kawasaki disease are typically discharged within 2 to 3 days of hospital admission. A 5-day course of intravenous corticosteroids presents logistical and financial difficulties. Hopefully, a study will be undertaken in which the intravenous route is switched to a high-dose oral route so this problem would be obviated.

Despite these disclaimers, this is a very important study. The trick now would be for investigators in the United States to define better techniques to identify high-risk patients then to repeat this study adding corticosteroids to intravenous immunoglobulin as part of the treatment of patients with Kawasaki disease.

J. A. Stockman III, MD

References

1. Newburger JW, Sleeper LA, McCrindle BW, et al. Randomized trial of pulsed corticosteroid therapy for primary treatment of Kawasaki disease. *N Engl J Med.* 2007;356:663-675.
2. Athappan G, Gale S, Ponniah T. Corticosteroid therapy for primary treatment of Kawasaki disease — weight of evidence: a meta-analysis and systematic review of the literature. *Cardiovasc J Afr.* 2009;20:233-236.
3. Son MB, Newburger JW. Management of Kawasaki disease: corticosteroids revisited. *Lancet.* 2012;379:1571-1572.
4. Sleeper LA, Minich LL, McCrindle BM, et al. Evaluation of Kawasaki disease risk-scoring systems for intravenous immunoglobulin resistance. *J Pediatr.* 2011;158: 831-835.

Relation Between Red Cell Distribution Width and Clinical Outcome After Surgery for Congenital Heart Disease in Children

Massin MM (Free Univ of Brussels (ULB), Belgium)
Pediatr Cardiol 33.1021-1025, 2012

Recent studies have reported a strong association between increased red cell distribution width (RDW) and the risk of adverse outcomes for adults with heart failure. This study investigated the association between preoperative RDW and postoperative clinical outcomes for children with cardiac disease. The relation between preoperative RDW and the length of postoperative stay was tested with 688 consecutive children undergoing surgery for congenital heart disease (CHD). The RDW was significantly higher in patients who died during the postoperative hospital stay (mean, 18.34 ± 4.69 vs 16.12 ± 2.84; $p = 0.004$). The risk of postoperative death was five times higher for patients with an RDW of 16% or more. In the general study population, RDW correlated with the intensive care unit (ICU) stay ($p < 0.0001$) and with the total hospital stay in the local population ($p < 0.0001$). The correlation between RDW and ICU stay was stronger for patients with acyanotic CHD ($p < 0.0001$) than for those with cyanotic CHD ($p = 0.0007$), and for the subpopulation of patients with acyanotic CHD and normal hemoglobin level ($p < 0.0001$) than for anemic patients with acyanotic CHD ($p = 0.025$). Preoperative RDW is a strong predictor of an adverse outcome in children undergoing surgery for CHD, especially in nonanemic patients, for whom it reflects an underlying inflammatory stress (Table).

▶ Red cell distribution width (RDW) is a quantitative way of measuring variation in red cell size of circulating red blood cells. More specifically, the RDW is the coefficient of variation of red cell size and is routinely reported by automated laboratory equipment when a complete blood count is performed. Historically,

TABLE.—Surgical Procedures

Surgical Procedure	n (deaths)
Repair of tetralogy of Fallot	111
Repair of ventricular septal defect	99 (2)
Repair of complete atrioventricular septal defect	79 (4)
Arterial switch operation	66 (2)
Repair of atrial septal defect	54
Bidirectional Glenn procedure	52
Total cavopulmonary connection	30
Conduit replacement	28
Repair of pulmonary atresia + ventricular septal defect	25 (2)
Rastelli procedure	24 (1)
Plastic correction of aortic valve incompetence	20
Relief of subvalvar aortic stenosis	20
Mitral valve repair or replacement	18
Repair of aortic coarctation + ventricular septal defect	15
Repair of truncus arteriosus communis	13
Ross procedure	10 (1)
Conduit repair of complex pulmonary stenosis or pulmonary regurgitation	7 (1)
Repair of total anomalous pulmonary venous return	6
Repair of anomalous origin of the left coronary artery from the pulmonary artery	3 (1)
Norwood procedure	3
Other procedures	5
Total	688 (14)

the RDW has been used in defining the differential diagnosis of anemia. For example, an elevated RDW in a patient with microcytosis indicates iron deficiency as opposed to a thalassemia trait disorder. Also, the RDW value can assist a clinician in determining whether iron deficiency is present when accurate determinations of serum ferritin are confusing in situations such as inflammation or malignancy. In such cases, for example, the serum ferritin may be normal or increased despite the fact the patient is iron deficient, but the RDW in such cases will be elevated as one would expect in the presence of iron deficiency.

In recent years, several clinical outcomes have been correlated with RDW values, specifically in adults with heart failure, stable coronary artery disease, acute myocardial infarction, and pulmonary hypertension. The mechanism underlying this association has remained unknown; nonetheless, the RDW does appear to be a powerful and independent predictor of mortality and adverse outcomes for a broad population of cardiovascular patients across a spectrum of risks.

Massin has helped fill a void because no information exists regarding the prognostic significance of RDW for children with cardiac disease. The author looked at data on all consecutive children undergoing open-heart surgery for congenital heart disease at a children's hospital in Brussels, Belgium between January 1, 2006, and December 31, 2010. Routine hematology parameters collected at the time of admission for surgery were correlated with various outcomes, including length of stay and postoperative death rates. Almost 700 youngsters younger than 16 years were enrolled in the study (mean age, 37.3 ± 43.1 months). The surgical procedures performed are noted in Table. The range of RDW was determined to vary between 11.6% and 31.7%. The mean RDW was significantly higher for 14 patients who died during the postoperative stay when compared with the 674 survivors (mean 18.3% ± 4.7% vs 16.1% ± 2.8%; $P = .004$). The risk of postoperative death was 5 times higher for those patients with an RDW of 16 or more than among those with an RDW value less than 16% (3.9% vs 0.8%). The strongest prognostic value of RDW was noted in the subpopulation of nonanemic patients with acyanotic congenital heart disease (18.4% ± 6.1%, n = 7 deaths vs 14.8% ± 1.9%, n = 81 survivors; $P = .000017$). The RDW also correlated directly with the length of intensive care unit (ICU) stay. The correlation between RDW and ICU stay was stronger for patients with acyanotic congenital heart disease.

This report suggests that the biomarker RDW, routinely reported in automated complete blood counts, is an integrative correlate for ineffective red cell production, inflammation, nutritional deficiencies and other comorbidities. The RDW is a novel and strong predictor of adverse outcomes in children undergoing cardiac surgery for congenital heart disease and could theoretically be considered a simple, noninvasive, inexpensive, and objective tool for detecting high-risk children who are going to undergo surgery.

The interesting question of course is why the RDW in children undergoing congenital heart disease surgery correlates so well with clinical outcomes. It is well known that the RDW is increased in children with cyanotic congenital heart disease largely because hypoxemia produces a macrocytosis. Nonetheless, as noted in this report, it was the group of children with acyanotic congenital heart disease who had the highest correlations between outcomes and elevations in RDW. In such circumstance, one can likely assume that inflammation, malnutrition, and the impact of comorbidities on RDW were the reasons for the increased values for RDW in correlation with poor outcomes. Also, it is possible that children who have abnormal vascular endothelium for whatever reason, as the result of structural heart disease, may have increased mechanical alterations of the red cells membrane, driving up the RDW. The authors of this report suggest that persistent inflammation (as a cause of elevated RDW) is a known pathophysiologic finding and a poor prognostic factor for heart failure and that RDW values may very well correlate with this finding of inflammation.

It would be interesting for other investigators to look at iron status and other biomarkers of inflammation in patients with high RDW values and congenital heart disease to determine what the precise mechanism is that allows the RDW to be a biomarker for less than positive outcomes.

As this is the Heart and Blood Vessel chapter, it seems appropriate to ask a question that has bothered cardiac transplant surgeons for some time: What happens if you transplant a heart that might be considered somewhat too small or two large for a recipient? The answer to this question is that, in the long run, it probably does not matter too much. At least, it appears that size does not matter when it comes to transplanting hearts into babies and children. The medical and echocardiographic records of 147 children who received transplanted hearts showed that, despite disparities in body surface area and heart size between donors and recipients, the hearts grew appropriately after transplantation, keeping pace with the physiological requirements of the growing child.[1]

J. A. Stockman III, MD

Reference

1. Walter EMD, Huebler M, Schubert S, et al. Influence of size disparity of transplanted hearts on cardiac growth in infants and children. *J Thorac Cardiovasc Surg.* 2012;143:168-177.

Prospective Trial of a Pediatric Ventricular Assist Device

Fraser CD Jr, for the Berlin Heart Study Investigators (Texas Children's Hosp, Houston; et al)

N Engl J Med 367:532-541, 2012

Background.—Options for mechanical circulatory support as a bridge to heart transplantation in children with severe heart failure are limited.

Methods.—We conducted a prospective, single-group trial of a ventricular assist device designed specifically for children as a bridge to heart transplantation. Patients 16 years of age or younger were divided into two cohorts according to body-surface area (cohort 1, <0.7 m^2; cohort 2, 0.7 to <1.5 m^2), with 24 patients in each group. Survival in the two cohorts receiving mechanical support (with data censored at the time of transplantation or weaning from the device owing to recovery) was compared with survival in two propensity-score—matched historical control groups (one for each cohort) undergoing extracorporeal membrane oxygenation (ECMO).

Results.—For participants in cohort 1, the median survival time had not been reached at 174 days, whereas in the matched ECMO group, the median survival was 13 days ($P < 0.001$ by the log-rank test). For participants in cohort 2 and the matched ECMO group, the median survival was 144 days and 10 days, respectively ($P < 0.001$ by the log-rank test). Serious adverse events in cohort 1 and cohort 2 included major bleeding (in 42% and 50% of patients, respectively), infection (in 63% and 50%), and stroke (in 29% and 29%).

Conclusions.—Our trial showed that survival rates were significantly higher with the ventricular assist device than with ECMO. Serious adverse events, including infection, stroke, and bleeding, occurred in a majority of study participants. (Funded by Berlin Heart and the Food and Drug Administration Office of Orphan Product Development; ClinicalTrials. gov number, NCT00583661.)

▶ It was in 2004, in response to the need for better ventricular assist options for young patients, that the National Heart, Lung, and Blood Institute awarded 5 contracts for the development of novel circulatory support systems for use in small children. These devices are already or soon will be ready for clinical trials through the Pumps for Kids, Infants and Neonates (PUMPKIN) program. While the development of these devices was underway, the Berlin Heart EXCOR Pediatric Ventricular Assist Device, designed for children with a body weight as low as 3 kg, was made available in the United States on a compassionate-use basis. There have been several single-institution reports of its utility. Data suggest survival rates between 70% and 86% among patients receiving this device as a bridge to transplantation. This rate is substantially better than the rates cited in many reports on the use of extracorporeal membrane oxygenation (ECMO), which is designed for short-term support for those in need of heart transplant.

The successes reported to date are now followed by information from the first prospective multicenter study of pediatric ventricular assist devices that has been undertaken in the United States. The study is sponsored by the Federal Food and Drug Administration Office of Orphan Product Development. The outcomes in 48 children who prospectively received the EXCOR Pediatric Ventricular Assist Device are the basis of the report of Fraser et al.

In the multicenter collaborative study as reported by Fraser et al, the children included in the trial were divided into 2 cohorts according to size; those in cohort 1 had a body surface area of less than 0.7 m^2. Those in cohort 2 had a body surface area of 0.7 m^2 to 1.5 m^2. The study was designed to evaluate the safety and risk-benefit profile of this pump in both groups. A randomized trial was not considered to be ethically feasible because of the mounting evidence of success with the device. Therefore, the decision was made to compare the prospective data with data from a historical control of groups of children who had received support with ECMO. The study showed that children survived longer than their counterparts who had received support with ECMO, validating the efficacy of the EXCOR Ventricular Assist Device in supporting patients during long waiting times for transplantation. However, at the end of device support, there was no significant difference in the rate of successful outcome (transplantation or successful weaning from the device) between the patients in cohort 1 and the matched ECMO group with an absolute advantage of only 13 percentage points for the children who received the ventricular assist device. In contrast, a significant advantage of 25 percentage points was found for the larger children in cohort 2. Thus, it may be that the device is preferentially better for larger children. There may be an inherent problem with miniaturizing a pulsatile system for the low flow rates required in the smallest of children.

It should be noted that the risk of any serious adverse event was 92% in cohort 1 (the smaller patients) and 79% in cohort 2 (the larger patients). The major events included bleeding and infection. The most worrisome outcomes were neurologic complications seen in 29% of those in both cohorts. Seventeen strokes occurred in 14 of 48 children. In 6 children, the strokes were severe enough that support was withdrawn.

The occurrence of strokes alone is enough to suggest that children should not be put on ventricular assist devices until it is absolutely necessary. Such devices can save lives and successfully provide a bridge to transplantation for children, but they should remain, at present, a last resort in small children. Kudos to Fraser et al for giving us a thorough assessment of a ventricular assist device from Europe. The newer devices under development in the United States will have to undergo equally rigorous evaluation. It is hoped that the PUMPKIN program will represent the greatest step forward that has been seen to date in this regard.

J. A. Stockman III, MD

Transplantation of an allogeneic vein bioengineered with autologous stem cells: a proof-of-concept study
Olausson M, Patil PB, Kuna VK, et al (Univ of Gothenburg, Sweden)
Lancet 379:230-237, 2012

Background.—Extrahepatic portal vein obstruction can have severe health consequences. Variceal bleeding associated with this disorder causes upper gastrointestinal bleeding, leading to substantial morbidity and mortality. We report the clinical transplantation of a deceased donor iliac vein graft repopulated with recipient autologous stem cells in a patient with extrahepatic portal vein obstruction.

Methods.—A 10 year old girl with extrahepatic portal vein obstruction was admitted to the Sahlgrenska University Hospital in Gothenburg, Sweden, for a bypass procedure between the superior mesenteric vein and the intrahepatic left portal vein (meso Rex bypass). A 9 cm segment of allogeneic donor iliac vein was decellularised and subsequently recellularised with endothelial and smooth muscle cells differentiated from stem cells obtained from the bone marrow of the recipient. This graft was used because the patient's umbilical vein was not suitable and other strategies (eg, liver transplantation) require lifelong immunosuppression.

Findings.—The graft immediately provided the recipient with a functional blood supply (25—30 cm/s in the portal vein and 40 mL/s in the artery was measured intraoperatively and confirmed with ultrasound). The patient had normal laboratory values for 9 months. However, at 1 year the blood flow was low and, on exploration, the shunt was patent but too narrow due to mechanical obstruction of tissue in the mesocolon. Once the tissue causing the compression was removed the graft dilated. We therefore used a second stem-cell populated vein graft to lengthen the previous graft. After this second operation, the portal pressure was reduced from 20 mm Hg to 13 mm Hg and blood flow was 25—40 cm/s in the portal vein. With restored portal circulation the patient has substantially improved physical and mental function and growth. The patient has no anti-endothelial cell antibodies and is receiving no immunosuppressive drugs.

Interpretation.—An acellularised deceased donor vein graft recellularised with autologous stem cells can be considered for patients in need of vascular vein shunts without the need for immunosuppression.

▶ Conventional approaches to replacing blood vessels have focused on the use of autologous tissue, particularly the use of the saphenous vein, and synthetic materials such as polyethylene terephthalate (Dacron) and expanded polytetrafluoroethylene. Finding vascular conduits for surgery in children poses extra-special difficulties because of a paucity of acceptable autologous conduits and poor patency and lack of growth in prosthetic conduits.

Olausson et al present the case of a child with a portal vein obstruction who was successfully treated with successive tissue-engineered vein grafts. A 2-week decellularization protocol, imposed on a graft from a deceased donor, was accompanied by the differentiation of bone marrow-derived mesenchymal stem cells into endothelial and smooth muscle cells that were then seeded onto 9 cm matrix. Stem cells are preferable to mature cells in this context because of their proliferative properties and the potential to manipulate differentiation with exogenous cytokines. The result was a perfectly engineered segment of vein that no longer had cells from the original donor, but was recomposed with tissue from stem cells, tissue that would not be rejected by the patient. This graft was used because the patient's umbilical vein was not suitable and other strategies such as liver transplantation would require lifelong immunosuppression. The graft, when inserted, immediately provided the recipient with a functional blood supply in the portal vein and subsequently in the related arteries. The patient had normal laboratory values for 9 months, but at 1 year the blood flow became low, and on exploration the shunt had narrowed because of mechanical obstruction of tissue in the surrounding areas. Once the tissue causing the compression was removed, the graft immediately dilated and a second stem-cell populated vein graft was added to lengthen the previous graft. With restored portal circulation, the patient substantially improved clinically and subsequently has shown no anti-endothelial cell antibodies and is receiving no immunosuppressive drugs.

Obviously, the approaches used in this report are hand-tailored to specific clinical applications for small numbers of children for whom conventional approaches are not possible or might otherwise be hazardous. Needless to say, difficulties in terms of finding sources of materials, the numbers of preparatory steps needed, and the time to prepare grafts mean that the present protocol is unlikely to be one that ultimately succeeds in the health care market. Nonetheless, various suppliers will ultimately provide decellularized matrices from human and animal sources. Decellularization protocols are shortening and simplifying. Furthermore, recruitment of circulating endothelial progenitor cells and inducible pluripotent cell protocols might remove the need for bone marrow aspirates to produce stem cells to repopulate the decellularized matrices of donor grafts.

The report of Olausson et al suggests that tissue-engineered vascular grafts are promising, albeit one-off experiences that need to be replicated in full clinical trials if at all possible. Nonetheless, in exceptional circumstances, these one-offs turn out to be one-off life-saving maneuvers.

J. A. Stockman III, MD

10 Infectious Diseases and Immunology

Respiratory Tract Illnesses During the First Year of Life: Effect of Dog and Cat Contacts

Bergroth E, Remes S, Pekkanen J, et al (Kuopio Univ Hosp, Finland; Natl Inst for Health and Welfare, Kuopio, Finland; et al)
Pediatrics 130:211-220, 2012

Objectives.—To investigate the effect of dog and cat contacts on the frequency of respiratory symptoms and infections during the first year of life.

Methods.—In this birth cohort study, 397 children were followed up from pregnancy onward, and the frequency of respiratory symptoms and infections together with information about dog and cat contacts during the first year of life were reported by using weekly diaries and a questionnaire at the age of 1 year. All the children were born in eastern or middle Finland between September 2002 and May 2005.

Results.—In multivariate analysis, children having dogs at home were healthier (ie, had fewer respiratory tract symptoms or infections) than children with no dog contacts (adjusted odds ratio, [aOR]: 1.31; 95% confidence interval [CI]: 1.13—1.52). Furthermore, children having dog contacts at home had less frequent otitis (aOR: 0.56; 95% CI: 0.38—0.81) and tended to need fewer courses of antibiotics (aOR: 0.71; 95% CI: 0.52—0.96) than children without such contacts. In univariate analysis, both the weekly amount of contact with dogs and cats and the average yearly amount of contact were associated with decreased respiratory infectious disease morbidity.

Conclusions.—These results suggest that dog contacts may have a protective effect on respiratory tract infections during the first year of life. Our findings support the theory that during the first year of life, animal contacts are important, possibly leading to better resistance to infectious respiratory illnesses during childhood.

▶ A number of factors are associated with variations in rates of respiratory infections in the first year of life. These include daycare attendance, older siblings, and lack of breastfeeding. Parent history of asthma and smoking also seem to have a role in a child's susceptibility to infections and to respiratory symptoms. Previous studies have suggested that dog contacts, not cat contacts, seem to decrease the number of common cold episodes during childhood. Data in this regard have been somewhat controversial. Nonetheless, in the last decade or so, a large body of literature has evaluated the role of early childhood animal exposure, including household pets, in the risk of asthma or allergy in children.

The authors of this report designed a study describing the effect of domestic animal contacts on respiratory tract infection morbidity during the first year of life. The study was a prospective birth cohort study using diary-based data on respiratory tract infections and exposure to animals during the first year of life. Families documented the frequency of respiratory tract symptomatologies and were asked in weekly questionnaires whether they had a dog or cat at home and how much time it had spent inside daily. According to the results of the study, dog and cat contacts during early infancy were associated with less morbidity in general (indicated as more healthy weeks) and had a protective effect on respiratory tract symptoms and infections.

In comparing dogs and cats, dog contact showed a much more significant protective role in respiratory infections. The authors showed that children who had dog contacts at home had less otitis media and rhinitis and more healthy weeks than children without a dog at home, although having a dog at home during the first postnatal year did not show any differences in occurrence of wheezing and cough, findings consistent with those of several other studies. Cat ownership did have some protective effect, although weaker than dog owner-ship. Other studies have suggested that cat contacts have no effect on infectious symptoms.

Curiously, the authors of this report show that children living in houses in which dogs spend only part of a day inside (defined as less than 6 hours a day) had the lowest risk of infectious symptoms and respiratory tract infections. They suggest that a possible explanation for this interesting finding is that the amount of dirt brought inside the home by dogs could be higher in families in which dogs spend part of a day outside.

The data from this report are clear. Dog ownership may pay for itself in the first year of life. It is time to get down and dirty with our tiny tots and the best way to do that, perhaps, is to acquire a pooch.

J. A. Stockman III, MD

Transplantation in patients with SCID: mismatched related stem cells or unrelated cord blood?

Fernandes JF, on behalf of Eurocord and Inborn Errors Working Party of European Group for Blood and Marrow Transplantation (Hôpital Saint Louis, Paris, France; et al)
Blood 119:2949-2955, 2012

Pediatric patients with SCID constitute medical emergencies. In the absence of an HLA-identical hematopoietic stem cell (HSC) donor, mis-matched related-donor transplantation (MMRDT) or unrelated-donor umbilical cord blood transplantation (UCBT) are valuable treatment options. To help transplantation centers choose the best treatment option, we retrospectively compared outcomes after 175 MMRDTs and 74 UCBTs in patients with SCID or Omenn syndrome. Median follow-up time was 83 months and 58 months for UCBT and MMRDT, respectively. Most UCB recipients received a myeloablative conditioning regimen; most MMRDT recipients did not. UCB recipients presented a higher frequency of complete donor chimerism ($P = .04$) and faster total lymphocyte count recovery ($P = .04$) without any statistically significance with the preparative regimen they received. The MMRDT and UCBT groups did not differ in terms of T-cell engraftment, CD4$^+$ and CD3$^+$ cell recoveries, while Ig replacement therapy was discontinued sooner after UCBT (adjusted $P = .02$). There was a trend toward a greater incidence of grades II-IV acute GVHD ($P = .06$) and more chronic GVHD ($P = .03$) after UCBT. The estimated 5-year overall survival rates were 62% ± 4% after MMRDT and 57% ± 6% after UCBT. For children with SCID and no HLA-identical sibling donor, both UCBT and MMRDT represent available HSC sources for transplantation with quite similar outcomes.

▶ Severe combined immunodeficiency (SCID) represents the most severe form of T-cell immune deficiency. Children affected with this are highly susceptible to infections and invariably die in the first year of life if left untreated. The first hematopoietic stem cell transplantation (HSCT) from an human leukocyte antigen (HLA)-identical sibling donor was used in 1968 to treat a patient with SCID and totally corrected the immune function deficiency. HSCT from an HLA-identical sibling donor has become the treatment of choice with overall survivals at 1 year approaching 90%. Unfortunately, because SCID is a genetic disease, less than 25% of affected children will have an HLA-matched sibling donor available for transplantation. The alternative is the use of a mismatched–related donor transplantation (MMRDT) using techniques for removing mature T cells from bone marrow grafts. A study examining the period between 2000 and 2005 has found that there is no significant difference in survival comparing a well-HLA-matched unrelated adult with a mismatched relative. The time needed to find an appropriate, unrelated donor is a serious limiting factor in this medical emergency setting.

The alternative to these sources of stem cells is umbilical cord blood transplantation, first reported in 1989. Over the next 25 years, more than 20 000 umbilical cord blood transplants have been performed worldwide, usually for hematologic disorders. One advantage of umbilical cord blood as a stem cell source is the acceptable degree of HLA mismatch, which increases the likelihood of finding a suitable unrelated donor. Given the urgency of the need to treat a newborn with SCID, umbilical cord blood constitutes a more readily available stem cell source than an HLA-matched, unrelated HSCT donor.

The study reported by Fernandes et al compares the outcomes (eg, survival, occurrence of graft vs host disease, engraftment, and immune recovery) after MMRDT and umbilical cord blood transplant in a large population of children with SCID. Data were collected from 2 European registries summarizing information from 32 centers. Almost 250 patients were included in the study. In this report, MMRDT and umbilical cord blood transplant groups had similar engraftment rates. However, a higher proportion of patients in the MMRDT group had to undergo repeat transplantation as the result of poor graft function compared with umbilical cord blood recipients. This finding could be related to the higher frequency of complete donor chimerism in myeloid cells in umbilical cord blood transplant recipients. Umbilical cord blood recipients also had higher total lymphocyte counts during the first year after transplantation. Total numbers of CD3+ and CD4+ T-cell numbers did not significantly differ at any point in time, however. Similar findings were found in these 2 groups with respect to neurologic development, growth, and school attendance. Also, small numbers of youngsters treated with MMRDT developed secondary malignancies including 1 with a posttransplantation lymphoproliferative disease and 2 with myelodysplastic syndrome. None of the patients treated with umbilical cord blood developed secondary malignancies.

The authors of this report concluded that MMRDT and umbilical cord blood transplantation are both valid options in SCID patients who lack an HLA-identical sibling donor. They suggest that each transplantation center choose a strategy based on their own experience and skills, considering the rapid availability of suitable umbilical cord blood or the availability of techniques for efficient removal of mature T cells from MMRD grafts. The good news is that there are now several options for infants affected with SCID, options that were not available a quarter of a century ago.

J. A. Stockman III, MD

Characteristics and outcome of early-onset, severe forms of Wiskott-Aldrich syndrome

Mahlaoui N, Pellier I, Mignot C, et al (Hôpital Universitaire Necker-Enfants Malades, Paris, France; Centre Hospitalier Universitaire Angers, France; et al)
Blood 121:1510-1516, 2013

On the basis of a nationwide database of 160 patients with Wiskott-Aldrich syndrome (WAS), we identified a subset of infants who were significantly more likely to be attributed with an Ochs score of 5 before the age of 2 (n = 26 of 47 [55%], $P = 2.8 \times 10^{-7}$). A retrospective analysis revealed that these patients often had severe refractory thrombocytopenia (n = 13), autoimmune hemolytic anemia (n = 15), and vasculitis (n = 6). One patient had developed 2 distinct cancers. Hemizygous mutations predictive of the absence of WAS protein were identified in 19 of the 24 tested patients, and the absence of WAS protein was confirmed in all 10 investigated cases. Allogeneic hematopoietic stem cell transplantation (HSCT) was found to be a curative treatment with a relatively good prognosis because it was successful in 17 of 22 patients. Nevertheless, 3 patients experienced significant disease sequelae and 4 patients died before HSCT. Therefore, the present study identifies a distinct subgroup of WAS patients with early-onset, life-threatening manifestations. We suggest that HSCT is a curative strategy in this subgroup of patients and should be performed as early in life as possible, even when a fully matched donor is lacking.

▶ Wiskott-Aldrich syndrome (WAS) can present in a variety of ways and at different ages. It is a rare X-linked primary immune deficiency that leads to the classical triad of eczema, microthrombocytopenia, and combined immunodeficiency. Only about one in 100 000 live births are affected. It is now known to be caused by the hemizygous mutation in the *WAS* gene (Xp11.22-23), which encodes the WAS protein. The latter protein is expressed solely in hematopoietic cells and has a major role in signal transduction and apoptosis. The most mild form of WAS is an X-linked thrombocytopenia, and the most severe form is true WAS with the triad described. The treatment of WAS is with allogenic hematopoietic stem cell transplantation (HSCT), which will cure the disease. Gene therapy protocols are also being developed now for those who do not have a potential transplantation donor. It is also known that the more severe the deficiency in expressing the WAS protein, the more severe the phenotype. It is not possible early on in the course of the disease to fully predict the clinical expression of the gene abnormality. Currently, the phenotypic expression is given a score range known as an Ochs range, which runs from a low (least penetrance) to 5 (full penetrance). Needless to say, a score of 5 is associated with severe disease, including autoimmunity or inflammation or malignancy. Autoimmune problems and malignancy can occur at any age and severe life-threatening issues can present during childhood.

Mahlaoui et al present data on the presentations and outcomes of patients assigned with the highest Ochs score (5) early in life. This study found that infants account for most patients with the severest form of WAS (an Ochs score of 5 with autoimmunity, inflammation, severe refractory thrombocytopenia, or malignancies). Autoimmune or cancerous complications in the course of WAS turn out to be relatively frequent. Also, a patient with a milder form of WAS could progress to a score of 5 at a later point in life. The investigators also documented many different mutations in the *WAS* gene in young patients with a severe form of WAS. None of the patients with a most advanced degree of WAS showed any detectable amounts of WAS protein.

In the most severely affected patients, the lack of efficacy of platelet transfusion indicated that the thrombocytopenia was not caused by bone marrow failure but rather to peripheral destruction, suggesting an autoimmune etiology, which was not possible to document in all cases. The finding of a refractory thrombocytopenia was an extremely strong risk factor for poor survival because therapeutic approaches other than transplantation are known to be poorly effective in such situations.

This report showed that when stem cell transplantation could be carried out, it seemed to be reasonably effective. When used for the most severe forms of WAS, long-term survival was in excess of 65%. Infants with Ochs score of 5 should undergo transplantation as soon as possible with the best available donor. Gene therapy for WAS patients lacking a suitable donor may also deliver further substantial improvements and may constitute a cure for patients with a severe WAS phenotype.

J. A. Stockman III, MD

Tetralogy of Fallot is an Uncommon Manifestation of Warts, Hypogammaglobulinemia, Infections, and Myelokathexis Syndrome

Badolato R, Dotta L, Tassone L, et al (Pediatric Clinic and A. Nocivelli Inst of Molecular Medicine, Brescia, Italy; et al)
J Pediatr 161:763-765, 2012

Warts, hypogammaglobulinemia, infections, and myelokathexis (WHIM) syndrome is a rare immunodeficiency disorder. We report three patients with WHIM syndrome who are affected by Tetralogy of Fallot (TOF). This observation suggests a possible increased risk of TOF in WHIM syndrome and that birth presentation of TOF and neutropenia should lead to suspect WHIM syndrome.

▶ If you have never heard of the WHIM syndrome, it is a rare immunodeficiency characterized by warts, hypogammaglobulinemia, infections, and myelokathexis. Myelokathexis relates to the abnormal retention and destruction of mature neutrophils in the bone marrow, resulting in a neutropenia. The disorder falls into multiple subspecialty bailiwicks including that of immunologists, infectious disease experts, and hematologists. The presenting signs may include warts, so dermatologists are often on the frontline as well. The neutropenia itself is associated with a B- and T-cell lymphopenia and hypogammaglobulinemia, the combination of which will result in a significantly increased risk of bacterial infections. In addition, certain viral infections may characterize WHIM syndrome. For example, those infected with human papillomavirus can present as not only with warts, but also with genital dysplasia and cervical cancer among other cancers. The disorder itself is the result of an autosomal dominant heterozygous mutation in the gene encoding the CXC chemokine receptor 4 (CXCR4) that leads to a gain of CXCR4 function. CXCR4 is a G-protein—coupled receptor, which together with a unique ligand helps to orchestrate leukocyte trafficking and is involved in the regulation of bone marrow homeostasis, hematopoiesis, and organogenesis.

The function of the gene that is defective in WHIM as it involves organogenesis is the subject of this report. It is well known that in addition to hematopoietic and central nervous system defects, animal models deficient in CXCR4 will exhibit cardiac defects indicating a role for this gene in the causation of cardiac malformations, including ventricular septal defects. The report by Badolato et al tells us about the interrelationship between WHIM and tetralogy of Fallot. Those who care for children know that tetralogy of Fallot is characterized by pulmonary outflow tract obstruction, ventricular septal defect, overriding aortic route, and right ventricular hypertrophy (the 4 elements of the tetralogy). The first 3 features represent abnormalities during cardiac formation in the embryo period, whereas the fourth one is merely the consequence of the obstruction of pulmonary blood flow. Tetralogy of Fallot represents 10% of all congenital defects and occurs with an incidence of 3 per 10 000 live births and often is seen in individuals with microdeletions of chromosome 22.

Badolato et al report 3 cases of WHIM syndrome in patients with tetralogy of Fallot. One patient was a 19-year-old man with a history of WHIM syndrome identified at 2.5 years of age manifesting as severe neutropenia and recurrent pneumonias resulting in bronchiectases. The teen had no evidence of hypogammaglobulinemia or warts, however. The CXCR4 gene was identified. At birth he had been diagnosed with tetralogy of Fallot. His neutropenia was able to be managed with granulocyte-colony stimulating factor. The second case was of a 15-year-old girl diagnosed with tetralogy of Fallot at birth, surgically corrected at 2 years of age. Neutropenia was discovered at 2 years of age and the bone marrow showed evidence of myelokathexis characterized by presence of mature neutrophils with morphologic abnormalities consistent with apoptosis. She too received lifelong granulocyte-stimulating factor and had genetic confirmation of WHIM syndrome following the onset of recurrent pulmonary infections. The third patient was a 7-year-old girl who had a diagnosis made of tetralogy of Fallot soon after birth and had surgical correction in the first several months of life. Neutropenia, lymphopenia, and hypogammaglobulinemia were present since infancy and again a similar bone marrow diagnosis made the likelihood of WHIM high, a diagnosis confirmed by genetic analysis of CXCR4. The child underwent treatment with intravenous immunoglobulins and had satisfactory control of infectious episodes.

I mention these cases to bring readers up to date with this interesting disorder called WHIM syndrome and its interlinks with congenital malformations, in this case, with tetralogy of Fallot. If you are ever involved with the care of a youngster with tetralogy of Fallot who begins to have recurrent infections, think about this syndrome. It is relatively easy now to diagnose with genetic testing.

J. A. Stockman III, MD

Vaccination Site and Risk of Local Reactions in Children 1 Through 6 Years of Age

Jackson LA, Peterson D, Nelson JC, et al (Group Health Res Inst, Seattle, WA; et al)
Pediatrics 131:283-289, 2013

Objective.—Our objective was to assess whether the occurrence of medically attended local reactions to intramuscularly administered vaccines varies by injection site (arm versus thigh) in children 1 to 6 years of age.

Methods.—This is a retrospective cohort study of children in the Vaccine Safety Datalink population from 2002 to 2009. Site of injection and the outcome of medically attended local reactions were identified from administrative data.

Results.—The study cohort of 1.4 million children received 6.0 million intramuscular (IM) vaccines during the study period. The primary analyses evaluated the IM vaccines most commonly administered alone, which included inactivated influenza, hepatitis A, and diphtheria-tetanus-acellular pertussis (DTaP) vaccines. For inactivated influenza and hepatitis A vaccines, local reactions were relatively uncommon, and there was no difference in risk of these events with arm versus thigh injections. The rate of local reactions after DTaP vaccines was higher, and vaccination in the arm was associated with a significantly greater risk of this outcome compared with vaccination in the thigh, both for children 12 to 35 months (relative risk: 1.88 [95% confidence interval: 1.34−2.65]) and 3 to 6 years of age (relative risk: 1.41 [95% confidence interval: 0.84−2.34]), although this difference was not statistically significant in the older age group.

Conclusions.—Injection in the thigh is associated with a significantly lower risk of a medically attended local reaction to a DTaP vaccination among children 12 to 35 months of age, supporting current recommendations to administer IM vaccinations in the thigh for children younger than 3 years of age.

▶ It has been a fairly common teaching that the choice of vaccination injection sites for children will affect the risk of local reactions after vaccination. Current recommendations of the US Advisory Committee on Immunization Practices indicate that intramuscular vaccinations given to children aged 3 years or older should be administered in the deltoid, and for toddlers aged 12 months to 2 years the anterior lateral thigh muscle is preferred, but the deltoid can be used if the muscle mass is adequate. In actual practice there is quite a bit of variability in the choice of vaccine injection site for children based on the preferences of the individuals giving the vaccine.

There have been relatively few data in the literature on the relationship between the site of vaccination and the risk of local reactions to other intramuscular vaccines recommended for children. These authors designed a study to evaluate the association between site of vaccination and the risk of medically attended local reactions by conducting a retrospective cohort study of intramuscular vaccinations administered to children aged 1 to 5 years in the Vaccine Safety Datalink (VSD) population.

The VSD is a collaborative project between the Centers for Disease Control and Prevention and 10 managed care organizations the United States. VSD was established in 1991 to monitor and evaluate vaccine safety. The VSD collects data, including information on demographics, health plan enrollment, vaccinations, and medical encounters, on more than 9 million managed care organization members annually. As part of the reporting, documentation of a child's body habitus is recorded with respect to height and weight.

The information from VSD shows that local reactions to intramuscularly administered vaccines occur more frequently after a diphtheria-tetanus-acellular pertussis (DTaP) vaccine than after an inactivated influenza or hepatitis A vaccine and that injection of a DTaP vaccine in the arm is associated with a significantly higher risk compared with administration in the thigh. No association of injection site and risk of local reaction was seen for influenza vaccine or hepatitis A vaccine. If DTaP vaccine was coadministered with another vaccine, again greater local reactions were seen when administered intermuscularly in the arm.

The results of this study support the current preference for thigh administration of intramuscular vaccinations for children aged 12 to 35 months, particularly for the DTaP vaccine. Among this age group, arm administration of DTaP vaccine was associated with a nearly 2-fold increase in the risk of medically attended local reactions compared with thigh administration, although the absolute risk of this outcome was relatively uncommon, occurring in less than 1% of vaccinated children. The results also suggest that a similar benefit may be derived from thigh administration of DTaP vaccine to children aged 3 to 6 years. Among the 3-year to 6-year age group, the investigators found a trend toward and increased risk of medically attended injection site reaction with arm administration of DTaP vaccine.

The findings from this article do support current recommendations for thigh administration of intramuscular injections in younger age children.

J. A. Stockman III, MD

Immunogenicity and safety of an investigational multicomponent, recombinant, meningococcal serogroup B vaccine (4CMenB) administered concomitantly with routine infant and child vaccinations: results of two randomised trials

Vesikari T, for the EU Meningococcal B Infant Vaccine Study group (Univ of Tampere Med School, Finland; et al)
Lancet 381:825-835, 2013

Background.—Meningococcal serogroup B disease disproportionately affects infants. We assessed lot-to-lot consistency, safety and immunogenicity, and the effect of concomitant vaccination on responses to routine vaccines of an investigational multicomponent vaccine (4CMenB) in this population.

Methods.—We did primary and booster phase 3 studies between March 31, 2008, and Aug 16, 2010, in 70 sites in Europe. We used two series of sponsor-supplied, computer-generated randomisation envelopes to allocate healthy 2 month-old infants to receive routine vaccinations (diphtheria-tetanus-acellular pertussis, inactivated poliovirus, hepatitis B plus *Haemophilus influenzae* type b, and seven-valent pneumococcal vaccine) wat 2, 4, and 6 months of age alone, or concomitantly with 4CMenB or serogroup C conjugate vaccine (MenC) in: 1) an open-label, lot-to-lot immunogenicity and safety substudy of three 4CMenB lots compared with routine vaccines alone (1:1:1:1, block size eight); or 2) an observer-blind, lot-to-lot safety substudy of three 4CMenB lots compared with MenC (1:1:1:3, block size six). At 12 months, 4CMenB-primed children from either substudy were randomised (1:1, block size two) to receive 4CMenB booster, with or without measles-mumps-rubella-varicella (MMRV) vaccine. Immunogenicity was assessed by serum bactericidal assay with human complement (hSBA) against serogroup B test strains, and on randomly selected subsets of serum samples for routine vaccines; laboratory personnel were masked to assignment. The first coprimary outcome was lot-to-lot consistency (hSBA geometric mean ratio of all lots between 0·5 and 2·0), and the second was an immune response (hSBA titre ≥5) for each of the three strains. The primary outcome for the booster study was immune response to booster dose. Immunogenicity data for 4CMenB were for the modified intention-totreat population, including all infants from the open-label substudy who provided serum samples. The safety population included all participants who contributed safety data after at least one dose of study vaccine. These trials are registered with ClinicalTrials.gov, numbers NCT00657709 and NCT00847145.

Findings.—We enrolled 2627 infants in the open-label phase, 1003 in the observer-blind phase, and 1555 in the booster study. Lot-to-lot consistency was shown for the three 4CMenB lots, with the lowest 95% lower confidence limit being 0·74 and the highest upper limit being 1·33. Of 1181−1184 infants tested 1 month after three 4CMenB doses (all lots pooled), 100% (95% CI 99−100) had hSBA titres of 5 or more against strains selective for factor H binding protein and neisserial adhesin A, and 84% (82−86) for New Zealand outer-membrane vesicle. In a subset (n = 100), 84% (75−91) of infants had hSBA titres of 5 or more against neisseria heparin binding antigen. At 12 months of age, waning titres were boosted by a fourth dose, such that 95−100% of children had hSBA titres of 5 or more for all antigens, with or without concomitant MMRV. Immune responses to routine vaccines were much the same with or without concomitant 4CMenB, but concomitant vaccination was associated with increased reactogenicity. 77% (1912 of 2478) of infants had fever of 38·5°C or higher after any 4CMenB dose, compared with 45% (295 of 659) after routine vaccines alone and 47% (228 of 490) with MenC, but only two febrile seizures were deemed probably related to 4CMenB.

Interpretation.—4CMenB is immunogenic in infants and children aged 12 months with no clinically relevant interference with routine vaccines, but increases reactogenicity when administered concomitantly with routine vaccines. This breakthrough vaccine offers an innovative solution to the major remaining cause of bacterial meningitis in infant and toddlers.

▶ Widespread use of glycoconjugate vaccines against *Haemophilus influenzae* type b, *Streptococcus pneumoniae*, and serogroup C *Neisseria meningitidis* has resulted in a substantial decrease in childhood meningitis in industrialized countries, but the persisting threat posed by serogroup B *N meningitidis* is an unwelcome anomaly as a result of the success of these other vaccines. In fact, meningococcal serogroup B is now the most prominent cause of infant bacterial meningitis and septicemia in Europe and increasingly so in the United States. This organism's external polysaccharide capsule is poorly immunogenic, sharing chemical and antigenic identity with human fetal neural-cell antigens and thus is unsuitable for use as a glycoconjugate vaccine.

These authors have hit upon a new methodology for developing a vaccine against meningococcal serogroup B organisms. The novel approach was to create a broadly protective vaccine against meningococcal serogroup B strains using identification of antigens by genome mining. The investigators report the first large-scale, phase 3 trials of primary doses of infants and a booster dose in children aged 12 months using an investigational formulation of the new meningococcal serogroup B vaccine. On the basis of this and other studies, this vaccine, known as 4CMenB, has recently been recommended for licensure by the European Medicines Agency and has been considered for approval in other countries including Canada and Australia. Although licensure in Europe will allow physicians to prescribe the vaccine, substantial benefit at a population level will only be achieved by incorporation of this vaccine into routine immunization approaches. The potential for the vaccine to induce herd immunity is unknown, and without this information, the cost-effectiveness analysis essential to inform immunization policy remains incomplete.

In an editorial that accompanied this article, Snape and Pollard[1] note that although several questions about the possible effect of the new meningococcal vaccine exist, it is certain that no disease will be prevented if the vaccine is not used. Licensure of the vaccine is only the first step in the gradual evolution of recommendations for its distribution and use.

J. A. Stockman III, MD

Reference

1. Snape MD, Pollard AJ. The beginning of the end for serogroup B meningococcus? *Lancet.* 2013;381:785-787.

Waning Protection after Fifth Dose of Acellular Pertussis Vaccine in Children

Klein NP, Bartlett J, Rowhani-Rahbar A, et al (Kaiser Permanente Vaccine Study Ctr, Oakland, CA)
N Engl J Med 367:1012-1019, 2012

Background.—In the United States, children receive five doses of diphtheria, tetanus, and acellular pertussis (DTaP) vaccine before 7 years of age. The duration of protection after five doses of DTaP is unknown.

Methods.—We assessed the risk of pertussis in children in California relative to the time since the fifth dose of DTaP from 2006 to 2011. This period included a large outbreak in 2010. We conducted a case–control study involving members of Kaiser Permanente Northern California who were vaccinated with DTaP at 47 to 84 months of age. We compared children with pertussis confirmed by a positive polymerase-chain-reaction (PCR) assay with two sets of controls: those who were PCR-negative for pertussis and closely matched controls from the general population of health-plan members. We used logistic regression to examine the risk of pertussis in relation to the duration of time since the fifth DTaP dose. Children who received whole-cell pertussis vaccine during infancy or who received any pertussis-containing vaccine after their fifth dose of DTaP were excluded.

Results.—We compared 277 children, 4 to 12 years of age, who were PCR-positive for pertussis with 3318 PCR-negative controls and 6086 matched controls. PCR-positive children were more likely to have received the fifth DTaP dose earlier than PCR-negative controls ($P < 0.001$) or matched controls ($P = 0.005$). Comparison with PCR-negative controls yielded an odds ratio of 1.42 (95% confidence interval, 1.21 to 1.66), indicating that after the fifth dose of DTaP, the odds of acquiring pertussis increased by an average of 42% per year.

Conclusions.—Protection against pertussis waned during the 5 years after the fifth dose of DTaP. (Funded by Kaiser Permanente).

▶ One would think that as much as has been written about pertussis that we would know essentially everything there is to know about this infectious disease, including its prevention via vaccination. Unfortunately, more than a quarter of a million cases of pertussis are diagnosed here in the United States. These cases result in approximately 10 000 deaths per year, largely among infants. Most care providers recall that the whole-cell pertussis vaccine, when administered as part of a combined diphtheria, tetanus toxoid in pertussis vaccine, was effective, but were also associated with adverse effects leading to the development of the diphtheria-tetanus acellular pertussis (DTaP) vaccine. The transition to DTaP began in the early 1990s, and within 10 years DTaP was being used for all 5 recommended doses. Despite high levels of vaccine coverage in children, we continue to see outbreaks of pertussis, generally occurring every 3 to 5 years. In 2010, for example, California had a large pertussis outbreak with the highest incidence rates since 1958.

Klein et al have undertaken a study to determine whether waning of DTaP protection against pertussis is occurring over time in a highly vaccinated population of school age children who had received only DTaP rather than the original whole-cell pertussis vaccine in California.

The study undertaken was carried out under the auspices of the Kaiser Permanente Northern California integrated health care delivery system that provides care to approximately 3.2 million members. In this health care system, DTaP was introduced for the first time for the fifth dose of pertussis vaccine in 1991 and completed the transition from whole-cell pertussis vaccine to DTaP for all 5 doses by 1999. The authors were able to assess the risk of pertussis in California in children relative to the time since their fifth dose of DTaP. It was determined that in the 2010 pertussis outbreak in California, a longer time since receipt of a fifth dose of DTaP was associated with an elevated risk of acquiring pertussis among children who had received all recommended acellular pertussis vaccines. In this study, the risk of pertussis increased by 42% each year after the fifth DTaP dose. The math shows that if DTaP effectiveness is initially 95%, so that the risk of pertussis in vaccinated children is only 5% that of unvaccinated children, then the risk would increase after 5 years to 29% that of unvaccinated children. The corresponding decrease in DTaP effectiveness would be from 95% to 71%. If the initial effectiveness of DTaP were only

90%, it would decrease to 42% after 5 years. Either way, regardless of the initial effectiveness, the protection from disease afforded by the fifth dose of DTaP among fully vaccinated children who had exclusively received DTaP vaccines waned substantially during the 5 years after vaccination.

So what does all this mean? It means that the findings from this report highlight the need to develop new pertussis-containing vaccines that will provide long-lasting immunity. It is clear that 5 doses of the vaccine simply do not cut it, at least not in the long haul.

J. A. Stockman III, MD

Association of Childhood Pertussis With Receipt of 5 Doses of Pertussis Vaccine by Time Since Last Vaccine Dose, California, 2010

Misegades LK, Winter K, Harriman K, et al (US Ctrs for Disease Control and Prevention, Atlanta, GA; California Dept of Public Health, Richmond)
JAMA 308:2126-2132, 2012

Context.—In 2010, California experienced its largest pertussis epidemic in more than 60 years; a substantial burden of disease was noted in the 7- to 10-year-old age group despite high diphtheria, tetanus, and acellular pertussis vaccine (DTaP) coverage, indicating the possibility of waning protection.

Objective.—To evaluate the association between pertussis and receipt of 5 DTaP doses by time since fifth DTaP dose.

Design, Setting, and Participants.—Case control evaluation conducted in 15 California counties. Cases (n = 682) were all suspected, probable, and confirmed pertussis cases among children aged 4 to 10 years reported from January through December 14, 2010; controls (n = 2016) were children in the same age group who received care from the clinicians reporting the cases. Three controls were selected per case. Vaccination histories were obtained from medical records and immunization registries.

Main Outcome Measures.—Primary outcomes were (1) odds ratios (ORs) for the association between pertussis and receipt of the 5-dose DTaP series and (2) ORs for the association between pertussis and time since completion (<12, 12-23, 24-35, 36-47, 48-59, or ≥60 months) of the 5-dose DTaP series. Logistic regression was used to calculate ORs, accounting for clustering by county and clinician, and vaccine effectiveness (VE) was estimated as $(1-OR) \times 100\%$.

Results.—Among cases and controls, 53 (7.8%) and 19 (0.9%) had not received any pertussis-containing vaccines, respectively. Compared with controls, children with pertussis had a lower odds of having received all 5 doses of DTaP (OR, 0.11; 95% CI, 0.06-0.21 [estimated VE, 88.7%; 95% CI, 79.4%-93.8%]). When children were categorized by time since completion of the DTaP series, using an unvaccinated reference group, children with pertussis compared with controls were less likely to have received their fifth dose within the prior 12 months (19 [2.8%] vs 354 [17.6%], respectively; OR, 0.02; 95% CI, 0.01-0.04 [estimated VE, 98.1%; 95%

CI, 96.1%-99.1%]). This association was evident with longer time since vaccination, with ORs increasing with time since the fifth dose. At 60 months or longer (n = 231 cases [33.9%] and n = 288 controls [14.3%]), the OR was 0.29 (95% CI, 0.15-0.54 [estimated VE, 71.2%; 95% CI, 45.8%-84.8%]). Accordingly, the estimated VE declined each year after receipt of the fifth dose of DTaP.

Conclusion.—Among children in 15 California counties, children with pertussis, compared with controls, had lower odds of having received the 5-dose DTaP series; as time since last DTaP dose increased, the odds increased, which is consistent with a progressive decrease in estimated vaccine effectiveness each year after the final dose of pertussis vaccine.

▶ This is another report documenting the impact of the change to acellular pertussis vaccine resulting in resurgence of pertussis. With the eventual widespread use diphtheria, tetanus, and acellular pertussis vaccine (DTaP) vaccine (the whole-cell vaccine), the national incidence of reported cases of pertussis decreased anywhere from 150- to 200-fold. Because of higher rates of both local and systemic adverse events associated with diphtheria, tetanus, and whole-cell pertussis (DTwP) vaccine, DTaP that contains a small number of purified antigens of *Bordetella pertussis* and have fewer adverse effects replaced DTwP vaccine in the 1990s. A DTaP vaccine is currently recommended for both primary (3 doses administered at 2, 4, and 6 months of age) and booster (2 doses administered at 15 to 18 months and 4 to 6 years of age) immunizations. In 2005, formulations suitable for adults as well as adolescents (Tdap vaccine) were approved, and an additional 1-time booster dose is now recommended.

Currently, epidemics of pertussis seem to occur every 2 to 5 years despite vaccine administration. This appears to be due to the emergence of a pool of susceptible individuals that increases with time because immunity to pertussis, whether induced by immunization or by natural infection, is not long lasting. Here in the United States, more than 25 000 and 27 000 cases were reported in 2005 and 2010, respectively. 2012 was also a banner year. Misegades et al have studied the 2010 epidemic of pertussis in California to determine whether an explanation could be found for the cause of the epidemic. The authors found that children with pertussis were less likely than controls to have received their fifth dose of DTaP within the prior 12 months, and the association increased with time after the fifth dose, from an odds ratio of 0.02 and an estimated vaccine effectiveness of 98% in the first 12 months to an odds ratio of 0.29 and an estimated vaccine effectiveness of just 71% by 60 months or later.

There is a growing consensus that acellular pertussis vaccines are less effective for controlling pertussis than whole-cell vaccine. In addition to poor immunogenicity with earlier waning of immunity with acellular vaccines, perhaps related either to the presence of more or different pertussis antigens or to nonspecific adjuvant effect from other substances and whole-cell vaccines, some have proposed that genetic changes in the bacteria might result in a degree of mismatch between the acellular vaccine antigens and the circulating strains of *Bordetella pertussis* that results in less effective vaccine-induced antibodies.

In an editorial that accompanied this report, Shapiro reminds us that although acellular vaccines may be suboptimal, they are still quite effective. The overall incidence of pertussis still remains a small fraction of what it had been in the prevaccine era. Shapiro also reminds us that the most important consideration in the management of outbreaks of pertussis is to try to protect infants, who have the most morbidity and mortality from the infection.[1] The highest rates of both hospitalizations for pertussis occur in children younger than 2 months of age. Immunization of all pregnant women and all household and daycare contacts (both adults and children) of children younger than 1 year is an important strategy to diminish the frequency of outbreaks of pertussis. Studies are badly needed to determine whether shorter intervals for booster immunizations would be helpful. Some have suggested reverting back to whole-cell vaccine for the first dose of vaccine and then switching to acellular pertussis vaccine for subsequent administrations. Obviously the pot of gold at the end of the rainbow is the development of a high-quality vaccine that has durable immunity. The search for this has yielded little in the way of additional fruits.

J. A. Stockman III, MD

Reference

1. Shapiro ED. Acellular vaccines and resurgence of pertussis. *JAMA.* 2012;308: 2149-2150.

California Pertussis Epidemic, 2010

Winter K, Harriman K, Zipprich J, et al (California Dept of Public Health, Richmond, CA; et al)
J Pediatr 161:1091-1096, 2012

Objective.—In 2010, California experienced the highest number of pertussis cases in >60 years, with >9000 cases, 809 hospitalizations, and 10 deaths. This report provides a descriptive epidemiologic analysis of this epidemic and describes public health mitigation strategies that were used, including expanded pertussis vaccine recommendations.

Study Design.—Clinical and demographic information were evaluated for all pertussis cases with onset from January 1, 2010, through December 31, 2010, and reported to the California Department of Public Health.

Results.—Hispanic infants younger than 6 months had the highest disease rates; all deaths and most hospitalizations occurred in infants younger than 3 months. Most pediatric cases were vaccinated according to national recommendations, although 9% of those aged 6 months to 18 years were completely unvaccinated against pertussis. High disease rates also were observed in fully vaccinated preadolescents, especially 10-year-olds. Mitigation strategies included expanded tetanus, diphtheria, and acellular pertussis vaccine recommendations, public and provider education, distribution of free vaccine for postpartum women and contacts of infants, and clinical guidance on diagnosis and treatment of pertussis in young infants.

Conclusions.—Infants too young to be fully vaccinated against pertussis remain at highest risk of severe disease and death. Data are needed to evaluate strategies offering direct protection of this vulnerable population, such as immunization of pregnant women and of newborns. The high rate of disease among preadolescents suggests waning of immunity from the diphtheria, tetanus, and acellular pertussis series; additional studies are warranted to evaluate the efficacy and duration of protection of the diphtheria, tetanus, and acellular pertussis series and the tetanus, diphtheria, and acellular pertussis series.

▶ There is a lot to be learned from outbreaks of disorders that constitute the definition of epidemics. Data from California indicate that vaccination plays only a part in the overall control of pertussis in this day and age. Every few years, we see either large or mini-epidemics of pertussis reported in the United States. Peak pertussis numbers were reported back in 1934 at more than a quarter of a million cases in the United States. The lowest number of cases reported occurred following extensive childhood immunizations back in 1976 with just 1010 cases reported. Since then, the number of cases of pertussis has actually increased rather than fallen. For example, during one of the cyclic epidemics occurring in 2005, more than 25 000 cases were reported in the United States. The reasons for pertussis vaccination failures are likely based on large birth cohorts of susceptible infants, the replacement of more reactogenic whole-cell vaccines with less effective acellular pertussis vaccines in the 1990s, more rapid waning of immunity conveyed by acellular pertussis vaccines, and increased detection of cases. Also, increased detection of cases is more prevalent secondary to the availability of more sensitive assays, including polymerase chain reaction testing for laboratory confirmation.

Winter et al tell us about an epidemic of pertussis that occurred in California in 2010, when more than 9000 cases of pertussis occurred, more than in any of the previous 60 years. In California in 2010, pertussis rates were highest in infants younger than 2 months of age and remained high until 6 months of age, when most infants had received all 3 doses of diphtheria, tetanus, and pertussis (DTaP). The highest rates were observed in Hispanic infants. There was also an increase in disease observed among children 7 to 10 years of age who had completed the DTaP series, but who had not yet received the tetanus, diphtheria, and pertussis (Tdap) booster recommended at 11 to 12 years, suggesting that this age group is susceptible to waning immunity. The decrease in numbers of cases observed among adolescents age 11 years to 14 years suggests that the adolescent Tdap recommendation is effective in protecting younger adolescents. Ninety percent of pertussis-related deaths were observed in Hispanic infants in California. This increased incidence in Hispanic infants is of unknown cause. Despite an increased disease risk during infancy, Hispanic children in California are estimated to have pertussis immunization rates similar to those of non-Hispanic white children. In general, Hispanic households are larger than non-Hispanic households and higher rates of pertussis in Hispanic infants might be related to an increased number of contacts and therefore more opportunities for exposure to pertussis in the household or elsewhere.

As expected, in California almost all severe pertussis disease occurred in infants. Household members most often are the source of transmission of pertussis to infants. Prevention strategies that provide direct protection to young infants such as passive transfer of pertussis antibodies to infants via immunization of pregnant women (as is done to prevent neonatal tetanus and influenza, and immunizing newborn infants, as is done to prevent transmission of hepatitis B virus) may be applicable to pertussis. In fact, in 2010 the California Department of Public Health did recommend the use of Tdap vaccine in pregnant women. The actual efficacy of this prepartum vaccination is not known.

Pertussis is almost as infectious as measles. Unfortunately, unlike measles, neither pertussis immunization nor actual disease confers lifelong immunity. It will be extremely difficult if not impossible to achieve and sustain levels of population immunity high enough to control pertussis using currently available vaccines. It is unfortunate that among adults, we still see very low Tdap immunization rates. Improvements in pertussis immunization levels may help to reduce endemic transmission of pertussis and reduce the numbers of infected infants. Until there is a vaccine that is more efficacious and confers lifelong immunity, however, one can expect that we will see continuing outbreaks from time to time.

J. A. Stockman III, MD

Measles-Containing Vaccines and Febrile Seizures in Children Age 4 to 6 Years
Klein NP, Lewis E, Baxter R, et al (Kaiser Permanente Vaccine Study Ctr, Oakland, CA; et al)
Pediatrics 129:809-814, 2012

Background.—In the United States, children receive 2 doses of measles-mumps-rubella vaccine (MMR) and varicella vaccine (V), the first between ages 1 to 2 years and the second between ages 4 to 6 years. Among 1- to 2-year-olds, the risk of febrile seizures 7 to 10 days after MMRV is double that after separate MMR + V. Whether MMRV or MMR + V affects risk for febrile seizure risk among 4- to 6-year-olds has not been reported.

Methods.—Among 4- to 6-year-old Vaccine Safety Datalink members, we identified seizures in the emergency department and hospital from 2000 to 2008 and outpatient visits for fever from 2006 to 2008 during days 7 to 10 and 0 to 42 after MMRV and MMR + V. Incorporating medical record reviews, we assessed seizure risk after MMRV and MMR + V.

Results.—From 2006 through 2008, 86 750 children received MMRV; from 2000 through 2008, 67 438 received same-day MMR + V. Seizures were rare throughout days 0 to 42 without peaking during days 7 to 10. There was 1 febrile seizure 7 to 10 days after MMRV and 0 after MMR + V. Febrile seizure risk was 1 per 86 750 MMRV doses (95% confidence interval, 1 per 3 426 441, 1 per 15 570) and 0 per 67 438 MMR + V doses (1 per 18 282).

Conclusions.—This study provides reassurance that MMRV and MMR + V were not associated with increased risk of febrile seizures among 4- to 6-year-olds. We can rule out with 95% confidence a risk greater than 1 febrile seizure per 15 500 MMRV doses and 1 per 18 000 MMR + V doses.

▶ This is an important study and should help convince vaccine naysayers that measles-mumps-rubella vaccine (MMRV) and MMR + varicella vaccine (V) are not associated with an elevated risk of febrile seizures. The data show that at most there would be only 1 febrile seizure for every 15 500 doses of measles vaccine of the MMRV type or 1 febrile seizure for every 18 000 doses of MMR + V administered.

In 2011, the United States had 222 cases of measles reported to the Centers for Disease Control and Prevention. Actually these numbers were very few compared with Europe, but it is its highest number since 1996. Interestingly, most importations of measles have come from Europe. In Europe, cases of measles have quadrupled since 2009. France alone had more than 15 000 cases in 2011. Measles' stubborn persistence in Europe is a stumbling block to any plan to eradicate the disease globally. In Europe, 1 in 3000 cases of measles results in a fatality.

Thus if one thinks it's bad in the United States with respect to eradication of measles, even the developed nations of Europe are facing a worse problem. Europe's failure has multiple and complex causes. To protect an entire population against measles, at least 95% of the population needs to be vaccinated. This has proven very difficult in Europe. Many parents underestimate the risk of the disease and overestimate the vaccine's side effects. Allegations by the British gastroenterologist, Andrew Wakefield, that MMRV can lead to autism were particularly damaging to vaccination rates in Western Europe. Such vaccination rates plummeted in the United Kingdom and Ireland as a result of the misinformation provided by Wakefield. Also, communities and certain Protestant churches are opposed to vaccinations on philosophical or religious grounds. The successes seen in the United States are largely because vaccination is required before entry into school. That is not necessarily true in all European countries.

In the United States, the combination MMRV vaccine as licensed in 2005 is recommended for administration by the Advisory Committee on Immunization Practices and is given at 1 to 2 years and 4 to 6 years of age. We now know that the risk of febrile seizures is extremely small, which is good news for parents who have had reservations about the use of this vaccine.

J. A. Stockman III, MD

Assessment of the 2010 global measles mortality reduction goal: results from a model of surveillance data

Simons E, Ferrari M, Fricks J, et al (WHO, Geneva, Switzerland; Pennsylvania State Univ, University Park; et al)
Lancet 379:2173-2178, 2012

Background.—In 2008 all WHO member states endorsed a target of 90% reduction in measles mortality by 2010 over 2000 levels. We developed a model to estimate progress made towards this goal.

Methods.—We constructed a state-space model with population and immunisation coverage estimates and reported surveillance data to estimate annual national measles cases, distributed across age classes. We estimated deaths by applying age-specific and country-specific case-fatality ratios to estimated cases in each age-country class.

Findings.—Estimated global measles mortality decreased 74% from 535 300 deaths (95% CI 347 200—976 400) in 2000 to 139 300 (71 200—447 800) in 2010. Measles mortality was reduced by more than three-quarters in all WHO regions except the WHO southeast Asia region. India accounted for 47% of estimated measles mortality in 2010, and the WHO African region accounted for 36%.

Interpretation.—Despite rapid progress in measles control from 2000 to 2007, delayed implementation of accelerated disease control in India and continued outbreaks in Africa stalled momentum towards the 2010 global measles mortality reduction goal. Intensified control measures and renewed political and financial commitment are needed to achieve mortality reduction targets and lay the foundation for future global eradication of measles.

▶ The eradication of measles globally is critical for health goals in the United States given that many cases of measles seen are imported from elsewhere in the world. A new report from the World Health Organization (WHO), the Centers for Disease Control and Prevention, and Penn State University estimates that global measles deaths declined dramatically between 2000 and 2007 thanks in part to a new partnership called the Measles Initiatives. Nonetheless, since 2007, the numbers of infections have remained flat. This report abstracted from Penn State University estimates that 139 000 children died of measles in 2010 worldwide, an impressive 74% reduction since 2000, but far short of the WHO's goal of 90%.

Some have speculated that part of the failure to achieve complete eradication is the result of the worldwide recession that has been under way. Measles vaccination campaigns have been delayed and funding has been curtailed.

Still, measles researchers feel confident that mortality from measles will drop further. Funding for the Measles Initiative has recently picked up along with adoption of a 2-dose vaccination strategy that provides optimal protection. Worldwide, Africa has seen the greatest reduction in mortality from measles—from 337 000 in 2000 to 50 000 in 2010. Deaths have dropped from an estimated 88 000 to 66 000 in India, a country that now accounts for almost half of the world's mortality resulting from measles.

Simons et al report crucial gaps in our ability to eradicate measles. Surveillance and vital record registrations are inadequate in much of the world, so we do not have a good heads-up on exactly how well we are doing. Because measles is considered for worldwide eradication, it will be crucial to improve surveillance to the point that deaths and cases will be actually measured, not estimated. It is also clear that measles' stubborn persistence in Europe is a stumbling block in any plan to eradicate the disease globally.

This commentary on the topic of measles closes with an interesting observation of how one can predict epidemic outbreaks of measles in parts of Africa by a simple method of calculating population density since measles outbreaks in that part of the world tend to occur with sudden periods of crowding. It turns out that the nighttime glow of lights picked up by satellite imaging from space predicts the spread of measles in West Africa.[1] In Niger, measles epidemics fluctuate dramatically from one season to the next. Suspecting that population density plays a part, as cities swell in numbers during the dry season and deflate when the rain starts, researchers used light sources from electric lights and fires at night as a measure of human occupancy. Measles transmission rates and population density were highly correlated. Such observations are important for tracking public health issues, for crisis management, and for improving intervention strategies.

J. A. Stockman III, MD

Reference

1. Barti M, Tatem AJ, Ferrari MJ, et al. Explaining Seasonal Fluctuations of Measles in Niger Using Nighttime Lights Images. *Science.* 2011;334:1424-1427.

Mumps Outbreak in Orthodox Jewish Communities in the United States

Barskey AE, Schulte C, Rosen JB, et al (Natl Ctr for Immunization and Respiratory Diseases, Atlanta, GA; New York State Dept of Health, Albany; New York City Dept of Health and Mental Hygiene; et al)
N Engl J Med 367:1704-1713, 2012

Background.—By 2005, vaccination had reduced the annual incidence of mumps in the United States by more than 99%, with few outbreaks reported. However, in 2006, a large outbreak occurred among highly vaccinated populations in the United States, and similar outbreaks have been reported worldwide. The outbreak described in this report occurred among U.S. Orthodox Jewish communities during 2009 and 2010.

Methods.—Cases of salivary-gland swelling and other symptoms clinically compatible with mumps were investigated, and demographic, clinical, laboratory, and vaccination data were evaluated.

Results.—From June 28, 2009, through June 27, 2010, a total of 3502 outbreak-related cases of mumps were reported in New York City, two upstate New York counties, and one New Jersey county. Of the 1648 cases for which clinical specimens were available, 50% were laboratory-confirmed. Orthodox Jewish persons accounted for 97% of case patients. Adolescents 13 to 17 years of age (27% of all patients) and males (78% of patients in that age group) were disproportionately affected. Among case patients 13 to 17 years of age with documented vaccination status, 89% had previously received two doses of a mumps containing vaccine, and 8% had received one dose. Transmission was focused within Jewish schools for boys, where students spend many hours daily in intense, face-to-face interaction. Orchitis was the most common complication (120 cases, 7% of male patients ≥12 years of age), with rates significantly higher among unvaccinated persons than among persons who had received two doses of vaccine.

Conclusions.—The epidemiologic features of this outbreak suggest that intense exposures, particularly among boys in schools, facilitated transmission and overcame vaccine-induced protection in these patients. High rates of two dose coverage reduced the severity of the disease and the transmission to persons in settings of less intense exposure.

▶ One would have thought that by this point in time, we would see few reports about outbreaks of mumps. The live attenuated mumps-virus vaccine first became available in this country in 1967. Ten years later, a single dose was recommended for children 12 months of age or older and a second dose of measles-mumps-rubella (MMR) vaccine, which was licensed in 1971, was recommended for children 4 years to 6 years of age. The widespread use of the MMR vaccine has been well-documented. Single-dose MMR vaccine coverage among children 19 months to 35 months of age during the period 1995 through 2010 ranges from 90% to 93% and 2-dose MMR vaccine coverage among adolescents 13 years to 17 years of age during the period from 2006 through 2010 range ranged from 87% to 91%. By 2005, the incidence of mumps in the United States had fallen by more than 99% in comparison to the prevaccine era.

Despite the widespread use of the mumps vaccine, in 2006 there was a national outbreak of mumps in a population of college-age persons in which the 2-dose mumps vaccination coverage had ranged from 79% to 99%. In subsequent years, outbreaks have been reported in other countries in populations that have had high 2-dose coverage. During 2009 and 2010, another outbreak occurred in the United States, this time affecting Orthodox Jewish communities. Members of these communities did not refuse vaccination and 2-dose coverage among adolescents 13 years to 17 years of age was not lower than the national average.

Barskey et al tell us about more than 1500 provisional cases of mumps occurring from June 2009 through January 2010 and also report 5 additional months of investigation, during which almost 2000 cases more were identified. These cases were largely in well-vaccinated, adolescent Orthodox Jewish males 13 years to 17 years of age, suggesting that Yeshivas (religious schools separated by sex in which Orthodox Jewish study religious text) for boys were the locus for the transmission of mumps virus during this outbreak just as colleges were locus of transmission during the 2006 mumps outbreak. It appears that intense exposure, particularly among boys in a school setting, overwhelms the protection afforded by the vaccine. In general, Orthodox girls received conventional schooling, whereas boys in Yeshivas receive intensive religious education starting at 12 years of age, with school days that are up to 15 hours long. Yeshiva study is typically interactive, involving a "chavrusa" (study partner). Partners face each other across narrow tables or lecterns to study religious text; the format is face-to-face, often with animated discussion. Frequently, several pairs of students study at a single table. A typical day involves a number of study sessions with students changing partners for each session. This chavrusa style of study may have allowed for a particularly efficient form of transmission of the mumps virus. Mumps is a respiratory infection, spread through droplets and requires closer exposure than other contagious respiratory infections transmitted by the airborne route, such as measles. The finding that transmission of mumps to non-Orthodox persons in the affected community occurred rarely and was not sustained in that population supports the conclusion that intense exposure is necessary to overcome an individual's vaccine-induced immunity. Exposures in an otherwise standard community setting would not typically be as intense as those in Yeshivas. The fact that the outbreak did not spread to surrounding communities highlights the relative effectiveness of the 2-dose MMR vaccine schedule in most settings.

This report is a fascinating one because it suggests a unique phenomenon, and that is that intense exposure to a particular virus in a vaccinated individual may overcome the immunity that is induced by routine vaccination. This editor is not aware that similar findings have been reported with other common childhood contagious illnesses for which we vaccinate.

J. A. Stockman III, MD

Clinicians' gut feeling about serious infections in children: observational study

Van den Bruel A, Thompson M, Buntinx F, et al (Radcliffe Observatory Quarter, Oxford, UK; Catholic Univ of Leuven, Belgium)
BMJ 345:e6144, 2012

Objective.—To investigate the basis and added value of clinicians' "gut feeling" that infections in children are more serious than suggested by clinical assessment.

Design.—Observational study.

Setting.—Primary care setting, Flanders, Belgium.

Participants.—Consecutive series of 3890 children and young people aged 0-16 years presenting in primary care.

Main Outcome Measures.—Presenting features, clinical assessment, doctors' intuitive response at first contact with children in primary care, and any subsequent diagnosis of serious infection determined from hospital records.

Results.—Of the 3369 children and young people assessed clinically as having a non-severe illness, six (0.2%) were subsequently admitted to hospital with a serious infection. Intuition that something was wrong despite the clinical assessment of non-severe illness substantially increased the risk of serious illness (likelihood ratio 25.5, 95% confidence interval 7.9 to 82.0) and acting on this gut feeling had the potential to prevent two of the six cases being missed (33%, 95% confidence interval 4.0% to 100%) at a cost of 44 false alarms (1.3%, 95% confidence interval 0.95% to 1.75%). The clinical features most strongly associated with gut feeling were the children's overall response (drowsiness, no laughing), abnormal breathing, weight loss, and convulsions. The strongest contextual factor was the parents' concern that the illness was different from their previous experience (odds ratio 36.3, 95% confidence interval 12.3 to 107).

Conclusions.—A gut feeling about the seriousness of illness in children is an instinctive response by clinicians to the concerns of the parents and the appearance of the children. It should trigger action such as seeking a second opinion or further investigations. The observed association between intuition and clinical markers of serious infection means that by reflecting on the genesis of their gut feeling, clinicians should be able to hone their clinical skills.

▶ This report underscores the fact that modern technology cannot replace a seasoned clinician relative to her or his own gut feeling about how sick a child is. The report of Van den Bruel et al is a fascinating one, as it represents a cross-sectional study that was originally designed to determine the accuracy of certain clinical findings to detect serious illness. The authors looked at the diagnostic accuracy of "gut feeling" for the presence of serious infections. The study was comprised of 3369 children who were seeing a primary care clinician. As one might suspect, gut feelings are strongly influenced by certain clinical features. The report showed, for example, that the presence of weight loss increased the likelihood of a clinician feeling a patient was seriously ill by a factor (odds ratio) of 10. The youngster who did not laugh increased the odds ratio by 3.8. Tachypnea produced an odds ratio of 13.6 and decreased consciousness, of course, had an odds ratio of 52. A parent concerned that the illness was different from anything they had seen before in their child produced an odds ratio of 36. Curiously, years of experience of the attending physician (years from medical school graduation) had an odds ratio for a gut feeling of serious illness of just 0.95.

The bottom line is that in children with an otherwise reassuring clinical presentation, gut feeling was associated with a sensitivity of 33%, a specificity of 99%, and a positive likely ratio of 25.5. The features most strongly associated with gut feeling were decreased consciousness, rapid breathing, and parent concern.

If one looks to Wikipedia to define gut feeling, you will find that a gut feeling, or gut reaction, is a visceral emotional reaction to something, often one of uneasiness. Gut feelings, it is said, are generally regarded as not modulated by conscious thought and are a reflection of intuition rather than rationality. They are thought to originate from the brain's insular cortex. The phrase *gut feeling* may also be used as a short-hand term for an individual's common sense perception of what is considered the right thing to do.

Wikipedia suggests that gut feelings, like all reflexive unconscious comparisons, can be reprogrammed by practice or experience. Interestingly, this report suggests that it probably does not take a lot of experience to develop gut feelings about a seriously ill child. Hopefully, that means that the ability to tell one sick child from another is well learned during residency training.

J. A. Stockman III, MD

Estimates of Illnesses, Hospitalizations and Deaths Caused by Major Bacterial Enteric Pathogens in Young Children in the United States

Scallan E, Mahon BE, Hoekstra RM, et al (Univ of Colorado Denver, Aurora; Natl Ctr for Emerging and Zoonotic Infectious Diseases, Atlanta, GA)
Pediatr Infect Dis J 32:217-221, 2013

Background.—Many enteric pathogens disproportionately affect young children. However, higher incidences of laboratory-confirmed illness may be explained, at least in part, by higher rates of medical care-seeking and stool sample submission in this age group. We estimated the overall number of bacterial enteric illnesses among children <5 years old in the United States caused by *Campylobacter, Escherichia coli* O157, nontyphoidal *Salmonella, Shigella* and *Yersinia enterocolitica.*

Materials and Methods.—We used a statistical model that scaled counts of laboratory-confirmed illnesses from the Foodborne Diseases Active Surveillance Network up to an estimated number of illnesses in the United States, adjusting for the surveillance steps needed for an illness to be laboratory diagnosed (medical care sought, stool sample submitted, bacterial culture performed, laboratory tested for pathogen, laboratory test sensitivity).

Results.—We estimated that 5 bacterial enteric pathogens caused 291,162 illnesses each year among children <5 years old, resulting in 102,746 physician visits, 7830 hospitalizations and 64 deaths. Nontyphoidal *Salmonella* caused most illnesses (42%), followed by *Campylobacter* (28%), *Shigella* (21%), *Y. enterocolitica* (5%) and *E. coli* O157 (3%). The estimated annual number of physician visits ranged from 3763 for *E. coli* O157 to 44,369 for nontyphoidal *Salmonella.* Nontyphoidal *Salmonella* was estimated to cause most hospitalizations (4670) and deaths (38).

Conclusions.—Bacterial enteric infections cause many illnesses in US children. Compared with the general population, enteric illnesses among children <5 years old are more likely to be diagnosed. However, overall rates of illness remain higher in children after adjusting for underdiagnosis in both groups.

▶ This is a fascinating report telling us how one can use reported cases of illness to extrapolate incidence and prevalence numbers. In this case, we are speaking about enteric pathogens that can cause mild to severe illness in children. We know that many enteric pathogens disproportionately affect young children. The Foodborne Diseases Active Surveillance Network (FoodNet), which conducts active, population-based surveillance in 10 US states, has consistently documented higher rates of laboratory-confirmed infection caused by *Campylobacter*, nontyphoidal *Salmonella*, *Shigella*, *Escherichia coli* O157, and *Yersinia enterocolitica* occurring in children less than 5 years old than in older children and adults. For illness to be included in the FoodNet surveillance, the ill individual must seek medical attention and submit a stool sample; the sample must be submitted for bacterial culture, and the clinical laboratory must test for and identify the causative agent. For this reason, FoodNet estimates that for every laboratory-confirmed case of infection with *E coli* O157, *Campylobacter*, nontyphoidal *Salmonella*, and *Shigella*, there are between 26 and 33 illnesses that are not laboratory confirmed, and 123 for every laboratory-confirmed *Y enterocolitica* illness. Because young children are more likely to seek medical care than their older peers, the rate of underdiagnoses may actually be lower in this age group.

Scallan et al attempted to estimate the number of illnesses, physician visits, hospitalizations, and deaths caused by these 5 bacterial pathogens here in the United States among children less than 5 years of age. They used a very interesting theoretical model to make their estimates using probability distributions to describe a range of plausible values for all model inputs. For the 5 pathogens included in this analysis, it was estimated that the organisms cause an estimated 291 162 illnesses resulting in 102 716 physician visits, 7830 hospitalizations, and 64 deaths annually among children less than 5 years of age. Nontyphoidal *Salmonella* was the leading cause of these bacterial illnesses, accounting for more than 40% of the estimated illnesses and physician visits and approximately 60% of estimated hospitalizations and deaths caused by these 5 pathogens. As suspected, the rate of underdiagnoses in children less than 5 years of age was less than half that of persons in the general population. For every one case of nontyphoidal *Salmonella* illness in children less than 5 years old, the investigators estimated 12 undiagnosed illnesses compared with 29 undiagnosed illnesses for every laboratory-confirmed illness in the general population. *Y enterocolitica* illnesses had the highest rate of underdiagnoses in both groups (48 and 123, respectively) because most clinical laboratories do not routinely test for this organism, and, of those that do, many do not use sensitive diagnostic techniques.

This report also reminds us that underdiagnoses generally occur in those who have nonbloody diarrhea. Blood in the stool usually is a trigger for a request for an enteric culture.

This commentary ends with a warning regarding a certain pet and the risk of *Salmonella* infection. It is not the common box turtle or a snake. It's the African dwarf frog (ADF), an aquatic frog part of the genus Hymenochirus, commonly kept in home aquariums. From April 1, 2009 to May 10, 2011, the CDC reported a total of 224 human infections in 42 states resulting from *S. Typhimurium*.[1] The average age of infected individuals was just 5 years. While no deaths were reported, the infection resulted in hospitalization in 30% of infected individuals. Sixty-five percent recalled contact with frogs, in particular, ADFs in the home. The median time from acquiring the frog to onset of illness was 15 days. The frogs in question came from a single breeder in California.

ADFs are currently unregulated by federal or state agencies. Persons at high-risk for *Salmonella* infection (children, pregnant women and the immune-compromised) should avoid contacts with frogs, water used by frogs, and their habitats.

J. A. Stockman III, MD

Reference

1. CDC Report. Outbreak of Human *Salmonella* Typhimurium Infections Associated with African Dwarf Frogs. 2011.

Outbreak of Salmonellosis Linked to Live Poultry From a Mail-Order Hatchery
Gaffga NH, Behravesh CB, Ettestad PJ, et al (Ctrs for Disease Control and Prevention, Atlanta, GA; New Mexico Dept of Health, Santa Fe; et al)
N Engl J Med 366:2065-2073, 2012

Background.—Outbreaks of human salmonella infections are increasingly associated with contact with live poultry, but effective control measures are elusive. In 2005, a cluster of human salmonella Montevideo infections with a rare pattern on pulsed-field gel electrophoresis (the outbreak strain) was identified by PulseNet, a national subtyping network.

Methods.—In cooperation with public health and animal health agencies, we conducted multistate investigations involving patient interviews, trace-back investigations, and environmental testing at a mail-order hatchery linked to the outbreak in order to identify the source of infections and prevent additional illnesses. A case was defined as an infection with the outbreak strain between 2004 and 2011.

Results.—From 2004 through 2011, we identified 316 cases in 43 states. The median age of the patient was 4 years. Interviews were completed with 156 patients (or their caretakers) (49%), and 36 of these patients (23%) were hospitalized. Among the 145 patients for whom information was available, 80 (55%) had bloody diarrhea. Information on contact with live young poultry was available for 159 patients, and 122 of these patients (77%) reported having such contact. A mail-order hatchery in the western United States was identified in 81% of the trace-back investigations, and the outbreak strain was isolated from samples collected at the hatchery. After interventions at the hatchery, the number of human infections declined, but transmission continued.

Conclusions.—We identified a prolonged multistate outbreak of salmonellosis, predominantly affecting young children and associated with contact with live young poultry from a mail-order hatchery. Interventions performed at the hatchery reduced, but did not eliminate, associated human infections, demonstrating the difficulty of eliminating salmonella transmission from live poultry.

▶ With all the emphasis on eating healthy these days, more and more chicken is being consumed, and the bulletin board ads of cows saying "Eat Mor Chikin" do not help these poor creatures. In the United States, approximately 50 million live poultry are sold by mail-order hatcheries annually, generating between $50 million and $70 million in sales. In 2009, 12 mail-order hatcheries sold poultry. Although the mail-order hatchery industry is smaller than the commercial poultry industry, which generates billions of dollars a year, hatcheries are encouraged to maintain the same standards of environmental hygiene as large commercial poultry and egg industries. Within 24 hours after hatching, live young poultry (eg, chickens, goslings, ducklings) are frequently shipped via the US Postal Service in cardboard boxes containing up to 100 birds to agriculture feed stores or private homes around the country. These birds can be purchased for $5 or less from agricultural stores or can be purchased directly from mail-order hatcheries. In the first half of 2009, the US Postal Service reported that it shipped approximately 1.2 million pounds of packages containing live poultry, a period during which mail-order hatcheries reported record sales because of an increased interest in raising backyard flocks.

So what does all this have to do with health-related issues? These authors report on an investigation of an ongoing multistate outbreak of human *Salmonella* Montevideo infection associated with contact with live young poultry. This report is from the Centers for Disease Control and Prevention (CDC) in Atlanta, Georgia. The investigators observed a prolonged and continuing outbreak of *Salmonella* infection primarily affecting young children and linked it firmly to contact with live young poultry from a single mail-order hatchery in the western United States. During an 8-year period from 2004 through 2011, 316 cases in 43 states were detected as part of the outbreak. Although the hatchery was working closely with the local state Departments of Public Health and Animal Health, a veterinary consultant with poultry expertise, the CDC, and other organizations to enhance and further implement *Salmonella* prevention and control recommendations, the outbreak continues. The investigation clearly showed the difficulty of reducing *Salmonella* transmission from live poultry. The particular hatchery that was investigated is not the only hatchery in the United States that has been linked to outbreaks of human *Salmonellosis* caused by infected poultry. Problems have also arisen from hatcheries in the East, the Midwest, the Southwest, and the Pacific Northwest.

Nontyphoidal *Salmonella* infections are associated with substantial morbidity and mortality in the United States, with an estimated 1 million illnesses, 19 000 hospitalizations, and 370 deaths occurring annually. Although the majority of these infections are foodborne, infection via contact with animals, including live poultry, is common. Poultry become infected with *Salmonella* through comingling with infected birds from different sources, vertical transmission from infected hens, or contaminated feed. Live poultry infected with *Salmonella* typically appear healthy and can shed bacteria intermittently, making sampling of individual birds an unreliable way to determine which birds are actually shedding the bacteria. Consumers who want to reduce their risk of illness should practice meticulous hand hygiene and encourage this behavior in children, because children younger than 5 years of age, along with elderly persons and the immunocompromised, are at highest risk of severe infection. No child should be permitted to handle or touch chicks, ducklings, or other live poultry. Live poultry should not be allowed inside a residence, bathrooms, or areas where food or drink is prepared, served, or consumed. The CDC also recommends prohibiting practices (eg, artificially coloring birds) that target the sale of birds to children. It is clear from this particular investigation that consumers are more often than not unaware of the risk of *Salmonellosis* from exposure to live poultry and are certainly not adequately warned at the time of purchase. Information warning customers about the risk of *Salmonella* infections from live poultry should be distributed by mail-order hatcheries with all shipments of live birds.

J. A. Stockman III, MD

A Phase 3 Trial of RTS,S/AS01 Malaria Vaccine in African Infants
The RTS,S Clinical Trials Partnership (Univ of Tübingen, Germany; et al)
N Engl J Med 367:2284-2295, 2012

Background.—The candidate malaria vaccine RTS,S/AS01 reduced episodes of both clinical and severe malaria in children 5 to 17 months of age by approximately 50% in an ongoing phase 3 trial. We studied infants 6 to 12 weeks of age recruited for the same trial.

Methods.—We administered RTS,S/AS01 or a comparator vaccine to 6537 infants who were 6 to 12 weeks of age at the time of the first vaccination in conjunction with Expanded Program on Immunization (EPI) vaccines in a three-dose monthly schedule. Vaccine efficacy against the first or only episode of clinical malaria during the 12 months after vaccination, a coprimary end point, was analyzed with the use of Cox regression. Vaccine efficacy against all malaria episodes, vaccine efficacy against severe malaria, safety, and immunogenicity were also assessed.

Results.—The incidence of the first or only episode of clinical malaria in the intention-to-treat population during the 14 months after the first dose of vaccine was 0.31 per person-year in the RTS,S/AS01 group and 0.40 per person-year in the control group, for a vaccine efficacy of 30.1% (95% confidence interval [CI], 23.6 to 36.1). Vaccine efficacy in the per-protocol population was 31.3% (97.5% CI, 23.6 to 38.3). Vaccine efficacy against severe malaria was 26.0% (95% CI, -7.4 to 48.6) in the intention-to-treat population and 36.6% (95% CI, 4.6 to 57.7) in the per-protocol population. Serious adverse events occurred with a similar frequency in the two study groups. One month after administration of the third dose of RTS,S/AS01, 99.7% of children were positive for anti-circumsporozoite antibodies, with a geometric mean titer of 209 EU per milliliter (95% CI, 197 to 222).

Conclusions.—The RTS,S/AS01 vaccine coadministered with EPI vaccines provided modest protection against both clinical and severe malaria in young infants. (Funded by GlaxoSmithKline Biologicals and the PATH Malaria Vaccine Initiative; RTS,S ClinicalTrials.gov number, NCT00866619.)

▶ This is an important study. Malaria continues to cause more than one million childhood deaths every year. In 2010 it was estimated that there were 216 million cases of malaria worldwide, and the deaths that have occurred are largely in children. We have been hearing about the potential for the development of a malaria vaccine for years. For example, the RTS, S/AS01 candidate malaria vaccine was designed to target the pre-erythrocyte stage of the *Plasmodium falciparum* parasite. In 2011, the authors of this report provided the results of the first ongoing phase 3 trial of this vaccine that showed that during 12 months of follow up, the vaccine had an efficacy against clinical and severe malaria, 56% among children who were 5 months to 17 months of age at the time of enrollment.[1]

This report tells us the results of the same study for children 6 weeks to 12 weeks of age comparing the vaccine with another vaccine against clinical malaria. The vaccine efficacy against clinical malaria turned out to be 31%, and the efficacy against severe malaria was 26%. This efficacy was much lower than that observed among older children.

Needless to say, the development of a malaria vaccine has been quite challenging. We do know that in subjects living in areas with high malaria infection rates, prior infection does provide partial protection for the development of severe malaria. What mediates this acquired partial protection is not known. Such partial protection may mitigate the full benefits of malaria vaccines. In fact, mechanisms of vaccine protection may be totally distinct from that of natural immunity. Nonetheless, the achievement of a vaccine efficacy against clinical malaria on the order of 56% among children 5 months to 17 months of age is indeed remarkable. The current study shows a much lower efficacy for both endpoints among children 6 weeks to 12 weeks of age, which means that the vaccines that are available now for study are not likely to be anywhere nearly as effective in this younger age group. There are probably good immunologic reasons why vaccine efficacy is significantly less at these young ages, but what is not known is why the vaccine is effective in some infants and not in others.

As of now, the results of this trial suggest that this candidate malaria vaccine is not ready to become part of the routine panel of immunizations in infants in high malaria infection areas. Several vaccine candidates are now in the pipeline that use alternative parasite targets and vaccination strategies. The results from this report suggest that attaining an effective malaria vaccine is possible, but we need to know a lot more about the effective host responses that are necessary to achieve full immunization. The work continues.

J. A. Stockman III, MD

Reference

1. Agnandji ST, Lell B, Soulanoudjingar SS, et al. The RTS, S Clinical Trials Partnership. First results of phase 3 trial of RTS, S/AS01 malaria vaccine in African children. *N Engl J Med.* 2011;365:1863-1875.

Differentiation of Reinfection from Relapse in Recurrent Lyme Disease

Nadelman RB, Hanincová K, Mukherjee P, et al (New York Med College, Valhalla; et al)
N Engl J Med 367:1883-1890, 2012

Background.—Erythema migrans is the most common manifestation of Lyme disease. Recurrences are not uncommon, and although they are usually attributed to reinfection rather than relapse of the original infection, this remains somewhat controversial. We used molecular typing of *Borrelia burgdorferi* isolates obtained from patients with culture-confirmed episodes of erythema migrans to distinguish between relapse and reinfection.

Methods.—We determined the genotype of the gene encoding outer-surface protein C (*ospC*) of *B. burgdorferi* strains detected in cultures of skin or blood specimens obtained from patients with consecutive episodes of erythema migrans. After polymerase-chain-reaction amplification, *ospC* genotyping was performed by means of reverse line-blot analysis or DNA sequencing of the nearly full-length gene. Most strains were further analyzed by determining the genotype according to the 16S–23S ribosomal RNA intergenic spacer type, multilocus sequence typing, or both. Patients received standard courses of antibiotics for erythema migrans.

Results.—B. *burgdorferi* isolates obtained from 17 patients who received a diagnosis of erythema migrans between 1991 and 2011 and who had 22 paired episodes of this lesion (initial and second episodes) were available for testing. The *ospC* genotype was found to be different at each initial and second episode. Apparently identical genotypes were identified on more than one occasion in only one patient, at the first and third episodes, 5 years apart, but different genotypes were identified at the second and fourth episodes.

Conclusions.—None of the 22 paired consecutive episodes of erythema migrans were associated with the same strain of *B. burgdorferi* on culture. Our data show that repeat episodes of erythema migrans in appropriately treated patients were due to reinfection and not relapse. (Funded by the National Institutes of Health and the William and Sylvia Silberstein Foundation.)

▶ Left to its own devices, untreated Lyme disease, caused by the tick-borne Spirochete *Borrelia burgdorferi*, starts with an expanding skin lesion, erythema migrans, followed later by neurologic involvement and/or cardiac involvement and, ultimately in some, arthritis. The latter may wax and wane for several years. Episodes of arthritis are frequently preceded by episodes of erythema migrans. Such prolonged illness was thought to be due to persistence and/or relapse of the original infection. This set of circumstances has been virtually eliminated with the use of antibiotic therapy given orally or intravenously for 2 to 4 weeks. Some patients, however, who were treated initially with antibiotics, will have recurrent erythema migrans at new body sites during subsequent Lyme disease seasons.

When a patient who has been fully treated with antibiotics has recurrence of the initial symptoms of Lyme disease such as erythema migrans during a subsequent Lyme disease transmission season, the explanation appears to be due to reinfection rather than relapse. Nadelman et al using several types of molecular typing systems to subtype strains of *B. burgdorferi* have found that in previously antibiotic treated patients if the organism can be identified a second time, it will be a different subtype of the spirochete. This will cause what appears to be "recurrent" infection. Thus the problem is reinfection, not relapse. In all cases of reinfection, virtually all recurrences took place 1 year or more apart, with the recurrence observed during June through August, paralleling the activity of nymphal ticks, the variety of which are responsible for more than 90% of cases of Lyme disease here in the United States. It is extremely unlikely that a relapse of a prior infection would have such a seasonal distribution given the delay of 1 year or more between episodes of erythema migrans.

The bottom line here is that if a patient presents with what looks like recurrent Lyme disease, chances are overwhelming that the patient has been bitten a second time by a tick and has developed a new case of Lyme disease, requiring antibiotic treatment all over again.

J. A. Stockman III, MD

Long-term Clinical Outcome After Lyme Neuroborreliosis in Childhood

Skogman BH, Glimåker K, Nordwall M, et al (Falun General Hosp, Sweden; Linköping Univ, Sweden; Vrinnevi General Hosp, Norrköping, Sweden)
Pediatrics 130:262-269, 2012

Objectives.—To determine long-term clinical outcome in children with confirmed Lyme neuroborreliosis (LNB) and to evaluate persistent subjective symptoms compared with a control group.

Methods.—After a median of 5 years, 84 children with confirmed LNB underwent a neurologic re-examination, including a questionnaire. Medical records were analyzed, and a control group ($n = 84$) was included.

Results.—The total recovery rate was 73% ($n = 61$). Objective neurologic findings, defined as "definite sequelae," were found in 16 patients (19%). The majority of these children had persistent facial nerve palsy ($n = 11$), but other motor or sensory deficits occurred ($n = 5$). Neurologic signs and/or symptoms defined as "possible sequelae" were found in another 7 patients (8%), mainly of sensory character. Nonspecific subjective symptoms were reported by 35 patients (42%) and 32 controls (38%) (nonsignificant). Affected daily activities or school performance were reported to the same extent in both groups (23% vs 20%, nonsignificant).

Conclusions.—The long-term clinical recovery rate was 73% in children with confirmed LNB. Persistent facial nerve palsy occurred in 13%, whereas other motor or sensory deficits were found in another 14%. Neurologic deficits did not affect daily activities or school performance more often among patients than controls and should be considered as mild. Furthermore, nonspecific subjective symptoms such as headache, fatigue, or memory or

TABLE 5.—Self-Reported Symptoms in Patients With LNB at Follow-Up and Controls

Major Subjective Symptoms[a]	Patients With LNB ($n = 84$), n (%)	Controls ($n = 84$), n (%)	P
Headache	28 (33)	32 (38)	NS
Fatigue	19 (23)	29 (34)	NS
Facial problems[b]	7 (8)	0 (0)	<.001
Neck pain or stiffness	9 (11)	5 (6)	NS
Vertigo	6 (7)	1 (1)	<.001
Pain, numbness, or weakness in limbs	6 (7)	1 (1)	<.001
Poor appetite or wt loss	4 (5)	5 (6)	NS
Memory or concentration problems	9 (11)	5 (6)	NS
Sleeping disorder	10 (12)	7 (8)	NS
Affected daily activities	14 (17)	12 (14)	NS
Affected school performance	12 (14)	8 (10)	NS
No reported symptoms	34 (40)	41 (49)	NS

LNB, lyme neuroborreliosis; NS, nonsignificant.
[a]Several individuals reported several symptoms.
[b]Symptoms associated with the persistent facial nerve palsy.

concentration problems were reported as often among patients as controls and should not be considered as sequelae after LNB (Table 5).

▶ This report reminds us that lyme borreliosis (LB) remains the most common tick-borne infection in the United States and most of Europe. It is caused by the spirochete *Borrelia burgdorferi*. The infection itself produces signs and symptoms in the skin, joints, heart muscles, and nervous system, although not all in individual patients. The hallmark usually is the onset of erythema migrans, the typical skin lesion of LB. The life-threatening problems with LB come when the heart is involved or when the nervous system is affected, including peripheral facial nerve palsy and subacute meningitis. Other cranial or peripheral neuropathies may occur. Joint problems can be chronic and debilitating.

Skogman et al looked at long-term outcomes in children affected by LB. This may occur even if initial therapy appears to be effective with antibiotics. For example, in children, persistent facial nerve palsy may occur in 15% to 20% of patients after lyme neuroborreliosis (LNB). Prognostic factors for this long-term problem have not been elucidated. Skogman et al designed a study to determine the long-term clinical outcome in children with confirmed LNB evaluating persistent subjective symptoms compared with control groups. The study was carried out in Sweden from 1996 through 2002. Some 84 patients were evaluated compared with control patients. The median age was 7 years (range, 2–14 years). All patients were treated with antibiotics for 10 to 14 days. A diagnosis of confirmed LNB was defined according to the European Clinical Case definition: neurologic symptoms attributable to LNB, pleocytosis in cerebrospinal fluid, and intrathecally produced immunoglobulin M (IgM) or IgG *Borrelia*-specific antibodies. The study results showed that long-term follow-up confirms that patients with neurologic manifestations of lyme disease have a recovery rate of 73%. The major finding of this report, however, was that persistent facial nerve palsy appeared in 21% of patients who had the onset of acute facial nerve palsy at the time of original diagnosis. The severity of the persistent facial nerve palsy among the patients observed was moderate. No patient was found to have a severe or total loss of facial nerve function. Patients with persistent facial nerve palsy did report subjective symptoms such as eye-closing impairment, excessive tear secretion, pronunciation difficulties, cosmetic complaints, and social problems. Other serious complications, such as persistent neuropathy, trigeminal neuropathy, hemiparesis after an associated stroke, polyneuropathy, and peroneal nerve palsy were observed in single patients with LND at follow-up. Table 5 shows the self-reported symptoms at long-term follow-up in affected individuals.

The authors of this report concluded that neurologic deficits after LB did not seem to affect daily activities and school performance and generally should be considered mild. Obviously, the truth of such a statement would be in the eye of the beholder.

J. A. Stockman III, MD

Dermatologic Manifestations of Human Parechovirus Type 3 Infection in Neonates and Infants

Shoji K, Komuro H, Miyata I, et al (Natl Ctr for Child Health and Development, Tokyo, Japan)
Pediatr Infect Dis J 32:233-236, 2013

Background.—Human parechovirus type 3 (HPeV3) infection can cause sepsis-like syndrome and meningoencephalitis in neonates and young infants. Although maculopapular rash is a reported clinical manifestation of HPeV3 infection, the frequency and detailed characteristics of rash in neonates and young infants with HPeV3 infection are unknown.

Methods.—We retrospectively reviewed the clinical characteristics of neonates and young infants who received a diagnosis of HPeV3 infection on the basis of real-time polymerase chain reaction analysis of serum and/or cerebrospinal fluid specimens at the National Center for Child Health and Development in Tokyo between November 2010 and September 2011.

Results.—Fifteen neonates and young infants were diagnosed as having HPeV3 infection; median age was 33 days (range: 10—81 days). The most common clinical presentation on admission was fever (80%), the median duration of which was 3 days (range: 1—4 days). Five (33%) children required admission to the intensive care unit for close observation, and 2 (13%) required mechanical ventilation for cardiovascular instability. After hospitalization, all children developed rash, mainly on the extremities, at a mean of 3 days (range: 1—5 days) after fever onset. The most striking finding was that 80% (12/15) of patients developed a distinctive palmar—plantar erythematous rash, which disappeared after a median of 3 days (range: 2—7 days). All patients were discharged from hospital without serious sequelae

Conclusions.—Palmar–plantar erythema in febrile neonates and young infants may be a diagnostic clue of HPeV3 infection.

▶ Most of us are very familiar with the common type of organisms that cause febrile illness in newborns and young infants. The human parechoviruses are part of a relatively newly recognized genus, *Parechovirus*, in the family Picornaviridae. Human parechovirus 1 and 2 were formerly classified in the echovirus genus as Echoviruses 22 and 23 but were reclassified because of their molecular and genetic differences. Thus far, some 16 parechoviruses have been identified with type 3 being a cause of sepsislike illness and meningoencephalitis in newborns. The latter viral infection can cause devastating neurologic damage and even death. Polymerase chain reaction (PCR) is diagnostic for parechovirus infection.

Shoji et al tell us more about the clinical manifestations of human parechovirus type 3 infection in newborns and in infants. The principal findings of sepsislike syndrome secondary to this virus in newborns and infants include fever, tachycardia, tachypnea, and rash. It is important to understand what the rash looks like. Although a maculopapular or erythematous rash is a symptom and sign of parechovirus 3 infection, until the report of Shoji et al appeared, there was little detailed description of how the dermatologic manifestations of the infection actually appear.

Shoji et al designed a study to investigate the clinical characteristics of parechovirus 3 infection in newborns and infants with emphasis on the dermatologic manifestations. The study was carried out in Japan, but the findings should apply to infants born in the United States. Parechovirus in this report was isolated from the stools of affected babies. Based on the findings from this report and others, it appears that the frequency of dermatologic manifestations in parechovirus 3 infection range from 50% to 100%. Eighty percent of children in this study had erythematous palmar-plantar rash. Rash limited to distal extremities and palmar-plantar rash are rare physical findings in neonates and infants and should initiate thinking about parechovirus and certain other enteroviruses. Needless to say, the differential diagnosis for parechovirus 3 infection includes sepsislike syndrome in neonates and young infants, which is caused by a variety of bacteria and a handful of viral pathogens. Unlike other viral pathogens, such as herpesvirus and some of the enteroviruses, hepatic enzyme elevation is relatively infrequent in parechovirus 3 infection. It should also be mentioned that the differential diagnosis must include Kawasaki disease because it too can present with palmar-plantar erythema and persistent fever unresponsive to antibiotics.

Please recognize that encephalitis is the most important clinical manifestation of parechovirus 3 infection. Data suggest that about 40% of affected infants will have neurologic sequelae after parechovirus 3 encephalitis, which highlights the importance of close developmental follow-up after hospital discharge.

Currently, PCR is not widely available for detecting parechovirus 3. Hopefully, it will be soon.

While on the topic of bacterial infections, three patients living in impoverished neighborhoods of Vancouver, British Columbia, Canada developed severe bacterial infections related to methicillin-resistant Staphylococcus aureus[1].

Investigators analyzed bed bugs taken from the patients' home. They found the same Staphylococcus aureus harbored in the bed bugs. The battle against the common bed bug has risen to an even higher level.

J. A. Stockman III, MD

Reference

1. Editorial comment. Bed bugs more than creep? *JAMA*. 2011;305:2279.

Trends in the Management of Viral Meningitis at United States Children's Hospitals

Nigrovic LE, Fine AM, Monuteaux MC, et al (Boston Children's Hosp and Harvard Med School, MA; et al)
Pediatrics 131:670 676, 2013

Objective.—To determine trends in the diagnosis and management of children with viral meningitis at US children's hospitals.

Methods.—We performed a multicenter cross sectional study of children presenting to the emergency department (ED) across the 41 pediatric tertiary-care hospitals participating in the Pediatric Health Information System between January 1, 2005, and December 31, 2011. A case of viral meningitis was defined by *International Classification of Diseases, Ninth Revision*, discharge diagnosis, and required performance of a lumbar puncture. We examined trends in diagnosis, antibiotic use, and resource utilization for children with viral meningitis over the study period.

Results.—We identified 7618 children with viral meningitis (0.05% of ED visits during the study period). Fifty-two percent of patients were <1 year of age, and 43% were female. The absolute number and the proportion of ED visits for children with viral meningitis declined from 0.98 cases per 1000 ED visits in 2005 to 0.25 cases in 2011 ($P < .001$). Most children with viral meningitis received a parenteral antibiotic (85%), and were hospitalized (91%). Overall costs for children for children with viral meningitis remain substantial (median cost per case $5056, interquartile range $3572–$7141).

Conclusions.—Between 2005 and 2011, viral meningitis diagnoses at US children's hospitals declined. However, most of these children are hospitalized, and the cost for caring for these children remains considerable.

▶ Be it fact or fiction, we seem to be seeing more patients with viral meningitis since the introduction of conjugate vaccines because there have been many fewer admissions for bacterial meningitis. A large percentage of infants and children with viral meningitis are hospitalized to receive antibiotic therapy while awaiting the results of bacterial culture. Unfortunately, there is not much written lately about rates of hospitalization for children with viral meningitis.

The authors of this article address this shortfall in our knowledge by determining whether the rate of diagnosis and management of children with viral gastroenteritis at children's hospitals has changed in recent years. Data for the article were gathered from information related to children presenting to the emergency department of a Pediatric Health Information System (PHIS) participating children's hospital. PHIS is an administrative database that contains inpatient, emergency department, ambulatory surgery, and observation data from tertiary care pediatric hospitals in the United States.

This particular study evaluated data from PHIS for children under 18 years of age who were seen in a participating hospital emergency room with a diagnosis of viral meningitis. Patients with "suspected" viral meningitis were defined by using the 6 discharge diagnosis codes from the International Clarification of Diseases Ninth Revision: meningitis due to coxsackie viruses, meningitis due to echoviruses, meningitis due to other specified enteroviruses, unspecified viral meningitis, meningitis due to adenovirus, and meningitis due to viruses not otherwise classified.

What we learn from this article is that 0.05% of emergency department visits of the participating hospitals resulted in a diagnosis of viral meningitis. Once the diagnosis was made, the average admission probability was 94%. The youngest of children were more likely to have a lumbar puncture performed, and the oldest of children were more likely to have a cranial CT performed as part of their diagnostic evaluation (43% for children ≥3 years vs 9% for children ≤3 years with respect to CT scans). Eighty-five percent of those with an "ultimate diagnosis" of viral meningitis were treated with parenteral antibiotics. The most commonly prescribed antibiotics were third-generation cephalosporins, ampicillin, and vancomycin. The most common frequently used antibiotic combinations were a third-generation cephalosporin with ampicillin, third-generation cephalosporin with vancomycin, and ampicillin with gentamicin. The youngest infants were more likely to receive acyclovir. A small minority of patients received steroids. The overall cost for the average admission was $5363. Thus, viral meningitis remains a common reason for hospitalization with the highest burden in the youngest children.

It seems clear that hospitals are being overused for admission for viral meningitis. Although some children may require hospitalization for hydration, pain control, or to ensure adequate follow-up, most children at low risk for bacterial meningitis based on signs, symptoms, and laboratory values can be appropriately managed as outpatients. For example, administration of a single dose of long-acting parenteral antibiotics such as ceftriaxone can provide coverage in the unlikely case of bacterial infection. It should be noted that the authors were surprised to observe a substantial decline in the number and proportion of patients with viral meningitis over the 7-year study period. One would have theorized that the rate of viral meningitis would not change substantially over time.

It seems that we need to reexamine the evidence-based clinical guidelines for the management of children with meningitis. This would help primary care providers and emergency medicine physicians establish better decision-making criteria to reduce hospitalization rates and antibiotic use for children with viral meningitis.

While on the topic of things viral, recognize that one virus in particular is rapidly re-emerging in one part of the world, Africa and now elsewhere. In the past decade, chikungunya — a virus transmitted by *Aedes* spp mosquitoes — has re-emerged in Africa, southern and southeastern Asia, and the Indian Ocean Islands as the cause of large outbreaks of human disease. This disease is characterized by fever, headache, myalgia, rash, and both acute and persistent arthralgia. The disease can cause severe morbidity and death. This virus is endemic to tropical regions, but the spread of *Aedes albopictus* into Europe and the Americas coupled with high viremia in infected travelers returning from endemic areas increases the risk that this virus could establish itself in new endemic regions.

Chikungunya was first isolated from a febrile patient during an outbreak in the southern province of Tanzania in 1952-1953. The name, chikungunya, which is used to describe both the virus and the disease, is derived from a Swahili or Makonde word Kun qunwala, meaning "to be contorted" or "that which bends up." The latter relates to one of the long-term consequences of the infection, a disabling arthritis that causes affected individuals to be bent over with a stooping posture.

J. A. Stockman III, MD

Risk of Fetal Death after Pandemic Influenza Virus Infection or Vaccination
Håberg SE, Trogstad L, Gunnes N, et al (Norwegian Inst of Public Health, Oslo, Norway; et al)
N Engl J Med 368:333-340, 2013

Background.—During the 2009 influenza A (H1N1) pandemic, pregnant women were at risk for severe influenza illness. This concern was complicated by questions about vaccine safety in pregnant women that were raised by anecdotal reports of fetal deaths after vaccination.

Methods.—We explored the safety of influenza vaccination of pregnant women by linking Norwegian national registries and medical consultation data to determine influenza diagnosis, vaccination status, birth outcomes, and background information for pregnant women before, during, and after the pandemic. We used Cox regression models to estimate hazard ratios for fetal death, with the gestational day as the time metric and vaccination and pandemic exposure as time-dependent exposure variables.

Results.—There were 117,347 eligible pregnancies in Norway from 2009 through 2010. Fetal mortality was 4.9 deaths per 1000 births. During the pandemic, 54% of pregnant women in their second or third trimester were vaccinated. Vaccination during pregnancy substantially reduced the risk of an influenza diagnosis (adjusted hazard ratio, 0.30; 95% confidence interval [CI], 0.25 to 0.34). Among pregnant women with a clinical diagnosis of influenza, the risk of fetal death was increased (adjusted hazard ratio, 1.91; 95% CI, 1.07 to 3.41). The risk of fetal death was reduced with vaccination during pregnancy, although this reduction was not significant (adjusted hazard ratio, 0.88; 95% CI, 0.66 to 1.17).

Conclusions.—Pandemic influenza virus infection in pregnancy was associated with an increased risk of fetal death. Vaccination during pregnancy reduced the risk of an influenza diagnosis. Vaccination itself was not associated with increased fetal mortality and may have reduced the risk of influenza-related fetal death during the pandemic. (Funded by the Norwegian Institute of Public Health.)

▶ It was well recognized during the 2009 influenza A (H1N1) pandemic that pregnant women are particularly vulnerable to severe influenza illness. Women were shown to have a heightened risk of adverse pregnancy outcomes and maternal death. These findings are consistent with prior pandemics. The World Health Organization's recommendation for administration of seasonal influenza vaccine, which includes vaccination of pregnant women, did not change during the H1N1 pandemic. Investigators in Norway thus were able to determine whether women who were vaccinated might in fact have a lower risk of severe complications or reduced fetal mortality.

These authors used National Health Registry data in Norway to assess these outcomes. In this study there were 117 347 births documented in Norway in 2009 and 2010 among women who had became pregnant during the eligible study time period. During the same period, there were 570 fetal deaths (4.9 per 1000 births). A total of 25 976 children were born after their mothers had been vaccinated during pregnancy. Almost all vaccinations had occurred during the second or third trimester. Among vaccinated women, there were 78 fetal deaths. Among 87 335 women who were pregnant during the pandemic but were unvaccinated, there were 414 fetal deaths. Vaccination during pregnancy substantially reduced the risk of influenza diagnosis (adjusted hazard ratio 0.30). Among pregnant women who did develop influenza, the risk of fetal death was increased (hazard ratio 1.91).

Given the danger posed by maternal influenza virus infection on fetal survival, this study adds to the growing evidence that vaccination of pregnant women during influenza pandemics does not harm—and may in fact benefit—the fetus. The study found absolutely no basis for withholding influenza vaccination from pregnant women in their second or third trimester, an important group, given that these women are particularly vulnerable to the severe effects of influenza virus infection.

While on the topic of disease outbreaks, those in practice should be aware that social media is helping greatly in defining the spread of disease outbreaks. Digital surveillance platforms such as HealthMap and BioCaster use software programs that assist web sites on the Internet to search and extract information, a process known as trawling and scraping. The software monitors news and social media sites, including blogs, to pick up clues about emerging public health threats. Reviews of such social media document that social media represent a new frontier in disease surveillance. For example, 1 study has shown that if Twitter had been monitored, one could have identified the spread of influenza into the London area in 2009 1 week before it emerged on the official records of public health officials.[1] Although mining of social media can be helpful in the detection of outbreaks, the methodology used is hardly perfect. It will be interesting to see how this plays out in the future.

J. A. Stockman III, MD

Reference

1. St Louis C, Zorlu G. Can Twitter predict disease outbreaks? *BMJ*. 2012;344: e2353.

Vaccination against pandemic A/H1N1 2009 influenza in pregnancy and risk of fetal death: cohort study in Denmark
Pasternak B, Svanström H, Mølgaard-Nielsen D, et al (Statens Serum Institut, Copenhagen, Denmark)
BMJ 344:e2794, 2012

Objective.—To investigate whether an adjuvanted pandemic A/H1N1 2009 influenza vaccine in pregnancy was associated with an increased risk of fetal death.
Design.—Nationwide register based cohort study.
Setting.—Denmark.
Participants.—All clinically recognised singleton pregnancies that ended between November 2009 and September 2010. Individual level data on exposure to an inactivated AS03 pandemic A/H1N1 2009 influenza vaccine (Pandemrix) and potential confounders were linked to the study cohort using a unique person identifier.
Main Outcome Measures.—The primary outcome measure was risk of fetal death (spontaneous abortion and stillbirth combined) in H1N1 vaccinated compared with unvaccinated pregnancies, adjusting for propensity scores. Secondary outcome measures were spontaneous abortion (between seven and 22 weeks' gestation) and stillbirth (after 22 completed weeks' gestation).
Results.—The cohort comprised 54 585 pregnancies; 7062 (12.9%) women were vaccinated against pandemic A/H1N1 2009 influenza during pregnancy. Overall, 1818 fetal deaths occurred (1678 spontaneous abortions and 140 stillbirths). Exposure to the H1N1 vaccine was not associated with an increased risk of fetal death (adjusted hazard ratio 0.79, 95% confidence interval 0.53 to 1.16), or the secondary outcomes of spontaneous abortion (1.11, 0.71 to 1.73) and stillbirth (0.44, 0.20 to 0.94). Estimates for fetal death were similar in pregnant women with (0.82, 0.44 to 1.53) and without comorbidities (0.77, 0.47 to 1.25).
Conclusion.—This large cohort study found no evidence of an increased risk of fetal death associated with exposure to an adjuvanted pandemic A/H1N1 2009 influenza vaccine during pregnancy.

▶ Pregnant women should be concerned about vaccines they might receive during pregnancy. However, when it comes to certain vaccines, such as the A/H1N1 vaccine, there is no need for concern. Although live vaccines are generally not recommended in pregnancy because they carry a theoretical risk to the fetus, the A/H1N1 and seasonal influenza vaccines are inactivated and do not pose this risk. Concern also exists about exposure to thimerosal in vaccines, which is used as a preservative. However, although trace amounts of thimerosal may be present in some vaccines, early exposure in utero or in infancy has not been associated with deficits in neuropsychological functioning in children. The safety of vaccine adjuvants has also raised issues for some. Adjuvants are included in vaccines to improve the immune response of a vaccine. Again, experience with adjuvanted seasonal influenza vaccines in pregnancy suggests there are no safety concerns.

The studies of influenza A/H1N1 rapidly found that infected pregnant women were at particularly high risk of severe illness. Studies showed that women were also at risk of poor perinatal outcomes should they become infected with the natural virus. Prior studies have additionally suggested that infection with seasonal influenza is associated with increased risks in pregnancy, although these risks are not as high as with A/H1N1. Thus, the prevention of infection through immunization is likely to reduce these risks. These authors present findings from an important new Danish national cohort study of women vaccinated against influenza A/H1N1 in 2009. The study suggests that women who are immunized in pregnancy will have a lower risk of fetal loss than nonimmunized women. The study provides reassuring information for people who are worried about the safety of the vaccine.

It is clear from multiple studies that women who are offered influenza vaccination by their health care professionals are more likely to be immunized and to have positive attitudes toward vaccine safety and effectiveness. In the United States and elsewhere, too few pregnant women receive the seasonal influenza vaccine. They should. In an editorial that accompanied this article, Knight and Lim[1] state that it is the duty of all professionals who care for pregnant women to be aware of the findings of this article documenting the safety of the influenza vaccine when administered during pregnancy.

J. A. Stockman III, MD

Reference

1. Knight M, Lim B. Immunization against influenza during pregnancy. *BMJ.* 2012; 344:e3091.

Risk of Adverse Fetal Outcomes Following Administration of a Pandemic Influenza A(H1N1) Vaccine During Pregnancy

Pasternak B, Svanström H, Mølgaard-Nielsen D, et al (Statens Serum Institut, Copenhagen, Denmark)

JAMA 308:165-174, 2012

Context.—Assessment of the fetal safety of vaccination against influenza A(H1N1)pdm09 in pregnancy has been limited.

Objective.—To investigate whether exposure to an adjuvanted influenza A(H1N1)pdm09 vaccine during pregnancy was associated with increased risk of adverse fetal outcomes.

Design, Setting, and Participants.—Registry-based cohort study based on all live-born singleton infants in Denmark, delivered between November

2, 2009, and September 30, 2010. In propensity score—matched analyses, we estimated prevalence odds ratios (PORs) of adverse fetal outcomes, comparing infants exposed and unexposed to an AS03-adjuvanted influenza A(H1N1)pdm09 vaccine during pregnancy.

Main Outcome Measures.—Major birth defects, preterm birth, and small size for gestational age.

Results.—From a cohort of 53 432 infants (6989 [13.1%] exposed to the influenza A[H1N1]pdm09 vaccine during pregnancy [345 in the first trimester and 6644 in the second or third trimester]), 660 (330 exposed) were included in propensity score—matched analyses of adverse fetal outcomes associated with first-trimester exposure. For analysis of small size for gestational age after second- or third-trimester exposure, 13 284 (6642 exposed) were included; for analyses of preterm birth, 12 909 (6543 exposed) were included. A major birth defect was diagnosed in 18 of 330 infants (5.5%) exposed to the vaccine in the first trimester, compared with 15 of 330 unexposed infants (4.5%) (POR, 1.21; 95% CI, 0.60-2.45). Preterm birth occurred in 31 of 330 infants (9.4%) exposed in the first trimester, compared with 24 of 330 unexposed infants (7.3%) (POR, 1.32; 95% CI, 0.76-2.31), and in 302 of 6543 infants (4.6%) with second- or third-trimester exposure, compared with 295 of 6366 unexposed infants (4.6%) (POR, 1.00; 95% CI, 0.84-1.17). Small size for gestational age was observed in 25 of 330 infants (7.6%) with first-trimester exposure compared with 31 of 330 unexposed infants (9.4%) (POR, 0.79; 95% CI, 0.46-1.37), and in 641 of 6642 infants (9.7%) with second- or third-trimester exposure, compared with 657 of 6642 unexposed infants (9.9%) (POR, 0.97; 95% CI, 0.87-1.09).

Conclusions.—In this Danish cohort, exposure to an adjuvanted influenza A(H1N1)pdm09 vaccine during pregnancy was not associated with a significantly increased risk of major birth defects, preterm birth, or fetal growth restriction.

▶ It is well known that pandemic influenza is associated with a remarkably increased morbidity and mortality during pregnancy. That was first noted at the time of the 1918 influenza epidemic. More recent studies have shown that non-pandemic seasonal influenza strains also lead to excess morbidity for pregnant women as well as for their infants. For example, in the 2009 worldwide pandemic of influenza A(H1N1), pregnant women were at high risk for severe complications, including death and intensive care admission. Thus antenatal influenza infection in pregnant women suggests a biological effect of influenza infection in the mother that compromises the fetus. These effects are rarely associated with direct infection of the fetus with the influenza virus, although fetal infection has been reported albeit infrequently during epidemics and pandemics. It appears that the normal pregnancy-associated immunologic changes many inhibit the inflammatory response to influenza virus during pregnancy, leading to increased risk to mother and infant. Because of these observations, pregnant women have been listed among high-risk groups for seasonal influenza vaccine in the United States since 1997. Safety data do suggest that these vaccines are safe in pregnancy. At the time of the 2009 influenza pandemic, women were prioritized for immunization.

Pasternak et al report on the results of an observational study on the safety in pregnancy of the monovalent inactivated influenza A(H1N1) vaccine. The authors were able to link several Danish National Registries to examine the outcomes in infants born during the 2009 epidemic. No statistically significant relationships were found between receipt of vaccine and a number of perinatal outcomes including major birth defects, preterm birth, and fetal growth restriction. The authors had sufficient sample size to exclude such adverse outcomes after vaccination in the second or third trimester, but could only exclude moderate to large risks after vaccination in the first trimester. The authors did not address the question of vaccine efficacy during pregnancy. The pandemic vaccine used in Denmark was an adjuvanted vaccine. In the United States, a nonadjuvanted vaccine was used during the same 2009 epidemic. Data from the United States suggest that this vaccine is safe.

Protection of mothers and their infants against pandemic or seasonal influenza through immunization of pregnant women remains a key strategy. If influenza infection does occur during pregnancy, treatment with antiviral agents is recommended. A recent report from Canada has shown that during the 2009 influenza epidemic, the use of the vaccine strain used at that time was associated with a small but significant risk in the incidence of Guillain-Barré syndrome, not as bad as was noted back in the 1970s, but still a risk.[1]

J. A. Stockman III, MD

Reference

1. De Wals P, Deceuninck G, Toth E. Risk of Guillain-Barré syndrome following H1N1 influenza vaccination in Quebec. *JAMA.* 2012;308:175-181.

The Burden of Influenza in Young Children, 2004—2009
Poehling KA, Edwards KM, Griffin MR, et al (Wake Forest School of Medicine, Winston-Salem, NC; Vanderbilt Univ, Med Ctr, Nashville TN; et al)
Pediatrics 131:207-216, 2013

Objective.—To characterize the health care burden of influenza from 2004 through 2009, years when influenza vaccine recommendations were expanded to all children aged ≥ 6 months.

Methods.—Population-based surveillance for laboratory-confirmed influenza was performed among children aged < 5 years presenting with fever and/or acute respiratory illness to inpatient and outpatient settings during 5 influenza seasons in 3 US counties. Enrolled children had nasal/throat swabs tested for influenza by reverse transcriptase-polymerase chain reaction and their medical records reviewed. Rates of influenza hospitalizations per 1000 population and proportions of outpatients (emergency department and clinic) with influenza were computed.

Results.—The study population comprised 2970, 2698, and 2920 children from inpatient, emergency department, and clinic settings, respectively. The single-season influenza hospitalization rates were 0.4 to 1.0 per 1000 children aged < 5 years and highest for infants < 6 months. The proportion of outpatient children with influenza ranged from 10% to 25% annually. Among children hospitalized with influenza, 58% had physician-ordered influenza testing, 35% had discharge diagnoses of influenza, and 2% received antiviral medication. Among outpatients with influenza, 7% were tested for influenza, 7% were diagnosed with influenza, and < 1% had antiviral treatment. Throughout the 5 study seasons, < 45% of influenza-negative children ≥6 months were fully vaccinated against influenza.

Conclusions.—Despite expanded vaccination recommendations, many children are insufficiently vaccinated, and substantial influenza burden remains. Antiviral use was low. Future studies need to evaluate trends in use of vaccine and antiviral agents and their impact on disease burden and identify strategies to prevent influenza in young infants.

▶ There has been much written about influenza in recent years, particularly related to the 2009 to 2010 H1N1 pandemic. Without question, influenza is a major cause of illness in young children. This is the reason the current recommendations are in place that have expanded influenza vaccine administration from children 6 months and older with underlying medical conditions to all children 6 months to 24 months in 2004, and to all children 6 months to 60 months in 2006, and finally to all children over the age of 6 months now. Unfortunately, there continues to be the problem of matching the vaccine strains to the circulating influenza virus strains that run each year. This makes it somewhat difficult to assess the disease burden over time to determine what the impact is of the new strategies for vaccination programs. Without question, in the past 10 years, several factors have affected the burden of influenza in young children, including expansion of the vaccine age recommendation, improved diagnostic tests, and the introduction of antiviral therapies.

These authors examined data from the New Vaccine Surveillance Network database to determine the burden of laboratory-confirmed influenza, vaccine coverage, and the frequency of physician-ordered, influenza-specific tests as well as influenza-specific discharge diagnoses and antiviral prescriptions. In a sense, this study packages various aspects of the burden of disease in a different way than has been reported previously because it includes diagnostic laboratory information and the writing of prescription for antiviral agents. This study targeted specific locales as typical examples of where influenza attacks affect children. For example, among almost 3600 eligible hospitalized children, data existed on 3000 who had adequate culture samples taken to package together the complete dataset. A similar number of children in emergency departments also had data collected on them.

What we learn from this article is that in the 5 influenza seasons spanning from 2004 through 2009, influenza vaccination coverage actually changed relatively little, whereas the rates of influenza hospitalization and the prevalence of influenza among outpatients did vary, as expected, annually. Most hospitalizations were for infants younger than 6 months of age. It seems very apparent that physician awareness of influenza increased among infants less than 6 months of age, but not so much among older children. During the 5 seasons under study, rates of hospitalization for influenza ranged from 0.4 to 1.0 per 1000 children aged less than 5 years. In children less than 5 years of age, complete vaccination still remained less than 50% and did not increase appreciably among hospitalized children over the later years of the study. Only in clinic population children did vaccination coverage increase significantly.

Despite the expanded age recommendations for influenza vaccination and the availability of antiviral therapy, seasonal influenza remains an important cause of hospitalization, emergency room visits, and outpatient visits among children. Vaccination and antiviral medications appear to be substantially underused. A strong focus on vaccinating children aged 6 months and older and pregnant women, as noted elsewhere, are badly needed.

J. A. Stockman III, MD

Hepatitis C Virus-Specific Cell-Mediated Immune Responses in Children Born to Mothers Infected with Hepatitis C Virus

El-Kamary SS, Hashem M, Saleh DA, et al (Univ of Maryland School of Medicine, Baltimore; Cairo Univ, Egypt; et al)
J Pediatr 162:148-154, 2013

Objective.—To investigate the association between hepatitis C virus (HCV)-specific cell-mediated immunity (CMI) responses and viral clearance in children born to mothers infected with HCV.

Study Design.—A cross-sectional study of children from a mother-infant cohort in Egypt were enrolled to detect CMI responses to recombinant core and nonstructural HCV antigens (nonstructural segments NS3, NS4a/b, and NS5 of the HCV genome) using an interferon-gamma enzyme-linked immunospot assay. Children born to mothers with chronic HCV were enrolled into 3 groups: transiently viremic (n = 5), aviremic (n = 36), and positive control (n = 6), which consisted of 1 child with chronic HCV from this cohort and another 5 children with chronic HCV from a companion study. Children without HCV born to mothers without HCV (n = 27) served as a negative control group. Wilcoxon rank sum test was used to compare the magnitude of CMI responses between groups.

Results.—None of the 6 control children who were positive for HCV responded to any HCV antigen, and 4 (80%) of 5 children with transient viremia responded to at least one HCV antigen, compared with 5 (14%) of 36 and 3 (11%) of 27 children in the aviremic and negative control groups, respectively. Children with transient viremia elicited stronger responses than did negative controls ($P = .005$), positive controls ($P = .011$), or children without HCV viremia ($P = .012$), particularly to nonstructural antigens.

Conclusions.—HCV-specific CMI responses were significantly higher in magnitude and frequency among transiently infected children compared with those persistently infected. This suggests CMI responses may be associated with past viral clearance and can identify children at high risk of infection, who can be targeted for health education, screening, and follow-up.

▶ Hepatitis C virus (HCV) infection affects a large number of children and adults throughout the world. Currently it is estimated that nearly 130 million children and adults worldwide carry this virus, which is a known major cause of liver cirrhosis and hepatic cancer. In most cases, the infection causes no symptoms and is not diagnosed until complications develop late in the course of the disease. Once detected, therapy is quite expensive and only moderately effective, with many individuals not able to tolerate the antiviral agents that are used to control infection. Some individuals will experience spontaneous eradication of HCV. We know that these individuals do so by developing neutralizing antibodies, but such antibodies correlate quite poorly with actual documentation of viral clearance. Better still is the development of cell-mediated immunity (CMI), which has also been shown to control HCV infection and to provide natural protective immunity. CMI may actually be the only biomarker of host contact with the virus when there is an absence of antibodies to HCV in infected individuals.

This study examined the relationship between HCV infection in children born of mothers with HCV infection. The infants were divided into 3 groups: transiently viremic, aviremic, and positive controls, which consisted of a child with chronic HCV from this cohort and another 5 children with chronic HCV from a companion study. Children without HCV born to mothers without HCV were included in the negative control group. The study demonstrated strong HCV-specific CMI responses among children born to mothers infected with HCV 3 to 8 years after birth. These broad HCV-specific CMI responses are similar to those detected among adults whose infection had in fact resolved and where there was loss of CMI responses in those associated with recurrent infection. The importance of CMI responses to resolving HCV infection in children is further strengthened by studies showing that humoral immunity is not necessary to clear infections in children, and that maternal neutralizing antibodies transplant subtly when transferred to the fetus and do not necessarily protect against vertical transmission of HCV.

These authors indicate that using only antibody seroconversion as a marker for past infection in HCV studies or in any patient population will miss a large number of individuals with prior HCV infection. On the other hand, CMI conversion now has been repeatedly proven to be a useful tool in detecting past exposure to the virus and can also be used to identify pediatric population at high risk of infection, thereby providing them with health education and closer follow-up in HCV screening.

Recently, the Centers for Disease Control and Prevention and a group of governmental and private sector partners developed specific recommendations regarding HCV testing of adults. Their recommendations indicate that any adult born between 1945 and 1965 should receive onetime testing for HCV without prior ascertainment of HCV risk. A second recommendation is that everyone with identified HCV infection should receive a brief alcohol screening and intervention as clinically indicated, followed by a referral to appropriate care and treatment services for HCV infection and related conditions. If these recommendations are followed, some of the issues related to vertical transmission will be minimized.[1] The reason for testing this specific age group is related to the statistic that more than three-quarters of all who are HIV infected in the United States fall within this age group.

J. A. Stockman III, MD

Reference

1. Smith BD, Morgan RL, Beckett GA, Falck-Ytter Y, Holtzman D, Ward JW. Hepatitis C virus testing of persons born during 1945–1965: recommendations from the Centers for Disease Control and Prevention. *Ann Intern Med.* 2012;157:817-822.

Nucleotide Polymerase Inhibitor Sofosbuvir plus Ribavirin for Hepatitis C

Gane EJ, Stedman CA, Hyland RH, et al (Auckland City Hosp, New Zealand; Univ of Otago, Christchurch, New Zealand; Pharmasset, Princeton, NJ; et al)
N Engl J Med 368:34-44, 2013

Background.—The standard treatment for hepatitis C virus (HCV) infection is interferon, which is administered subcutaneously and can have troublesome side effects. We evaluated sofosbuvir, an oral nucleotide inhibitor of HCV polymerase, in interferon-sparing and interferon-free regimens for the treatment of HCV infection.

Methods.—We provided open-label treatment to eight groups of patients. A total of 40 previously untreated patients with HCV genotype 2 or 3 infection were randomly assigned to four groups; all four groups received sofosbuvir (at a dose of 400 mg once daily) plus ribavirin for 12 weeks. Three of these groups also received peginterferon alfa-2a for 4, 8, or 12 weeks. Two additional groups of previously untreated patients with HCV genotype 2 or 3 infection received sofosbuvir monotherapy for 12 weeks or sofosbuvir plus peginterferon alfa-2a and ribavirin for 8 weeks. Two groups of patients with HCV genotype 1 infection received sofosbuvir and ribavirin for 12 weeks: 10 patients with no response to prior treatment and 25 with no previous treatment. We report the rate of sustained virologic response 24 weeks after therapy.

Results.—Of the 40 patients who underwent randomization, all 10 (100%) who received sofosbuvir plus ribavirin without interferon and all 30 (100%) who received sofosbuvir plus ribavirin for 12 weeks and interferon for 4, 8, or 12 weeks had a sustained virologic response at 24 weeks. For the other patients with HCV genotype 2 or 3 infection, all 10 (100%) who received sofosbuvir plus peginterferon alfa-2a and ribavirin for 8 weeks had a sustained virologic response at 24 weeks, as did 6 of 10 (60%) who received sofosbuvir monotherapy. Among patients with HCV genotype 1 infection, 21 of 25 previously untreated patients (84%) and 1 of 10 with no response to previous therapy (10%) had a sustained virologic response at 24 weeks. The most common adverse events were headache, fatigue, insomnia, nausea, rash, and anemia.

Conclusions.—Sofosbuvir plus ribavirin for 12 weeks may be effective in previously untreated patients with HCV genotype 1, 2, or 3 infection. (Funded by Pharmasset and Gilead Sciences; ClinicalTrials.gov number, NCT01260350.)

▶ Hepatitis C virus (HCV) remains a problem in both children and adults, although most infections are in adults with children becoming infected from their older counterparts. This article, therefore, is important, although it largely deals with an older age population. When it comes to children, there are an estimated 40 000 children born to HCV-positive women each year. Mother-to-infant (vertical) transmission is the main route of childhood HCV infection. Estimates for the rate of vertical transmission range from a low of 3% to a high of 10%. Risk for transmission is highest among women with a high viral load at the time of delivery and also those who may be coinfected with human immunodeficiency virus. Although antiviral therapies are contraindicated in pregnancy because of teratogenic risk, prenatal HCV screening to identify HCV-infected women unaware of their status could theoretically lead to other interventions during labor and delivery or in the perinatal period that might reduce the risk of vertical transmission.

Recently, Cottrell et al[1] produced a systematic review for the US Preventive Services Task Force on methods to reduce vertical transmission of HCV. These investigators found that 18 observational studies have evaluated the association between mode of delivery, labor management strategies, or breastfeeding practices and risk for vertical HCV transmission. Fourteen of these studies found no clear association between mode of delivery (vaginal vs cesarean delivery) and risk for transmission. Two studies reported an association between prolonged duration of ruptured membranes and increased risk for transmission. Fourteen studies found no association between breastfeeding and risk for transmission. Only English language articles were included. The meta-analysis and systematic review showed that no intervention has been clearly demonstrated to reduce the risk for vertical HCV transmission. Avoidance of breastfeeding does not seem to be indicated for reducing transmission risk.

We remain saddled with the problem of how to treat infants and older children who are HCV-positive, thus the importance of this article. These investigators evaluated the role of sofosbuvir, an oral nucleotide inhibitor of HCV polymerase, in interferon-sparing and interferon-free regimens for the treatment of HCV infection. This article follows progress in recent years on the treatment of chronic HCV infection with the first-generation protease inhibitors telaprevir and boceprevir, which has benefited many but unfortunately not all patients with HCV infection. One-quarter of all age patients with HCV genotype 1 infection who have not received previous therapy and 71% of those with no response to previous therapy do not have a sustained virologic response with protease-inhibitor—based regimens. Unfortunately, no direct-acting antiviral agents have yet been approved for patients with HCV genome type 2 or 3 infection.

These authors note that the standard of care for patients with HCV infection continues to include 24 to 48 weeks of treatment with peginterferon-alfa 2a.

Treatment with interferon unfortunately has a number of side effects, including influenza-like symptoms, depression, fatigue, neutropenia, and thrombocytopenia. Interferon must be given by weekly subcutaneous injections. As a result, a fair percentage of patients who are so treated drop out of therapy. Needless to say, the development of an interferon-free all-oral treatment regimen would represent an important advance in the management of such patients. The agent reported in this study, sofosbuvir, is a direct-acting nucleotide polymerase inhibitor that has been developed as an oral drug for the treatment of chronic HCV infection. This article provides results from a multipart phase 2a study that was designed to test the safety and efficacy of sofosbuvir and ribavirin in various regimens for the treatment of patients with HCV genotype 1, 2, or 3 infections. It appeared that sofosbuvir plus ribavirin for 12 weeks is effective in previously untreated patients with all three genotypes. These early results potentially pave the way to address several unmet medical needs for such patients who may benefit from a short-duration, all-oral regimen for HCV infection that does not include interferon with all of its complications.

It should be noted that another study appeared simultaneously in the *New England Journal of Medicine*. Investigators from San Antonio and Seattle have also shown that 12 weeks of therapy with a combination of protease inhibitor, a nonnucleoside polymerase inhibitor, and ribavirin may also be effective for treatment of HCV genotype 1 infection.[2]

J. A. Stockman III, MD

References

1. Cottrell EB, Chou R, Wasson N, Rahman B, Guise JM. Reducing risk for mother-to-infant transmission of hepatitis C virus: a systematic review for the U.S. Preventive Services Task Force. *Ann Intern Med.* 2013;158:109-113.
2. Poordad F, Lawitz E, Kowdley KV, et al. Exploratory study of oral combination antiviral therapy for hepatitis C. *N Engl J Med.* 2013;368:45-53.

Effect of Vitamin D_3 Supplementation on Upper Respiratory Tract Infections in Healthy Adults: The VIDARIS Randomized Controlled Trial
Murdoch DR, Slow S, Chambers ST, et al (Univ of Otago, Christchurch, New Zealand; et al)
JAMA 308:1333-1339, 2012

Context.—Observational studies have reported an inverse association between serum 25-hydroxyvitamin D (25-OHD) levels and incidence of upper respiratory tract infections (URTIs). However, results of clinical trials of vitamin D supplementation have been inconclusive.

Objective.—To determine the effect of vitamin D supplementation on incidence and severity of URTIs in healthy adults.

Design, Setting, and Participants.—Randomized, double-blind, placebo-controlled trial conducted among 322 healthy adults between February 2010 and November 2011 in Christchurch, New Zealand.

Intervention.—Participants were randomly assigned to receive an initial dose of 200 000 IU oral vitamin D_3, then 200 000 IU 1 month later, then 100 000 IU monthly (n = 161), or placebo administered in an identical dosing regimen (n = 161), for a total of 18 months.

Main Outcome Measures.—The primary end point was number of URTI episodes. Secondary end points were duration of URTI episodes, severity of URTI episodes, and number of days of missed work due to URTI episodes.

Results.—The mean baseline 25-OHD level of participants was 29 (SD, 9) ng/mL. Vitamin D supplementation resulted in an increase in serum 25-OHD levels that was maintained at greater than 48 ng/mL throughout the study. There were 593 URTI episodes in the vitamin D group and 611 in the placebo group, with no statistically significant differences in the number of URTIs per participant (mean, 3.7 per person in the vitamin D group and 3.8 per person in the placebo group; risk ratio, 0.97; 95% CI, 0.85-1.11), number of days of missed work as a result of URTIs (mean, 0.76 days in each group; risk ratio, 1.03; 95% CI, 0.81-1.30), duration of symptoms per episode (mean, 12 days in each group; risk ratio, 0.96; 95% CI, 0.73-1.25), or severity of URTI episodes. These findings remained unchanged when the analysis was repeated by season and by baseline 25-OHD levels.

Conclusion.—In this trial, monthly administration of 100 000 IU of vitamin D did not reduce the incidence or severity of URTIs in healthy adults.

Trial Registration.—anzctr.org.au Identifier: ACTRN12609000486224.

▶ To date, there has been no Nobel Prize awarded for the cure of the common cold. Reviews by the Cochrane Collaboration show 13 potential therapeutic or preventive interventions that have been documented to be ineffective, have questionable benefits, or are associated with adverse effects, including the use of Echinacea, zinc, steam inhalation, vitamin C, garlic, antihistamines, Chinese medicinal herbs, intranasal steroids, intranasal ipratropium, *Pelargonium sidoides* herbal extract, saline nasal irrigation, increasing fluid intake, and the administration of antivirals. Needless to say, antibiotic prescriptions are ineffective and costly, promote antibiotic-resistant bacteria, and expose patients to adverse drug effects. So is vitamin D another alternative?

The use of vitamin D to prevent the common cold or to treat it is appealing because basic research points to a protective role of vitamin D in the immune system. Vitamin D itself acts on the innate immune system, increasing production of human cathelicidin antimicrobial peptide and the adaptive immune system and modulating cytokine responses and T helper cell balance. There is research to suggest that vitamin D can enhance the clearance of bacteria, strengthen epithelial barriers to infection, and enhance the function of antigen-presenting cells. Vitamin D deficiency in children is associated with a higher rate of pneumonia and upper respiratory tract infections.[1] Also, the seasonal variation seen in 25-hydroxy vitamin D levels mirrors the seasonality of upper respiratory tract infections. There is some correlation between levels of 25-hydroxy vitamin D and the prevalence of respiratory tract infections in the overall population.

Murdoch et al report the result of a randomized clinical trial in which the investigators rigorously address the question of whether vitamin D supplementation can prevent upper respiratory tract infections. The investigators used a double-blind clinical trial that enrolled 322 healthy adults with mean 25-hydroxy vitamin D levels of 21 ng/mL who were given 100 000 IU of vitamin D_3 monthly versus placebo with follow-up for 18 months through 2 southern hemisphere winter seasons. The study was of sufficient size to detect meaningful differences. Therapy in the intervention group resulted in a rapid increase in vitamin D levels. However, the primary outcome of number of upper respiratory tract infections was not different between those receiving vitamin D and those receiving placebo.

In an editorial that accompanied this report by Linder,[2] it was noted that Clinicaltrials.gov lists at least 8 randomized, placebo-controlled trials of vitamin D to prevent respiratory tract infections. These trials vary in participant age, sample size, and vitamin D form, dosage, and frequency. The largest study that includes respiratory tract infections as a primary outcome is projected to enroll 720 senior housing residents and staff and follow them up for 1 year (Clinicaltrials.gov identifier: NCT01069874). On a much larger scale, the ongoing VITAL is a placebo-controlled, 2×2 factorial trial randomizing 20 000 men age 50 years or older and women age 55 years or older to determine whether 2000 IU/d of vitamin D or omega-3 fatty acid reduce cancer or cardiovascular outcomes over 5 years.[3] Respiratory diseases and infections are ancillary outcomes of the trial.

The Institute of Medicine back in 2011 called for additional research to determine whether vitamin D therapy reduces the incidence of respiratory tract infection. The trial abstracted has rigorously addressed this question and the results suggest that vitamin D should join the therapies listed in the Cochrane Reviews as being ineffective for preventing or treating upper respiratory tract infections in healthy adults. Presumably if such a trial were ever carried out in children, one would see the same results, but that is speculation. As an aside, a recent report showed that vitamin D supplementation does not improve depression scores of patients with low levels of vitamin D.[4] The randomized study took patients with low levels of vitamin D and administered placebo or 40 000 units of vitamin D per week for 6 months. There was no effect on depression scores.

Vitamin D may be good for your heart and bone, but it does not help your brain, at least when it comes to one's psyche, nor will it protect your chest at the time of an upcoming viral season.

J. A. Stockman III, MD

References

1. Linder JA, Singer DE. Health-related quality of life of adults with upper respiratory tract infections. *J Gen Intern Med.* 2003;18:802-807.
2. Linder JA. Vitamin D and the cure for the common cold. *JAMA.* 2012;308:1375-1376.
3. Institute of Medicine. *Dietary Reference Intakes for Calcium and Vitamin D.* Washington, DC: National Academies Press; 2011.
4. Kjærgaard M, Waterloo K, Wang CE, et al. Effect of vitamin D supplement on depression scores in people with low levels of serum 25-hydroxyvitamin D: nested case-control study and randomised clinical trial. *Br J Psychiatry.* 2012;201:360-368.

Burden of Human Metapneumovirus Infection in Young Children

Edwards KM, for the New Vaccine Surveillance Network (Vanderbilt Univ School of Medicine, Nashville, TN; et al)
N Engl J Med 368:633-643, 2013

Background.—The inpatient and outpatient burden of human metapneumovirus (HMPV) infection among young children has not been well established.

Methods.—We conducted prospective, population-based surveillance for acute respiratory illness or fever among inpatient and outpatient children less than 5 years of age in three U.S. counties from 2003 through 2009. Clinical and demographic data were obtained from parents and medical records, HMPV was detected by means of a reverse-transcriptase polymerase-chain-reaction assay, and population-based rates of hospitalization and estimated rates of outpatient visits associated with HMPV infection were determined.

Results.—HMPV was detected in 200 of 3490 hospitalized children (6%), 222 of 3257 children in outpatient clinics (7%), 224 of 3001 children in the emergency department (7%), and 10 of 770 asymptomatic controls (1%). Overall annual rates of hospitalization associated with HMPV infection were 1 per 1000 children less than 5 years of age, 3 per 1000 infants less than 6 months of age, and 2 per 1000 children 6 to 11 months of age. Children hospitalized with HMPV infection, as compared with those hospitalized without HMPV infection, were older and more likely to receive a diagnosis of pneumonia or asthma, to require supplemental oxygen, and to have a longer stay in the intensive care unit. The estimated annual burden of outpatient visits associated with HMPV infection was 55 clinic visits and 13 emergency department visits per 1000 children. The majority of HMPV-positive inpatient and outpatient children had no underlying medical conditions, although premature birth and asthma were more frequent among hospitalized children with HMPV infection than among those without HMPV infection.

Conclusions.—HMPV infection is associated with a substantial burden of hospitalizations and outpatient visits among children throughout the first 5 years of life, especially during the first year. Most children with HMPV infection were previously healthy. (Funded by the Centers for Disease Control and Prevention and the National Institutes of Health.)

▶ Metapneumovirus is a paramyxovirus that was discovered in 2001. It is associated with a significant acute respiratory illness in infants and children. The virus itself is a negative single-stranded RNA virus that is closely related to the avian metapneumovirus subgroup C. It was first isolated in the Netherlands, and in the intervening dozen years until now, it has become what is thought to be the second most common cause, after respiratory syncytial virus, of lower respiratory tract infections in young children. Compared with respiratory syncytial virus, infection with human metapneumovirus tends to occur in slightly older children and to produce disease that is somewhat less severe. If coinfection occurs with both metapneumovirus and respiratory syncytial virus, a real occurrence at times, this is generally associated with worse disease than with either virus infection alone. The virus itself is found worldwide and seems to have a seasonal distribution comparable to that seen with the common influenza viruses during winter months. The virus can be identified using polymerase chain reaction techniques. Transmission of the virus is usually the result of contact with contaminated secretions via droplet, aerosol, or fomite vectors. No treatment is known at the present time.

This article gives us much new information about the inpatient and outpatient burden of human metapneumovirus as it affects young children. The investigators designed a prospective population-based surveillance for acute respiratory illnesses in inpatient and outpatient children aged less than 5 years in three counties. The surveillance covered a 6-year period and detected metapneumovirus in 200 of almost 3500 hospitalized children.

The findings from this study document that the rate of hospitalization associated with human metapneumovirus is 1 per 1000 children, roughly the same as the rate of hospitalization associated with influenza virus and the combined parainfluenza types. The admission rate, however, is lower than the rate for respiratory syncytial virus, which currently runs about 3 per 1000 children. To say this differently, the inpatient burden of disease from metapneumovirus is roughly similar to that associated with other common respiratory viruses. If we extrapolate the numbers found in the counties surveyed in this study to the nation as a whole, we would expect about 20 000 hospitalizations to be associated annually with a diagnosis of metapneumovirus. We also learn from this article that about 40% of children hospitalized with this particular virus infection have an underlying high-risk condition such as premature birth or reactive airway disease. Conversely, about two-thirds of inpatients and three-quarters of outpatients with metapneumovirus infection are otherwise healthy, suggesting that all children are at risk for metapneumovirus infection requiring medical attention, not just those who might be at high risk for viral respiratory tract infections.

As for the clinical course of those infected with metapneumovirus, for hospitalized children, a higher rate of oxygen requirement seems to be the case as opposed to other respiratory tract viral infections. Fortunately, in this article, there were no deaths associated with human metapneumovirus infection, respiratory syncytial virus infection, or influenza. Nonetheless, other data show that human metapneumovirus is capable of causing severe disease and even fatal infection. As with other common respiratory viruses, although the peak of human metapneumovirus detection varies from year to year, the prevalence of this viral infection generally overlaps with the circulation of other common respiratory viruses.

J. A. Stockman III, MD

A New Phlebovirus Associated with Severe Febrile Illness in Missouri

McMullan LK, Folk SM, Kelly AJ, et al (Ctrs for Disease Control and Prevention, Atlanta, GA; Heartland Regional Med Ctr, St Joseph, MO)
N Engl J Med 367:834-841, 2012

Two men from northwestern Missouri independently presented to a medical facility with fever, fatigue, diarrhea, thrombocytopenia, and leukopenia, and both had been bitten by ticks 5 to 7 days before the onset of illness. *Ehrlichia chaffeensis* was suspected as the causal agent but was not found on serologic analysis, polymerase-chain-reaction (PCR) assay, or cell culture. Electron microscopy revealed viruses consistent with members of the Bunyaviridae family. Next-generation sequencing and phylogenetic analysis identified the viruses as novel members of the phlebovirus genus. Although Koch's postulates have not been completely fulfilled, we believe that this phlebovirus, which is novel in the Americas, is the cause of this clinical syndrome.

▶ This report was the first in a peer-reviewed journal to tell us about a new viral infection related to an organism in the genus Phlebovirus. This genus contains more than 70 antigenically distinct viruses that are borne by sandflies, mosquitoes, or ticks. It is known that sandfly-borne viruses are found in the Americas, Asia, Africa, and the Mediterranean regions. Infections with these viruses commonly result in a self-limited 3-day fever with the exception of *Toscana* virus, which can cause aseptic meningitis. The most well-known mosquito-borne Phlebovirus is Rift Valley Fever virus, which causes large-scale epizootics. Although most human infection with the latter results in a self-limited febrile process, the infection can progress to hepatitis, encephalitis, or hemorrhagic fever. Until now, the only tick-borne Phlebovirus known to cause human disease is "severe fever with thrombocytopenia syndrome" virus, which has been identified in central and northeastern China. Now we know that there is at least one other form of tick-borne Phlebovirus with the report of 2 men from northwestern Missouri who independently developed similar signs and symptoms.

The first patient was a 59-year-old man who lived on a 70-acre farm. In June 2009, he noticed a small nymphal tick embedded on his abdomen that he removed with tweezers. There was no rash or localized itching. The following day, the man developed a fever that was followed by severe fatigue, headache, anorexia, nausea, and nonbloodied diarrhea. He was admitted to the hospital, and laboratory tests showed a low white cell count (1900 cells per cubic millimeter) and a low platelet count of 115 000 cells per cubic millimeter. The patient was hospitalized for 10 days, during which his platelet count dropped to 37 000 cells per cubic millimeter on day 5. Leukopenia continued throughout the hospitalization with notable lymphopenia and mild neutropenia. The latter progressed to moderate neutropenia by 1 week. The patient also had elevations in hepatic enzymes. He was empirically placed on doxycycline, administered intravenously twice daily for 14 days for suspected ehrlichiosis even though this organism could never be identified. While gradually getting better, the patient still reported fatigue and recurrent headaches for 2 years from the time of his hospitalization.

The second patient was a 67-year-old man who also lived on a moderate-sized farm. He noted that in early 2009 he received an average of 20 tick bites daily for almost 2 weeks, also removing the embedded ticks with his fingers and tweezers. He developed symptoms virtually identical to the first patient. Laboratory findings were quite similar. He was hospitalized for 12 days. He gradually got better, but after hospital discharge he noted fatigue, short-term memory difficulty and anorexia that lasted for approximately 6 months.

In both cases, leukocytes were collected and total RNA was isolated from infected culture media. Full-length genome sequences were found to be identical to those of phleboviruses.

The authors of this report note that although Koch's postulates have not been completely fulfilled in these 2 cases, the findings are consistent with the identification of a new pathogenic virus here in the United States. This novel virus has been dubbed the "Heartland Virus." It is a distinct member of the Phlebovirus genus and is most closely related to tick-borne phleboviruses, notably those isolated recently in China. Common laboratory findings are leukopenia with moderate neutropenia, thrombocytopenia, and elevated hepatic enzymes. Viremia appears by day 7 after the onset of symptoms. Although the liver was involved as well as several cell lines in the blood, clinical evidence did not suggest respiratory or kidney involvement in either patient. Unfortunately, tick specimens from the 2 patients were not available, but it is suspected that the lone star tick, *Amblyomma americanum*, was the culprit. In central and southern Missouri, 99.9% of captured ticks are of this particular type. These are also abundant in northwestern Missouri and are found throughout the southeastern and south central United States, extending up the Atlantic coast to Maine.

Needless to say, 2 cases do not a series make, and therefore we do not know the full range of severity of this new and novel viral infection. Epidemiologic and ecologic studies are needed to identify disease burden, risk factors for infection, and the natural hosts of this new virus.

This commentary closes with mention of a recently implemented CalciNet, a national electronic norovirus outbreak surveillance network. The network detected a recent norovirus outbreak when several friends came down with nausea and diarrhea 24-48 hours after a meal that involved consumption of raw oysters.[1] These had been shipped frozen from South Korea. Samples of the oysters from the restaurant freezer documented the presence of norovirus. With the assistance of CalciNet, those receiving oysters from the south Asian supplier were readily notified and the shipped products recalled.

J. A. Stockman III, MD

Reference

1. Brucker R, Bui T, Kwan-Gett T, et al. Norovirus infections associated with frozen raw oysters — Washington, 2011. *MMWR*. 2012;61:109.

HIV in Persons Born Outside the United States, 2007-2010

Prosser AT, Tang T, Irene Hall H (Ctrs for Disease Control and Prevention, Atlanta, GA; ICF International Inc, Atlanta, GA)
JAMA 308:601-607, 2012

Context.—Persons born outside the United States comprise about 13% of the US population, and the challenges these persons face in accessing health care may lead to poorer human immunodeficiency virus (HIV) disease outcomes.

Objective.—To describe the epidemiology of HIV among persons born outside the United States and among US-born persons diagnosed in the United States.

Design, Setting, and Participants.—Analysis of the estimated number of US-born persons and persons born outside the United States diagnosed with HIV from 2007 through 2010 in 46 states and 5 US territories, the demographic characteristics, and the HIV transmission risk factors reported to the National HIV Surveillance System. Foreign-born persons were defined as persons born outside the United States and its territories, inclusive of naturalized citizens.

Main Outcome Measure.—Diagnosis of HIV infection.

Results.—From 2007 through 2010, HIV was diagnosed in 191 697 persons in the US population; of these, 16.2% (95% CI, 16.0%-16.3%) (n = 30 995) were born outside the United States. Of the 25 255 persons with a specified country or region of birth outside the United States, 14.5% (n = 3656) were from Africa, 41.0% (n = 10 343) were from Central America (including Mexico), and 21.5% (n = 5418) were from the Caribbean. The 4 states (California, Florida, New York, and Texas) reporting the highest numbers of persons born outside the United States and diagnosed with HIV were also the top 4 reporters of HIV cases overall. Among persons born outside the United States with HIV, 73.5% (n = 22 773) were male. Among whites, 1841 of 55 574 (3.3%) of HIV diagnoses were in persons born outside the United States; in blacks, 8614 of 86 547 diagnoses (10.0%); in Hispanics, 17 913 of 42 431 diagnoses (42.2%); and in Asians, 1987 of 3088 diagnoses (64.3%). The percentage infected through heterosexual contact was 39.4% among persons born outside the United States vs 27.2% for US-born persons.

Conclusions.—Among persons in 46 US states and 5 US territories who received a diagnosis of HIV from 2007 through 2010, 16.2% were born outside the United States. Compared with US-born persons diagnosed with HIV, persons born outside the United States had different epidemiologic characteristics.

▶ Prosser et al provide data on human immunodeficiency virus (HIV) infection among people living in, but born outside, the United States. The issue of imported infection overall is a major one in the United States. For example, in 2011, the incidence of tuberculosis among people born outside the United States was 12 times greater than that in people born in the United States. The prevalence of hepatitis B infection is at least 10 times higher among those born outside but living in the United States compared with those born in the United States. An estimated 300 000 people born in Latin America and living in the United States are infected with *Trypanosoma cruzi*, the causative organism of Chagas disease. There are fewer than 10 new cases of infection occurring de novo in the United States since 1955.

Prosser et al, using data from 46 states and 5 US territories reported through the HIV Surveillance System from 207 through 2010, identified 191 697 people who had HIV diagnosed and for whom a country or continent of birth was reported. The authors showed that of these people with HIV infection, 30 995 (16.2%) of infections occurred among those born outside the United States. The countries of birth origin with the highest number of persons diagnosed with HIV were Mexico, Haiti, Cuba, and El Salvador. Moreover, the 4 states with the highest proportion of persons born outside the United States and diagnosed with HIV (California, Florida, New York, and Texas) were also the 4 states with the highest numbers of HIV cases reported overall. The findings show that the epidemiology of HIV among those born outside the United States is different and more complicated than for other infectious diseases, such as tuberculosis, hepatitis B, or Chagas disease. For these infections, the substantially higher prevalence of infection among those born outside the United States is primarily caused by the high prevalence of these infections in the immigrant's country of origin; however, with the exception of Africa, this is not necessarily so with HIV. For example, the authors report that the largest proportion of HIV diagnoses among those born outside the United States was among those from Central America (including Mexico; 41%) where HIV is not particularly highly prevalent. In fact, the estimated adult HIV prevalence in Mexico is half (0.3) that of the United States (0.6). Although selective migration of HIV-infected people from these other countries to the United States cannot be excluded, it is likely that the majority of those who immigrated from Mexico and other areas of the world where HIV infection is uncommon among adults, such as South and Southeast Asia and East Asia, acquired their infections in the United States. In contrast, it is likely that a higher proportion of HIV infections among those of Caribbean descent, for whom the adult prevalence of infection is 1.0%, may have occurred in the country of birth. Overall, this suggests that immigrants are more likely to contract HIV once they get to the United States than its citizens, presumably for sociological reasons such as poverty.

It should be noted that even though HIV carries no casual risk of transmission, the United States has a very strict policy regarding entry of people with HIV. In 1987, the United States prohibited entry of HIV-infected travelers or those wishing legal residence. In 1991, the ban was lifted for travelers, but remained in place until 2010 for those wishing to reside in the United States. During this time, the United States did not ban people with latent tuberculosis infection or evidence of hepatitis B infection from traveling or immigrating to the United States, and reentry testing was not required for US travelers returning home after having visited high-prevalence HIV areas. A ban on entry of HIV-infected people to the United States is not consistent with public health principles and may have negative consequences. For those hoping to reside permanently in the United States, the ban raises concerns about HIV testing. Concerns about deportation or inability to reenter the United States may have dissuaded those who test positive with anonymous testing from obtaining needed medical care.

Although the United States historically is a nation of immigrants, it has been fearful and discriminatory against later generations of immigrants. The debate surrounding whether undocumented immigrants are entitled to benefits, such as health insurance, driver licenses, and publicly supported higher education, remains contentious and physicians are also caught in the middle. An editorial that accompanied this report by Katz reminds us that a central tenet of medicine is to provide care to all of those in need.[1] There is a lesson in that for the United States, a nation of immigrants.

J. A. Stockman III, MD

Reference

1. Katz MH. HIV infection among persons born outside the United States. *JAMA*. 2012;308:623-624.

Nevirapine versus Ritonavir-Boosted Lopinavir for HIV-Infected Children

Violari A, Paed FC, Lindsey JC, et al (Univ of the Witwatersrand, Johannesburg, South Africa; Harvard School of Public Health, Boston, MA; et al)
N Engl J Med 366:2380-2389, 2012

Background.—Nevirapine-based antiretroviral therapy is the predominant (and often the only) regimen available for children in resource-limited settings. Nevirapine resistance after exposure to the drug for prevention of maternal-to-child human immunodeficiency virus (HIV) transmission is common, a problem that has led to the recommendation of ritonavir-boosted lopinavir in such settings. Regardless of whether there has been prior exposure to nevirapine, the performance of nevirapine versus ritonavir-boosted lopinavir in young children has not been rigorously established.

Methods.—In a randomized trial conducted in six African countries and India, we compared the initiation of HIV treatment with zidovudine, lamivudine, and either nevirapine or ritonavir-boosted lopinavir in HIV-infected children 2 to 36 months of age who had no prior exposure to nevirapine. The primary end point was virologic failure or discontinuation of treatment by study week 24.

Results.—A total of 288 children were enrolled; the median percentage of CD4+ T cells was 15%, and the median plasma HIV type 1 (HIV-1) RNA level was 5.7 $\log_{10}$ copies per milliliter. The percentage of children who reached the primary end point was significantly higher in the nevirapine group than in the ritonavir-boosted lopinavir group (40.8% vs. 19.3%; $P < 0.001$). Among the nevirapine-treated children with virologic failure for whom data on resistance were available, more than half (19 of 32) had resistance at the time of virologic failure. In addition, the time to a protocol-defined toxicity end point was shorter in the nevirapine group ($P = 0.04$), as was the time to death ($P = 0.06$).

Conclusions.—Outcomes were superior with ritonavir-boosted lopinavir among young children with no prior exposure to nevirapine. Factors that may have contributed to the suboptimal results with nevirapine include elevated viral load at baseline, selection for nevirapine resistance, background regimen of nucleoside reverse-transcriptase inhibitors, and the standard ramp-up dosing strategy. The results of this trial present policy-makers with difficult choices. (Funded by the National Institute of Allergy and Infectious Diseases and others; P1060 ClinicalTrials.gov number, NCT00307151.)

▶ The World Health Organization (WHO) guidelines for antiretroviral treatment (ART) now recommend ritonavir-boosted lopinavir for the initial treatment of HIV-positive children younger than 2 years of age who have been previously exposed to single-dose nevirapine. The latter drug continues to be recommended for initial therapy in children without prior exposure to nevirapine; however, there has been no randomized trial comparing ritonavir-boosted lopinavir ART and nevirapine-based ART in such children. Such a comparison is important because nevirapine if effective is highly desired because it is stable at high temperatures, available in fixed-dose combinations and relatively inexpensive. Its use has also been based on extensive experience and its acceptable safety profile in the pediatric population. Often it is the only option available for infants and children.

The authors of this report tell us about a randomized trial conducted in 6 African countries and India comparing the initiation of HIV treatment with zidovudine, lamivudine, and either nevirapine or ritonavir-boosted lopinavir in HIV-infected children 2 to 36 months of age who had had no prior exposure to nevirapine. A total of 288 children were enrolled. The primary endpoint of the study was treatment failure by 24 weeks, defined as virologic failure or permanent discontinuation of the nevirapine or ritonavir-boosted lopinavir component of the treatment regimen for any reason such as the need for tuberculosis therapy, death, or another reason.

The results of this randomized clinical trial clearly will influence future therapeutic regimens. The data show that for infants and young children, regardless of whether they were previously exposed to nevirapine, clear evidence exists of the superiority of ritonavir-boosted lopinavir-based regimens over nevirapine-based regimens in terms of both safety and efficacy. These findings are important because the nevirapine-based treatment is currently the choice for first-line ART in most countries where resources are limited and is often the only readily available option.

The important issue is why the nevirapine fared less well than ritonavir-boosted lopinavir among infants in this study when in most other studies nevirapine alone seems to have been effective. The authors of this report suggest that 1 important factor may be the high plasma HIV-1 RNA levels commonly seen during infancy, which makes viral suppression much more difficult. This also tends to make the time to achievement of an undetectable plasma virus level quite a bit longer in infants than for older children and adults who have lower viral loads. It is plausible, therefore, that the use of agents for which single-gene mutations result in resistance (eg, nevirapine) may be suboptimal in the presence of high viral replication and a prolonged time to viral suppression that may confer a predisposition to the emergence of resistance. Another problem is that nevirapine is usually given in a ramped up dosing strategy in order to minimize dermatologic reactions during the initiation of therapy. This slow increase in dosage occurs over several weeks. This could also result in suboptimal levels of drug therapy during the ramp-up period, a time when viral levels in infected infants are profoundly elevated.

The data from this report clearly support ritonavir-boosted lopinavir as the basis for first-line ART in all children younger than 3 years of age, regardless of whether they have had prior drug exposure. The authors of this report note that enthusiasm for such an approach, however, may be tempered by the inherent challenges to its implementation worldwide. For example, the liquid formulation of ritonavir-boosted lopinavir has an unpleasant taste and it does not withstand high temperatures. Also, the cost of this drug combination is approximately twice that of a nevirapine-based regimen. Needless to say, policy makers are left with the usual conundrum of weighing cost versus benefit with these 2 different first-line regimens.

This report was accompanied by another looking at antiretroviral regimens to prevent intrapartum HIV infection.[1] This study of 1684 infants enrolled in the Americas and South Africa showed that in neonates whose mothers did not receive ART during pregnancy, prophylaxis with a 2- or 3-drug ART regimen is superior to a zidovudine alone for the prevention of intrapartum HIV transmission. The study also showed that the 2-drug regimen had less toxicity than the 3-drug regimen. Single-drug therapy was used in prior reports initiated within 24 hours after birth and continued for 6 weeks in neonates born to untreated mothers with HIV type 1. Transmission rates ran as high as 12% to 26%. Clearly this is not the way to go.

J. A. Stockman III, MD

Reference

1. Nielsen-Saines K, Watts DH, Veloso VG, et al. Three postpartum antiretroviral regimens to prevent intrapartum HIV infection. *N Engl J Med.* 2012;366:2368-2379.

Inhibition of HIV-1 Disease Progression by Contemporaneous HIV-2 Infection

Esbjörnsson J, Månsson F, Kvist A, et al (Lund Univ and Skåne Univ Hosp, Sweden; Lund Univ, Malmö, Sweden)
N Engl J Med 367:224-232, 2012

Background.—Progressive immune dysfunction and the acquired immunodeficiency syndrome (AIDS) develop in most persons with untreated infection with human immunodeficiency virus type 1 (HIV-1) but in only approximately 20 to 30% of persons infected with HIV type 2 (HIV-2);

among persons infected with both types, the natural history of disease progression is poorly understood.

Methods.—We analyzed data from 223 participants who were infected with HIV-1 after enrollment (with either HIV-1 infection alone or HIV-1 and HIV-2 infection) in a cohort with a long follow-up duration (approximately 20 years), according to whether HIV-2 infection occurred first, the time to the development of AIDS (time to AIDS), CD4+ and CD8+ T-cell counts, and measures of viral evolution.

Results.—The median time to AIDS was 104 months (95% confidence interval [CI], 75 to 133) in participants with dual infection and 68 months (95% CI, 60 to 76) in participants infected with HIV-1 only ($P = 0.003$). CD4+ T-cell levels were higher and CD8+ T-cell levels increased at a lower rate among participants with dual infection, reflecting slower disease progression. Participants with dual infection with HIV-2 infection preceding HIV-1 infection had the longest time to AIDS and highest levels of CD4+ T-cell counts. HIV-1 genetic diversity was significantly lower in participants with dual infections than in those with HIV-1 infection alone at similar time points after infection.

Conclusions.—Our results suggest that HIV-1 disease progression is inhibited by concomitant HIV-2 infection and that dual infection is associated with slower disease progression. The slower rate of disease progression was most evident in participants with dual infection in whom HIV-2 infection preceded HIV-1 infection. These findings could have implications for the development of HIV-1 vaccines and therapeutics. (Funded by the Swedish International Development Cooperation Agency—Swedish Agency for Research Cooperation with Developing Countries and others.)

▶ This report provides fascinating new information about what factors can help to inhibit the progression of human immunodeficiency virus type 1 (HIV-1) disease. It is well known that the natural course of HIV infection involves 3 stages. The acute infection stage is characterized by viremia, a rapid decrease in the CD4+ T-cell count, and the development of influenzalike symptoms. In the asymptomatic stage, a continuous and moderate decline in T-cell counts is seen. Finally, in the acquired immunodeficiency syndrome (AIDS) stage, opportunistic diseases develop, owing to a dysfunctional immune system. The duration of these 3 stages, particularly the asymptomatic stage, can vary widely among infected individuals. HIV-1 and HIV-2 can have similar transmission routes, cellular targets, and AIDS-defining HIV-related symptoms. However, compared with HIV-1 infection, HIV-2 infection is characterized by lower transmission rates, a longer asymptomatic stage, a slower decline in CD4+ T-cell counts, and a lower mortality rate. Progressive immune dysfunction and AIDS develop in most persons who have untreated HIV infection with HIV-1 only compared with only 20% to 30% of persons infected with HIV-2 only. HIV-2 infection largely is confined to individuals living in West Africa. In West Africa, the prevalence of dual infection with HIV-1 and HIV-2 has been reported to be 0% to 3.2%.

It was almost 2 decades ago that a possible protective effect of HIV-2 against subsequent HIV-1 infection was noted in commercial sex workers in Senegal.[1]

Unfortunately, studies of natural disease progression among persons with HIV-1 and HIV-2 infection have been limited by low numbers of study participants, short follow-up times, and lack of data on the actual time of infection.

Esbjörnsson et al analyzed data from 223 individuals who were infected with HIV and studied the impact of co-infection with HIV-2. The investigators found that HIV-2 has an inhibitory effect on the rate of HIV-1 disease progression. This inhibition was evident in the time to AIDS, at the cellular level of the immune system, and at the molecular level of HIV-1 evolution. In vitro findings have suggested that HIV-2 infection generates higher levels of β-chemokines (the natural ligands of the HIV receptor in peripheral blood cells). It is suggested that this can inhibit HIV infection and replication.

It is not clear exactly what the implications are of the data from this report, but they could be quite important. It is clear that patients with dual infection in whom HIV-2 infection preceded the HIV-1 infection will have a longer time to the development of AIDS than individuals infected only with HIV-1. This slower disease progression results in higher levels of CD4+ T cells in participants with dual infection than in those with HIV-1 alone at similar time points. Further investigation of this interplay between HIV-1 and HIV-2 could reveal new and critical mechanisms important for the development of future HIV interventions. We do not know, for example, whether vaccine development against HIV-2 could additionally help prevent the onset of either infection with HIV-1 or slow the progression of newly acquired HIV-1 infection.

J. A. Stockman III, MD

Reference

1. Travers K, Mboup S, Marlink R, et al. Natural protection against HIV-1 infection provided by HIV-2. *Science.* 1995;268:1612-1615.

Antiretroviral Prophylaxis for HIV Prevention in Heterosexual Men and Women
Baeten JM, for the Partners PrEP Study Team (Univ of Washington, Seattle; et al)
N Engl J Med 367:399-410, 2012

Background.—Antiretroviral preexposure prophylaxis is a promising approach for preventing human immunodeficiency virus type 1 (HIV-1) infection in heterosexual populations.

Methods.—We conducted a randomized trial of oral antiretroviral therapy for use as preexposure prophylaxis among HIV-1—serodiscordant heterosexual couples from Kenya and Uganda. The HIV-1—seronegative partner in each couple was randomly assigned to one of three study regimens—once-daily tenofovir (TDF), combination tenofovir—emtricitabine (TDF—FTC), or matching placebo—and followed monthly for up to 36 months. At enrollment, the HIV-1—seropositive partners were not eligible for antiretroviral therapy, according to national guidelines. All couples received standard HIV-1 treatment and prevention services.

Results.—We enrolled 4758 couples, of whom 4747 were followed: 1584 randomly assigned to TDF, 1579 to TDF—FTC, and 1584 to placebo. For 62% of the couples followed, the HIV-1—seronegative partner was male. Among HIV-1—seropositive participants, the median CD4 count was 495 cells per cubic millimeter (interquartile range, 375 to 662). A total of 82 HIV-1 infections occurred in seronegative participants during the study, 17 in the TDF group (incidence, 0.65 per 100 person-years), 13 in the TDF—FTC group (incidence, 0.50 per 100 person-years), and 52 in the placebo group (incidence, 1.99 per 100 person-years), indicating a relative reduction of 67% in the incidence of HIV-1 with TDF (95% confidence interval [CI], 44 to 81; $P < 0.001$) and of 75% with TDF—FTC (95% CI, 55 to 87; $P < 0.001$). Protective effects of TDF—FTC and TDF alone against HIV-1 were not significantly different ($P = 0.23$), and both study medications significantly reduced the HIV-1 incidence among both men and women. The rate of serious adverse events was similar across the study groups. Eight participants receiving active treatment were found to have been infected with HIV-1 at baseline, and among these eight, antiretroviral resistance developed in two during the study.

Conclusions.—Oral TDF and TDF—FTC both protect against HIV-1 infection in heterosexual men and women. (Funded by the Bill and Melinda Gates Foundation; Partners PrEP ClinicalTrials.gov number, NCT00557245.)

▶ The use of antiretroviral agents by HIV-uninfected persons before potential sexual exposure to HIV-infected partners, known as preexposure prophylaxis, is a new approach to HIV prevention. Several studies have begun to explore the possibility of preexposure prophylaxis in other parts of the world. The results of these trials are reported by Baeten et al. This report comes at a time when an Food and Drug Administration panel on the topic of preexposure prophylaxis has recommended approval of a combination antiretroviral drug for this purpose.

The results of this trial show effectiveness of antiretroviral prophylaxis against HIV infection in heterosexual men and women. The trial raises a number of issues as one might suspect. Although no evidence of increased risky sexual behavior or decreased condom usage was reported in the studies examined, it will be necessary to ensure that preexposure prophylaxis does not indirectly encourage such behavior. The high rate of pregnancies reported actually demonstrates the occurrence of unprotected intercourse and the need for increased family planning and it raises a concern about the inadvertent use of these medications in the first trimester of pregnancy. We will need to know more about how long preexposure prophylaxis should be given. We need to develop messages that health care workers can provide to patients who wish to use these drugs. Most importantly, the drugs used have the potential to affect kidney and liver function and to reduce bone density. It is also possible that HIV infection acquired during preexposure prophylaxis has the potential to develop resistance to the antiretroviral agents used, jeopardizing the therapeutic use of these drugs for both the patient in his or her subsequent treatment and for the community at large if resistance to the agents spreads more broadly. This risk is highest if preexposure of prophylaxis is started during unrecognized acute HIV infection, but can also be a risk with subsequent HIV acquisition.

To read more about preexposure prophylaxis for HIV, see the excellent editorial by Cohen and Baden.[1]

J. A. Stockman III, MD

Reference

1. Cohen MS, Baden LR. Preexposure prophylaxis for HIV — where do we go from here? *N Engl J Med.* 2012;367:459-461.

11 Miscellaneous

A Randomized Study of How Physicians Interpret Research Funding Disclosures
Kesselhoim AS, Robertson CI, Myers JA, et al (Brigham and Women's Hosp and Harvard Med School, Boston, MA; Edmond J. Safra Ctr for Ethics at Harvard Univ, Cambridge, MA; et al)
N Engl J Med 367:1119-1127, 2012

Background.—The effects of clinical-trial funding on the interpretation of trial results are poorly understood. We examined how such support affects physicians' reactions to trials with a high, medium, or low level of methodologic rigor.

Methods.—We presented 503 board-certified internists with abstracts that we designed describing clinical trials of three hypothetical drugs. The trials had high, medium, or low methodologic rigor, and each report included one of three support disclosures: funding from a pharmaceutical company, NIH funding, or none. For both factors studied (rigor and funding), one of the three possible variations was randomly selected for inclusion in the abstracts. Follow-up questions assessed the physicians' impressions of the trials' rigor, their confidence in the results, and their willingness to prescribe the drugs.

Results.—The 269 respondents (53.5% response rate) perceived the level of study rigor accurately. Physicians reported that they would be less willing to prescribe drugs tested in low-rigor trials than those tested in medium-rigor trials (odds ratio, 0.64; 95% confidence interval [CI], 0.46 to 0.89; $P = 0.008$) and would be more willing to prescribe drugs tested in high-rigor trials than those tested in medium-rigor trials (odds ratio, 3.07; 95% CI, 2.18 to 4.32; $P < 0.001$). Disclosure of industry funding, as compared with no disclosure of funding, led physicians to downgrade the rigor of a trial (odds ratio, 0.63; 95% CI, 0.46 to 0.87; $P = 0.006$), their confidence in the results (odds ratio, 0.71; 95% CI, 0.51 to 0.98; $P = 0.04$), and their willingness to prescribe the hypothetical drugs (odds ratio, 0.68; 95% CI, 0.49 to 0.94; $P = 0.02$). Physicians were half as willing to prescribe drugs studied in industry-funded trials as they were to prescribe drugs studied in NIH-funded trials (odds ratio, 0.52; 95% CI, 0.37 to 0.71; $P < 0.001$). These effects were consistent across all levels of methodologic rigor.

Conclusions.—Physicians discriminate among trials of varying degrees of rigor, but industry sponsorship negatively influences their perception of methodologic quality and reduces their willingness to believe and act on trial findings, independently of the trial's quality. These effects may influence the translation of clinical research into practice.

▶ This is a fascinating report that tells us how we as physicians interpret research funding disclosures when we read medical journals. The investigators created 27 abstracts describing hypothetical research studies on 3 fictitious drugs, 1 for diabetes, 1 for hyperlipidemia, and 1 for angina pectoris. These abstracts were sent to groups of randomly selected internists with active outpatient practices. Each received 3 abstracts, 1 for each drug, describing hypothetical studies. One abstract described a large double-blind active-comparator, randomized, controlled trial with high patient retention and long follow-up; the second a medium size, single-blind, active-comparator trial with modest patient retention and moderate follow-up; the third, an open-labeled poorly controlled trial with small numbers of participants. Given only the abstracts, the internists then answered questions about the strength of the evidence presented and their willingness to prescribe each drug on the basis of that information alone. As would be hopefully expected, they put much more faith in the blinded, randomized, controlled trials than in the open-label poorly controlled trials. But that was not the only aspect of the study. The investigators also randomly varied the attributed source of support for each study. Of the abstracts submitted to each participant, 1 abstract listed the National Institutes of Health (NIH) as the source of support, 1 listed no support source, and 1 listed a fictitious pharmaceutical company as supporting both the study and the principal investigator. When the data were analyzed according to funding source, the investigators found that for studies of equivalent rigor, the internist put much less faith in those supported by the pharmaceutical industry than in those supported by the NIH.

This report was accompanied by an editorial by Jeffrey Drazen, editor of the *New England Journal of Medicine*.[1] Drazen notes that it seems logical that clinicians might be suspicious of a solidly done study supported by pharmaceutical companies that would have a financial stake in the outcome of a study, but at the same time it is noted that investigators in NIH-sponsored studies also have substantial incentives, including academic promotion and recognition. The editor of the *New England Journal of Medicine* believes that decisions about how trials influence practice should be based on the quality of the information conveyed in the full study report. This particular journal also posts study protocols accompanying published articles involving randomized controlled trials to provide a better definition of each trial's study design. Also to ensure full transparency, the journal posts all the financial associations of each study author. With these facts in hand, the reader of a research study should be able to judge a trial's validity on the basis of study design, the quality of data accrual analytic processes used, and the fairness of the results reporting. Drazen suggests that ideally these factors—not the funding source—should be the criteria for deciding clinical utility. He suggests that patients who put themselves at risk to provide research data should earn the respect of all of us and the courtesy of believing the data produced from their efforts no matter what the funding source, assuming the design and execution of the study is bulletproof.

This commentary closes with the observation that doctors are held in high esteem, at least in Spain.[2] Doctors, scientists, and public health workers were rated highest among the most trusted in a poll of who are the most trusted professionals, institutions and public officials by the Spanish lay public. In the poll, they were rated 7.4, 7.4 and 6.8 points (of a maximum of 10), respectively, above King (5.6), the Catholic Church (4), judges (3.5), unions (3.3) and politicians (2.6). It would be interesting to see the same poll taken in the US. The "King" would likely win; Elvis, that is.

J. A. Stockman III, MD

References

1. Drazen JM. Believe the data. *N Engl J Med.* 2012;367:1152-1153.
2. Editorial comment. Spaniards rate doctors. *BMJ.* 2011;343:556.

Validation of Search Filters for Identifying Pediatric Studies in PubMed
Leclercq E, Leeflang MMG, van Dalen EC, et al (Emma Children's Hosp/ Academic Med Ctr, Amsterdam, The Netherlands; Univ of Amsterdam, The Netherlands)
J Pediatr 162:629-634.e2, 2013

Objective.—To identify and validate PubMed search filters for retrieving studies including children and to develop a new pediatric search filter for PubMed.

Study Design.—We developed 2 different datasets of studies to evaluate the performance of the identified pediatric search filters, expressed in terms of sensitivity, precision, specificity, accuracy, and number needed to read (NNR). An optimal search filter will have a high sensitivity and high precision with a low NNR.

Results.—In addition to the PubMed Limits: All Child: 0-18 years filter (in May 2012 renamed to PubMed Filter Child: 0-18 years), 6 search filters for identifying studies including children were identified: 3 developed by Kastner et al, 1 developed by BestBets, one by the Child Health Field, and 1 by the Cochrane Childhood Cancer Group. Three search filters (Cochrane Childhood Cancer Group, Child Health Field, and BestBets) had the highest sensitivity (99.3%, 99.5%, and 99.3%, respectively) but a lower precision (64.5%, 68.4%, and 66.6% respectively) compared with the other search filters. Two Kastner search filters had a high precision (93.0% and 93.7%, respectively) but a low sensitivity (58.5% and 44.8%, respectively). They failed to identify many pediatric studies in our datasets. The search terms responsible for false-positive results in the reference dataset were determined. With these data, we developed a new search filter for identifying studies with children in PubMed with an optimal sensitivity (99.5%) and precision (69.0%).

Conclusion.—Search filters to identify studies including children either have a low sensitivity or a low precision with a high NNR. A new pediatric search filter with a high sensitivity and a low NNR has been developed.

▶ Most know about PubMed, which is a free database accessing primarily the MEDLINE database of references and abstracts on life sciences and biomedical topics. The US National Library of Medicine at the Institutes of Health maintains the database as part of the Entrez system of information retrieval. PubMed was first released in early 1996. The Entrez Global Query system is an integrated search and retrieval system that provides access to all databases simultaneously with a single query string and user interface. Entrez can efficiently retrieve related sequences, structures, and references. Entrez also has access to some textbooks online. By the way, if you are an aficionado of word meanings, Entrez happens to be the second person plural form of the French verb *entrer* (meaning to enter), providing the invitation "come in," or as we say here in North Carolina, "Ya'll come visit."

Most physicians use PubMed to keep up to date with the latest developments in their field and to practice in an evidence-based manner. Pediatric health care professionals can target literature searches in medical databases looking for primary studies and systematic reviews in children. There are specific search filters for identifying only pediatric studies using PubMed and MEDLINE/Ovid. These search features vary with respect to the number of search terms that can be used, but the existing search filters for identifying studies of children in PubMed have not been validated. It is therefore not clear how well the different search filters are able to identify all studies in PubMed that involve children.

These authors remind us that the performance of literature search filters can be expressed in terms of sensitivity, precision, specificity, accuracy, and number needed to read (NNR). These investigators have developed a study to advise pediatric health care professionals about the usefulness of the different available search filters for identifying studies that include children. They outline 3 objectives as part of their study. The first objective was to identify all available search filters. The second objective was to evaluate the performance of the search filters focusing on identifying all relevant studies (sensitivity of the filters) and the effort needed to obtain these results (expressed as NNR to identify one relative article). The third objective was to develop and improve search filters for identifying studies in PubMed that include children. The goal was to find an optimum search filter that would have the high sensitivity and high precision with a low NNR.

It would be important for most clinicians who are deeply invested in practicing evidence-based medicine to read this article in detail including the methodologies used. The methodologies used are a bit complicated, but the conclusion of the article is fairly clear. There are 3 search filters that work extremely well in identifying studies with children. They are the Cochrane Childhood Cancer Group, the Cochrane Child Health Field, and BestBets.[1-3] The likelihood of missing relevant studies with any one of these filters is quite low.

PubMed remains one of the most widely used medical databases among health care professionals. It spans over 21 million records representing articles in the biol-iterature. In this day and age, to be able to keep up to date with relevant findings in the literature, health care professionals must be able to search filters that are both sensitive (ie, retrieving as many relevant publications as possible) and precise (ie, identifying as few irrelevant studies as possible). This article is the first in which the performance of all available search filters identifying studies including children was evaluated. It is worth reading this article in detail to see how it could help improve the care you provide to your patients. The authors specifically recommend using the new and improved Cochrane Childhood Cancer Group search filter for retrieving studies involving children in PubMed. The search filter is not restricted to oncology patients. It has high sensitivity and high precision with low NNR, exactly what the average person would be looking for.

This commentary closes with a question. How long on average does it take research evidence to change clinical practice? The answer appears to be 17 years based on a review of 23 studies that quantified time lags in the translation of research information.[4]

J. A. Stockman III, MD

References

1. Kremer LCM, van Dalen EC, Moher D, Caron HN. Childhood cancer group. About the Cochrane Collaboration (Cochrane Review Groups). 2008; 4. http://onlinelibrary.wiley.com/o/cochrane/clabout/articles/childca/frame.html. Accessed April 6, 2013.
2. Boluyt N, Tjosvold L, Lefebvre C, Klassen TP, Offringa M. Usefulness of systematic review search strategies in finding child health systematic reviews in MEDLINE. *Arch Pediatr Adolesc Med.* 2008;162:111-116.
3. BestBets. Best evidence topics. Manchester: Best Evidence Topics. Best Search Strategies. http://www.bestbets.org/links/search-strategies.php. Accessed April 6, 2013.
4. Editorial Comment. Time for research information to inform clinical practice. *BMJ.* 2012;344:344.

A Preliminary Screening Instrument for Early Detection of Medical Child Abuse

Greiner MV, Palusci VJ, Keeshin BR, et al (Cincinnati Children's Hosp Med Ctr, OH; New York Univ School of Medicine; et al)
Hospital Pediatrics 3:39-44, 2013

Objective.—The goal of this research was to develop a screening instrument for early identification among hospitalized children of medical child abuse (MCA).

Methods.—We developed a preliminary screening instrument for the early identification of MCA. Items were chosen based on published characteristics of MCA, including caregiver, patient, and illness information. Each item in the instrument was scored with 1 point if positive. This instrument was tested by reviewing the hospital charts of child protective services—confirmed MCA patients and comparing the results with charts of children with admissions for apnea, vomiting/diarrhea, and seizures who were not diagnosed with MCA. Nineteen cases and 389 controls were used for analysis. We used receiver operating characteristic curves, starting with items most highly associated with MCA in our sample. Predictive values and strengths of association were assessed by using χ^2 and Fisher's exact tests, as appropriate.

Results.—From an initial 46 questions, we determined that 26 items showed a statistically significant difference between cases and control patients. From these, an instrument with 15 items maximized the area under the receiver operating characteristic curve, and a score of ≥ 4 had a sensitivity of 0.947 and a specificity of 0.956 ($P < .05$) in detecting MCA.

Conclusions.—This chart review screening instrument identified differences in characteristics of children, caregivers, and illness during hospitalization that may allow for earlier detection of MCA and referral for further assessment to the multidisciplinary team.

▶ There has been a great deal written about screening for child abuse. This report that appeared in the *Annals of Internal Medicine* tells us about a screening instrument for the identification of that form of child abuse known as *medical child abuse*, also called *Munchausen syndrome by proxy*, first described by Meadow in 1977.[1] Very recently, a report appeared, also in the *Annals of Internal Medicine*, summarizing the United States Preventive Services Task Force recommendations on behavioral interventions and counseling to prevent child abuse and neglect.[2]

The US Preventive Task Force in 2004 found, on the basis of a previous review of the literature, insufficient evidence to recommend for or against routine screening of parents or caregivers for child abuse or neglect. Based on the current systematic review that appeared in 2013, the US Preventive Services Task Force notes that risk assessment and behavioral interventions in pediatric clinics do reduce abuse and neglect outcomes for young children and that early childhood home visitation also reduces abuse and neglect, even though the data from the literature are somewhat inconsistent. The report notes that approximately 695 000 children in the United States were victim of child abuse and neglect in 2010, and 1537 died. Most of these deaths were in infants and toddlers. In survivors, associated long-term physical conditions occurred in many youngsters who were abused. These long-term problems have included neurologic and musculoskeletal disorders, gastrointestinal problems, metabolic conditions including diabetes, autoimmune disorders, obesity, chronic pain, teen pregnancy and pregnancy complications, and others.

Greiner et al note that the diagnosis of medical child abuse is often very difficult, with an average time from onset of symptoms to diagnosis of 15 months and 22 months, respectively, in two large series.[3,4] Greiner et al described the development of a preliminary screening instrument for medical child abuse that differentiates children at risk for this disorder compared with otherwise normal children hospitalized for evaluation of 3 common pediatric conditions (apnea, vomiting/diarrhea, and seizures). The investigators developed a 15-question screening instrument for the purpose of detecting medical child abuse. They designed a mathematical instrument to see which elements added the most value in distinguishing youngsters affected by medical child abuse from otherwise normal children. The most predictive caregiver items included a personal history of child abuse (odds ratio [OR], 72), features of Munchausen syndrome (OR, 46), and mental illness (OR, 8.9). Additional caregiver predictive factors were request to leave the hospital against medical advice or by transfer (OR, 18) and caregiver request for apnea monitors (OR, 9.4). The most predictive patient items included illness abatement out of care of the primary caregiver (OR, 89), care at more than one hospital (OR, 3.5), and consultation with more than subspecialist (OR, 8.8). The most predictive illness characteristics included bruising of the face/neck (OR, 73), toxic appearance (OR, 46), and erratic drug levels (OR, 2.8) as well as chronic vomiting and diarrhea without an alternative diagnosis (OR, 2.1). Items excluded from the final tool because they did not assist in distinguishing medical child abuse from control cases were sibling deaths and hospitalizations for more than 30 days, both of which were as common in control patients. Symptoms such as lethargy, fever, and pain were also not useful in distinguishing medical child abuse from nonmedical child abuse children.

The authors of this report suggest that their preliminary screening tool would best be used for hospitalized children who have apnea, chronic vomiting/diarrhea, or seizures of unknown etiology not responsive to standard medical care. They note that a positive screening result using their tool is neither diagnostic of medical child abuse, nor the basis for a referral to children's services. Nonetheless, a positive screening test result should increase the suspicion of medical child abuse.

The authors of this report should be congratulated on publishing their data in a medical journal largely targeted to internal medicine and family medicine physicians who are frequently in contact with the parents of these abused children. Clearly, the preliminary tool described should be evaluated further and larger, multicenter prospective trials with multiple reviewers undertaken to confirm the evidence of the tool's clinical utility and interrater reliability. Nonetheless, this report is a valuable contribution to the medical literature.

We close this commentary with information that was recently published concerning the costs associated with the care of children who have been abused. Each year it costs about $74 000 000 to hospitalize more than 4500 children with injuries caused by physical abuse.[5] This is likely an underestimate and pales by comparison to the ultimate cost of such care. Researchers have estimated that the lifetime cost of 1740 fatal and 579 000 nonfatal cases reported in 2008 topped $200 000 per child, including health care during childhood, special education, adult medical care, lost productivity, child welfare system cost and criminal justice system costs.

J. A. Stockman III, MD

References

1. Meadow R. Munchausen syndrome by proxy. The hinterland of child abuse. *Lancet*. 1977;2:343-345.
2. Selph SS, Bougatsos C, Blazina I, Nelson HD. Behavioral interventions and counseling to prevent child abuse and neglect: a systematic review to update the US Preventive services task force recommendation. *Ann Intern Med*. 2013;158:179-190.
3. Rosenberg DA. Web of deceit: a literature review of Munchausen syndrome by proxy. *Child Abuse Negl*. 1987;11:547-563.
4. Sheridan MS. The deceit continues: an updated literature review of Munchausen Syndrome by Proxy. *Child Abuse Negl*. 2003;27:431-451.
5. Editorial comment. Child abuse common, costly. *JAMA*. 2011;307:1014.

Utility of Hepatic Transaminases in Children With Concern for Abuse

Lindberg DM, for the ExSTRA investigators (Brigham & Women's Hosp, Boston, MA; et al)

Pediatrics 131:268-275, 2013

Objective.—Routine testing of hepatic transaminases, amylase, and lipase has been recommended for all children evaluated for physical abuse, but rates of screening are widely variable, even among abuse specialists, and data for amylase and lipase testing are lacking. A previous study of screening in centers that endorsed routine transaminase screening suggested that using a transaminase threshold of 80 IU/L could improve injury detection. Our objectives were to prospectively validate the test characteristics of the 80-IU/L threshold and to determine the utility of amylase and lipase to detect occult abdominal injury.

Methods.—This was a retrospective secondary analysis of the Examining Siblings To Recognize Abuse research network, a multicenter study in children younger than 10 years old who underwent subspecialty evaluation for physical abuse. We determined rates of identified abdominal injuries and results of transaminase, amylase, and lipase testing. Screening studies were compared by using basic test characteristics (sensitivity, specificity) and the area under the receiver operating characteristic curve.

Results.—Abdominal injuries were identified in 82 of 2890 subjects (2.8%; 95% confidence interval: 2.3%–3.5%). Hepatic transaminases were obtained in 1538 (53%) subjects. Hepatic transaminases had an area under the receiver operating characteristic curve of 0.87. A threshold of 80 IU/L yielded sensitivity of 83.8% and specificity of 83.1%. The areas under the curve for amylase and lipase were 0.67 and 0.72, respectively.

Conclusions.—Children evaluated for physical abuse with transaminase levels >80 IU/L should undergo definitive testing for abdominal injury.

▶ Expert statements have recommended routine transaminase testing, with or without amylase and lipase testing, in children with concern for physical abuse.[1] The report of Lindberg et al evaluated the test characteristics of an 80-IU/L threshold for transaminases to detect occult intraabdominal injury in children evaluated for physical abuse. The study also attempted to determine rates of abdominal screening after publication of an earlier previous study recommending transaminases be used to screen for abdominal injury.

In this multicenter cohort of children less than 10 years of age being evaluated for physical abuse, 2.8% had an intraabdominal injury identified. Among children with an initial transaminase level less than 80 IU/L, the posttest probability for intra-abdominal injury was 20.0%. These data support the use of a transaminase threshold of 80 IU/L as an indicator for further definitive testing for abdominal injury in children with concern about physical abuse.

It is clear that intra-abdominal injuries, while uncommon among children evaluated for physical abuse, do carry significant risk of morbidity and mortality. Measurement of hepatic transaminases will increase the sensitivity for occult intra-abdominal injury relative to clinical examination alone. It seems reasonable to accept the recommendations of these investigators that children with elevated transaminases (>80 IU/L) should undergo definitive testing for abdominal injury, such as the use of a computed tomography scan.

J. A. Stockman III, MD

Reference

1. Lindberg D, Makoroff K, Harper N, et al; ULTRA investigators. Utility of hepatic transaminases to recognize abuse in children. *Pediatrics*. 2009;124:509-516.

Abusive Head Trauma in Young Children: A Population-Based study
Selassie AW, Borg K, Busch C, et al (Med Univ of South Carolina, Charleston)
Pediatr Emerg Care 29:283-291, 2013

Objective.—The objectives of this study were to provide population-based incidence estimate of abusive head trauma (AHT) in children aged 0 to 5 years from inpatient and emergency department (ED) and identify risk characteristics for recognizing high-risk children to improve public health surveillance.

Methods.—This was a retrospective cohort study based on children's first encounter in ED or hospital admission with a diagnosis of head trauma (HT), 2000–2010. The relationship between clinical markers and AHT was examined controlling for covariables in the model using Cox hazards regression. Kaplan-Meier incidence probability was plotted, and the number of weeks elapsing from date of birth to the first encounter with HT established the survival time (T).

Results.—Twenty-six thousand six hundred eighty-one children had HT, 502 (1.8%) resulted from abuse; 42.4% was captured from ED. Incidence varied from 28.9 (95% confidence interval [CI], 27.9–37.4) in infants to 4.1 (95% CI, 2.4–5.7) in 5-year-olds per 100,000 per year. Adjusted hazard ratio was 20.3 (95% CI, 10.9–38.0) for intracranial bleeding and 11.4 (95% CI, 8.57–15.21) for retinal hemorrhage.

Conclusions.—Incidence estimates of AHT are incomplete without including ED. Intracranial bleeding is a cardinal feature of AHT to be considered in case ascertainment to improve public health surveillance.

▶ Abusive head trauma has a very high case fatality rate, and many childhood survivors succumb to lifelong disability. Most case series show that the fatality rate is reported to be in the range of 1 in 5 in infants through 3 years of age and over 53% in infants, toddlers, and older children admitted to pediatric intensive care units. A number of studies have identified demographic, socioeconomic, and clinical factors associated with abusive head trauma in young children. Most of these studies have shown a higher risk of such trauma in boys than girls, blacks than whites, and children from families with low incomes. Loss of employment and economic distress in the family, natural disasters, poor social support and family cohesion, and single parenthood are also risk factors. Clinical factors strongly suggestive of abusive head trauma include retinal bleeding and retinal detachment, subdural hematomas, and specific fracture patterns.

This article provides a population-based incidence estimate of abusive head trauma in youngsters 0 to 5 years of age based on information from inpatient services and emergency department evaluations. This article may be the first population-based incidence estimate of all severity abusive head trauma from hospital and emergency departments' sources that provides a comprehensive risk profile of children with abusive head trauma. The study hypothesizes that intracranial bleeding and retinal hemorrhage in children with head trauma are significantly more likely to be associated with abuse than other causes. The study itself was a retrospective cohort study examining demographic, socioeconomic, and clinical characteristics of children 0 through 5 years of age based on their first encounter in an emergency department or hospital inpatient service with a diagnosis of head trauma. The record review spanned January 1, 2000, through December 31, 2010.

The results of this study show that abusive head trauma is indeed a significant public health problem, with an incidence rate of 13.7 per 100 000 per year in the State of South Carolina. These data mean that about 1 infant per 3450 will experience a brain insult as a result of abusive trauma before his or her first birthday. This study confirms the hypothesis that intracranial hemorrhage and retinal bleeding are strong indicators of abusive head trauma. The authors also note that although a large portion of abusive head trauma is severe, mild or moderate cases are probably more common and much more difficult and challenging to identify.

We learn from this article that high-risk groups for abusive head trauma include children with indigent insurance, multiple injuries, and children from rural underserved communities.

J. A. Stockman III, MD

Nondepressed Linear Skull Fractures in Children Younger Than 2 Years: Is Computed Tomography Always Necessary?
Reid SR, Liu M, Ortega HW (Childrens Hosp and Clinics of Minnesota, St Paul)
Clin Pediatr 51:745-749, 2012

Background.—Current recommendations are that young children with a skull fracture following head injury undergo computed tomography (CT) examination of their head to exclude significant intracranial injury. Recent reports, however, have raised concern that radiation exposure from CT scanning may cause malignancies.

Objective.—To estimate the proportion of children with nondisplaced linear skull fractures who have clinically significant intracranial injury.

Methods.—Retrospective review of patients younger than 2 years who presented to an emergency department and received a diagnosis of skull fracture.

Results.—Ninety-two patients met the criteria for inclusion in the study; all had a head CT scan performed. None suffered a clinically significant intracranial injury.

Conclusion.—Observation, rather than CT, may be a reasonable management option for head-injured children younger than 2 years who have a non-displaced linear skull fracture on plain radiography but no clinical signs of intracranial injury.

▶ Recent reports have raised concerns about the safety of computed tomography (CT) examinations, particularly in early childhood. The radiation doses delivered by CT scanning have been linked with the subsequent development of a number of different malignancies. Everything that can be done to reduce radiation exposure would seem wise. Currently, protocols for closed head injury frequently call for the use of CT examination to exclude the possibility of intracranial injury. In children younger than 2 years, some authorities recommend a CT examination for any skin injury suggestive of skull fracture. Recently published decision rules for the prediction of clinically important intracranial injuries in young head-injured children include scalp hematoma as an indication for CT scanning.[1]

Reid et al examined whether a simple nondepressed linear skull fracture in a child younger than 2 years, without other clinical symptoms, would necessitate the performance of a CT scan. They conducted a retrospective review of patients younger than 2 years who presented to the emergency department of the Children's Hospital and Clinics of Minnesota. Patients were excluded if they suffered a depressed, diastatic, or open fracture; sustained a significant noncranial injury; or had received some initial care at an outside hospital. A nondepressed linear skull fracture was diagnosed with simple head x-rays. The main outcome from the study was the presence of significant intracranial injury defined as death as a result of head injury, requirement for neurosurgical intervention, tracheal intubation for a neurologic indication, or hospitalization of more than 2 days because of concerns related to head injury.

In this report, the presence of a nondepressed linear skull fracture in children younger than 2 years was not associated with a significant intracranial injury. Given the recent concern as to the long-term sequelae of radiation exposure from CT scanning, especially in young children, the data from this report prove helpful to clinicians hoping to minimize radiation exposure to their patients. In otherwise asymptomatic children with skull x-ray findings of a nondepressed linear skull fracture, observation rather than CT scanning may be a reasonable management option for children younger than 2 years. It should be noted that all patients in this study were without altered consciousness. It was clear that nondepressed linear skull fractures were not associated with clinically significant intracranial injury in an otherwise well-appearing child.

J. A. Stockman III, MD

Reference

1. Dunning J, Daly JP, Lomas JP, Lecky F, Batchelor J, Mackway-Jones K; Children's head injury algorithm for the prediction of important clinical events study group. Derivation of the children's head injury algorithm for the prediction of important clinical events decision rule for head injury in children. *Arch Dis Child.* 2006;91: 885-891.

Ultrasound Evaluation of Skull Fractures in Children: A Feasibility Study

Riera A, Chen L (Yale Univ School of Medicine, New Haven, CT)
Pediatr Emerg Care 28:420-425, 2012

Objective.—The objective of this study was to investigate feasibility and evaluate test characteristics of bedside ultrasound for the detection of skull fractures in children with closed head injury (CHI).

Methods.—This was a prospective, observational study conducted in a pediatric emergency department of an urban tertiary care children's hospital. A convenience sample of children younger than 18 years were enrolled if they presented with an acute CHI, and a computed tomography (CT) scan was performed. Ultrasound was performed by pediatric emergency medicine physicians with at least 1 month of training in bedside ultrasound. Ultrasound interpretation as either positive or negative for the presence of skull fracture was compared with attending radiologist CT scan dictation. Test characteristics (sensitivity, specificity, and positive and negative predictive values) were calculated.

Results.—Forty-six patients were enrolled. The median age was 2 years (range, 2 months to 17 years). Eleven patients (24%) were diagnosed with skull fractures on CT scan. Bedside ultrasound had a sensitivity of 82% (95% confidence interval [CI], 48%−97%), specificity of 94% (95% CI, 79%−99%), positive predictive value of 82% (95% CI, 48%− 97%), and negative predictive value of 94% (95% CI, 79%−99%).

Conclusions.—Bedside ultrasonography can be used by pediatric emergency medicine physicians to detect skull fractures in children with acute CHI. Larger studies are needed to validate these findings. Future studies should investigate the role of this modality as an adjunct to clinical decision rules to reduce unnecessary CT scans in the evaluation of acute CHI in children (Fig 2).

▶ Multiple studies have been conducted to establish clinical prediction rules to identify patients at low risk for traumatic brain injury, thereby obviating the need for a head CT scan. In general, these decision pathways yield high sensitivity scores in the range of 98% to 99%, but at the expense of lower specificity. These same studies have shown poor interobserver agreement with parameters that define the need for a CT scan. For this reason, a large number of CT scans are still performed in children after blunt head trauma, with the vast majority revealing no abnormalities. Emergency department physicians must weigh the benefits of early diagnosis of intracranial pathology with the increased cost and long-term risks of CT scans, including the child's exposure to radiation and the potential adverse effects of sedative medications.

These authors have undertaken a prospective observational study at Yale Hospital to evaluate the test characteristics of bedside ultrasound for the detection of skull fractures in children with closed head injury. They have demonstrated that ultrasound can be used to detect skull fractures (Fig 2). They did so showing high specificity but lower sensitivity. There are several advantages of ultrasound for detection of skull fractures. Bedside ultrasound can usually

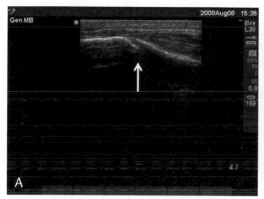
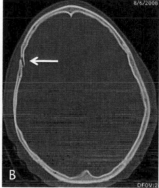

FIGURE 2.—A, Linear temporal skull fracture in an 11-year-old child as seen on bedside ultrasound. B, Linear temporal skull fracture in an 11-year-old child as seen on corresponding CT scan. (Reprinted from Riera A, Chen L. Ultrasound evaluation of skull fractures in children: a feasibility study. *Pediatr Emerg Care.* 2012;28:420-425, with permission from Lippincott Williams & Wilkins.)

be performed quicker than obtaining a CT scan, and earlier detection of skull pathology might lead to prioritization of getting into a CT scanner. The question is whether it can further reduce head CT imaging in young patients after closed head injury. The diagnostic conundrum for the emergency physician is that the youngest patient with intracranial injury is often asymptomatic early in the course of his or her injury, yet these patients are the most sensitive to the effects of ionizing radiation by CT scan.

This article, appearing in *Pediatric Emergency Care*, should be read by anyone who works in emergency room settings. Only time will tell whether it is worthwhile adding performance of a bedside ultrasound into the diagnostic schema for closed head injury. The authors of this article indicate that it can be used by a pediatric emergency medicine physician to detect skull fractures in children with acute head injury, but larger studies are needed to validate the findings from this article, and future studies should investigate the role of this modality as an adjunct to the clinical decision rules to reduce unnecessary CT scans in the evaluation of acute closed head injury in children.

J. A. Stockman III, MD

Countdown to 2015: changes in official development assistance to maternal, newborn, and child health in 2009—10, and assessment of progress since 2003

Hsu J, Pitt C, Greco G, et al (London School of Hygiene and Tropical Medicine, UK; et al)
Lancet 380:1157-1168, 2012

Background.—Tracking of financial resources to maternal, newborn, and child health provides crucial information to assess accountability of donors. We analysed official development assistance (ODA) flows to maternal, newborn, and child health for 2009 and 2010, and assessed progress since our monitoring began in 2003.

Methods.—We coded and analysed all 2009 and 2010 aid activities from the database of the Organisation for Economic Co-operation and Development, according to a functional classification of activities and whether all or a proportion of the value of the disbursement contributed towards maternal, newborn, and child health. We analysed trends since 2003, and reported two indicators for monitoring donor disbursements: ODA to child health per child and ODA to maternal and newborn health per live-birth. We analysed the degree to which donors allocated ODA to 74 countries with the highest maternal and child mortality rates (Countdown priority countries) with time and by type of donor.

Findings.—Donor disbursements to maternal, newborn, and child health activities in all countries continued to increase, to $6511 million in 2009, but slightly decreased for the first time since our monitoring started, to $6480 million in 2010. ODA for such activities to the 74 Countdown priority countries continued to increase in real terms, but its rate of increase has been slowing since 2008. We identified strong evidence that targeting of ODA to countries with high rates of maternal mortality improved from 2005 to 2010. Targeting of ODA to child health also improved but to a lesser degree. The share of multilateral funding continued to decrease but, relative to bilaterals and global health initiatives, was better targeted.

Interpretation.—The recent slowdown in the rate of funding increases is worrying and likely to partly result from the present financial crisis. Tracking of donor aid should continue, to encourage donor accountability and to monitor performance in targeting aid flows to those in most need (Fig 2).

▶ This is the last entry in a trilogy of reports telling us how well we are doing toward the achievement of the Millennium Development Goals (MDGs) for

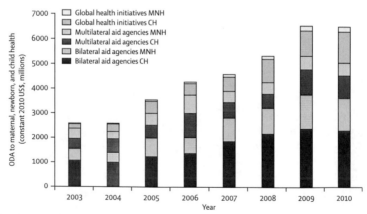

FIGURE 2.—Worldwide official development assistance to maternal, newborn, and child health, by source of aid flows, 2003–10. ODA=official development assistance. MNH=maternal and newborn health. CH=child health. (Reprinted from Hsu J, Pitt C, Greco G, et al. Countdown to 2015: changes in official development assistance to maternal, newborn, and child health in 2009–10, and assessment of progress since 2003. *Lancet.* 2012;380:1157-1168, Copyright 2012, with permission from Elsevier.)

childhood survival (MDG 4) and maternal health (MDG 5A). This report specifically attempts to correlate the degree of financial assistance over time with rates of improvement in maternal and child health. There is concern that the financial crisis that began in 2008, which rapidly spread worldwide, may have affected the rate of maternal and child health improvements. The concern is that donors may have found it difficult to provide funding beyond what they are spending domestically on global health issues. A 2009 estimate places the additional requirements to achieve health-related MDGs (with a focus on maternal and child health) in 49 low-income countries at $10 billion per year.[1] Others have estimated additional required funding to be as much as $34 billion per year.[2]

Hsu et al have examined data from the Organization for Economic Cooperation and Development to determine the value of the worldwide disbursements to help the MDGs. The data show a slight decline for the first time in world assistance in 2010, with a decrease in such assistance to $6.48 billion. It is clear that the overall rate of increase in funding has been slowing since 2008. Fig 2 shows the worldwide official development assistance to maternal, newborn, and child health by source of aid over an 8-year period. The greatest increases in aid were seen before 2008, although we are still, in recent years, at a fairly high level of support. In fact, the total volume of worldwide aid to maternal, newborn, and child health activities more than doubled during the 8-year period, increasing from $2.566 billion in 2003 to $6.480 billion in 2010, although the trend of increasing aid volume drifted downward in 2010 as noted. This recent slow-down in the rate of increases, both worldwide and in priority countries, probably results partly from the financial crisis that rapidly became worldwide in the last half-dozen years. Although the absolute amount of money being targeted for maternal and child health-related issues is higher over the last 8 years, the rate of increase has been slowing since 2008.

J. A. Stockman III, MD

References

1. Task Force on Innovative International Financing for Health Systems. *More Money for Health, and More Health for the Money.* Geneva, Switzerland: World Health Organization; 2009.
2. PMNCH. *Background Paper for Global Strategy for Women's and Children's Health: Financial Estimates in the Global Strategy.* Geneva, Switzerland: The Partnership for Maternal, Newborn and Child Health; 2010.

Global, regional, and national causes of child mortality: an updated systematic analysis for 2010 with time trends since 2000

Liu L, for the Child Health Epidemiology Reference Group of WHO and UNICEF (Johns Hopkins Bloomberg School of Public Health, Baltimore, MD; et al)
Lancet 379.2151-2161, 2012

Background.—Information about the distribution of causes of and time trends for child mortality should be periodically updated. We report the latest estimates of causes of child mortality in 2010 with time trends since 2000.

Methods.—Updated total numbers of deaths in children aged 0—27 days and 1—59 months were applied to the corresponding country-specific distribution of deaths by cause. We did the following to derive the number of deaths in children aged 1—59 months: we used vital registration data for countries with an adequate vital registration system; we applied a multinomial logistic regression model to vital registration data for low-mortality countries without adequate vital registration; we used a similar multinomial logistic regression with verbal autopsy data for high-mortality countries; for India and China, we developed national models. We aggregated country results to generate regional and global estimates.

Findings.—Of 7·6 million deaths in children younger than 5 years in 2010, 64·0% (4·879 million) were attributable to infectious causes and 40·3% (3·072 million) occurred in neonates. Preterm birth complications (14·1%; 1·078 million, uncertainty range [UR] 0·916—1·325), intrapartum-related complications (9·4%; 0·717 million, 0·610—0·876), and sepsis or meningitis (5·2%; 0·393 million, 0·252—0·552) were the leading causes of neonatal death. In older children, pneumonia (14·1%; 1·071 million, 0·977—1·176), diarrhoea (9·9%; 0·751 million, 0·538—1·031), and malaria (7·4%; 0·564 million, 0·432—0·709) claimed the most lives. Despite tremendous efforts to identify relevant data, the causes of only 2·7% (0·205 million) of deaths in children younger than 5 years were medically certified in 2010. Between 2000 and 2010, the global burden of deaths in children younger than 5 years decreased by 2 million, of which pneumonia, measles, and diarrhoea contributed the most to the overall reduction (0·451 million [0·339—0·547], 0·363 million [0·283—0·419], and 0·359 million [0·215—0·476], respectively). However, only tetanus, measles, AIDS, and malaria (in Africa) decreased at an annual rate sufficient to attain the Millennium Development Goal 4.

Interpretation.—Child survival strategies should direct resources toward the leading causes of child mortality, with attention focusing on infectious and neonatal causes. More rapid decreases from 2010—15 will need accelerated reduction for the most common causes of death, notably pneumonia and preterm birth complications. Continued efforts to gather high-quality data and enhance estimation methods are essential for the improvement of future estimates.

▶ This report reminds us that in 2010, between 7 and 8 million children died before reaching school age, although this number was a decrease from the 9.6 million in 2000. The mortality rate per 1000 live births in children younger than 5 years of age decreased from 73 to 57 over the same period. There is less than 3 years left to reach the deadline for the Millennium Development Goal (MDG) 4 to reduce child mortality by two-thirds between 1990 and 2015. Thus far, relatively few countries are on track to achieve this aggressive goal.

The report of Liu et al is important because it allows us to guide global and national programs as well as research efforts to continue the progress that has been made to date and hopefully to accelerate that progress based on information concerning the distribution of causes of childhood deaths. Without such a barometer, we would otherwise be shooting in the dark. Liu et al report updated estimates of the distribution of child deaths by cause in 2010 as well as time trends of childhood deaths by cause since the year 2000. The investigators used vital registration data for countries with an adequate vital registration system and applied various statistical analyses to estimate the number of deaths and causes of deaths. Of 7.6 million children who died before their fifth birthday in 2010, almost two-thirds died of infectious causes, nearly all of which could have been prevented. Forty percent of deaths in children younger than 5 years of age occurred in the first 28 days of life, showing that targeting a reduction in neonatal deaths is critical for countries to achieve MDG 4. Preterm birth remains the second leading cause of death after pneumonia and is likely to become number 1 on the cause of death by 2015. If there is good news in these data, there have been continued decreases in the percentage of deaths in children younger than 5 years. The average decrease was 26%. Infectious diseases decreased more rapidly than noncommunicable causes with fairly significant reductions in deaths caused by pneumonia, diarrhea, and measles. Only a few causes of death, including tetanus, measles, and AIDS, were reduced at a rate that was sufficient to achieve MDG 4. These causes, however, contribute only a small fraction of the overall burden of deaths in children younger than 5 years of age.

Five countries—India, Nigeria, Democratic Republic of the Congo, Pakistan, and China—contributed to almost half of the world's deaths in children younger than 5 years. They also had half of the mortality attributable to infections and more than half from neonatal causes worldwide. Thus, these countries should also be heavily targeted, and must be, to achieve MDG 4. Deaths from other disorders in children age 1 to 59 months caused 18% of global deaths in children younger than 5 years of age in 2010. These disorders included noncommunicable entities such as cancer and infectious causes (eg, pertussis). They also include severe malnutrition and perinatal disorders such as prematurity and intrapartum-related complications.

The data from this report allow policy makers to fine tune efforts that will be continued for the next couple of years regarding the work of MDG 4. The authors of this report, one funded by the Bill and Melinda Gates Foundation, challenge countries in the entire global health community to promote registration and medical certification of deaths in order to strengthen national health information systems to enable better accountability for the survival of children. The report that follows tells us how changes in health coverage affect equity in maternal and child health interventions.[1]

This commentary closes with an observation about the risks of vacationing. See how you would answer the following question. You are planning a vacation to Africa that will include a safari in Tanzania. You are told about the hazards related to lions that prey at night on tourists and local villagers. The question is, were you to attempt to minimize the risks of being eaten, would you plan the safari with its overnight camp outs in the 10 days before a full moon or in the 10 days following a full moon?

The answer to this curious query comes from an analysis of records of more that 1000 lion attacks on Tanzanian villagers that occurred from 1988 to 2009, as performed by researchers from the University of Minnesota.[2] The analysis showed that lion attacks on humans occur 2-4 times more often during the 10 days after a full moon than the 10 days prior to a full moon. This appears to relate to the fact that lions hunt best in darkness and are most hungry after periods of non-hunting during full moon periods. The researchers were also able to pinpoint the times of greatest risk. Lions prefer to hunt most often between 6 p.m. and 9:45 p.m. By the way, if attacked by a lion, the chance of dying is 66%! The lion does not sleep at night ... it feeds tonight.

J. A. Stockman III, MD

References

1. Victora CG, Barros AJ, Axelson H, et al. How changes in coverage affect equity in maternal and child health interventions in 35 countdown to 2015 countries: an analysis of national surveys. *Lancet.* 2012;380:1149-1156.
2. Drake N. The lion eats tonight. *Science News.* 2011;8:10.

How changes in coverage affect equity in maternal and child health interventions in 35 Countdown to 2015 countries: an analysis of national surveys

Victora CG, Barros AJD, Axelson H, et al (Federal Univ of Pelotas, Brazil; Lund Univ, Sweden; et al)
Lancet 380:1149-1156, 2012

Background.—Achievement of global health goals will require assessment of progress not only nationally but also for population subgroups. We aimed to assess how the magnitude of socioeconomic inequalities in health changes in relation to different rates of national progress in coverage of interventions for the health of mothers and children.

Methods.—We assessed coverage in low-income and middle-income countries for which two Demographic Health Surveys or Multiple Indicator Cluster Surveys were available. We calculated changes in overall coverage of skilled birth attendants, measles vaccination, and a composite coverage index, and examined coverage of a newly introduced intervention, use of insecticide-treated bednets by children. We stratified coverage data according to asset-based wealth quintiles, and calculated relative and absolute indices of inequality. We adjusted correlation analyses for time between surveys and baseline coverage levels.

Findings.—We included 35 countries with surveys done an average of 9·1 years apart. Pro-rich inequalities were very prevalent. We noted increased coverage of skilled birth attendants, measles vaccination, and the composite index in most countries from the first to the second survey, while inequalities were reduced. Rapid changes in overall coverage were associated with improved equity. These findings were not due to a capping effect associated with limited scope for improvement in rich households. For use of insecticide-treated bednets, coverage was high for the richest households, but countries making rapid progress did almost as well in reaching the poorest groups. National increases in coverage were primarily driven by how rapidly coverage increased in the poorest quintiles.

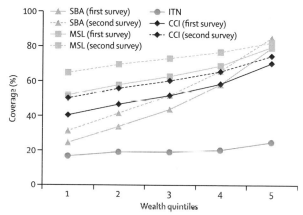

FIGURE 1.—Unweighted mean coverage levels by wealth quintile in the first and second surveys SBA=skilled birth attendants. MSL =measles vaccination. ITN=use of insecticide treated bednets. CCI=composite coverage index. (Reprinted from Victora CG, Barros AJD, Axelson H, et al. How changes in coverage affect equity in maternal and child health interventions in 35 Countdown to 2015 countries: an analysis of national surveys. *Lancet.* 2012;380:1149-1156, Copyright 2012, with permission from Elsevier.)

Interpretation.—Equity should be accounted for when planning the scaling up of interventions and assessing national progress (Fig 1).

▶ This report contains data from a collaboration that monitors 75 countries that account for more than 95% of all global deaths of mothers and children. The study itself investigated the relationship between coverage change and socio-economic inequalities from 1990 to present.

Fig 1 shows the mean coverage levels by wealth quintile in 2 surveys that spanned more than 10 years. Absolute inequalities in care seem to have decreased with time with fewer improvements for the poor than for the rich. It is clear that in recent years, issues related to accountability for health have brought to the forefront the global maternal and child health problems, including the notion that progress should be measured not only by overall rates of change, but also by how well the poorest and most deprived subgroups of the population are being reached. Countries making rapid overall progress, such as Brazil, Thailand, and China, are examples of what can be achieved in short timeframes. Conversely, in some countries, inequalities have actually increased. One such country is Zimbabwe.

This report stands out as the first systematic investigation of time trends in inequalities according to changes in health coverage levels in all low-income and middle-income countries that have data that can be analyzed. It is clear that countries making faster gains in coverage were able to increase coverage among the poorest at a faster rate than for better-off persons. The conclusion reached from these results is that there is a need to give special emphasis to reach the poorest segments of the population to achieve rapid gains in intervention coverage. Equity must be taken into account when assessing overall progress in health coverage and improvement of health at a country level.

While on the topic of life expectancy, some countries have run out of places to bury people. In the absence of cremation, Shanghai, with an extreme shortage of useable land, has addressed this problem by subsidizing sea burials for willing families.[1] What a way to go!

J. A. Stockman III, MD

Reference

1. Editorial comment. Sea burial. *Lancet.* 2012;379.

Racial and Ethnic Health Disparities among Fifth-Graders in Three Cities
Schuster MA, Elliott MN, Kanouse DE, et al (Boston Children's Hosp, MA; RAND, Santa Monica, CA; et al)
N Engl J Med 367:735-745, 2012

Background.—For many health-related behaviors and outcomes, racial and ethnic disparities among adolescents are well documented, but less is known about health-related disparities during preadolescence.

Methods.—We studied 5119 randomly selected public-school fifth-graders and their parents in three metropolitan areas in the United States. We examined differences among black, Latino, and white children on 16 measures, including witnessing of violence, peer victimization, perpetration of aggression, seat-belt use, bike-helmet use, substance use, discrimination, terrorism worries, vigorous exercise, obesity, and self-rated health status and psychological and physical quality of life. We tested potential mediators of racial and ethnic disparities (i.e., sociodemographic characteristics and the child's school) using partially adjusted models.

Results.—There were significant differences between black children and white children for all 16 measures and between Latino children and white children for 12 of 16 measures, although adjusted analyses reduced many of these disparities. For example, in unadjusted analysis, the rate of witnessing a threat or injury with a gun was higher among blacks (20%) and Latinos (11%) than among whites (5%), and the number of days per week on which the student performed vigorous exercise was lower among blacks (3.56 days) and Latinos (3.77 days) than among whites (4.33 days) ($P < 0.001$ for all comparisons). After statistical adjustment, these differences were reduced by about half between blacks and whites and were eliminated between Latinos and whites. Household income, household highest education level, and the child's school were the most substantial mediators of racial and ethnic disparities.

Conclusions.—We found that harmful health behaviors, experiences, and outcomes were more common among black children and Latino children than among white children. Adjustment for socioeconomic status and the child's school substantially reduced most of these differences. Interventions that address potentially detrimental consequences of low socioeconomic status and adverse school environments may help reduce racial and ethnic differences in child health. (Funded by the Centers for Disease Control and Prevention.) (Table 2).

▶ This report reminds us that racial and ethnic disparities, although well-documented among adolescents, have not been looked at carefully in preadolescents when it comes to health-related behaviors. In the older age group, behaviors such as use of bike helmets, the witnessing of violence, the experience of victimization and perpetration of violence, the experience of discrimination, and differences in perceived health status and obesity have all been looked at. Schuster et al have conducted a study of racial and ethnic disparities in a broad range of health-related measures in children in 5th grade. The study was designed to assess whether disparities that are typically associated with adolescents, such as violence peer victimization and substance abuse, emerge during adolescence or are already

TABLE 2.— Unadjusted Health Related Measures, According to the Child's Racial and Ethnic Group*

Measure[†]	White Non-Latino (N = 1249)	Black Non-Latino (N = 1748)	Latino (N = 1615)
Witnessed violence in past 12 mo (%)			
Saw physical assault without weapon "lots of times"	4	19[‡]	7[§]
Saw threat or injury with a gun	5	20[‡]	11[†]
Victimized by peers in past 12 mo (z score)	−0.08	0.12[‡]	−0.02
Aggression in past 30 days (z score)			
Perpetrated nonphysical aggression	−0.17	0.25[‡]	−0.07[§]
Perpetrated physical aggression	−0.14	0.24[‡]	−0.08
Substance use (%)			
Smoked cigarette (ever)	5	10[¶]	6
Drank alcohol (past 12 mo)	5	7[§]	5
Injury prevention (%)			
Always wears seat belt	76	61[‡]	66[‡]
Always wears bike helmet	49	14[‡]	18[‡]
Social issues (z score)			
Experienced discrimination	−0.17	0.14[‡]	−0.02[¶]
Worried about terrorist attacks	−0.74	0.06[‡]	0.39[‡]
Exercise and obesity			
Classified as obese (%)	17	29[‡]	32[‡]
No. of days of performing vigorous exercise in past 7 days	4.33	3.56[‡]	3.77[‡]
Health status and quality of life			
Reported fair or poor health (%)	7	15[‡]	27[‡]
Psychological quality of life in past 30 days (z score)	0.23	−0.06[‡]	−0.11[‡]
Physical quality of life in past 30 days (z score)	0.26	0.02[‡]	−0.16[‡]

*All measures except for obesity were reported by the child. Complete data were available except for bike-helmet use (number of children who have ridden a bicycle: whites, 1106; blacks, 1481; and Latinos, 1306) and obesity (reliable height and weight available for 1192 whites, 1627 blacks, and 1476 Latinos). The reference group for comparisons among racial and ethnic groups is non-Latino white. P values were calculated with the use of a logistic or linear regression predicting each outcome with racial or ethnic group.

[†]Responses are reported as either percentages of participants (for dichotomous measures) or z scores with a mean of 0 and a standard deviation of 1 (for continuous measures). (Details about scoring and instruments of measurement are provided in Table S1 in the Supplementary Appendix.) Higher values indicate a greater level of response to each measure.

[‡]$P < 0.001$.

[§]$P < 0.05$.

[¶]$P < 0.01$.

present during preadolescence. The study is important in understanding the mediators of such disparity allowing identification of the most promising policies for addressing them. Childhood morbidity and mortality related to health behaviors and other behaviors in childhood can have lifelong implications, patterning youngsters with habits that persist into adulthood, habits such as cigarette use and creating long-term biologic difficulties, such as obesity.

The study reported took place between August 2004 and September 2006 and examined 5th graders at public schools in and around Birmingham, Alabama; Houston, Texas; and Los Angeles County, California. The study looked at differences between black 5th graders, Latino 5th graders, and white 5th graders. More than 5000 children participated in the study. Sixteen health-related measures were evaluated. These included witnessing of physical assault without a weapon, witnessing of a threat or injury with a gun, victimization by peers, perpetration of nonphysical aggression, perpetration of physical aggression, cigarette smoking, alcohol use, seatbelt use, bike helmet use, experience of discrimination, worrying about terrorism, obesity, vigorous exercise, health status, psychological quality of life, and physical quality of life. Also examined were variables that might mediate the relationship between racial and ethnic disparities with respect to health-related measures. Factors such as age, sex, parent marital status, socioeconomic status, including household income and highest household education level, and the child's school environment were characterized. Table 2 shows the unadjusted health-related measures according to a child's racial and ethnic group. By every measure, black children compared with white children in the 5th grade had many more adverse health-related risk factors. With respect to Latino children, these youngsters was not quite as bad off as their peers in the black population, but were not doing anywhere near as well as white children.

What was interesting about this report is that for nearly all health-related measures that were examined, adjustment for available socioeconomic characteristics and the child's school eliminated a sizable portion of these disparities and in some cases it counted fully for the disparities. In general, adjustment for these factors affected disparities between Latino children and white children more substantially than disparities between black children and white children. Significantly fewer disparities between Latino children and white children persisted after adjustment and significant differences emerged in a favorable direction for Latino children for several variables (experiencing peer victimization and perpetrating physical and nonphysical aggression). These findings are consistent with previous research in adults that has identified socioeconomic status in neighborhood characteristics as important mediators of racial and ethnic health disparities. One finding, however, stood out in contrast. Parent marital status appeared to have little independent association with racial and ethnic disparities in health-related problems.

It should be noted that the prevalence of obesity was high among children in this study with a prevalence ranging from 1 in 6 among whites to 1 in 3 among blacks and Latinos. The disparities in obesity were not well explained by sociodemographic or contextual factors.

It is clear that disparities and health behaviors are closely associated with socioeconomic status, even behaviors such as bike helmet use and much less cigarette smoking. Hopefully these risk factors might be ameliorated through educational interventions targeted at parental health literacy or subsidization of safety equipment. The authors note that disparities tied to school (eg, peer victimization, perpetration of nonphysical aggression) might be improved through efforts to change the school environment such as school-based antibullying programs. Last, given that substantial disparities sometimes remain even after adjustment, a good example is obesity. Additional research is needed to identify remaining factors that might be associated with such disparities. In any event, that disparities are prevalent among preadolescents and in many cases mirror disparities found in older age groups suggests intervention efforts beginning relatively earlier in life need to be undertaken.

J. A. Stockman III, MD

Improving Patient Handovers From Hospital to Primary Care: A Systematic Review

Hesselink G, Schoonhoven L, Barach P, et al (Radboud Univ Nijmegen Med Centre, the Netherlands; Univ Med Ctr Utrecht, the Netherlands)
Ann Intern Med 157:417-428, 2012

Background.—Evidence shows that suboptimum handovers at hospital discharge lead to increased rehospitalizations and decreased quality of health care.

Purpose.—To systematically review interventions that aim to improve patient discharge from hospital to primary care.

Data Sources.—PubMed, CINAHL, PsycInfo, the Cochrane Library, and EMBASE were searched for studies published between January 1990 and March 2011.

Study Selection.—Randomized, controlled trials of interventions that aimed to improve handovers between hospital and primary care providers at hospital discharge.

Data Extraction.—Two reviewers independently abstracted data on study objectives, setting and design, intervention characteristics, and outcomes. Studies were categorized according to methodological quality, sample size, intervention characteristics, outcome, statistical significance, and direction of effects.

Data Synthesis.—Of the 36 included studies, 25 (69.4%) had statistically significant effects in favor of the intervention group and 34 (94.4%) described multicomponent interventions. Effective interventions included medication reconciliation; electronic tools to facilitate quick, clear, and structured summary generation; discharge planning; shared involvement in follow-up by hospital and community care providers; use of electronic discharge notifications; and Web-based access to discharge information for general practitioners. Statistically significant effects were mostly found in reducing hospital use (for example, rehospitalizations), improvement of continuity of care (for example, accurate discharge information), and improvement of patient status after discharge (for example, satisfaction).

Limitations.—Heterogeneity of the interventions and study characteristics made meta-analysis impossible. Most studies had diffuse aims and poor descriptions of the specific intervention components.

Conclusion.—Many interventions have positive effects on patient care. However, given the complexity of interventions and outcome measures, the literature does not permit firm conclusions about which interventions have these effects.

▶ There is only a modest amount of literature in pediatrics dealing with handoffs and transitions of care. Most of the literature dealing with this comes from our adult counterparts. There is much to be learned from them that can be applied to pediatric care. The authors of this report point out that when a patient's transition from hospital to home is suboptimal, the repercussions can be far reaching— rehospitalization, adverse medical events, and even death. Ineffective handovers at hospital discharge seriously impede the quality and safety of patient care. The trend toward shorter and shorter hospital stays means more of the aftercare will be given in the community after hospitalization. Most studies have found that single-shot solutions to the problem rarely are effective. Interventions to solve the problem need to be multiple and integrated.

Hesselink et al did a systematic review of the literature to assess what interventions seem to be effective in improving the transition of care from hospital to the primary care community setting. The investigators searched the English-language studies published between 1990 and 2011 to find reports dealing with interventions that explicitly describe one or more components that aim to improve the handover of care from hospital and primary care providers during hospital discharge (before, during, and after physical transition of the patient). The studies that were accepted into the systematic review had to have at least one outcome measure addressing the quality or safety of the handover process or outcomes of handovers within the first 3 months after discharge from the hospital.

This review was the first systematic study of randomized, controlled trials evaluating the effects of interventions to improve patient handovers between hospital and primary care providers at discharge. The systematic review found that most interventions were multicomponent, and most studies had statistically significant effects in favor of the intervention group in one or more outcomes. Most of the interventions were primarily aimed at facilitating the coordination of care and communication between hospital and primary care providers and pharmacists. Limited evidence suggests that effective discharge interventions consist of components or activities that focus on structuring and reconciling discharge information, coordinating follow-up to care, and direct and timely communication between providers. Discharge interventions were mainly effective for reducing hospital use (eg, rehospitalizations or emergency department visits), aspects related to the improvement of continuity of care after discharge (eg, timeliness and accuracy of discharge information received by or accessible to the generalist physician), and improvement of patient's status (eg, quality of life and satisfaction). There was no strong indication that any one single intervention was regularly associated with positive effects on a specific outcome measure.

In recent years, many interventions aimed at improving hospital discharge handovers between hospital and primary care providers have had a positive effect on improving patient care. These are increasingly being embraced as best practices by hospitals. If there is a weakness on the pediatric side, it tends to be with community hospitals that are not as "hooked in" with the specific issues that are unique to pediatrics. Most children's hospitals have begun to figure out how to do better discharge planning and transition of care.

For more on the topic of transition of care, the American Board of Pediatrics Foundation sponsored a number of studies on this specific topic. To find these and related articles, go to *www.abp.org* (select "Research").

This commentary closes with a question. If you live in England, what is the worst day to be admitted to the hospital? If you answered on a Sunday, you would be correct. A comprehensive study of 14.2 million admissions to the National Health Service Hospitals was carried out in 2009 and 2010.[1] Deaths during a hospitalization ran 16% higher if admitted on a Sunday compared to 8% less on average if admitted on a Wednesday! Presumably, this relates to the lesser staffing that takes place in NHS hospitals on weekends. It would be interesting to see this study repeated in the US. We all know that the worst day of all to be admitted here to University hospitals is on or about July 1, the annual resident changeover day.

J. A. Stockman III, MD

Reference

1. Wise J. New evidence of worse outcomes for weekend patients reignites call for seven day hospitals. *BMJ.* 2012;344:3.

Does Performance-Based Remuneration for Individual Health Care Practitioners Affect Patient Care? A Systematic Review
Houle SKD, McAlister FA, Jackevicius CA, et al (Univ of Alberta, Edmonton, Canada; Western Univ of Health Sciences, Pomona, CA)
Ann Intern Med 157:889-899, 2012

Background.—Pay-for-performance (P4P) is increasingly touted as a means to improve health care quality.

Purpose.—To evaluate the effect of P4P remuneration targeting individual health care providers.

Data Sources.—MEDLINE, EMBASE, Cochrane Library, OpenSIGLE, Canadian Evaluation Society Unpublished Literature Bank, New York Academy of Medicine Library Grey Literature Collection, and reference lists were searched up until June 2012.

Study Selection.—Two reviewers independently identified original research papers (randomized, controlled trials; interrupted time series; uncontrolled and controlled before–after studies; and cohort comparisons).

Data Extraction.—Two reviewers independently extracted the data.

Data Synthesis.—The literature search identified 4 randomized, controlled trials; 5 interrupted time series; 3 controlled before–after studies;

1 nonrandomized, controlled study; 15 uncontrolled before–after studies; and 2 uncontrolled cohort studies. The variation in study quality, target conditions, and reported outcomes precluded meta-analysis. Uncontrolled studies (15 before–after studies, 2 cohort comparisons) suggested that P4P improves quality of care, but higher-quality studies with contemporaneous controls failed to confirm these findings. Two of the 4 randomized trials were negative, and the 2 statistically significant trials reported small incremental improvements in vaccination rates over usual care (absolute differences, 8.4 and 7.8 percentage points). Of the 5 interrupted time series, 2 did not detect any improvements in processes of care or clinical outcomes after P4P implementation, 1 reported initial statistically significant improvements in guideline adherence that dissipated over time, and 2 reported statistically significant improvements in blood pressure control in patients with diabetes balanced against statistically significant declines in hemoglobin A1c control.

Limitation.—Few methodologically robust studies compare P4P with other payment models for individual practitioners; most are small observational studies of variable quality.

Conclusion.—The effect of P4P targeting individual practitioners on quality of care and outcomes remains largely uncertain. Implementation of P4P models should be accompanied by robust evaluation plans.

▶ The Affordable Care Act called for expansion of pay-for-performance (P4P) programs within US health care. An outstanding issue, however, is whether P4P actually improves health care. A recent Cochrane review on the effect of financial incentives for primary care physicians included 7 studies and concluded that "there is insufficient evidence to support or not support the use of financial incentives to improve the quality of primary healthcare."[1] There are very few data about the impact of P4P in pediatrics.

This systematic review was designed to evaluate the effect of P4P remuneration among individual health care providers examining large electronic databases for information in this regard. The review identified 30 original research articles comparing P4P programs that targeted individual performance with other remuneration models for health care practitioners. Although uncontrolled before and after studies suggest that P4P improves adherence to quality-of-care indicators for chronic illnesses (such as ordering of laboratory tests in patients with diabetes, measurement and achievement of target blood pressure, adherence to prescribing guidelines for patients with heart failure), higher-quality studies with contemporaneous control groups or analyses that considered secular trends failed to confirm these benefits. Despite this paucity of studies on P4P, several hundred commentaries or editorials in support of P4P have appeared in the literature in the past 10 years or so. Clearly, evaluation of P4P initiatives has not kept pace with the rush to implement them. Although evidence does suggest modest effectiveness for P4P in improving preventive activities such as immunization rates, there seems to be little evidence that P4P is effective for other outcomes at least at this time.

These authors believe that implementation of P4P models in health care should be considered still experimental and not yet evidence based. Randomized, controlled trials may not be feasible or generalizable to study the effects of P4P. Despite the fact that performance incentives originally arose from the principal agent theory in economics and have been shown in some instances to affect behavior (eg, annual bonuses tied to sales or cost savings in the business sector), the optimal P4P scheme for health care remains an unresolved question. As we might suspect, the use of P4P can have a number of unintended consequences. One of these is the negative effect on job satisfaction on the part of clinicians. There has also been a trend to change health care provider focus from quality of care provision to quality of record keeping and also the potential for some for gaming.

As noted, there is very little information about the impact of P4P in pediatrics. One can assume, however, based on adult related studies that the enthusiasm for P4P as a driver of quality improvement is disproportionate to the amount and quality of the current evidence.

This commentary closes with a quiz. See if you can name the surgeon. This individual (1852-1922) was the first Surgeon-in-Chief at Johns Hopkins Hospital. He was one of the early surgeons to remove a gall bladder for cholecystitis, the patient being his own mother whom he also transfused using his own blood. He also devised the first radical mastectomy procedure, one still bearing his own name. He is credited with establishing the first surgical residency in the US and was the first to recommend the use of rubber gloves, not because of concerns for sepsis but because his wife, a surgical nurse, complained about the harsh antiseptics used during surgical preps that hurt her hands. He made casts of her hands so the Good Year Tire Company could devise a way to produce surgical gloves that were tight fitting.

Perhaps this surgeon's greatest gift to medicine was his development of cocaine formulations that could be injected under the skin to allow local surgical procedures, in particular dental extractions, to be performed without pain. Unfortunately, he took his own cocaine and became addicted to it. His retreats into rehab only served to convert a cocaine addiction to a morphine addiction. Despite this addiction, he continued to practice successfully for years and is commonly called "The Father of Modern Surgery."

In case you have not guessed correctly by this point, the surgeon was Dr William Stewart Halsted.[2]

J. A. Stockman III, MD

References

1. Scott A, Sivey P, Ait Ouakrim D, et al. The effect of financial incentives on the quality of healthcare provided by primary care physicians. *Cochrane Database Syst Rev.* 2011;(9):CD008451.
2. Imber G. *Genius in the Edge: the Bizarre Story of William Steward Halsted, the Father of Modern Surgery.* Kaplan Publishing; 2010.

Pediatric Readmission Prevalence and Variability Across Hospitals

Berry JG, Toomey SL, Zaslavsky AM, et al (Boston Children's Hosp, MA; Harvard Med School, Boston, MA; et al)
JAMA 309:372-380, 2013

Importance.—Readmission rates are used as an indicator of the quality of care that patients receive during a hospital admission and after discharge.

Objective.—To determine the prevalence of pediatric readmissions and the magnitude of variation in pediatric readmission rates across hospitals.

Design, Setting, and Patients.—We analyzed 568 845 admissions at 72 children's hospitals between July 1, 2009, and June 30, 2010, in the National Association of Children's Hospitals and Related Institutions Case Mix Comparative data set. We estimated hierarchical regression models for 30-day readmission rates by hospital, accounting for age and Chronic Condition Indicators. Hospitals with adjusted readmission rates that were 1 SD above and below the mean were defined as having "high" and "low" rates, respectively.

Main Outcome Measures.—Thirty-day unplanned readmissions following admission for any diagnosis and for the 10 admission diagnoses with the highest readmission prevalence. Planned readmissions were identified with procedure codes from the *International Classification of Diseases, Ninth Revision, Clinical Modification.*

Results.—The 30-day unadjusted readmission rate for all hospitalized children was 6.5% (n = 36 734). Adjusted rates were 28.6% greater in hospitals with high vs low readmission rates (7.2% [95% CI, 7.1%-7.2%] vs 5.6% [95% CI, 5.6%-5.6%]). For the 10 admission diagnoses with the highest readmission prevalence, the adjusted rates were 17.0% to 66.0% greater in hospitals with high vs low readmission rates. For example, sickle cell rates were 20.1% (95% CI, 20.0%-20.3%) vs 12.7% (95% CI, 12.6%-12.8%) in high vs low hospitals, respectively.

Conclusions and Relevance.—Among patients admitted to acute care pediatric hospitals, the rate of unplanned readmissions at 30 days was 6.5%. There was significant variability in readmission rates across conditions and hospitals. These data may be useful for hospitals' quality improvement efforts.

▶ The Centers for Medicare and Medicaid Services (CMS) Hospital Readmissions Reduction Program initiated a major shift in hospitals' attitude toward coordinating transitions of care in October 2012 when more than 2000 hospitals began losing money (a national total of about $300 million in the first year) to financial penalties for excessive readmissions. The design of the regulations that were put in place at that time triples the penalty for some hospitals by 2014 under provisions of the Affordable Care Act. Although the absolute amount of money related to the penalties is just a tiny fraction of 1% of the overall CMS budget, the penalties themselves are driving major changes in hospital philosophy about how to improve their quality of transition of care.

To date, hospitals that care for children have not been targeted by the Affordable Care Act's Hospital Readmissions Reduction Program, but often policies that start in adult hospitals gradually migrate to hospitals that care principally for children. If that happens, then this study takes on substantial significance.

Unlike adults, most children are hospitalized only once in their childhood, that is when they are born. Only a small percentage of children account for the majority of hospital admissions of children, and these are mostly children with complex medical problems. This study provides the most comprehensive description of readmissions for hospitalized children in the United States. The authors found an overall 30-day readmission rate of only 6.5% when analyzing 72 children's hospitals and more than half a million admissions. There was wide variation among hospitals, however. The range of variation was 28.6%.

In an editorial that accompanied this article, it was noted that these differences in readmission rates across hospital and conditions, while possibly caused by defects in quality, could very well be from additional factors particular to children that influence the pediatric readmission rate.[1] Unfortunately, the current article does not help to distinguish between these 2 plausible reasons for the differences. Readmission rates can vary with a parent's health status, family and caregiver resources, and the patient—parent relationship, an ever-changing process with age. Other factors include access to the medical home and family socioeconomic resources to care for a youngster. Without question, the child with a medical illness that is very complex and whose family resources are maximally challenged may end up being readmitted to the hospital more frequently to properly manage the youngster's illness.[1]

More research is needed to understand to what extent pediatric readmissions are caused by poor adherence to evidence-based best practices as opposed to patient and family resources and capabilities or some combination thereof. Without a better understanding of these factors that influence pediatric readmissions, it seems premature to hold pediatric hospitals that care for children entirely accountable for readmission rates. At least as of now, it is not reasonable to hamstring children's hospitals with penalties that are being used for adult-type hospitals.

J. A. Stockman III, MD

Reference

1. Srivastava R, Keren R. Pediatric readmissions as a hospital quality measure. *JAMA*. 2013;309:396-398.

Improved Survival Among Children with Spina Bifida in the United States
Shin M, Kucik JE, Siffel C, et al (Ctrs for Disease Control and Prevention, Atlanta, GA; et al)
J Pediatr 161:1132-1137.e3, 2012

Objective.—To evaluate trends in survival among children with spina bifida by race/ethnicity and possible prognostic factors in 10 regions of the United States.

Study Design.—A retrospective cohort study was conducted of 5165 infants with spina bifida born during 1979-2003, identified by 10 birth defects registries in the United States. Survival probabilities and adjusted hazard ratios were estimated for race/ethnicity and other characteristics using the Cox proportional hazard model.

Results.—During the study period, the 1-year survival probability among infants with spina bifida showed improvements for whites (from 88% to 96%), blacks (from 79% to 88%), and Hispanics (from 88% to 93%). The impact of race/ethnicity on survival varied by birth weight, which was the strongest predictor of survival through age 8. There was little racial/ethnic variation in survival among children born of very low birth weight. Among children born of low birth weight, the increased risk of mortality to Hispanics was approximately 4-6 times that of whites. The black-white disparity was greatest among children born of normal birth weight. Congenital heart defects did not affect the risk of mortality among very low birth weight children but increased the risk of mortality 4-fold among children born of normal birth weight.

Conclusions.—The survival of infants born with spina bifida has improved; however, improvements in survival varied by race/ethnicity, and blacks and Hispanics continued to have poorer survival than whites in the most recent birth cohort from 1998-2002. Further studies are warranted to elucidate possible reasons for the observed differences in survival.

▶ There is no question that the prevalence of spina bifida has decreased in the United States with the introduction of mandatory fortification of enriched grain products with folic acid. The prevalence of spina bifida now runs 3 to 4 cases per 10000 live births. Along with the decreasing prevalence of spina bifida, there has been an increasing survival rate from better surgical and other medical advances. Unfortunately, improvements in survival rates have not been uniform across socioeconomic groups and races in the United Sates.

Shin et al conducted a study of more than 5000 infants born with spina bifida to determine survival rates across varying ethnicities. A 20-year period was studied. The authors observed that the 1-year survival rate probability improves significantly over time for all children with spina bifida, but the magnitude of improvements varies quite significantly by race and ethnicity. Children with spina bifida born to nonwhite mothers have a lower probability of survival compared with children born to white mothers. The pooled survival probability at 1 year of age was 92.8%, a significant improvement over the past 20-year period of time, suggesting that medical and surgical medical advances are working and that folic acid fortification may have improved survival by reducing the risk of severe types of spina bifida. The data from this report do show that survival rates improve after fortification with folic acid. Survival rates among blacks and Hispanics with spina bifida did improve over time, but were consistently lower compared with that of whites. Hispanic babies of low birth weight had an increased risk of up to 6 times that of whites in terms of survival.

Thus, survival rates in infants and children with spina bifida are a good news/bad news story. Whereas survival rates have improved, racial and ethnic disparities still exist. Newborns with spina bifida and other congenital anomalies, particularly congenital heart disease, are at high risk of mortality, remarkably so if also black or Hispanic.

J. A. Stockman III, MD

Inpatient Hospital Care of Children With Trisomy 13 and Trisomy 18 in the United States
Nelson KE, Hexem KR, Feudtner C (Children's Hosp Boston, MA; The Children's Hosp of Philadelphia, PA)
Pediatrics 129:869-876, 2012

Background and Objective.—Trisomy 13 and trisomy 18 are generally considered fatal anomalies, with a majority of infants dying in the first year after birth. The inpatient hospital care that these patients receive has not been adequately described. This study characterized inpatient hospitalizations of children with trisomy 13 and trisomy 18 in the United States, including number and types of procedures performed.

Methods.—Retrospective repeated cross-sectional assessment of hospitalization data from the nationally representative US Kids' Inpatient Database, for the years 1997, 2000, 2003, 2006, and 2009. Included hospitalizations were of patients aged 0 to 20 years with a diagnosis of trisomy 13 or trisomy 18.

Results.—The number of hospitalizations for each trisomy type ranged from 846 to 907 per year for trisomy 13 ($P = .77$ for temporal trend) and 1036 to 1616 per year for trisomy 18 ($P < .001$ for temporal trend). Over one-third (36%) of the hospitalizations were of patients older than 1 year of age. Patients underwent a total of 2765 major therapeutic procedures, including creation of esophageal sphincter (6% of hospitalizations; mean age 23 months), repair of atrial and ventricular septal defects (4%; mean age 9 months), and procedures on tendons (4%; mean age 8 years).

Conclusions.—Children with trisomy 13 and trisomy 18 receive significant inpatient hospital care. Despite the conventional understanding of these syndromes as lethal, a substantial number of children are living longer than 1 year and undergoing medical and surgical procedures as part of their treatment.

▶ This report reminds us that the most common chromosomal abnormalities noted in live-born infants are trisomy 21, trisomy 18, and trisomy 13. The latter 2 abnormalities have been considered fatal given that the significant majority of affected infants will die in the first year of life. Death usually occurs from problems with multiple organ systems including the cardiovascular system, central nervous system anomalies, and gastrointestinal and abdominal wall defects, etc. The mean survival for both syndromes is generally thought to be on the order of days. Population studies and multiple single case reports have identified some long-term survivors. Mosaicism has been suggested as 1 possible reason for longer term survivorship.

Nelson et al undertook a study analyzing data from a multiyear national repository containing a representative sample of inpatient discharge data to evaluate the medical and surgical inpatient care that children with trisomy 13 and trisomy 18 receive in the United States. They assessed factors likely to be associated with short- and long-term survivorship. Despite the fact that the literature suggests a mean survivorship of only days, in the series reported by Nelson et al, about half of infants with trisomy 13 and 18 were discharged alive after an average stay of 7.8 days. In fact, the authors identified that 41% and 32% of hospital records of children with trisomy 13 and 18 were of children older than 1 year of age. Slightly over 10% of hospital discharges were of youngsters 8 years of age. These longer term survivors had multiple surgical and other medical interventions performed to sustain life. It was not clear whether mosaicism did indeed contribute to longer survivorship.

This study reveals that at least in the United States, a significant number of children with trisomy 13 and 18 will undergo surgical procedures as part of their inpatient medical care and that these procedures may increase the lifespan of affected individuals. The authors suggest that because we are currently unable to identify which children might be long-term survivors, universal application of the term "lethal" to the diagnosis of trisomy 13 or 18 is no longer appropriate.

Another study recently appeared from the Vermont Oxford Network that also looked at major chromosomal anomalies among very low-birth-weight infants.[1] It was clear that among very low-birth-weight infants with trisomy 13 and trisomy 18, survival was extremely poor. By 1 week of age, more than two-thirds of infants with these 2 trisomies had died. Survivorship at 1 year of age was well under 1%. These mortality rates might have been affected by withholding medical treatment from these infants, given the dual risk of major chromosomal anomaly and very low birth weight. As one might therefore suspect, being born very low birth weight with trisomy 13 and 18 contributes very negatively to survivorship.

J. A. Stockman III, MD

Reference

1. Boghossian NS, Horbar JD, Carpenter JH, Murray JC, Bell EF; Vermont Oxford Network. Major chromosomal anomalies among very low birth weight infants in the Vermont Oxford Network. *J Pediatr.* 2012;160:774-780.

Natural history of fetal trisomy 18 after prenatal diagnosis
Burke AL, Field K, Morrison JJ (Galway Univ Hosp, Ireland)
Arch Dis Child Fetal Neonatal Ed 98:F152-F154, 2013

Objective.—To evaluate the natural fetal and neonatal outcome for pregnancies with an established prenatal diagnosis of fetal trisomy 18, and a parental decision for continuation of the pregnancy.

Methods.—The obstetric and neonatal outcome data for 23 such pregnancies, diagnosed at a single referral Fetal Medicine Centre, were retrospectively obtained.

Results.—The overall intrauterine fetal death rate was 61%, with a progressive decline in live fetuses up to 39 weeks gestation. For fetuses diagnosed before 20 weeks gestation, there was a trend towards a higher intrauterine fetal death rate (88%), in comparison to those diagnosed after this period (44%) ($p = 0.06$). For live births, the preterm delivery rate was 44%. All infants born alive died within 48 h of birth.

Conclusion.—These data provide reliable information for parental counselling pertaining to risk of intrauterine death when trisomy 18 is diagnosed prenatally. These findings suggest that long-term survival implications for trisomy 18 are different when it is diagnosed prenatally (Fig).

▶ Trisomy 18 remains the most common autosomal trisomy after Down syndrome. There has been an increase in prenatal diagnosis of trisomy 18 as a result of advances in prenatal screening tests and high-definition prenatal ultrasound scanning. Although infant survival has largely remained unchanged, there has been an increase in the number of live born newborns with trisomy 18 as a result of improved perinatal care. There is a small minority of parents who do elect to continue pregnancy. Prior to this article, there was little information available to counsel such parents about the natural history of those who are live born with trisomy 18.

These authors carried out a retrospective study in Ireland about the natural history of those who are live born with trisomy 18. Over the period 2000 to 2009, 23 pregnancies were given a prenatal diagnosis of trisomy 18 where a continuation of the pregnancy took place beyond the period of diagnosis. The overall rate of intrauterine fetal death was 61%, and the live birth rate was 39%. Fetal losses were seen through 39 weeks' gestation. In this study, all infants

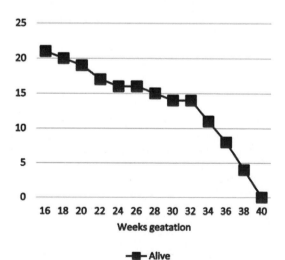

Weeks geatation

—■— Alive

FIGURE.—Demonstrates the number of live fetuses present for each 2-week period of gestation, from 16 to 40 weeks, after prenatal diagnosis with trisomy 18. (Reprinted from Burke AL, Field K, Morrison JJ. Natural history of fetal trisomy 18 after prenatal diagnosis. *Arch Dis Child Fetal Neonatal Ed.* 2013;98:F152-F154, with permission from the BMJ Publishing Group Ltd.)

born alive died within 48 hours of birth, that is, there was a 100% perinatal mortality. For live born infants, the preterm delivery rate at less than 37 weeks was 44% with 56% delivering at term. For fetuses diagnosed before 20 weeks' gestation, there was a trend toward a higher intrauterine fetal death rate, which was 88%. For those diagnosed before 20 weeks' gestation, fetal demise occurred between 16 and 33 weeks' gestation.

This article adds significantly to our understanding about the "natural history" of trisomy 18. The findings from this article are based on the natural outcome for trisomy 18 from 20 pregnancies in which the diagnosis was made prenatally and clearly provide useful figures for management of such patients in a fetal medicine service. Parents can be informed that if the pregnancy continues postdiagnosis, the overall intrauterine death rate will be slightly over 60%, and the likelihood of survivorship beyond the perinatal period is extremely small. Fig illustrates the number of fetuses and when they were lost during pregnancy or died shortly after birth.

J. A. Stockman III, MD

Injuries Associated With Bottles, Pacifiers, and Sippy Cups in the United States, 1991–2010

Keim SA, Fletcher EN, TePoel MRW, et al (Nationwide Children's Hosp, Columbus, OH; et al)
Pediatrics 129:1104-1110, 2012

Objective.—To describe the epidemiology of injuries related to bottles, pacifiers, and sippy cups among young children in the United States.

Methods.—A retrospective analysis was conducted by using data from the National Electronic Injury Surveillance System for children < 3 years of age treated in emergency departments (1991–2010) for an injury associated with a bottle, pacifier, or sippy cup.

Results.—An estimated 45 398 (95% confidence interval: 38 770–52 026) children aged < 3 years were treated in emergency departments for injuries related to these products during the study period, an average of 2270 cases per year. Most injuries involved bottles (65.8%), followed by pacifiers (19.9%) and sippy cups (14.3%). The most common mechanism was a fall while using the product (86.1% of injuries). Lacerations comprised the most common diagnosis (70.4%), and the most frequently injured body region was the mouth (71.0%). One-year-old children were injured most often. Children who were aged 1 or 2 years were nearly 2.99 times (95% confidence interval: 2.07–4.33) more likely to sustain a laceration compared with any other diagnosis. Product malfunctions were relatively uncommon (4.4% of cases).

Conclusions.—This study is the first to use a nationally representative sample to examine injuries associated with these products. Given the number of injuries, particularly those associated with falls while using the product, greater efforts are needed to promote proper usage, ensure safety in product design, and increase awareness of American Academy of

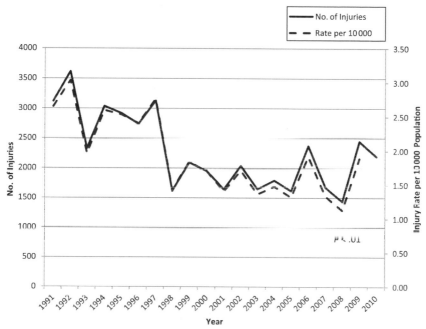

FIGURE 1.—Number of bottle-, pacifier-, and sippy cup—related injuries and prevalence per 10 000 US children, 1991 to 2010. Prevalence per 10 000 US children ≤2 years of age based on intercensal population estimates.[17,18] Estimate not available for 2010. *Editor's Note:* Please refer to original journal article for full references. (Reproduced with permission from Pediatrics, Keim SA, Fletcher EN, TePoel MRW, et al. Injuries associated with bottles, pacifiers, and sippy cups in the United States, 1991–2010. *Pediatrics*. 2012;129:1104-1110. Copyright © 2012 by the American Academy of Pediatrics.)

Pediatrics' recommendations for transitioning to a cup and discontinuing pacifier use (Figs 1 and 2).

▶ Who would have thought that baby bottles, pacifiers, and sippy cups would be so dangerous? There have been occasional reports, however, of pacifier or baby bottle-related injuries going back more than half a century. Most of these were related to airway obstruction from bottle nipples or pacifier parts or burns from bottle warming. Product design improvements have made such safety concerns much less. Given that no manufacturing process is perfect, more than 16 million pacifiers and 1 million sippy cups have been recalled by the US Consumer Product Safety Commission (USPSC) since 1991, documenting that baby bottles, pacifiers, and sippy cups are not always as safe as parents or care providers might believe.

Keim et al designed a research project to educate parents, other care providers, and health care professionals about the potential injury risk from baby bottles, pacifiers, and sippy cups. They examined data from the National Electronic Injury Surveillance System. This information source provides data on consumer product-related and sports-related injuries treated in emergency departments in the United States. The surveillance system was put into place in 1972. Figs 1 and 2 show the absolute number of bottle-, pacifier-, and sippy cup-related

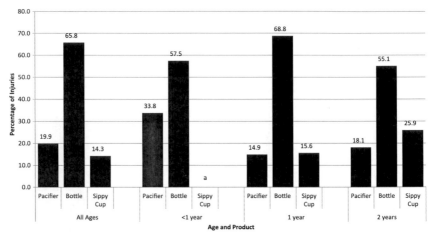

FIGURE 2.—Percent of injuries involving pacifiers, bottles, and sippy cups according to age among US children ages 0 to 2 years, 1991 to 2010. [a]Injuries from sippy cups in the < 1-year-old age group were too rare to provide reliable national estimates. (Reproduced with permission from Pediatrics, Keim SA, Fletcher EN, TePoel MRW, et al. Injuries associated with bottles, pacifiers, and sippy cups in the United States, 1991–2010. *Pediatrics*. 2012;129:1104-1110. Copyright © 2012 by the American Academy of Pediatrics.)

injuries and their prevalence per 10 000 US children between 1991 and 2010. The age group looked at was 0 to 2 years. Interestingly, falls were the most common mechanism of injury, with most occurring using a bottle (64.7%); however, pacifiers (19.3%) and sippy cups (15.9%) were also involved. The most commonly injured body parts were the mouth (71%), followed by the head, face, or neck (19.6%). There were 1321 cases of aspiration and ingestion. A total of 1895 burns were reported and 1821 miscellaneous diagnoses such as fractures and dislocations. Over the 20-year period, a total of 45 391 cases of injuries related to bottle, sippy cups, and pacifiers were treated in emergency departments.

This report appears to be the first to tell us about national estimates, rates, and trends of injuries of the types described. There was an increasing trend downward in the rates over time of injuries from baby bottles, pacifiers, and sippy cups. Presumably this is because of more stringent requirements from the USPSC, which in 1978 issued requirements for pacifiers intended to protect infants from choking or suffocating and required that the pacifiers not have sharp edges. A recall in 1991 of more than 16 million pacifiers was based on failure of manufacturers to meet these requirements. The USPSC also recalled more than 1 million sippy cups for reasons that include a risk of choking, laceration, or poisoning from cup materials. Most visits to emergency rooms now are not due to defective products, but rather infants and toddlers falling as a result of the use of these products during developmental periods when such a risk is highest. Children who are just learning to walk and run are at highest risk of such injuries. The authors of this report suggest that parents might wish to consider the potential for injury in deciding when to help their child give up the pacifier and transition to a cup. Encouraging children to remain seated while drinking may also reduce injury.

While on the topic of household contents and injuries to children, a recent report appeared from British Columbia about television-related injuries in children.[1] In

Canada, mortality from falling televisions is the 15th leading cause of childhood death. This injury severity appears to be higher in First Nations and recent immigrant families. Television tip-overs are not unique to Canada. The USPSC ranks the television as one of the top 5 hazards in a home and lists televisions as the third highest cause of mortality and morbidity from household injuries.

J. A. Stockman III, MD

Reference

1. Mills J, Grushka J, Butterworth S. Television-related injuries in children—the British Columbia experience. *J Pediatr Surg.* 2012;47:991-995.

Pediatric Battery-Related Emergency Department Visits in the United States, 1990—2009
Sharpe SJ, Rochette LM, Smith GA (The Res Inst at Nationwide Children's Hosp, Columbus, OH)
Pediatrics 129:1111-1117, 2012

Objective.—To investigate the epidemiology of battery-related emergency department (ED) visits among children < 18 years of age in the United States.

Methods.—Using a nationally representative sample from the National Electronic Injury Surveillance System, battery-related ED visits in the United States from 1990 to 2009 were analyzed. Four battery exposure routes for patients were determined from diagnosis codes and case narratives: ingestion, mouth exposure, ear canal insertion, and nasal cavity insertion.

Results.—An estimated 65 788 (95% confidence interval: 54 498—77 078) patients < 18 years of age presented to US EDs due to a battery-related exposure during the 20-year study period, averaging 3289 battery-related ED visits annually. The average annual battery-related ED visit rate was 4.6 visits per 100 000 children. The number ($P < .001$) and rate ($P = .002$) of visits increased significantly during the study period, with substantial increases during the last 8 study years. The mean age was 3.9 years (95% confidence interval: 3.5—4.2), and 60.2% of patients were boys. Battery ingestion accounted for 76.6% of ED visits, followed by nasal cavity insertion (10.2%), mouth exposure (7.5%), and ear canal insertion (5.7%). Button batteries were implicated in 83.8% of patient visits caused by a known battery type. Most children (91.8%) were treated and released from the ED.

Conclusions.—This study evaluated battery-related ED visits among US children using a nationally representative sample. Batteries pose an important hazard to children, especially those ≤ 5 years of age. The increasing number and rate of battery-related ED visits among children underscore the need for increased prevention efforts (Fig 2).

▶ One would think that there is not much left to learn about button battery-related injuries, but as this report shows, there is. Most button battery ingestions are benign, but severe complications and even death have been reported,

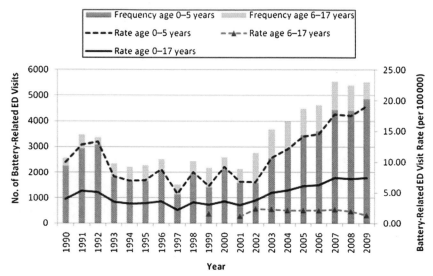

FIGURE 2.—Annual number and rate of battery-related ED visits according to age group and year in the United States, 1990—2009. Due to small sample size, national estimates for the age group 6 to 17 years were unstable for the years 1990—1998 and 2000; therefore, rates for these years are not represented. (Reproduced with permission from Pediatrics, Sharpe SJ, Rochette LM, Smith GA. Pediatric battery-related emergency department visits in the United States, 1990—2009. *Pediatrics.* 2012;129:1111-1117. Copyright © 2012 by the American Academy of Pediatrics.)

particularly if a button battery becomes lodged in the esophagus. Severe injuries related to button battery ingestions appear to be increasing, largely as the result of the more widespread use of 3-B 20-mm lithium button batteries. The esophagus is not the only area where these small items can cause great harm. If lodged in the nasal cavity or the external auditory canal, these can cause serious localized damage. Less common are injuries caused by cylindrical batteries. These contain alkaline corrosives that can cause burns if the integrity of the battery becomes damaged.

Sharpe et al now report on the epidemiology of battery-related emergency department visits using information from the National Electronic Injury Surveillance System (NEISS) of the Consumer Product Safety Commission. NEISS samples data from approximately 100 US hospital emergency departments, including 7 children's hospitals. The NEISS database is updated daily. Sharpe et al looked at information from this database for children younger than 18 years of age who visited an emergency department between 1990 and 2009. Over this interval, 65 788 visits to emergency departments occurred related to battery-related problems. The mean age of presentation was 3.9 years. Eighty-percent of presentations were in children younger than 5 years of age and 60% were in boys. Over the interval reviewed, the number of visits of children younger than 18 years of age for battery-related medical complications doubled (Fig 2). There was no seasonal variation noted.

Data from this report show that when the battery's intended use was mentioned in the records, 29% involved toys/games, 15.9% hearing aids, 13.7% watches, 12.4% calculators, 8.8% flashlights, 5.5% remote controls, and 14.7% other.

Ingestion of batteries accounted for three-quarters of all battery-related emergency department visits, followed by nasal cavity insertion (10.2%), mouth exposure (7.5%), and ear canal insertion (5.7%).

This is an important report. If one looks at the statistics from the study carefully, one will see that every 3 hours somewhere in the United States a person younger than 18 years of age will present with a battery-related problem to an emergency room in the United States. Of greatest concern are those youngsters presenting with ingestions. Most of ingestions appear to occur in children younger than 5 years of age. Although most batteries will pass through the gastrointestinal tract spontaneously without adverse consequences, severe morbidity and mortality can occur, particularly if the battery lodges in the esophagus. If a button battery lodges in the esophagus, surrounding tissue injury can occur in as short a period as 2 hours. The mechanism of injury is multifold. When placed in a conductive medium, a button battery gives rise to an external current, causing electrolysis of tissue fluids and the generation of hydroxide at the battery's negative pole. Leakage of alkaline electrolyte from an alkaline battery will cause liquefactive necrosis and pressure necrosis. Current discharge appears to be the most important problem, especially for 20-mm lithium batteries that do not contain an alkaline electrolyte and generate much more current because they have twice the voltage and higher capacitance compared with other button batteries. Delayed complications include esophageal perforation, esophageal stricture, vocal cord paralysis from recurrent laryngeal nerve damage, and development of tracheoesophageal or aortoesophageal fistulas that can lead to exsanguination and death.

Given the increasing number and rate of battery-related emergency department visits among children, an ounce of prevention on parents' part is critical. It is incumbent upon pediatricians to inform parents of the risks of such batteries and to tell parents to make sure that grandparents who have hearing aids to keep their hearing aid batteries in a secure location where tiny tots cannot get them.

J. A. Stockman III, MD

Safety Effects of Drawstring Requirements for Children's Upper Outerwear Garments

Rodgers GB, Topping JC III (US Consumer Product Safety Commission, Bethesda, MD)
Arch Pediatr Adolesc Med 166:651-655, 2012

Objective.—To evaluate the effectiveness of the requirements of the voluntary safety standard for drawstrings on children's upper outerwear garments in preventing child deaths resulting from drawstring entanglement.

Design.—An interrupted time series design. Annual estimates of drawstring-related child deaths were developed for the study period of January 1985 to December 2009. A Poisson regression model for rate data was used to evaluate the effectiveness of the drawstring requirements during the postintervention period.

Setting.—United States.

Subjects.—Children aged 14 years and younger.

Intervention.—The application of the drawstring requirements of the voluntary standard that were adopted in 1997.

Main Outcome Measure.—The estimated percentage reduction in the drawstring-related child mortality rate associated with the application of the drawstring requirements.

Results.—The drawstring requirements of the voluntary standard were associated with a 90.9% (95% CI, 83.8%-96.1%) reduction in the drawstring-related mortality rate. This suggests the prevention of about 50 child deaths from 1997, when the voluntary standard was adopted, through the end of our study period in 2009.

Conclusions.—The requirements of the voluntary safety standard for drawstrings have been highly effective in preventing deaths resulting from the entanglement of drawstrings in children's upper outerwear garments.

▶ Until this article appeared, I had not thought very much about the risks of injury related to drawstrings commonly used in upper outerwear garments. Drawstrings commonly appear on jackets and sweatshirts. Drawstrings in the neck and hood areas of outerwear garments present a strangulation hazard when they become caught in gaps or on protuberances from objects such as playground slides. Other drawstrings can also be a problem. Waist-level drawstrings can become entangled in a school bus handrail, for example, presenting a hazard to children when buses pull away after a stop. During the period January 1985 through September 1995, the US Consumer Product Safety Commission (CPSC) received reports of 17 fatal injuries and 42 cases of nonfatal injuries or potential injuries involving children whose hood or waist-level drawstrings had became entangled on playground equipment, school bus handrails, or other common items.[1]

It was in 1995 that the CPSC issued recommendations to address the hazards of injury related to drawstrings. As an alternative to neck-level drawstrings, the CPSC recommended the use of other closures such as snaps, buttons, Velcro, or elastic. At the waist level, the CPSC recommended that the ends of waist-level drawstrings measure no more than 3 inches from where the strings extend from the garment, reasoning that this limitation, among others, would reduce the risk of waist-level drawstring entanglements. At the same time these recommendations were coming forward, the National Highway Traffic Safety Administration issued recommendations to reduce injuries related to school bus handrails and doors so that drawstrings could not easily snag on school bus handrails and doors. The garment industry also adopted safety standards for drawstrings on children's upper outerwear. The standards prohibit the use of drawstrings in the neck area of garments sizes 2T to 12. It also requires that nonretractable drawstrings at the waist level of garment sizes 2T to 16 be limited to no more than 3 inches outside the drawstring channel when the garment is expanded to its fullest width, have no toggles, knots, or other attachments at free ends, and be bar tacked if the drawstring is a continuous string. The same guidelines indicate that fully retractable drawstrings can be exempt from these requirements. Obviously the garment sizes chosen were to protect the highest risk group of youngsters: those aged 18 months to 10 years for neck-level drawstrings and children aged 18 months to 14 years for waist-level drawstrings.

The purpose of this study was to see whether the recommendations that have been put in place over the past decade to 2 decades have been effective in preventing child deaths. The major source of information used in this study was the CPSC's Injury and Potential Injury Incidence Database. This database was culled for its information from January 1985 through December 2009. During that period, a total of 29 drawstring entanglement deaths were identified. Twenty-three of the reported deaths occurred before the voluntary standards were put in place in 1997. During the prestandard period, there were about 3.3 deaths per year from 1994 through 1996, but only 1.4 deaths per year from 1985 through 1993. The lower rate from 1985 through 1993 was probably related to underreporting. When the recommendations were gradually put in place in the 1990s, the number of deaths from drawstring injuries fell dramatically.

It appears that the garment industry has extensively conformed to the recommendations of the CPSC. There are probably very good reasons for this compliance. First and most obvious is the fact that substituting alternative closures such as snaps, buttons, Velcro, or elastic is relatively inexpensive. Also, the liability of not conforming is tremendous. Finally, the CPSC enforcement policies have encouraged conformance. The CPSP has told manufacturers to recall certain outwear garments that do not comply with their recommendations. These recalls are potentially extremely costly to firms that do not comply.

All in all it is not possible to say with a high degree of assurance that the recommendations emanating from the CPSC have made the remarkable differences that have been seen over time in the reduction of drawstring-related fatalities because it is possible that the growing popularity of Velcro or other closures on children's outerwear garments might have reduced these injuries even without such recommendations. Nonetheless, we should be proud of the CPSC for having paid attention to what is a serious problem for our teenagers and preteenagers.

J. A. Stockman III, MD

Reference

1. US Consumer Product Safety Commission. *Child's Death Spurs Effort to Release Guidelines for Drawstrings on Children's Jackets and Sweatshirts.* Bethesda, MD: US Consumer Product Safety Commission; 1995.

Pediatric Inflatable Bouncer—Related Injuries in the United States, 1990—2010

Thompson MC, Chounthirath T, Xiang H, et al (The Res Inst at Nationwide Children's Hosp, Columbus, OH)
Pediatrics 130:1076-1083, 2012

Objective.—To investigate inflatable bouncer—related injuries to children in the United States.

Methods.—Records were analyzed from the National Electronic Injury Surveillance System for patients ≤17 years old treated in US emergency departments (EDs) for inflatable bouncer—related injuries from 1990 to 2010.

Results.—An estimated 64 657 (95% confidence interval [CI]: 32 420—96 893) children ≤17 years of age with inflatable bouncer—related injuries were treated in US EDs from 1990 to 2010. From 1995 to 2010, there was a statistically significant 15-fold increase in the number and rate of these injuries, with an average annual rate of 5.28 injuries per 100 000 US children (95% CI: 2.62—7.95). The increase was more rapid during recent years, with the annual injury number and rate more than doubling between 2008 and 2010. In 2010, a total of 31 children per day were treated in US EDs for an inflatable bouncer—related injury, which equals a child every 46 minutes nationally. A majority of patients were male (54.6%), and the mean patient age was 7.50 years (95% CI: 7.17—7.83). Most injuries were fractures (27.5%) and strains or sprains (27.3%), and most injuries occurred to the lower (32.9%) or upper (29.7%) extremities. Most injuries occurred at a place of sports or recreation (43.7%) or at home (37.5%), and 3.4% of injured children were hospitalized or kept for <24 hours for observation.

Conclusions.—The number and rate of pediatric inflatable bouncer—related injuries have increased rapidly in recent years. This increase, along with similarities to trampoline-related injuries, underscores the need for guidelines for safer bouncer usage and improvements in bouncer design to prevent these injuries among children.

▶ There is not a parent around who is not familiar with inflatable bouncers, such as bounce houses and moonwalks. If you have been on the moon yourself, however, and missed the surge of interest in these inflatables, be aware that the bouncy castle started it all. One little inflatable bouncy house sparked an entire industry that keeps growing every day. A *bouncehouse*, also known as a *moonwalk, moonbounce, bouncy house, bouncy castle, bounce house, bouncer*, or *jumper*, is an enclosed inflatable structure usually cube shaped, in which children or even adults may enjoy bounce-around effects as they would on a trampoline. An inflatable bounce house has become a staple of almost every child's birthday party. At least once in their life, most youngsters have enjoyed bounce houses, whether at their own party or someone else's. The number of party rental companies that have these things has become ubiquitous.

What we learn from this report is that the rate of reported increases in injuries associated with pediatric inflatable bouncer-related items has increased fairly dramatically. Thompson et al have mined data from the National Electronic Injury Surveillance System to analyze data related to inflatable bouncer-related injuries. The surveillance system is a nationally representative database that has collected data from approximately 100 hospital emergency rooms in the United States and its territories. Information from the surveys performed at these hospitals shows that between the ages of 3 years and 12 years, one sees the largest numbers of all injuries associated with inflatable bouncers. Fig 2 in the original article shows a literal explosion in injury rates per 100 000 US consumers as a result of the increasing popularity of these fun objects. We learn from this report that boys slightly outnumber girls in the overall percentage of injuries. Most injuries observed in emergency departments relate to strains/sprains and fractures.

A minority of injuries relates to soft tissue injuries, lacerations, and concussion/closed head injuries. These injuries usually result from falling inside or on the bouncer or colliding with another user.

It is clear that with the increased number of inflatable bouncer-related injuries, there is a strong need for better guidelines for safer bouncer usage and improvements in bouncer design to prevent these injuries among children. There are international published standards for inflatable amusement devices. These voluntary standards include design, manufacturer, installation, operation, and maintenance guidelines that are aimed at manufacturers, owners, and operators of inflatable amusement devices. These guidelines relate to the installation of the devices and recommend that operators follow manufacturer specifications regarding the maximum capacity by weight or number of users as well as the physical requirements for users, including age, height, and weight. These same standards also call for the prohibition of bodily contact, flips, and dropkicks by users in accordance with manufacturer specifications. There must be trained operators supervising all play as well. Unfortunately, most safety guidelines are still determined by individual manufacturers. The medical and public health community has not provided recommendations regarding pediatric use of inflatable bouncers.

It should also be noted that although most rental companies of these inflatable bouncers carry liability insurance, not all do so because not all are required to do so. A quick search of the Internet indicates that the most common insurer of inflatable bouncers is a company called "Insure My Jumper." If you are giving a birthday party that involves children, and if you are interested in protecting yourself, liability-wise, you as a parent and/or homeowner might want to look toward getting your own temporary insurance. The Web site for this is http://www.insuremyjumper.com (this is not a paid promo!).

J. A. Stockman III, MD

Booster Seat Laws and Fatalities in Children 4 to 7 Years of Age

Mannix R, Fleegler E, Meehan WP III, et al (Children's Hosp Boston, MA)
Pediatrics 130:996-1002, 2012

Objective.—To determine whether state booster seat laws were associated with decreased fatality rates in children 4 to 7 years of age in the United States.

Methods.—Retrospective, longitudinal analysis of all motor vehicle occupant crashes involving children 4 to 7 years of age identified in the Fatality Analysis Reporting System from January 1999 through December 2009. The main outcome measure was fatality rates of motor vehicle occupants aged 4 to 7 years. Because most booster laws exclude children 6 to 7 years of age, we performed separate analyses for children 4 to 5, 6, and 7 years of age.

Results.—When controlling for other motor vehicle legislation, temporal and economic factors, states with booster seat laws had a lower risk of fatalities in 4- to 5-year-olds than states without booster seat laws (adjusted incidence rate ratio 0.89; 95% confidence interval [CI] 0.81−0.99). States with booster seat laws that included 6-year-olds had an adjusted incidence rate ratio of 0.77 (95% CI 0.65—0.91) for motor vehicle collision fatalities of 6-year-olds and those that included 7-year-olds had an adjusted incidence rate ratio of 0.75 (95% CI, 0.62—0.91) for motor vehicle collision fatalities of 7-year-olds.

Conclusions.—Booster seat laws are associated with decreased fatalities in children 4 to 7 years of age, with the strongest association seen in children 6 to 7 years of age. Future legislative efforts should extend current laws to children aged 6 to 7 years.

▶ There is no question that the appropriate use of car seats for children 4 years and under has resulted in a remarkable decrease in the risk of injury or death related to motor vehicle collisions. Every state and the District of Columbia has passed legislation requiring car seats for children 4 years and younger. This has been true for 30 years. After a child outgrows a car seat, it is recommended that children over 4 years of age and up to 8 years of age or a height of up to 4 feet 9 inches be placed in booster seats. These too have been highly effective in preventing injuries and death in motor vehicle collisions.

Unfortunately, information provided by the National Highway Traffic Safety Administration shows that less than half of 4-year-olds to 5-year-olds and only one-third of 6-year-olds to 7-year-olds are routinely restrained in booster seats. Between 2001 and 2009, legislation requiring the use of booster seats for children 4 years of age and older has been passed in 47 states and the District of Columbia, but unfortunately the age requirements for booster seat use vary somewhat from state to state. The national effect of booster seat legislation, while controlling for additional factors known to influence motor vehicle fatality rates, has not been previously described nor has there been a study that has evaluated the effect of legislation on older children with the use of data on the national level.

These authors undertook a study using data from the Fatality Analysis Reporting System to evaluate the effectiveness of booster seat laws and proper booster seat restraint on motor vehicle collision-related fatalities sustained by children aged 4 to 7 years after accounting for other factors that are known to influence motor vehicle fatality rates. Between 1999 and 2009, a total of 3639 motor vehicle collision-related fatalities were sustained by children aged 4 to 7 years. At the start of the study period, no states had enacted laws regarding booster seat use, and the rate of motor vehicle fatalities in children aged 4 to 7 years in the United States was 2.8 per 100 000 children. During the 11-year study period, 47 states and the District of Columbia passed booster seat legislation. This represents 219 state-years of booster seat legislation for children aged 4 to 5 years and 126 and 77 state-years for children aged 6 to 7 years, respectively. In 1999, at the start of the study period, 9% of 4-year-old to 5-year-old children involved in a motor vehicle collision were properly restrained in a booster seat; by 2009, the rate of proper booster seat restraint had increased to 41% in this age group. In states that enacted a booster seat law during the study period, the mean unadjusted rates of fatal injuries sustained by children aged 4 to 5 years before legislation was 5.7 per 100 000 children, with state-specific rates ranging from 0.4 per 100 000 to 18 children per 100 000. After enacting legislation, the mean fatality rate of 4-year-olds to 5-year-olds decreased to 4.2 per 100 000 children, with state-specific rates ranging from 0 per 100 000 to 10.8 per 100 000 children. For states that enacted legislation, there was no question that the decline in death rates was greater after the legislation than before. Similar findings were seen in other age groups. In states where there was no booster seat legislation, there have been no statistically significant changes in fatality rates for any childhood age group.

Obviously there is still much room for improvement since the use of booster seats by parents is not 100%, not even close to it. Typically a booster seat should be used from the age of 4 years until the child is between the ages of 8 years and 12 years and is 4 feet 9 inches in height. Legislation that reflects the best-practice recommendations can help guide parents in the most effective ways to protect their children while riding in a motor vehicle.

Please note that legislation alone will not suffice in solving the problem described. Barriers to booster seat use include parental lack of knowledge about booster seat recommendations, difficulty using booster seats, children refusing to use booster seats, the cost of the seats, and lack of knowledge regarding booster seat effectiveness in reducing death and injury rates. There are solutions to these impediments that can be found with public awareness campaigns, incentives to manufacturers for including built-in booster seats in motor vehicles, and financial assistance for those who cannot afford a booster seat. This article is worthy of every pediatrician's reading.

J. A. Stockman III, MD

Subungual Wooden Splinter Visualized With Bedside Sonography
Teng M, Doniger SJ (Stanford Univ, CA; Children's Hosp and Res Ctr Oakland, CA)
Pediatr Emerg Care 28:392-394, 2012

Bedside ultrasound has become increasingly important as an adjunct to clinical diagnosis and procedures in the emergency department. It is only recently that this modality, which involves no ionizing radiation, has become incorporated into the pediatric emergency department. We report a case of a 10-year-old boy with a suspected subungual wooden foreign body. Bedside ultrasound was used to identify and characterize the foreign body before removal and then to evaluate for any residual foreign body after removal. A brief review of the technique is presented, including the use of a water bath to enhance visualization of the object and decrease the patient's discomfort. This case highlights the utility of ultrasound in detecting radiolucent soft tissue foreign bodies (Fig 2).

▶ These authors report on a 10-year-old boy who sustained an injury to his right index finger. The injury occurred as the patient ran his finger against the edge of a wooden dresser. When seen in an emergency room, there was a suspicion of an embedded subungual foreign body. The attending physician decided to use ultrasound to make a diagnosis. He identified a hyperechoic linear structure running superficial to and parallel to the distal phalanx consistent with a foreign body such as a wood splinter. This was removed with needle-tip forceps.

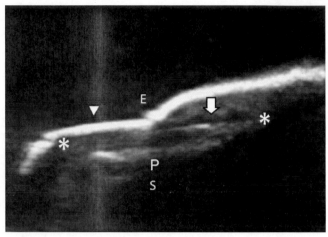

FIGURE 2.—Bedside ultrasound demonstrating hyperechoic foreign body (*) beneath the nail and extending proximally past the eponychium (E) of the nail. Wooden foreign bodies often are surrounded by a hypoechoic halo (arrow). The foreign body lies between the nail (arrowhead) and the hyperechoic phalanx (P). Of note, there is shadowing (S) posterior to the phalanx. (Reprinted from Teng M, Doniger SJ. Subungual wooden splinter visualized with bedside sonography. *Pediatr Emerg Care.* 2012;28:392-394, with permission from Lippincott Williams & Wilkins.)

Historically, plain x-rays have been the preferred imaging modality to detect retained foreign bodies. Metal, glass, and stone can be seen with standard x-rays. Plastic, rubber, and organic or vegetables materials such as wood, thorns, or cactus spines are not likely to show on x-ray. Ultrasound, however, can detect a soft tissue foreign body, regardless of whether it is radiopaque or radiolucent. Not surprisingly, ultrasound is superior to x-ray in certain situations.

Bedside ultrasound is an easily accessible modality, which is able to provide real-time localization of embedded foreign material. It can demonstrate surrounding anatomical structures. It is important to remember that bedside ultra-sonography merely complements a well-performed history and physical examination. It is no substitute. Also, it is recommended that ultrasound be repeated after foreign body extraction to ensure adequate removal. We are seeing more and more use of bedside ultrasound. Like all other technologies, it does require experience and skill.

J. A. Stockman III, MD

Practices of Unregulated Tanning Facilities in Missouri: Implications for Statewide Legislation

Balaraman B, Biesbroeck LK, Lickerman SH, et al (Washington Univ School of Medicine, St Louis, MO; Univ of Washington School of Medicine, Seattle; Saint Louis Univ School of Medicine, MO)
Pediatrics 131:415-422, 2013

Background.—The incidence of skin cancer has increased in the United States, concomitant with increased UV radiation (UVR) exposure among young adults. We examined whether tanning facilities in Missouri, a state without indoor-tanning regulations, acted in accordance with the Food and Drug Administration's recommendations and consistently imparted information to potential clients about the known risks of UVR.

Methods.—We conducted a statewide telephone survey of randomly selected tanning facilities in Missouri. Each tanning facility was surveyed twice, in the morning (7 AM–3 PM) and evening (3–10 PM), on different days, to determine intrasalon consistency of information provided to potential clients at different times.

Results.—On average, 65% of 243 tanning-facility operators would allow children as young as 10 or 12 years old to use indoortanning devices, 80% claimed that indoor tanning would prevent future sunburns, and 43% claimed that there were no risks associated with indoor tanning. Intrasalon inconsistencies involved allowable age of use, and UVR exposure type and duration. Morning tanning-facility employees were more likely to allow consumers to start with maximum exposure times and UV-A–emitting devices ($P < .001$), whereas evening employees were more likely to allow 10- or 12-year-old children to use indoor-tanning devices ($P = .008$).

Conclusions.—Despite increasing evidence that UVR exposure in indoor-tanning devices is associated with skin cancer, ocular damage, and premature photoaging, tanning facilities in Missouri often misinformed consumers regarding these risks and lack of health benefits and inconsistently provided information about the Food and Drug Administration's guidelines for tanning devices.

▶ Given that at least 1 in 5 Americans will have skin cancer some time in their lifetime, this report takes on added significance. It is clear that ultraviolet radiation is the single most common cause of nonmelanoma skin cancer (particularly basal cell and squamous cell carcinomas) in the United States. Some of this is caused by indoor tanning. Tanning bed use has been associated with a 1.5-fold increased risk of basal cell carcinoma and a 2.5-fold increased risk of squamous cell carcinoma and up to a 3-fold increased risk of melanoma, particularly in young people who are so exposed.

The report by Balaraman et al tells us about indoor tanning practices in the state of Missouri. This is a state in which there are no regulations regarding a minor's use of a tanning facility. There are 16 other states that also have no such regulations. As can be seen in this study, children as young as 10 to 12 years of age are permitted to tan in at least two-thirds of the tanning facilities surveyed. In many instances, this can be done without a parent's consent. Almost half of the tanning facilities told their clients that there were no health risks associated with the use of the tanning facility.

In a commentary that accompanied this report, we are reminded that indoor tanning remains a $5-billion-a-year industry and that there are at least 19 000 freestanding salons employing over 160 000 individuals here in the United States.[1] The use of such tanning facilities seems to be very popular with teenage girls and young women, and there is ready access to these given the fact that there are more tanning salons in an average city than there are Starbucks or McDonalds.

The International Agency for Research on Cancer has stated that ultraviolet radiating tanning devices are carcinogenic to humans.[2] Here in the United States, the US Food and Drug Administration does regulate tanning beds as a class I medical device, the same category as tongue depressors and elastic bandages. The agency itself places no age restrictions on the use of tanning beds, leaving it to state governments to regulate minors' use of these devices. As of November 2012, 33 states had some kind of restriction regarding salon use by teens. Some states placed bans at 14, 15, or 16 years of age. New York State passed an under-17 ban in July 2012. Some states require that a parent accompany his or her child younger than a certain age, and some require written consent of a parent or guardian or a physician's order or prescription.

Unfortunately, the regulation of tanning facilities has become a state's rights issue. It will take a long time before every one of our states and territories bellies up to the problem of indoor tanning salons. Entire nations have banned teen tanning. The United Kingdom, France, and Germany are among such countries. Some countries, such as Brazil, for example, have totally banned indoor tanning for everyone except for medical purposes. The role of pediatric care providers is clear. In our offices we can discuss indoor tanning with teens and families. At the advocacy level we can speak to the need for new and enforceable age bans and advocate for stronger laws in this regard.

J. A. Stockman III, MD

References

1. Balk SJ, Fisher DE, Geller AC. Stronger laws are needed to protect teens from indoor tanning. *Pediatr.* 2013;131:586-588.
2. The International Agency for Research on Cancer. Sun beds and UV radiation: www.iarc.fr/en/media-centre/iarcnews/2009/sunbeds_uvradiation.php. Accessed April 6, 2013.

12 Musculoskeletal

How Many Referrals to a Pediatric Orthopaedic Hospital Specialty Clinic Are Primary Care Problems?
Hsu EY, Schwend RM, Julia L (Univ of Missouri Kansas City School of Medicine; Univ of Missouri School of Medicine; Children's Mercy Hosp, Kansas City, MO)
J Pediatr Orthop 32:732-736 2012

Purpose.—Many primary care physicians believe that there are too few pediatric orthopaedic specialists available to meet their patients' needs. However, a recent survey by the Practice Management Committee of the Pediatric Orthopaedic Society of North America found that new referrals were often for cases that could have been managed by primary care practitioners. We wished to determine how many new referral cases seen by pediatric orthopaedic surgeons are in fact conditions that can be readily managed by a primary care physician should he/she chose to do so.

Methods.—We prospectively studied all new referrals to our hospital-based orthopaedic clinic during August 2010. Each new referral was evaluated for whether it met the American Board of Pediatrics criteria for being a condition that could be managed by a primary care pediatrician. Each referral was also evaluated for whether it met the American Academy of Pediatrics Surgery Advisory Panel guidelines recommending referral to an orthopaedic specialist, regardless of whether it is for general orthopaedics or pediatric orthopaedics. On the basis of these criteria, we classified conditions as either a condition manageable by primary care physicians or a condition that should be referred to an orthopaedic surgeon or a pediatric orthopaedic surgeon. We used these guidelines not to identify diagnosis that primary care physicians should treat but, rather, to compare the guideline-delineated referrals with the actual referrals our specialty pediatric orthopaedic clinic received over a period of 1 month.

Results.—A total of 529 new patient referrals were seen during August 2010. A total of 246 (47%) were considered primary care conditions and 283 (53%) orthopaedic specialty conditions. The most common primary care condition was a nondisplaced phalanx fracture (25/246, 10.1%) and the most common specialty condition was a displaced single-bone upper extremity fracture needing reduction (36/283, 13%). Only 77 (14.6%) of the total cases met the strict American Academy of Pediatrics Surgery Advisory Panel guidelines recommending referral to pediatric orthopaedics, with scoliosis being the most frequent condition. For 38 (7.2%) cases, surgical treatment was required or recommended. Patient age, referral source, or

TABLE 1.—Conditions That Should Be Referred to Pediatric Orthopaedics (AAP Surgery Advisory Panel Recommendations)

Specialty Problem	N	Percent of 77
Scoliosis	35	45.5
Bone lesion	11	14.3
Spine anomaly, spondylolysis	7	9.1
Developmental dysplasia of hip	7	9.1
Syndactyly	3	3.9
Other	14	18.1
Total	77	100.0

Other problems, 1 each (1.2%): achondroplasia, synostosis, lumbar gibbus, Kabuki syndrome, slipped capital femoral epiphysis, 1q36 deletion syndrome, Noonan syndrome, McCune-Albright syndrome, Splengel deformity, Scheuermann disease, Perthes disease, spondylocostal dysostosis, and Van Der Wonde, San Filippo, Hurler, Ehler Danlos syndromes.
AAP indicates American Academy of Pediatrics.

type of insurance did not influence whether the condition was a primary care or a specialty care case. A total of 134 (25%) cases were referred without having an initial diagnosis made by the referring clinician. These patients were more likely to have been referred from a primary care practitioner than from a tertiary care practitioner whether the diagnosis eventually made was considered to be a primary care condition ($P = 0.03$; relative risk, 1.9; 95% confidence interval, 96-3.86).

Conclusions.—Almost half of all new referrals to a tertiary pediatric orthopaedic clinic were for conditions considered to be manageable by primary care physicians should they chose to do so.

Significance.—This has implications for pediatric orthopaedic work-force availability, reimbursement under the Affordable Care Act, and pediatric musculoskeletal training needs for providers of primary care (Tables 1-3).

▶ This report emanating from Kansas reminds us of how we, at times, tend to overuse our subspecialty consultants for problems they think we should be able to manage as pediatricians. It is suggested in this report that common conditions or normal variants with very low requirement for surgical management should remain in the bailiwick of the generalist physician/pediatrician. The authors suggest that although pediatric orthopedic surgeons have traditionally been willing to see all comers, there is a severe shortage of pediatric orthopedic surgeons; as a result, having a large number of referrals for primary care types of problems can lead to longer wait times, making it difficult for children with urgent pediatric orthopedic specialty problems to be seen.

Hsu et al designed a study to determine how many cases referred patients to orthopedic surgeons would be considered manageable by primary care physicians. The authors of the report examined guidelines of major pediatric organizations that provide information on referral information to pediatric orthopedic surgeons. A review of 529 new patient referrals was undertaken at the Children's Mercy Hospital in Kansas City. It was determined that 47% of newly referred cases were thought to be a primary care condition not in need of referral to a pediatric orthopedic surgical clinic. Tables 1-3 illustrate the conditions that should be

TABLE 2.—Specialty Care Problems: Conditions That Should Be Referred to Orthopaedics (Either Pediatric Orthopaedics or General Orthopaedics)

Problem	N	Percent of 283
Displaced upper extremity single-bone fracture	36	13.0
Both-bone displaced fracture	31	11.0
Scoliosis	31	11.0
Lower extremity fracture requiring long-leg cast	24	8.5
Knee injury	20	7.1
Bone lesion requiring surgery	11	3.9
Spasticity of lower extremity	9	3.2
Deformity requiring surgery (upper and lower)	8	2.8
Cyst removal, surgical	7	2.5
Developmental dysplasia of hip	7	2.5
Phalanx fracture, displaced	7	2.5
Displaced metacarpal fracture	7	2.5
Spine anomaly/vertebral fracture/spondylosis/spondylolisthesis	7	2.5
Clubfoot	5	1.8
Trigger thumbs	6	2.1
Spondylolisthesis	1	1.4
Avulsion, displaced	4	1.4
Foreign body requiring surgical excision	3	1.1
Toddler fracture of tibia requiring long-leg cast	3	1.1
Tibial triplane injury	3	1.1
Syndactyly	3	1.1
Arthrogryposis	2	0.7
Metaphyseal fracture	2	0.7
Left wrist fracture	2	0.7
Cavovarus, severe	2	0.7
Leg length discrepancy	2	0.7
Tight heel cord	2	0.7
Scaphoid fracture	2	0.7
Other	33	11.0
Total	283	100.0

Other problem, 1 each (0.4%): metatarsal fracture, achondroplasia, avascular necrosis, hallux valgus requiring surgery, synostosis, pseudoarthrosis, equinous contracture, fibrous subtalar coalition, lumbar gibbus, Kabuki syndrome, slipped capital femoral epiphysis, severe metatarsal adductus requiring surgery, monteggia fracture, muscle contracture requiring surgery, 1q36 deletion syndrome, Noonan, cortical irregularity, osteopenia, mandible fracture, McCune-Albright syndrome, Splengel deformity, crush injury/displaced/angulated requiring surgery, Scheuermann disease, Perthes disease, spondylocostal dysostosis, shoulder dislocation, tillaux fracture, torticollis, degenerative joint disease/trochlear dysplasia/idiopathic erosion, right cervical rib, and Van Der Wonde, San Filippo, Hurler, Ehler Danlos syndromes.

referred to pediatric orthopedics and conditions that should be managed by primary care physicians.

The authors of this report remind us that a recent survey by the Practice Management Committee of the Pediatric Orthopedic Society of North America found that up to 95% of new referrals to an orthopedic surgeon were for common conditions or normal variants. Relatively few (3%) of such referrals resulted in a requirement for surgical management. The authors suggest that with a shortage of pediatric orthopedic specialists, primary care physicians should be careful about who they refer; otherwise, there will be longer waiting times for the most urgent of cases.[1,2]

The authors of this report comment that "the Affordable Health Care Act 2010 may have several effects on the practice of pediatric orthopedics. Because almost half of the conditions seen in our ambulatory specialty setting are considered

TABLE 3.—Conditions That Can Be Readily Managed by Primary Care Physicians

Problem	N	Percent of 246
Phalanx fracture	25	10.2
Femoral anteversion	24	9.8
Single-bone fracture upper extremity	22	8.9
Normal examination	17	6.9
Radius buckle fracture	13	5.3
Metatarsal fracture	12	4.9
Minor knee injury	11	4.5
Sprain	9	3.7
Tibia torsion	9	3.7
Planovalgus foot	9	3.7
Humerus fracture	8	3.3
Bow legs	7	2.9
Both-bone fracture forearm, nondisplaced	7	2.9
Tibia fracture	6	2.4
Simple laceration injury	5	2.0
Ankle fracture	5	2.0
Clavicle fracture	5	2.0
Deformity, minimal function inhibition	4	1.6
Hip flexor	4	1.6
Crush injury	4	1.6
Idiopathic pain	3	1.2
Chronic back pain	3	1.2
Contusion	3	1.2
Metacarpal fracture	3	1.2
Postural kyphosis	3	1.2
Avulsion fracture	2	0.8
Benign cyst	2	0.8
Metatarsus adductus	2	0.8
Cervical spine injury	2	0.8
Curly toe	2	0.8
Other	15	6.1
Total	246	100.0

Remaining problems, 1 each (0.4%): axial distance increase, mild bunion, capillary malformation, fascia hernia, fight bite, foreign body of foot, idiopathic lesion requiring no management, wound care, mild shoulder instability, corner fracture, rotator cuff strain, granuloma annulare, Osgood-Schlatter, Sinding-Larson-Johansson syndromes, enthesopathy.

primary care conditions, pediatric orthopedics may need consideration as a primary care specialty, as is the case for obstetrics and gynecology." Although that would be a stretch, the point is well taken.

J. A. Stockman III, MD

References

1. Schwend RM. The pediatric orthopaedics workforce demands, needs, and resources. *J Pediatr Orthop*. 2009;29:653-660.
2. Reeder BM, Lyne ED, Patel DR, Cucos DR. Referral patterns to a pediatric ortho- pedic clinic: implications for education and practice. *Pediatrics*. 2004;113: e163-e167.

Conditions Found Among Pediatric Survivors During the Early Response to Natural Disaster: A Prospective Case Study

Gamulin A, Armenter-Duran J, Assal M, et al (Univ Hosps of Geneva, Switzerland)

J Pediatr Orthop 32:327-333, 2012

Background.—Major natural disasters may provoke a mass casualty situation, and children tend to represent an important proportion of the victims. The purpose of this study was to prospectively record medical conditions presented by pediatric survivors of a major natural disaster to determine the type of medical specialists most needed during the acute phase of relief response.

Methods.—After the 2010 Haiti earthquake, age, sex, date of presentation, diagnosis, and treatment provided were prospectively recorded for all patients less than 18 years old treated by a medical relief team. Patients were then allocated to 1 of the 2 groups: surgical (traumatism or surgical disorder) and medical (medical disorder). Medical activity lasted for 43 days.

Results.—Four hundred seventy-one of the 796 treated patients were less than 18 years old. Two hundred forty-four (52%) were assigned to the surgical group and 227 (48%) to the medical group. As there was a substantial decrease in the number of new surgical patients registered on day 11 of activity, we arbitrarily defined an early period (until day 10 of activity) and a late period (beginning on day 11 of activity). Data obtained from the 147 new patients registered during the early period revealed 134 (91%) surgical patients and 13 (9%) medical patients. Eighty-eight percent of patients needed specialized care for traumatic orthopaedic lesions, and procedures under anesthesia or sedation were mainly (98%) performed for traumatic conditions. Data obtained for the 324 new patients registered during the late period revealed 110 (34%) surgical patients and 214 (66%) medical patients. There was a switch from high surgical needs to more routine medical and surgical care, with less procedures (88%) for the treatment of traumatic lesions.

Conclusions.—Pediatric orthopaedic surgeons have a major role to play in the acute phase of relief response to potentially minimize long-term physical and psychosocial disability associated with these complex injuries in growing patients.

Level of Evidence.—Economic or decision analyses, level II (Table 1).

▶ This report summarizes many of the medical consequences of the disaster reaped on Haiti in 2010. It is written from the viewpoint of orthopedic surgeons who bore much of the early brunt of the provision of care for injured patients. Recall that the Haiti earthquake, occurring on January 12, 2010, was graded a 7.0 on the Richter scale. The estimated death toll was 300 000, with more than 300 000 injured. Table 1 shows the demographic characteristics of the types of injuries that were sustained and that reached medical services in the first 10 days after the earthquake. The study was reported from a typical emergency unit that was set up by teams of individuals under the umbrella of the

TABLE 1.—Demographic Characteristics of Early Period Medical and Surgical Patients According to Type of Diagnosis

Diagnosis	Patients N (%)	F/M	Age (y)
Extremity crush injury	62 (42)	31/31	7.3 ± 4.2 (0-17)
Wound	47 (32)	28/19	6.8 ± 4.1 (0-15)
Open fracture	47 (32)	28/19	7.6 ± 4.4 (1-17)
Closed fracture	43 (29)	29/14	6.4 ± 3.9 (0-15)
Axial wound (head, neck, thorax, abdomen, pelvis)	33 (22)	15/18	7.7 ± 4.3 (1-15)
Soft-tissue infection	14 (9.5)	8/6	7.4 ± 3.7 (0-15)
Medical condition	13 (8.8)	4/9	2.5 ± 4.2 (0-14)
Other musculoskeletal condition	10 (6.8)	7/3	6 ± 2.7 (2-10)
Head open fracture	5 (3.4)	1/4	8 ± 4 (2-13)
Compartment syndrome	4 (2.7)	1/3	9 ± 3.9 (4-15)
Nonmusculoskeletal surgical condition	4 (2.7)	2/2	8 ± 5 (0-14)
Total	147 (100)	78/69	6.7 ± 4.4 (0-17)

Values are means ± SD (range) unless otherwise specified.

Some patients may have more than one diagnosis. Medical condition includes dehydration, undernutrition, diarrhea, infectious disease, and neonates needing monitoring. Other musculoskeletal condition includes contusion and sprain. Head open fracture includes skull, facial, and maxillary fracture. Nonmusculoskeletal surgical condition includes nontraumatic hollow viscus perforation and incarcerated hernia requiring surgery; there were no abdominal or thoracic traumatic lesion requiring laparotomy or thoracotomy.

Swiss Confederation. As one might suspect, 88% of the injuries were orthopedic in nature. That said, there were clearly 2 different periods of medical care provision. The early period—the first 2 weeks after the earthquake—consisted mostly of surgical patients (91%). After that, 66% of the care provided was medical and 34% surgical. This transition was consistent with data from the 1999 Marmara Region earthquake in Turkey.

Others have reported similar findings from the Haiti earthquake of 2010. Kreiss analyzed 1041 general population patients during the first 14 days after the earthquake and found that 25% of the patients had fractures, 18% open wounds, 12% superficial wounds, 10% crush injuries, and 9% contusions. In all reports from Haiti, orthopedists did what they had to deal with large volumes of patients. For example, during the first 10 days, most fractures seen were treated with casts because this was the only immobilization device available. Axial traction replaced casts for lower extremity long bone fractures partway through this period (about day 5) when things had settled down and shelters and beds had been installed to accommodate patients. Because of logistical issues, external fixators were available only beginning on day 9. X-rays became only available 5 days after the disaster; intraoperative fluoroscopy was not possible, thus making proper fracture alignment difficult. In any other circumstance, sterile external fixators and ideally fluoroscopy would have been available on the first day of surgical activity. Fasciotomy for compartment syndrome was rarely performed. Fasciotomy in an unfavorable environment is indicated only for early compartment syndrome in the first 6 to 8 hours when muscles are still viable and virtually all patients who would have benefitted from this approach frequently took days to be seen. Most patients with severe enough a crush injury to require fasciotomy died before arrival at the medical care facilities.

This study confirms that pediatric survivors of a major earthquake are predominantly affected by traumatic orthopedic lesions. Pediatric orthopedic surgeons are the most appropriately trained specialists to treat these injuries. The Haiti experience demonstrated a frustrating lack of basic medical supplies. Wise predisaster planning based on previous experience and smart onsite use of orthopedic treatments would have overcome this. Hindsight, though, has 20/20 vision.

J. A. Stockman III, MD

Racial Disparity in Fracture Risk between White and Nonwhite Children in the United States

Wren TAL, Shepherd JA, Kalkwarf HJ, et al (Children's Hosp Los Angeles, CA; Univ of California, San Francisco; Cincinnati Children's Hosp Med Ctr, OH; et al)
J Pediatr 161:1035-1040.e2, 2012

Objectives.—To examine risk factors for fracture in a racially diverse cohort of healthy children in the US.

Study Design.—A total of 1470 healthy children, aged 6-17 years, underwent yearly evaluations of height, weight, body mass index, skeletal age, sexual maturation, calcium intake, physical activity levels, and dual-energy x-ray absorptiometry (DXA) bone and fat measurements for up to 6 years. Fracture information was obtained at each annual visit, and risk factors for fracture were examined using the time-dependent Cox proportional hazards model.

Results.—The overall fracture incidence was 0.034 fracture per person-year with 212 children reporting a total of 257 fractures. Being white (hazard ratio [HR] = 2.1), being male (HR = 1.8), and having skeletal age of 10-14 years (HR = 2.2) were the strongest risk factors for fracture (all $P \leq .001$). Increased sports participation (HR = 1.4), lower body fat percentage (HR = 0.97), and previous fracture in white girls (HR = 2.1) were also significant risk factors (all $P \leq .04$). Overall, fracture risk decreased with higher DXA z scores, except in white boys, who had increased fracture risk with higher DXA z scores (HR = 1.7, $P < .001$).

Conclusions.—Boys and girls of European descent had double the fracture risk of children from other backgrounds, suggesting that the genetic predisposition to fractures seen in elderly adults also manifests in children.

▶ This report reminds us that the foundation for a strong adult skeleton begins in childhood. We also know that there is a difference in the likelihood of the development of fractures depending on one's racial background. Fractures, for example, in adults are much less likely among older black individuals than older white individuals. Little has been written, however, about the effects of race on the probability of developing a bone fracture during childhood. This topic was examined by the Bone Mineral Density in Childhood Study Group. The group undertook a multicenter longitudinal study examining bone accretion in a racially diverse group of more than 1500 healthy boys and girls, ages 6 to 17 years, recruited from several medical centers in the United States. Participants in this study were evaluated annually for a 6-year period. Documentation of height, weight, and body mass index scores were obtained. All subjects underwent a physical examination by a pediatrician or a pediatric endocrinologist to determine their stage of sexual development based on Tanner stages. Skeletal maturity was assessed by x-rays of the left hand and wrist. Dietary calcium intake was determined based on dietary history. Bone densitometry was periodically obtained. At each visit, participants also were asked whether they had any broken bones in the previous year.

In this study, the overall fracture rate incidence was 0.034 fractures per person-year (257 fractures over 7472 person-years of follow-up). Most fractures involved the upper extremities (64%) or lower extremities (28%). Most of the fractures occurred during medium-impact sporting activities (72%). The most common sports-related fractures involved basketball (19%), football (15%), soccer (11%), and skating (16%). Fracture rates were higher in boys than in girls and higher in white children than in other racial/ethnic groups. The greatest risk of fracture was observed in the 10- to 14-year age group. Fracture risk was higher during puberty Tanner stages 2 to 4 than in Tanner stage 1 or Tanner stage 5. There was also a greater risk of fracture for taller, thinner subjects. The risk of fractures decreased proportionately with higher bone densities.

This report underscores that healthy boys and girls of European descent have more than twice the risk of development of fractures in comparison with healthy children from other backgrounds. This study also documents that most pediatric factures occur predominantly during physical activities such as sports and are more common in boys and during adolescence. There is also a strong inverse relationship between bone density measurements and the risk of fracture. If one looks specifically at adolescent males, however, the opposite is true—that is, higher bone density values are associated with a higher fracture risk. There is no relationship in this study between fracture risk and calcium intake.

To learn more about osteoporosis and its origins in childhood, see the excellent medical progress article by Ma and Gordon.[1] Although primary causes of pediatric osteoporosis remain rare (such as osteogenesis imperfecta and idiopathic juvenile osteoporosis), the numerous forms of secondary osteoporosis seem to be on the increase. The latter include neuromuscular disease associated with osteopenia, chronic illnesses, malabsorption syndrome, anorexia nervosa, steroid-induced osteoporosis, etc. Front-line therapies to prevent osteoporosis include optimizing dietary calcium and vitamin D intake and implementing a regular routine of weight-bearing exercise. There are no specific guidelines for the use of bisphosphonates in children. Their use may be appropriate in specific situations, however.

J. A. Stockman III, MD

Reference

1. Ma NS, Gordon CM. Pediatric osteoporosis: where are we now? *J Pediatr.* 2012; 161:983-990.

Range of motion of the healthy pediatric elbow: cross-sectional study of a large population
Barad JH, Kim RS, Ebramzadeh E, et al (Univ of California, Los Angeles; Los Angeles Orthopaedic Hosp, CA)
J Pediatr Orthop B 22:117-122, 2013

To evaluate normative data on elbow range of motion (ROM) in the pediatric population. The passive ROM of 1361 healthy pediatric elbows was measured using a small goniometer calibrated in 1° increments, and recorded. The mean amount of flexion, extension, and arc of motion was 142°, −11°, and 153°, respectively. Our data indicated no meaningful correlation between patient sex, age, or weight and the amount of flexion, extension, or the total arc of motion. It appears that elbow ROM in this population is not affected by sex, age, or weight. Normative data are critical when setting the goals of a particular therapeutic approach.

▶ If you have ever wondered what the normal range of motion (ROM) should be for healthy kids, this report is for you. Before this report, there had been an extraordinary paucity of normative information on elbow ROM in the young population. The authors of this report analyzed the ROM in a large population of normal pediatric elbows to determine their normative values and how these values relate to patient characteristics. In this report, the arc of motion of the normal elbow was measured using a small goniometer calibrated in 1° increments.

This report turns out to be the largest study to date of normative values of elbow ROM in the pediatric population. Some 1361 healthy elbows were evaluated, which showed normal average range of pediatric elbow flexion, extension, and total arc of motion to be approximately 142°, −11°, and 153°, respectively. The study also showed small but statistically significant differences in ROM about the elbow on the basis of sex, with girls being slightly more flexible than boys. There was no correlation of pediatric elbow ROM with age. Other than the very modest difference seen between boys and girls, data from this report suggest that elbow motion is not affected by age or participant weight.

J. A. Stockman III, MD

Rotator cuff injuries in adolescent athletes
Weiss JM, Arkader A, Wells LM, et al (Univ of Southern California, Los Angeles, CA; Children's Hosp Philadelphia, PA)
J Pediatr Orthop B 22:133-137, 2013

The cause of rotator cuff injuries in the young athlete has been described as an overuse injury related to internal impingement. Abduction coupled with external rotation is believed to impinge on the rotator cuff, specifically the supraspinatus, and lead to undersurface tears that can progress to full-thickness tears. This impingement is believed to be worsened with increased range of motion and instability in overhead athletes. A retrospective review of seven patients diagnosed with rotator cuff injuries was performed to better understand this shoulder injury pattern. The type of sport played, a history of trauma, diagnosis, treatment method, and outcome were noted. Six patients were male and one was a female. Baseball was the primary sport for four patients, basketball for one, gymnastics for one, and wrestling for one. The following injury patterns were observed: two patients tore their subscapularis tendon, two sustained avulsion fractures of their lesser tuberosity, one tore his rotator interval, one tore his supraspinatus, and one avulsed his greater tuberosity. Only four patients recalled a specific traumatic event. Three patients were treated with arthroscopic rotator cuff repair, three with miniopen repair, and one was treated with rehabilitation. Six of the seven patients returned to their preinjury level of sport after treatment. Rotator cuff tears are rare in the adolescent age group. The injury patterns suggest that acute trauma likely accounts for many rotator cuff tears and their equivalents in the young patient. Adolescents with rotator cuff tears reliably return to sports after treatment. The possibility of rotator cuff tears in skeletally immature athletes should be considered. The prognosis is very good once this injury is identified and treated.

▶ This article tells us a lot about rotator cuff injuries in adolescent athletes. The investigators undertook a retrospective review of patients diagnosed with rotator cuff injuries in order to better understand the type of injuries athletes sustain. They reviewed in detail 7 athletes who had rotator cuff injuries. Six of the 7 were boys. The female athlete was a gymnast. Of the 6 male patients, 4 played baseball as their primary sport, 1 played basketball, and 1 was a wrestler. All but 1 injured their dominant arm.

Examination of the injury pattern of the athletes that were included in this article confirms that impingement of the supraspinatus in abduction coupled with external rotation does not account for the majority of these rotator cuff injuries and avulsion fractures. The authors did decide to include avulsion fractures of the greater and lesser tuberosities of the humerus in this study as "rotator cuff tear equivalents." Overuse in these young athletes most likely placed these patients at risk for their injuries. Such overuse tends to cause decreased stability and lesser strength in and about the shoulder.

These authors note that overuse injuries are increasing in the pediatric population and are responsible for up to about 70% of visits to pediatric sports medicine clinics. This most likely results from pressure to enhance performance at a young age, particularly in baseball. Whereas professional managers have the luxury of having 10 or 11 man pitching staffs, most coaches at the high school level rely on just 3 or 4 of their top arms to carry them through a 20-plus game season. Also, many, if not all, of today's youth pitchers are using their arms at other positions on the field when they are not on the mound.

The cases in this article help to provide an awareness of the growing trend of overuse injuries in the pediatric and adolescent population. The possibility of rotator cuff tears in skeletally immature athletes should be considered during physical examination and prevention programs should be emphasized to at-risk patients to help reverse the current trend in overuse injuries in this young age population. Treatment of these types of injuries requires a prospective study on operative versus nonoperative care in order to determine for whom surgical intervention is most appropriate. Conservative rehabilitation and activity modification may continue to be appropriate for the majority of these patients.

While on the topic of things athletic, are you aware of one activity that the British Olympic Association has warned athletes against during the 2012 Olympics? It's handshaking. The organization has emphasized that hand hygiene was paramount during the games to minimize the risk of contagion from a performance robbing viral illness in the intensely competitive environment of the Olympic Village.[1] No "high fives," either, but friendly hellos and verbal thank yous were considered to be OK.

J. A. Stockman III, MD

Reference

1. Editorial comment. Non-contact sports. *Lancet.* 2012;379.

School children's backpacks, back pain and back pathologies
Rodríguez-Oviedo P, Ruano-Ravina A, Pérez-Ríos M, et al (Hospital da Costa, Burela, Spain; University of Santiago de Compostela, Spain; et al)
Arch Dis Child 97:730-732, 2012

Objective.—To investigate whether backpack weight is associated with back pain and back pathology in school children.

Design.—Cross-sectional study.

Setting.—Schools in Northern Galicia, Spain.

Patients.—All children aged 12–17.

Interventions.—Backpack weight along with body mass index, age and gender.

Main Outcome Measures.—Back pain and back pathology.

Results.—1403 school children were analysed. Of these, 61.4% had backpacks exceeding 10% of their body weight. Those carrying the heaviest backpacks had a 50% higher risk of back pain (OR 1.50 CI 95% 1.06 to 2.12) and a 42% higher risk of back pathology, although this last result was not statistically significant (OR 1.42 CI 95% 0.86 to 2.32). Girls presented a higher risk of back pain compared with boys.

Conclusions.—Carrying backpacks increases the risk of back pain and possibly the risk of back pathology. The prevalence of school children carrying heavy backpacks is extremely high. Preventive and educational activities should be implemented in this age group.

▶ Here is another article describing how problematic children's backpacks can be, particularly when overloaded. This article emanates from Spain, a country that seems to have the same problems we have with children and their backpacks. These authors undertook a study to analyze the influence of backpack weight on back pain and various back pathologies by undertaking a cross-sectional analytic study among school-age children (aged 12 to 17 years) during the academic years of 2005 to 2006 in northern Spain. The sample included 1403 children; 92.2% of the youngsters used a backpack with 2 shoulder straps. The mean school bag weight was nearly 7 kg. Approximately two-thirds of participants carried school bags exceeding 10% of their body weight and 18% exceeded 15% of their body weight, with 26% reporting back pain for more than 15 days in the previous year.

Without question, children carrying the heaviest backpacks were at the greatest risk of suffering from back pain and showing a higher risk of back pathology including the presence of some degree of scoliosis, low back pain, and contractures. It appeared that backpacks did alter posture and gait and also head-neck angles. Some children suffered with shoulder asymmetry and lumbar lordosis. Such biomechanical alterations could readily induce chronic back pain. In this article, girls appeared to be more prone to experience back pain and back pathology than boys, although there was no difference in backpack weight by sex.

J. A. Stockman III, MD

Magnetically controlled growing rods for severe spinal curvature in young children: a prospective case series

Cheung KM-C, Cheung JP-Y, Samartzis D, et al (The Univ of Hong Kong, China; et al)
Lancet 379:1967-1974, 2012

Background.—Scoliosis in skeletally immature children is often treated by implantation of a rod to straighten the spine. Rods can be distracted (lengthened) as the spine grows, but patients need many invasive operations under general anaesthesia. Such operations are costly and associated with negative psychosocial outcomes. We assessed the effectiveness and safety of a new magnetically controlled growing rod (MCGR) for non-invasive outpatient distractions.

Methods.—We implanted the MCGR in five patients, two of whom have now reached 24 months' follow-up. Each patient underwent monthly outpatient distractions. We used radiography to measure the magnitude of the spinal curvature, rod distraction length, and spinal length. We assessed clinical outcome by measuring the degree of pain, function, mental health, satisfaction with treatment, and procedure-related complications.

Findings.—In the two patients with 24 months' follow-up, the mean degree of scoliosis, measured by Cobb angle, was 67° (SD 10°) before implantation and 29° (4°) at 24 months. Length of the instrumented segment of the spine increased by a mean of 1·9 mm (0·4 mm) with each distraction. Mean predicted versus actual rod distraction lengths were 2·3 mm (1·2 mm) versus 1·4 mm (0·7 mm) for patient 1, and 2·0 mm (0·2 mm) and 2·1 mm (0·7 mm) versus 1·9 mm (0·6 mm) and 1·7 mm (0·8 mm) for patient 2's right and left rods, respectively. Throughout follow-up, both patients had no pain, had good functional outcome, and were satisfied with the procedure. No MCGR-related complications were noted.

Interpretation.—The MCGR procedure can be safely and effectively used in outpatient settings, and minimises surgical scarring and psychological distress, improves quality of life, and is more cost-effective than is the traditional growing rod procedure. The technique could be used for non-invasive correction of abnormalities in other disorders (Fig 1).

▶ Most will agree that the best possible treatment for early-onset scoliosis remains elusive. Nonetheless, the past decade or 2 has seen quite a bit of

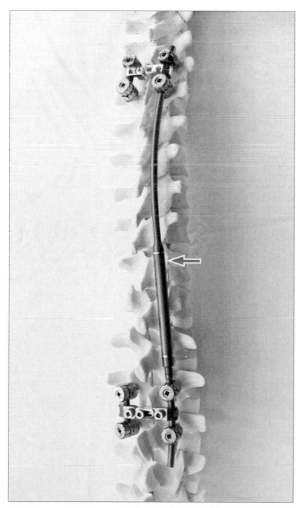

FIGURE 1.—A single magnetically controlled growing rod fixed to a spine model. Cervical vertebrae at top, sacrum at bottom. Arrow shows enlarged portion containing the distraction mechanism. (Reprinted from The Lancet, Cheung KM-C, Cheung JP-Y, Samartzis D, et al. Magnetically controlled growing rods for severe spinal curvature in young children: a prospective case series. *Lancet*. 2012;379:1967-1974. © 2012, with permission from Elsevier.)

movement forward in growth-sparing spine therapy in children with severe spinal deformities. Using techniques such as casting, bracing, growing rods, vertical expandible prosthetic titanium ribs, vertebral stapling and tethers has substantially increased. In addition, the negative outcomes of early fusion on pulmonary function and quality of life are now much better understood, so alternative approaches to fusion have become more commonplace. The latter techniques aim to preserve growth, but tend to have high complication rates and might necessitate repetitive surgical procedures throughout childhood. In many parts of the world, these treatment options are restricted by poor access to medical care and cost and the availability of the newer technologies. Repetitive surgeries in developing countries are often not practical or safe, resulting in the need for better forms of noninvasive approaches.

The report of Cheung et al tells us about one of these newer approaches. They report for the first time the use of noninvasive magnetically controlled growing rods to manage early-onset scoliosis. The technique described obviates one of the major drawbacks to growing-rod treatment: the need for several operations to lengthen the implant. Under anesthesia, the traditional growing rod is inserted across the segment of spine curvature, without the need for spinal fusion. Distraction of the growing rods is done approximately every 6 months, during which the surgeon reopens the surgical incision site to distract the rod to mimic and maintain normal spine growth. This approach historically has been effective in controlling the progression of spinal curvature and gradually straightens the spine. However, limitations of this method include the need for general anesthesia, the invasiveness of repeated distractions during surgery, and the associated anesthetic and wound complications. The traditional growing-rod surgery also has socioeconomic drawbacks, including missing school and the need for parents to take time off from work to support their child during and after each of the surgical procedures. The cost associated with repeated operations obviously also creates a substantial burden on health care systems.

What Cheung et al have done is to devise a more advanced and less invasive method that facilitates distraction of rods and overcomes many of the drawbacks described previously. They have developed a remotely distractible magnetically controlled growing rod system that allows frequent noninvasive distractions of the rod. The technology was validated in animals before first being used in humans in Hong Kong, China, where the report emanates from. The instrument itself is a single-use sterile titanium spinal distraction rod within a large midportion containing a magnetically drivable lengthening mechanism. One end of the rod is inserted and tethered above the curvature and the other end below the curvature of the spine. This is similar to the insertion of a traditional growing rod. Patients must wear a brace for approximately 3 months postoperatively to promote fusion of the upper end and lower end of the rods to the spine. In approximately monthly intervals, the patients are seen again and a hand-held magnetic external remote controller is placed over the internal magnet of the rod. A rotating mechanism within the rod causes the rod to lengthen and thus to distract or expand the spine. The predicted lengthening is displayed on the external distraction device. The device can also be used to retract the rod if the patient experiences unusual degrees of discomfort.

Although only 2 patients were reported from this study, the results were quite remarkable. In a 24-month follow-up, the mean degree of scoliosis, measured by Cobb angle, was 67° before implantation and 29° at 24 months. The length of the instrumented segment of the spine increased by a mean of 1.9 mm at each distraction; thus, spinal length approximated what might be seen in an otherwise normal child. Throughout the 2-year period, the patients experienced little or no pain, had good functional outcomes, and appeared to be satisfied with the procedure. There were no reported complications.

The procedure described was entirely developed outside the United States, where such a new pathway to implement such technology would face extensive barriers because growing rods remain unapproved by the US Food and Drug Administration. When and if this technology becomes available in the United States, it is suggested that it would rapidly be applied by orthopedic surgeons to avoid repetitive surgeries and improve the quality of life for children with spinal deformity.[1] We should be grateful to our colleagues in China for the development of a technology that may very well spread worldwide in the near future.

J. A. Stockman III, MD

Reference

1. Smith JT, Campbell RM Jr. Magnetically controlled growing rods for spinal deformity. *Lancet.* 2012;379:1930-1931.

Hip pathology in Hutchinson–Gilford progeria syndrome: a report of two children

Akhbari P, Jha S, James KD, et al (Conquest Hosp, East Sussex, UK)
J Pediatr Orthop B 21:563-566, 2012

Hutchinson—Gilford progeria syndrome (HGPS) is a rare genetic disorder. The estimated incidence is one in 4 million births. Orthopaedic manifestations include abnormality of the hips occurring early in the disease process. Severe coxa valga can be apparent by the age of 2 years. We report two cases of HGPS, one in a 7-year-old girl with avascular necrosis of the left hip and the second in a 13-year-old girl with recurrent traumatic hip dislocations. We demonstrate the pathoanatomical changes in the hip with HGPS using a combination of imaging modalities including radiographic, computed tomographic and MRI scans. These include coxa magna, coxa valga and acetabular dysplasia. We also comment on how these would affect the surgical management of this high-risk group of patients.

▶ We have known about the Hutchinson-Gilford progeria syndrome since it was first described by Hutchinson back in 1886 the growth pathologic characteristics of which were further elucidated by Gilford in 1904. It is a rare disorder affecting 1 in 4 million births. Most know about its clinical features that include premature aging, often occurring after the first year of life, growth retardation, loss of dermal appendages and subcutaneous fat, alopecia, restricted joint mobility, and osteopenia and osteolysis of the distal phalanges. Death usually occurs as a result of various factors related to advanced aging, including myocardial infarction, stroke, and other aspects of generalized atherosclerosis.

The report by Akhbari et al reminds us of the extensive orthopedic manifestations of progeria. Degenerative changes in hips can be a major problem in these kids. Severe coxa valga can be apparent by as early as 2 years, manifesting as a wide-based shuffling gait. As the authors of this report show, youngsters with progeria can experience avascular necrosis of the hips at a young age. Few generalist pediatricians will be involved with the care of children with progeria, but if you are, remember that orthopedic problems are one of the major concerns that affect quality of life.

Progeria is caused by a mutation in the gene called *LMNA*, when it encodes a protein called prelamin A. In healthy people, prelamin A is altered by an enzyme, farnesyltransferase, that begins its conversion into lamin A, which ultimately helps provide support to the cell nucleus. In progeria, however, a mutation truncates prelamin A, the critical conversion to lamin A fails, and patients experience buildup of abnormal protein in their cells. Among other things, the affected prelamin A distorts the nucleus and alters gene expression. Youngsters with progeria look normal at birth but as toddlers do not grow properly and, just like elderly people, they begin to lose hair and body fat and suffer joint stiffness and atherosclerosis. The average age at time of death is 13 years. Recently, a novel approach is being studied to see if the onset of the aging process in patients with progeria might be successfully slowed. In 2005, a group led by Steven Young, a cardiologist at the University of California, Los Angeles, showed that a class of drugs called *farnesyltransferase inhibitors* (FTIs) seemed to normalize cells from progeria patients. Interestingly, FTIs had recently been through cancer treatment trials without success, but the maker of the FTI product, lonafarnib, was willing to support production of the drug for compassionate use purposes as part of research in the treatment of patients with progeria. One of the key findings in the clinical trial of this agent was that patients with progeria started on this drug early in life seemed to gain weight. A total of 25 children on lonafarnib were closely tracked for more than 2 years. In the end, 9 had a median weight gain of 0.52 kg per year or just more than a pound, an improvement over essentially no weight gain the year before. Another 16 had no significant change in their rate of weight gain or lost weight during the study. Also, 17 of 18 children had a decrease in their carotid-femoral pulse wave velocity of between 26% and 48%, indicating these blood vessels grew more flexible over time on the experimental drug.

To learn more about what is going on, researchwise, in the field of aging with specific reference to the Hutchison-Gilford progeria syndrome, see the excellent editorial by Kouzin-Frankel.[1]

J. A. Stockman III, MD

Reference

1. Couzin-Frankel J. Drug trial offers uncertain start in race to save children with progeria. *Science*. 2012;337:1594-1595.

The Prevalence and Course of Idiopathic Toe-Walking in 5-Year-Old Children

Engström P, Tedroff K (Karolinska Institutet, Stockholm, Sweden)
Pediatrics 130:279-284, 2012

Background.—Children walking on their toes instead of with a typical gait, without evidence of an underlying medical condition, are defined as idiopathic toe-walkers. The prevalence of idiopathic toe-walking is unknown.

Methods.—A cross-sectional prevalence study of 5.5-year-old children (n = 1436) living in Blekinge County, Sweden, was performed at the regular 5.5-year visit to the local child welfare center. Children were assessed for a history of toe-walking or whether they still walked on their toes. Additionally, all 5.5-year-old children (n − 35) admitted to the clinic for children with special needs in the county were assessed.

Results.—Of the 1436 children in the cohort (750 boys, 686 girls), 30 children (2.1%, 20 boys and 10 girls) still walked on their toes at age 5.5 years and were considered as active toe-walkers. Forty children (2.8%, 22 boys and 18 girls) had previously walked on their toes but had stopped before the 5.5-year visit and were considered as inactive toe-walkers. At age 5.5 years, the total prevalence of toe-walking was 70 (4.9%) of 1436. For children with a neuropsychiatric diagnosis or developmental delay, the total prevalence for active or inactive toe-walking was 7 (41.2%) of 17.

Conclusions.—This study establishes the prevalence and- early spontaneous course of idiopathic toe-walking in 5.5-year-old children. At this age, more than half of the children have spontaneously ceased to walk on their toes. The study confirms earlier findings that toe-walking has a high prevalence among children with a cognitive disorder.

▶ Toe-walking is a common diagnosis, but must be made by exclusion of other conditions such as cerebral palsy. Unfortunately, there is no clear-cut definition of idiopathic toe-walking. Contractures of the Achilles tendon may or may not be present. Most parents do not seem to be very concerned about it, at least when the child is of preschool age, but in a school setting these youngsters can experience bullying and inability to join in a range of sporting activities. When the diagnosis is made, the patient is frequently referred to pediatric orthopedist or child neurologist. Most pediatricians do not get serious about idiopathic toe-walking until the child is about 5 or 6 years of age.

This report is from Sweden and was designed to elucidate the prevalence of idiopathic toe-walking in 5- to 6-year-old children. The study looked at both ongoing toe-walking and toe-walking that had ceased before the age of 5.5 years. The study showed that at 5.5 years of age, just over 2% of youngsters in Sweden were toe-walkers and an additional almost 3% of children had previously been toe-walkers. These numbers are somewhat lower than others that have appeared in the literature, but many of these studies were not of the rigor of this report from Sweden. The Swedish report also showed that 40% of children with active toe-walking had a first- or second-degree relative who had also been a toe-walker. Children with autism spectrum disorder or a communication/language disorder had a much higher prevalence of idiopathic toe-walking. The typical toe-walker began to toe-walk at the start of walking, although there was a small subset of children who did not start to toe walk until later. The typical toe-walker spent 25% of time on his or her toes while walking barefoot at 5.5 years.

Thus it appears that about half of toe-walkers will cease doing so between 5 and 6 years of age. As for the remainder, some will continue to toe-walk and experience a range of complaints including ankle and heel pain, particularly after activity, reduced ankle dorsiflexion precluding the use of skates or downhill skiing boots as well as difficulties walking uphill and an odd-walking pattern that attracts unfavorable comments from peers.

This is the first study that has looked at large numbers of children reported to have idiopathic toe-walking. There is a great deal to learn from this report, so it is well worth reading in detail. Perhaps the most important message is that when seeing a toddler with toe-walking, assuming underlying neurologic disorders have been ruled out, one can tell parents that about half the time this problem will go away prior to the start of school.

J. A. Stockman III, MD

Nail-Fold Excision for the Treatment of Ingrown Toenail in Children
Haricharan RN, Masquijo J, Bettolli M (Univ of Ottawa, Ontario, Canada; Dept of Infant Orthopedics and Trauma, Cöordoba, Argentina)
J Pediatr 162:398-402, 2013

Objective.—To evaluate the effectiveness of the nail-fold excision procedure in children.

Study Design.—Prospectively collected data on patients less than 18 years of age who underwent a nail-fold excision for symptomatic ingrown toenail were analyzed. Patients were seen in 2 centers and data collected included demographics, site of ingrown toenail, complications (including recurrence), patient satisfaction, and duration of follow-up.

Results.—Overall, 67 procedures were performed on 50 patients between June 2009 and July 2011 at the 2 institutions. The mean age was 14 years (range, 9-18 years) and 30 were male patients. No recurrences were seen after a follow-up for a median of 14 months (range 6-28 months). Patients were very satisfied with the cosmetic outcomes. Six minor complications occurred, including 3 patients with bleeding requiring dressing change, 2 with excessive granulation tissue, and 1 with nail growth abnormality.

Conclusions.—The nail-fold excision technique is highly effective in the pediatric population, with no recurrence, excellent cosmesis, and very high patient satisfaction (Fig 1).

▶ Before this report appeared, I had not run across the medical term for an ingrown toenail. The term is "onychocryptosis." Aficionados of onychocryptosis will tell you that the disorder is classified into whether the etiologic factor is

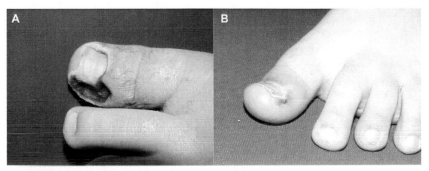

FIGURE 1.—A, Surgical site following nail-fold excision. The incision must include all the nail-fold skin to prevent recurrence, with preservation of the nail and nail matrix to prevent nail growth abnormality. B, Complete epithelialization after 8 weeks following nail-fold excision procedure. (Reprinted from Journal Pediatrics. Haricharan RN, Masquijo J, Bettolli M. Nail-fold excision for the treatment of ingrown toenail in children. *J Pediatr.* 2013;162:398-402, Copyright 2013, with permission from Elsevier.)

considered to be the nail itself or the soft tissues at the side of the nail. When the problem occurs and is sufficiently symptomatic, surgical techniques are generally used that target the nail, the nail fold, or both. Although ingrown toenails are largely a problem of adults, they do occur in children, and thus the value of the report of Haricharan et al.

This report reminds us that the most widely used surgical treatment for ingrown toenails in both adults and children is wedged excision of the nail with matricectomy (surgical or chemical) focusing on the nail. Recurrence rates in excess of 10% with poor cosmetic results caused by nail deformities are common with this procedure. Nail fold excision as a procedure was first described by Vandenbos and Bowers in 1959 and was published in the *US Armed Services Medical Journal.*[1] The procedure itself consists of an excision of the lateral or medial nail fold leaving a soft tissue defect to close by secondary intention. Unlike other techniques, the Vandenbos procedure does not excise any part of the nail or its matrix. Although the outcomes of this procedure have been studied in adults, it was not until the report abstracted appeared that there has been an evaluation of the effectiveness of this nail fold excision procedure in the pediatric age group.

This report tells us about the outcomes of nail fold excision in 2 medical centers, one in Canada and one in Argentina. Sixty-seven procedures were performed on 50 patients ranging in age from 9 to 18 years (median age, 14 years). The great toe was the toe most commonly involved. Usually the problem was unilateral. The procedure itself consisted of cleansing the toe with an antiseptic and instilling a 2% Xylocaine ring/digital block. An elastic Penrose drain tourniquet was applied around the base of the toe for a hemostasis. The incision started at the nail base cutting out toward the side and then up to the tip of the toe (Fig 1). The incision, the authors note, must be generous and adequate including all of the nail fold skin. Special care must be taken not to damage the nail matrix at the proximal area of the incision. After removal of the nail fold, the open skin edge and the subcutaneous tissue along the wound are cauterized to minimize bleeding. The nail bed matrix is not cauterized. An antibiotic ointment is applied followed by a nonadhesive gauze bandage. Normal ambulation tends to occur within a week and normal activities some 3 to 4 weeks later. Complete epithelialization occurs in about 2 months. The healing process generally results in no scar and a good cosmetic outcome. Recurrence rates were very low.

If you have any interest in caring for children with ingrown toenails in your practice, this report is well worth reading. The procedure described looks like a relatively straightforward one, one that could be performed in office setting, although it might be wiser to suggest to a referring surgeon given the fact that some technical equipment is needed to accomplish the cautery. Tell the surgeon to read this article before operating, however.

J. A. Stockman III, MD

Reference

1. Vandenbos KQ, Bowers WF. Ingrown toenail: a result of weight bearing on soft tissue. *US Armed Services Med J.* 1959;10:1168-1173.

A New Era in the Treatment of Systemic Juvenile Idiopathic Arthritis
Sandborg C, Mellins ED (Stanford Univ School of Medicine, CA)
N Engl J Med 367:2439-2440, 2012

Background.—Two new biologic agents have been evaluated for the treatment of systemic juvenile idiopathic arthritis (JIA). The interleukin-1 inhibitor canakinumab and the interleukin-6 inhibitor tocilizumab were tested in pediatric patients with severe systemic JIA. The results and implications of these studies were discussed.

Methods.—Both studies involved an initial randomized, placebo-controlled phase with the primary end point of absence of fever and a JIA American College of Rheumatology (ACR) 30 response, indicating improvement of 30% or more in at least three of the six core criteria for JIA and worsening of more than 30% in no more than one criterion. Both studies also had open-label phases, then the canakinumab study had a third phase with a patient-friendly randomized withdrawal designed to test efficacy.

Results.—More than 80% of the study participants reached the primary end point for the placebo-controlled phase within the first 2 to 6 weeks. The number of participants who had even greater improvement was notable. After 12 weeks, 71% of those who received tocilizumab had no fever and a JIA ACR 70 response compared to 8% of those in the placebo group. Of those treated with canakinumab, 67% had a JIA ACR 70 response and no fever after 4 weeks compared to 2% of the placebo group. In the open-label phases, sustained JIA ACR 30 responses were achieved in over 70% of patients, as was the ability to undergo glucocorticoid tapering. The magnitude and timing of responses to the two agents were similar, suggesting that interleukin-1 and interleukin-6 may be in the same pathway in systemic JIA. Partial or no responses in a significant minority of patients suggest that genetic or environmental factors may alter systemic JIA.

The severe underlying disease of participants, the high percentage of patients exposed to biologic agents previously, and the relatively short placebo exposure times made it difficult to assess safety profiles for the two agents. Both had apparently increased risks of infection, neutropenia, and liver dysfunction, and a small number of patients in both the placebo and treatment groups developed the macrophage activation syndrome. One canakinumab patient and two tocilizumab patients developed pulmonary hypertension.

Conclusions.—These two agents signal a new era in treating systemic JIA. The results of these studies suggest mechanisms that may be driving this infrequent and confusing disorder. Current findings suggest that systemic JIA should be considered an autoinflammatory disease, since it lacks the classic features of autoimmune disease and cells of the innate immune system are strongly implicated in the disorder. Further study should improve the understanding of other multigenic autoinflammatory diseases and the regulation of inflammation.

► Systemic juvenile idiopathic arthritis (JIA) is characterized by chronic arthritis; intermittently high, spiking temperatures; maculopapular rash; hepatosplenomegaly; lymphadenopathy; serositis; and a marked increase in the level of acute-phase reactants. The disease is also associated with a number of complications, including growth impairment, osteoporosis, and the potentially lethal disorder known as *macrophage activation syndrome.*

Unfortunately, systemic JIA has been considered a therapeutic orphan in the sense that the only effective treatment has seemed to be glucocorticoids, the latter associated with many side effects and toxicities. Over the years, several other therapeutic agents have been introduced in an attempt to modulate disease severity. These have included nonsteroidal antiinflammatory agents, methotrexate, and biological agents. Two studies appeared in the same issue of the *New England Journal of Medicine*, addressing agents that might be capable of modifying the natural course of systemic JIA.[1,2] These studies examined the biologic effects of the interleukin-1 inhibitor, canakinumab, and the interleukin-6 inhibitor, tocilizumab. These studies represent the culmination of work begun in a small but encouraging set of studies involving patients with systemic JIA who received treatment with interleukin-1 or interleukin-6 inhibitors some time ago. Before these agents were studied, it was fair to say that there was no effective therapy for children and young adults with systemic JIA, particularly those with severe forms of the disease despite the successful management of other types of JIA with methotrexate and tumor necrosis factor alpha inhibitors.

The studies that appeared in the *New England Journal of Medicine* had an initial, randomized, placebo-controlled phase with the same primary endpoint (absence of fever) and a JIA American College of Rheumatology 30 response, indicating improvement in 30% or more in at least 3 of the 6 core criteria for JIA and worsening of more than 30% in no more than one of the criterion. With both interleukin inhibitors, the primary endpoint for the placebo-controlled phase was reached in more than 80% of study participants within the first 4 to 6 weeks, and the number of participants who had even greater improvement was quite remarkable. At 12 weeks, 71% of patients who had received tocilizumab had absence of fever and a JIA score of 70 response (defined as improvement of

70% or more in at least 3 of the 6 core criteria for JIA and worsening of more than 30% in no more than one of the criterion) vs 8% of those in the placebo group. In the randomized, placebo-controlled phase of the canakinumab study, 67% of patients treated for this agent had a JIA score of 70 and an absence of fever at 4 weeks compared with 2% of those in the placebo group.

Safety profiles were difficult to assess in this report given the severe underlying disease of the study participants and the high percentage of patients with previous exposure to other biological agents. Also, there was a relatively short exposure to placebo in the control group. The authors of these reports indicate that the therapeutic benefits of these biologic agents will need to be weighed against the apparent risks of infection, neutropenia, and liver dysfunction. The macrophage activation syndrome developed in a small number of patients in both the placebo and active-treatment groups in these trials. An understanding of the overall effect of these agents on the macrophage activation syndrome will require additional studies over a longer period.

Curiously, the patients in these trials had marked similarities in the magnitude and timing of their responses, suggesting that interleukin-1 and interleukin-6 may be in the same pathway in systemic JIA. Despite a number of outstanding questions about how regulation of inflammation relates to the pathogenesis of JIA, it is obvious that the agents tested in these trials herald a new era in the treatment of systemic JIA. Interleukin-1 and interleukin-6 are being studied in other multigenetic auto inflammatory diseases, such as type 2 diabetes and inflammatory bowel disease. The more these agents are used, the more we will learn about their benefits and risks.

J. A. Stockman III, MD

References

1. De Benedetti F, Brunner HI, Ruperto N, et al. Randomized trial of tocilizumab in systemic juvenile idiopathic arthritis. *N Engl J Med.* 2012;367:2385-2395.
2. Ruperto N, Brunner HI, Quartier P, et al. Two randomized trials of canakinumab in systemic juvenile idiopathic arthritis. *N Engl J Med.* 2012;367:2396-2406.

The Value of Hip Aspiration in Pediatric Transient Synovitis
Liberman B, Herman A, Schindler A, et al (Edmond and Lilly Safra Hosp for Children, Tel-Hashomer, Israel; Tel Aviv Univ, Israel)
J Pediatr Orthop 33:124-127, 2013

Introduction.—Hip transient synovitis (TS) is a common pediatric orthopaedic problem. Although a self-limiting illness, it often makes the patient temporarily disabled and poses a diagnostic difficulty because of its similarity to septic arthritis in clinical manifestations. The aim of this study was to evaluate the use of a single ultrasound-guided hip aspiration as a treatment modality for TS.

Methods.—Between the years 1984 and 1989, 112 children with TS were treated through bed rest and using nonsteroidal anti-inflammatory drugs (group 1). Between the years 1990 and 1999, 119 children diagnosed with

TS were treated using hip aspiration, bed rest, and nonsteroidal anti-inflammatory drugs (group 2). Recovery parameters were compared between these patient groups.

Results.—Twenty-four hours after admission, limping was noted in 92% and 10% of the patients in groups 1 and 2, respectively, ($P < 0.001$). Refusal to bear weight was observed in 14% and 1% in groups 1 and 2, respectively, ($P < 0.001$), and hip joint pain was reported in 81% and 6% in groups 1 and 2, respectively, ($P < 0.001$). Larger joint effusions were found to be the reason behind the inability to bear weight.

Conclusions.—Pain due to TS may be because of capsule stretching owing to the accumulation of joint effusion. Ultrasound-guided hip aspiration relieves pain and limitation in movement and provides rapid differential diagnosis from septic arthritis of the hip joint.

▶ Children with hip pain not caused by trauma present with a typical differential diagnosis that includes transient synovitis, infection (such as osteomyelitis), septic arthritis, discitis, sacroiliitis (Legg-Calvé-Perthes disease), slipped capital femoral epiphysis, juvenile idiopathic arthritis, or tumor. Fortunately, most youngsters presenting with nontraumatic hip pain will ultimately receive a diagnosis of transient synovitis of the hip. The ratio of transient synovitis to septic arthritis runs roughly 8 to 1. A combination of hip pain, fever, high white blood cell count, elevated C-reactive protein level, and an increased erythrocyte sedimentation rate are reasonably good predictors for diagnosing septic arthritis as opposed to transient synovitis. The rub comes with youngsters who have overlapping signs and symptoms, and that is where hip aspiration under ultrasound guidance assists the clinician in making a correct diagnosis.

Liberman et al undertook a retrospective study comparing the clinical outcome in children with transient synovitis who underwent a single ultrasound-guided hip aspiration with that of historical controls with transient synovitis who were treated using only oral nonsteroidal anti-inflammatory drugs. The question addressed is whether ultrasound guidance adds anything to the currently accepted treatment for transient synovitis that includes bed rest along with the administration of anti-inflammatory medications.

Newly diagnosed patients with transient synovitis underwent aspiration using ultrasound guidance and were compared with a historical group of youngsters diagnosed with transient synovitis who did not undergo ultrasound-guided joint aspiration. The aim of the study was to evaluate the efficacy of hip joint aspiration in treating transient synovitis. It was clear that joint aspiration added valuable therapeutic benefits. Hip joint aspiration was associated with better and faster resolution of pain and limping in patients with transient synovitis and a significantly shorter length of stay in the hospital. For example, aspirated joints were associated with limping 24 hours after admission in only 10% of instances, whereas joints that were not aspirated were associated with limping in 92% of cases. Refusal to bear weight was seen in only 0.8% of those with aspirated joints versus 14.3% of those whose joints were not aspirated. The duration of hospitalization was just 2.5 days in those with joints that were aspirated compared with 3.9 days in those with unaspirated joints.

The authors of this report did not recommend routine joint aspiration for every patient with transient synovitis, as hip aspiration carries a small but not a nonexistent risk of inducing infection. They suggest that hip aspiration should be limited to patients who are unable to bear weight at all or to patients who pose a significant diagnostic problem, such as a high level of suspicion for septic arthritis or a rheumatologic disorder. One might think, however, that hip joint aspiration is warranted to save hospital costs and to more rapidly improve symptomatology.

J. A. Stockman III, MD

13 Neurology Psychiatry

Neurocognitive Development of Children 4 Years After Critical Illness and Treatment With Tight Glucose Control: A Randomized Controlled Trial
Mesotten D, Gielen M, Sterken C, et al (Catholic Univ of Leuven, Belgium)
JAMA 308:1641-1650, 2012

Context.—A large randomized controlled trial revealed that tight glucose control (TGC) to age adjusted normoglycemia (50-80 mg/dL at age < 1 year and 70-100 mg/dL at age 1-16 years) reduced intensive care morbidity and mortality compared with usual care (UC), but increased hypoglycemia (≤ 40 mg/dL) (25% vs 1%).

Objective.—As both hyperglycemia and hypoglycemia may adversely affect the developing brain, long-term follow-up was required to exclude harm and validate shortterm benefits of TGC.

Design, Setting, and Patients.—A prospective, randomized controlled trial of 700 patients aged 16 years or younger who were admitted to the pediatric intensive care unit (ICU) of the University Hospitals in Leuven, Belgium, between October 2004 and December 2007. Follow-up was scheduled after 3 years with infants assessed at 4 years old between August 2008 and January 2012. Assessment was performed blinded for treatment allocation, in-hospital (83%) or at home/school (17%). For comparison, 216 healthy siblings and unrelated children were tested.

Main Outcome Measures.—Intelligence (full-scale intelligence quotient [IQ]), as assessed with age-adjusted tests (Wechsler IQ scales). Further neurodevelopmental testing encompassed tests for visual-motor integration (Beery-Buktenica Developmental Test of Visual-Motor Integration); attention, motor coordination, and executive functions (Amsterdam Neuropsychological Tasks); memory (Children's Memory Scale); and behavior (Child Behavior Checklist).

Results.—Sixteen percent of patients declined participation or could not be reached (n = 113), resulting in 569 patients being alive and testable at follow-up. At a median (interquartile range [IQR]) of 3.9 (3.8-4.1) years after randomization, TGC in the ICU did not affect full-scale IQ score (median [IQR], 88.0 [74.0-100.0] vs 88.5 [74.3-99.0] for UC; $P = .73$) and had not increased incidence of poor outcomes (death or severe disability precluding neurocognitive testing: 19%[68/349] vs 18%[63/351] with UC; risk-adjusted odds ratio, 0.93; 95% CI, 0.60-1.46; $P = .72$). Other scores for intelligence, visual-motor integration, and memory also did not differ between groups. Tight glucose control improved motor coordination (9% [95% CI, 0%-18%] to 20% [95% CI, 5%-35%] better, all $P \leq .03$) and cognitive flexibility (19% [95% CI, 5%-33%] better, $P = .02$). Brief hypoglycemia evoked by TGC was not associated with worse neurocognitive outcome.

Conclusion.—At follow-up, children who had been treated with TGC during an ICU admission did not have a worse measure of intelligence than those who had received UC.

Trial Registration.—clinicaltrials.gov Identifier NCT00214916.

▶ For those who have not been in a pediatric intensive care unit (PICU) lately, one of the most hotly debated issues these days is how tightly one should manage hyperglycemia. Hyperglycemia is fairly common in critically ill children, and researchers have been asking by how much and with what effort should blood glucose levels be reduced or "normalized." Too loose a control has been suggested to deleteriously effect brain integration and cognition. A recent study, for example, on brain specimens of human patients and experimental animals has shown that hyperglycemia during critical illness causes brain inflammation, impaired astrocyte function, and neuronal damage in the hippocampus and frontal cortex.[1] Unfortunately, too tight a control of glucose can have the unintended consequence of the development of hypoglycemia, with equally potentially devastating consequences.

These authors have studied this issue in managing to follow-up 456 children (80% postoperative cardiac cases) some 4 years after PICU discharge. The result is the largest late outcome study of neurocognitive outcomes in a PICU or postoperative congenital heart disease practice. The data show that critically ill children with "brief" biochemical episodes of hypoglycemia but do not appear to have increased mortality, nor do they have worse neurocognitive performance when compared with critically ill children not experiencing hypoglycemia. This is very different from the outcomes seen with hypoglycemic episodes during critical illnesses in adults. There are several explanations as to why children seem to get into less long-term difficulties in such circumstances than do adults.[2]

The data of these authors indicating that children seem to tolerate brief periods of hypoglycemia raise the issue of whether one can safely "tightly" manage hyperglycemia in pediatric patients in critical care units. The study does not actually answer this question, but it does provide some assurance to those who get uncomfortable when blood sugars run unusually high and feel there is a need to effectively manage such periods of hyperglycemia.

J. A. Stockman III, MD

References

1. Sonneville R, den Hertog HM, Güiza F, et al. Impact of hyperglycemia on neuropathological alterations during critical illness. *J Clin Endocrinol Metab.* 2012;97: 2113-2123.
2. Tasker RC. Pediatric critical care, glycemic control, and hypoglycemia: what is the real target? *JAMA.* 2012;308:1687-1688.

Exercise Improves Behavioral, Neurocognitive, and Scholastic Performance in Children with Attention-Deficit/Hyperactivity Disorder

Pontifex MB, Saliba BJ, Raine LB, et al (Univ of Illinois at Urbana-Champaign)
J Pediatr 162:543-551, 2013

Objective.—To examine the effect of a single bout of moderate-intensity aerobic exercise on preadolescent children with attention-deficit/hyperactivity disorder (ADHD) using objective measures of attention, brain neurophysiology, and academic performance.

Study Design.—Using a within-participants design, task performance and event-related brain potentials were assessed while participants performed an attentional-control task following a bout of exercise or seated reading during 2 separate, counterbalanced sessions.

Results —Following a single 20-minute bout of exercise, both children with ADHD and healthy match control children exhibited greater response accuracy and stimulus-related processing, with the children with ADHD also exhibiting selective enhancements in regulatory processes, compared with after a similar duration of seated reading. In addition, greater performance in the areas of reading and arithmetic were observed following exercise in both groups.

Conclusion.—These findings indicate that single bouts of moderately intense aerobic exercise may have positive implications for aspects of neurocognitive function and inhibitory control in children with ADHD.

▶ Score one for exercise! As difficult as it is for this editor to admit, perhaps exercise does have one beneficial effect. This study documents that exercise can improve behavioral, neurocognitive, and scholastic performance in children with attention-deficit/hyperactivity disorder (ADHD).

Pontifex et al remind us that parents, teachers, and investigators for some time have suggested that kids with ADHD who wear themselves out tend to perform better after exercising than before. In fact, a wide body of literature suggests that this may be true.

Pontifex et al decided to test the hypothesis of whether exercise does improve processing in children with ADHD. They exposed children with ADHD to 20 minutes of either seated reading or aerobic exercise on a motor-driven treadmill at an intensity of 65% to 75% of maximum heart rate. On completion of the experimental conditions, participants were outfitted with an electrode cap and provided very specific task instructions. Once the heart rate returned within 10% of the pre-experimental conditions, the tasks then were administered. Enhancements were observed in inhibitory control and allocation of attentional resources, coupled with selective enhancement and stimulus classification and processing speed. Exercise also appeared to have an added benefit for children with ADHD who exhibited exercise-induced facilitations in action monitoring processes and regulatory adjustments in behavior. These acute exercise-induced enhancements in response to production and neurocognitive function could also have relevance for maximizing scholastic performance in all children because even healthy matched control children showed improvements after exercise.

This report does not give us any follow-up information regarding the half-life of the benefits of a single bout of exercise. Nonetheless, because it is known that children with ADHD are less likely to participate in vigorous physical activity and organized sports, the findings from this report do suggest that motivating children with ADHD to be physically active could have positive effects on aspects of neurocognitive function and inhibitory control. If the data hold up from this report, we might soon see ADHD-affected kids and even otherwise normal kids going on treadmills before they take their SATs.

J. A. Stockman III, MD

Does Childhood Attention-Deficit/Hyperactivity Disorder Predict Risk-Taking and Medical Illnesses in Adulthood?

Ramos Olazagasti MA, Klein RG, Mannuzza S, et al (New York Univ Med Ctr; et al)
J Am Acad Child Adolesc Psychiatry 52:153-162.e4, 2013

Objective.—To test whether children with attention-deficit/hyperactivity disorder (ADHD), free of conduct disorder (CD) in childhood (mean = 8 years), have elevated risk-taking, accidents, and medical illnesses in adulthood (mean = 41 years); whether development of CD influences risk-taking during adulthood; and whether exposure to psychostimulants in childhood predicts cardiovascular disease. We hypothesized positive relationships between childhood ADHD and risky driving (in the past 5 years), risky sex (in the past year), and between risk-taking and medical conditions in adulthood; and that development of CD/antisocial personality (APD) would account for the link between ADHD and risk-taking. We report causes of death.

Method.—Prospective 33-year follow-up of 135 boys of white ethnicity with ADHD in childhood and without CD (probands), and 136 matched male comparison subjects without ADHD (comparison subjects; mean = 41 years), blindly interviewed by clinicians.

Results.—In adulthood, probands had relatively more risky driving, sexually transmitted disease, head injury, and emergency department admissions ($p < .05-.01$). Groups did not differ on other medical outcomes. Lifetime risk-taking was associated with negative health outcomes ($p = .01-.001$). Development of CD/APD accounted for the relationship between ADHD and risk-taking. Probands without CD/APD did not differ from comparison subjects in lifetime risky behaviors. Psychostimulant treatment did not predict cardiac illness ($p = .55$). Probands had more deaths not related to specific medical conditions ($p = .01$).

Conclusions.—Overall, among children with ADHD, it is those who develop CD/APD who have elevated risky behaviors as adults. Over their lifetime, those who did not develop CD/APD did not differ from comparison subjects in risk-taking behaviors. Findings also provide support for long-term safety of early psychostimulant treatment.

▶ This report provides a comprehensive view of attention-deficit/hyperactivity disorder (ADHD) across the lifespan of affected individuals. The authors address the relationships between ADHD in childhood and risk taking, accidents, and medical illnesses later in middle adulthood. It additionally examines the role of conduct disorder on risk taking during adulthood when it coexists with ADHD.

The study itself described by Ramos Olazagasti et al is a 33-year follow-up composed of 135 boys with childhood ADHD. Matched controls are used in this report. The individuals were assessed again at 41 years of age. The report itself is among the very first studies to prospectively examine the relationship between ADHD and risk behaviors, accidents, and nonpsychiatric hospitalizations and emergency department visits and is the first study to follow long term outcomes of children with ADHD over 30 years, well into the fourth and fifth decades of affected individuals' lives. In a sense, the study is pioneering in examining the long-term effects of psychostimulants on cardiovascular health as well.

This study does indicate that the risky behaviors sometimes seen in those with ADHD continue into adulthood and are largely accounted for by coexisting conduct disorder along with antisocial personality disorders rather than being caused by ADHD itself. Overall health outcomes in study subjects were similar to those in the control group except for a somewhat higher mortality rate in subjects with ADHD. Those with childhood ADHD showed higher rates of premature deaths unrelated to medical conditions. Regarding the effects of exposure to psychostimulant drugs, the authors found no evidence that children exposed to relatively high stimulant doses were at higher risk of cardiovascular diseases.

The potential association between ADHD and conduct disorder is well known from prior studies, but this study indicates that one-third of subjects with ADHD but without conduct disorder during childhood may develop antisocial personality disorder by middle adulthood. Prevention strategies aimed at lowering the risk of the development of conduct disorder in children with ADHD are a key learning point from this report. If such targeted approaches to the management of ADHD (elimination of the development of conduct disorder) were achieved, many of the negative life outcomes associated with childhood ADHD could be prevented—an important message from this report.

If there is good news from the study of Ramos Olazagasti, it is that uncomplicated ADHD in adulthood is not associated with a significant increase in health problems. Second, it appears that psychostimulant medications seem not to be associated with an increased risk of cardiovascular disease as has been suggested in other studies. Hopefully, Ramos Olazagasti et al will continue their longitudinal study. Perhaps we will find out what happens to 80-year-olds who are diagnosed with ADHD in childhood.

J. A. Stockman III, MD

Medication for Attention Deficit–Hyperactivity Disorder and Criminality

Lichtenstein P, Halldner L, Zetterqvist J, et al (Karolinska Institutet, Stockholm, Sweden; et al)

N Engl J Med 367:2006-2014, 2012

Background.—Attention deficit–hyperactivity disorder (ADHD) is a common disorder that has been associated with criminal behavior in some studies. Pharmacologic treatment is available for ADHD and may reduce the risk of criminality.

Methods.—Using Swedish national registers, we gathered information on 25,656 patients with a diagnosis of ADHD, their pharmacologic treatment, and subsequent criminal convictions in Sweden from 2006 through 2009. We used stratified Cox regression analyses to compare the rate of criminality while the patients were receiving ADHD medication, as compared with the rate for the same patients while not receiving medication.

Results.—As compared with nonmedication periods, among patients receiving ADHD medication, there was a significant reduction of 32% in the criminality rate for men (adjusted hazard ratio, 0.68; 95% confidence interval [CI], 0.63 to 0.73) and 41% for women (hazard ratio, 0.59; 95% CI, 0.50 to 0.70). The rate reduction remained between 17% and 46% in sensitivity analyses among men, with factors that included different types of drugs (e.g., stimulant vs. nonstimulant) and outcomes (e.g., type of crime).

Conclusions.—Among patients with ADHD, rates of criminality were lower during periods when they were receiving ADHD medication. These findings raise the possibility that the use of medication reduces the risk of criminality among patients with ADHD. (Funded by the Swedish Research Council and others.)

▶ This study regarding the implications of attention deficit-hyperactivity disorder (ADHD) on criminal behavior was performed in Stockholm, Sweden. The study examined more than 25 000 individuals born prior to 1990 who had a diagnosis of ADHD. The study was able to define exposure to ADHD medications over time and correlated the diagnosis and its treatment with criminal activity as identified through the National Crime Register. All persons suspected of a crime after a completed investigation by police, customs authority, or prosecution service were identified. The intent was to determine criminal activity for appropriately diagnosed individuals on and off ADHD medications. Treatment periods were defined as a sequence of ADHD medication prescriptions filled with no more than 6 months between 2 consecutive prescriptions. During intervals of 6 months or more without any prescriptions, a patient was considered not to be receiving treatment. The ability to track such information in Sweden is far better than the situation here in the United States.

The data from this study show that, among the men in whom ADHD was diagnosed, 53.6% had taken an ADHD medication and 36.6% have been convicted of at least one crime during follow-up. The corresponding numbers in a matched population of non-ADHD individuals were 0.2% and 8.9%, respectively. Among female patients, 62.7% had taken an ADHD medication and 15.4% had been convicted of a crime as compared with 0.1% and 2.2% among controls. In patients with ADHD, crimes were less often noted during periods in which the individual was receiving an ADHD medication. These data indicate that medication use was associated with a significantly lower criminality rate. Because patients receiving medication might be different from untreated patients, a critical test of the association was whether there were differences in crime rates in the same person during treatment periods as compared with nontreatment periods. It was documented that the use of ADHD medications reduced the criminality rate in specific individuals by 32% to 41%. It did not matter whether the ADHD medication was a stimulant or a nonstimulant.

Over the years, there has been considerable waxing and waning about the pros and cons of the pharmacological treatment of patients with ADHD and debate about whether benefits outweigh the risk of side effects, potential overprescription, and the development of tolerance, dependence, or addiction. This report from Sweden does show a protective effect for the use of ADHD medications on concurrent rates of all types of criminality and no significant long-term reduction in the crime rate after termination of medication, findings that corroborate the results of prior smaller studies. These data apply to both women and to men. The suggestion is that pharmacologic ADHD treatment helps an individual to better organize their lives or contributes to enduring changes at the neuronal level. Another possibility is that concomitant associations with treatment do not persist, which could be an explanation for previous findings of the lack of long-term effects. In line with the latter possibility, these investigators found no significantly persistent association between medication use in a particular year and the crime rate several years later, an interpretation also supported by the findings of an association between medication use and criminality regardless of whether it was the first or second time that patients had changed their medication status.

So what do these data mean for the situation here in the United States? Sweden does not appear to be unusual in its rates of ADHD or its use of ADHD medications, so the information from this report may very well apply to the situation here in our country. Potential beneficial effects of ADHD medications do have to be carefully weighed against the potential adverse effects of medication, including overprescription and side effects. Nonetheless, in severe cases of ADHD, it is likely that medication therapy does reduce rates of criminality.

J. A. Stockman III, MD

Medications for Adolescents and Young Adults With Autism Spectrum Disorders: A Systematic Review

Dove D, Warren Z, McPheeters ML, et al (Vanderbilt Univ Med Ctr, Nashville, TN)
Pediatrics 130:717-726, 2012

Background and Objective.—Although many treatments have been studied in children with autism spectrum disorders (ASDs), less attention has focused on interventions that may be helpful in adolescents and young adults with ASD. The goal of this study was to systematically review evidence regarding medication treatments for individuals between the ages of 13 and 30 years with ASD.

Methods.—The Medline, PsycINFO, and ERIC databases were searched (1980–December 2011), as were reference lists of included articles. Two investigators independently assessed studies against predetermined inclusion/exclusion criteria. Two investigators independently extracted data regarding participant and intervention characteristics, assessment techniques, and outcomes and assigned overall quality and strength of evidence ratings on the basis of predetermined criteria.

Results.—Eight studies of medications were identified that focused on 13- to 30-year-olds with ASD; 4 of the studies were of fair quality. The strength of evidence was insufficient for all outcomes associated with medications tested in this population; however, the 2 available studies of the atypical antipsychotic medication risperidone in this age range were consistent with the moderate evidence in children with ASD for treating problem behavior, including aggression, and high strength of evidence for adverse events, including sedation and weight gain.

Conclusions.—There is a marked lack of data on use of medication treatments for adolescents and young adults with ASD. The evidence on the use of risperidone in this age range is insufficient when considered alone but is consistent with the data in the population of children with ASD.

▶ Any study dealing with autism spectrum disorder (ASD) would be timely in this day and age. This particular study by Dove et al from Vanderbilt University Medical Center was designed to give us information from a systematic review of therapies for adolescents and young adults (ages 13 to 30 years) with ASD. There also was additional information obtained as part of the review on nonmedicinal treatments including behavioral, educational, and allied health approaches to the management of ASD that can be found at http://www.effectivehealthcare. ahrq.gov. The study showed that the use of medications in adolescents and young adults with ASD is extremely common. As common as these medications are, there are few data, however, that really tell us how effective the medications are or what harms may be associated with the use of medications in this specific population. The closest we come to good data appears to be related to the use of antipsychotic medications. For example, a randomized controlled trial studying risperidone found improvements in aggression, repetitive behavior, sensory motor behaviors, and overall behavioral symptoms and did so with a high degree of validity.[1] A similarly designed study of fluvoxamine showed decreases in repetitive behavior, aggression, autistic symptoms, and language usage.[2] The data from this study were not quite as strong as the data related to risperidone.

The bottom line from this report is that based on studies in adolescents and adults with ASD, the strength of evidence is insufficient to draw conclusions regarding adverse events associated with medications tested in this population. The authors note that, as in the case of efficacy, the data on adverse events associated with risperidone, including sedation and weight gain, are consistent with an association of treatment with these adverse events in children with ASD. Unfortunately, there is a dearth of evidence in all areas of care for adolescents and young adults with ASD. The authors of this report remind us that a basic understanding of the effects of aging on health, cognitive skills, and other domains of functioning is absent and the lack of randomized controlled trials of medication adverse events is quite notable. It is critical to understand the age appropriateness of potential medication treatments with respect to social, physiologic, pharmacologic, and functional characteristics of the populations cared for by pediatricians. This report closes with the statement that although studies conducted to date have focused on the use of medications to address specific challenging behaviors, the effectiveness of medications on irritability and agitation in this age group remain largely unknown and can at best be inferred from studies including mostly younger children. ASD is a disorder that cries out for high-quality randomized controlled trials asking specific and critical questions.

J. A. Stockman III, MD

References

1. McDougle CJ, Holmes JP, Carlson DC, Pelton GH, Cohen DJ, Price LH. A double-blind, placebo-controlled study of risperidone in adults with autistic disorder and other pervasive developmental disorders. *Arch Gen Psychiatry.* 1998;55:633-641.
2. McDougle CJ, Naylor ST, Cohen DJ, Volkmar FR, Heninger GR, Price LH. A double-blind, placebo-controlled study of fluvoxamine in adults with autistic disorder. *Arch Gen Psychiatry.* 1996;53:1001-1008.

Diagnostic Exome Sequencing in Persons with Severe Intellectual Disability

de Ligt J, Willemsen MH, van Bon BWM, et al (Radboud Univ Nijmegen Med Ctr, the Netherlands)
N Engl J Med 367:1921-1929, 2012

Background.—The causes of intellectual disability remain largely unknown because of extensive clinical and genetic heterogeneity.

Methods.—We evaluated patients with intellectual disability to exclude known causes of the disorder. We then sequenced the coding regions of more than 21,000 genes obtained from 100 patients with an IQ below 50 and their unaffected parents. A data-analysis procedure was developed to identify and classify de novo, autosomal recessive, and X-linked mutations. In addition, we used high-throughput resequencing to confirm new candidate genes in 765 persons with intellectual disability (a confirmation series). All mutations were evaluated by molecular geneticists and clinicians in the context of the patients' clinical presentation.

Results.—We identified 79 de novo mutations in 53 of 100 patients. A total of 10 de novo mutations and 3 X-linked (maternally inherited) mutations that had been previously predicted to compromise the function of known intellectual-disability genes were found in 13 patients. Potentially causative de novo mutations in novel candidate genes were detected in 22 patients. Additional de novo mutations in 3 of these candidate genes were identified in patients with similar phenotypes in the confirmation series, providing support for mutations in these genes as the cause of intellectual disability. We detected no causative autosomal recessive inherited mutations in the discovery series. Thus, the total diagnostic yield was 16%, mostly involving de novo mutations.

Conclusions.—De novo mutations represent an important cause of intellectual disability; exome sequencing was used as an effective diagnostic strategy for their detection. (Funded by the European Union and others.)

▶ The authors of this study previously reported evidence supporting the theory that rare de novo point mutations can be a major cause of severe intellectual disability.[1] A clinical diagnosis of severe intellectual disability is generally based on an IQ of less than 50 and substantial limitations in activities of daily living. The diagnosis is supported by the findings of substantial developmental delays, including motor, cognitive, and speech delays, occurring in children without specific syndromes. Although intellectual disability can be caused by nongenetic factors such as infections and perinatal insults, in developed countries most forms of significant intellectual disability are likely caused by a genetic etiology. The latter has remained unidentified in the majority of cases. Fortunately, it is now possible to determine the sequence of essentially all genes in an individual's genome—referred to as the exome—within a matter of just days. This technology became widely available in 2005, and using such technology, investigators have been testing the hypothesis that sporadic intellectual disability is caused by de novo mutations (genetic changes that are present in affected individuals but not in the parents).

These authors were able to analyze DNA from intellectually disabled children and compared their DNA with both parents and thus were able to identify de novo sequence variants in the children. The authors were able to identify the genetic cause of intellectual disability in 16% of patients, with the majority of cases caused by a mutation in a gene that was already known to cause intellectual disability. A diagnostic yield of 16% in patients with intellectual disability is encouraging and similar to the yield that can be obtained by chromosome microarrays to detect deletions and duplications (15%-20%). Other de novo variants were also observed, but one could not say with confidence that they may have been the cause of the youngster's intellectual disability.

In an editorial that accompanied this article, Mefford[2] states that genomic technologies are rapidly evolving and that routine whole-genome sequencing is on the horizon. With advances in our understanding of regulatory DNA, it is conceivable that mutations that are noncoding will soon be identified in another subset of patients. An understanding of the genetic causes of intellectual disability can benefit patients and their families. A diagnosis may provide information on the prognosis, preclude further unnecessary invasive testing, and lead to an appropriate therapy. Family members may benefit from knowledge of the risk of recurrence, reproductive counseling, and possible prenatal diagnosis. It is clear that the genome project of more than a decade ago is now rapidly yielding fruit.

J. A. Stockman III, MD

References

1. Vissers LE, de Ligt J, Gilissen C, et al. A de novo paradigm for mental retardation. *Nat Genet.* 2010;42:1109-1112.
2. Mefford HC. Diagnostic exome sequencing—are we there yet? *N Engl J Med.* 2012;367:1951-1953.

Cerebrospinal Fluid Reference Ranges in Term and Preterm Infants in the Neonatal Intensive Care Unit

Srinivasan L, Shah SS, Padula MA, et al (The Children's Hosp of Philadelphia, PA, Cincinnati Children's Hosp Med Ctr, OH; et al)
J Pediatr 161:729-734, 2012

Objective.—To determine reference ranges of cerebrospinal fluid (CSF) laboratory findings in term and preterm infants in the neonatal intensive care unit.

Study Design.—Data were collected prospectively as part of a multisite study of infants aged <6 months undergoing lumbar puncture for evaluation of suspected sepsis. Infants with a red blood cell count >500 cells/μL or a known cause of CSF pleocytosis were excluded from the analysis.

Results.—A total of 318 infants met the inclusion criteria. Of these, 148 infants (47%) were preterm, and 229 (72%) received antibiotics before undergoing lumbar puncture. The upper reference limit of the CSF white blood cell (WBC) count was 12 cells/μL in preterm infants and 14 cells/μL in term infants. CSF protein levels were significantly higher in preterm infants (upper reference limit, 209 mg/dL vs 159 mg/dL in term infants; $P < .001$), and declined with advancing postnatal age in both groups (preterm, $P = .008$; term, $P < .001$). CSF glucose levels did not differ in term and preterm infants. Antibiotic exposure did not significantly affect CSF WBC, protein, or glucose values.

Conclusions.—CSF WBC counts are not significantly different in preterm and term infants. CSF protein levels are higher and decline more slowly with postnatal age in preterm infants compared with term infants. This study provides CSF reference ranges for hospitalized preterm and term infants, particularly in the first month of life (Table 3).

▶ It is clear that one table is worth a thousand words. This table (Table 3) from the report of Srinivasan et al tells us the normal ranges for cerebrospinal fluid (CSF) findings in preterm and term infants. The authors designed a study to characterize clinically relevant reference ranges for CSF laboratory findings in term and preterm infants hospitalized in a neonatal intensive care unit using prospectively collected data. Infants less than 6 months of age undergoing a lumbar puncture for evaluation of sepsis were eligible for inclusion. Preterm infants were those defined as being born at gestational age less than 37 weeks. A total of 318 patients were included in the study.

Study data showed that CSF white blood cell counts did not differ between preterm and term infants during the first week of life and beyond (median, 3

TABLE 3.—CSF Findings in Preterm and Term Infants

	Preterm Infants			Term Infants		
Value	All (n = 148)	≤7 days (n = 66)	>7 days (n = 82)	All (n = 170)	≤7 days (n = 130)	>7 days (n = 40)
CSF WBC, cells/μL						
All infants						
Median (IQR)	3 (1-6)	3 (1-7)	3 (1-4)	3 (1-6)	3 (1-6)	2 (1-4)
95th percentile	16	18	12	26	23	32
Upper IQR bound + 1.5 × IQR	14	16	9	14	14	9
Antibiotic-unexposed						
95th percentile	11	17	10	32	31	53
Upper IQR bound + 1.5 × IQR	9	17	9	20	20	21
CSF protein, mg/dL*						
All infants						
Median (IQR)	104 (79-131)	116 (93-138)	93 (69-122)	74 (54-96)	78 (60-100)	57 (42-77)
95th percentile	203	213	203	137	137	158
Upper IQR bound + 1.5 × IQR	209	206	202	159	160	130
Antibiotic-unexposed						
95th percentile	195	195	136	136	136	284
Upper IQR bound + 1.5 × IQR	175	245	143	172	188	105
CSF glucose, mg/dL						
All infants						
Median (IQR)	49 (42-62)	53 (43-65)	47 (40-58)	51 (44-57)	50 (44-56)	52 (45-64)
5th percentile	33	33	33	36	35	38
Lower IQR bound − 1.5 × IQR	12	10	13	24	26	17
Antibiotic-unexposed						
5th percentile	33	33	35	33	33	33
Lower IQR bound − 1.5 × IQR	19	25	18	21	26	21

Eight infants were excluded from the analysis because of unknown CSF WBC (n = 1), extremely outlying value (n = 1; CSF WBC 850), unknown CSF protein concentration (n = 4), and unknown CSF glucose concentration (n = 2).

*CSF protein values: $P < .001$, term versus preterm, term age ≤7 days versus preterm age ≤7 days, and term age >7 days versus preterm age >7 days.

cells per microliter). CSF white blood cell values did not decline significantly with increasing postnatal age in either preterm infants or term infants. CSF protein values were significantly higher in preterm infants compared with term infants (median, 104 mg/dL vs 74 mg/dL). CSF protein values decreased significantly with increasing postnatal age in both term and preterm infants. The rate of decline was greater in term infants (4.8 mg/dL/wk) compared with preterm infants (3.1 mg/dL/wk). Glucose values were similar in preterm and term infants both early and later in life. Infants with CSF red blood cell counts greater than 500 cells per microliter were excluded from analysis in this study.

Although many previous studies characterize reference ranges for CSF findings in infants, controversy has persisted, especially regarding appropriate values in hospitalized preterm infants and in the context of antibiotic pretreatment. Normative CSF values are of special importance in identifying infants with central nervous system infection, particularly in settings in which CSF cultures may yield false-negative results.

For the clinician, the most useful information from this study is the upper and lower limits of the CSF reference ranges. It should be noted that this study does have several limitations. The data were obtained from infants evaluated for sepsis in the neonatal intensive care unit and thus might not be applicable to febrile infants evaluated in the emergency department.

J. A. Stockman III, MD

Cerebrospinal Fluid Findings in Children with Fever-Associated Status Epilepticus: Results of the Consequences of Prolonged Febrile Seizures (FEBSTAT) Study
Frank LM, on behalf of the FEBSTAT Study Team (Children's Hosp of The King's Daughters and Eastern Virginia Med School, Norfolk, VA; et al)
J Pediatr 161;1169-1171.e1, 2012

This prospective multicenter study of 200 patients with fever-associated status epilepticus (FSE), of whom 136 underwent a nontraumatic lumbar puncture, confirms that FSE rarely causes cerebrospinal fluid (CSF) pleocytosis. CSF glucose and protein levels were unremarkable. Temperature, age, seizure focality, and seizure duration did not affect results. CSF pleocytosis should not be attributed to FSE.

▶ The Febrile Status Epilepticus Study is a prospective multicenter study that has examined the long-term consequences of febrile status epilepticus. Children entered into this study have had a single seizure or a series of seizures without interim recovery lasting 30 minutes or more that otherwise meet the definition of a febrile seizure as defined as a provoked seizure in which the sole identifiable provocation is fever (temperature > 38.4°C, 101.0°F).

In the study reported by Frank et al, data from the Febrile Status Epilepticus Study were used to tell us about cerebrospinal fluid (CSF) findings in children with fever-associated status epilepticus. In this population of patients, the mean CSF protein levels in children who had a nontraumatic lumbar puncture was 22 mg/dL with values ranging from 8 mg/dL to 137 mg/dL. A total of 29% of children had protein levels ≤15 mg/dL, 50% had ≤19 mg/dL, and 76% had ≤24 mg/dL. Only 2.3% of children had a CSF protein level of > 60 mg/dL. There was no correlation between protein levels and seizure duration. There is also no correlation between the age of febrile seizure and protein levels. The mean glucose level for children with a nontraumatic lumbar puncture was 89.6 mg/dL, with values ranging between 46 mg/dL and 201 mg/dL.

The American Academy of Neurology Practice Parameter on the diagnostic evaluation of the child with status epilepticus supports the diagnostic utility of a lumbar puncture.[1] The data from the report of Frank et al suggest that a simple febrile seizure is unlikely to be associated with a significant risk of serious infection. There is growing consensus that unexplained CSF pleocytosis after seizures in children should prompt a careful search for possible medical explanations other than simply being attributed to an ictal phenomenon, a position clearly supported by the present findings. Specific reports of CSF pleocytosis in children with status epilepticus, both complex febrile seizures and simple febrile seizures, support the impression that excess numbers of white blood cells in the CSF should not be dismissed as a seizure-related phenomenon in and of themselves. In young infants, a higher degree of clinical suspicion may be needed, even in the absence of clear pleocytosis because young infants are recognized to be at greater risk for presentation with central nervous system infection while showing minimal clinical and laboratory signs. The American Academy of Pediatrics Practice Parameter for the Diagnostic Evaluation of the child with a simple febrile seizure, specifically excludes children less than 6 months of age.[2] In a report published in the *Journal of the American Medical Association* several years back, investigators approached this topic from the perspective of abnormal cerebrospinal fluid results and concluded that the occurrence of seizures with an abnormal CSF finding (10 or greater white blood cells) increased the risk for meningitis in children.[3]

The authors of this report conclude that CSF findings are usually normal in children with febrile status epilepticus and that abnormal CSF results should prompt close clinical scrutiny and additional testing and treatment as indicated. They also note that normal CSF counts and chemistry results, although reassuring, do not in and of themselves eliminate the possibility of central nervous system infection, particularly in the youngest of patients.

J. A. Stockman III, MD

References

1. Riviello JJ Jr, Ashwal S, Hirtz D, et al. American Academy of Neurology Subcommittee, Practice Committee of the Child Neurology Society. Practice parameter: diagnostic assessment of the child with status epilepticus (an evidence-based review): report of the Quality Standards Subcommittee of the American Academy of Neurology and the Practice Committee of the Child Neurology Society. *Neurology.* 2006;67:1542-1550.
2. Subcommittee on Febrile Seizures, American Academy of Pediatrics. Neurodiagnostic evaluation of the child with a simple febrile seizure. *Pediatrics.* 2011;127: 389-394.
3. Nigrovic LE, Kuppermann N, Macias CG, et al. Clinical prediction rule for identifying children with cerebrospinal fluid pleocytosis at very low risk of bacterial meningitis. *JAMA.* 2007;297:52-60.

Structural Brain Changes in Migraine

Palm-Meinders IH, Koppen H, Terwindt GM, et al (Leiden Univ Med Ctr, the Netherlands; et al)
JAMA 308:1889-1897, 2012

Context.—A previous cross-sectional study showed an association of migraine with a higher prevalence of magnetic resonance imaging (MRI)—measured ischemic lesions in the brain.

Objective.—To determine whether women or men with migraine (with and without aura) have a higher incidence of brain lesions 9 years after initial MRI, whether migraine frequency was associated with progression of brain lesions, and whether progression of brain lesions was associated with cognitive decline.

Design, Setting, and Participants.—In a follow-up of the 2000 Cerebral Abnormalities in Migraine, an Epidemiological Risk Analysis cohort, a prospective population-based observational study of Dutch participants with migraine and an age- and sex-matched control group, 203 of the 295 baseline participants in the migraine group and 83 of 140 in the control group underwent MRI scan in 2009 to identify progression of MRI-measured brain lesions. Comparisons were adjusted for age, sex, hypertension, diabetes, and educational level. The participants in the migraine group were a mean 57 years (range, 43-72 years), and 71% were women. Those in the control group were a mean 55 years (range, 44-71 years), and 69% were women.

Main Outcome Measures.—Progression of MRI-measured cerebral deep white matter hyperintensities, intratentorial hyperintensities, and posterior circulation territory infarctlike lesions. Change in cognition was also measured.

Results.—Of the 145 women in the migraine group, 112 (77%) vs 33 of 55 women (60%) in the control group had progression of deep white matter hyperintensities (adjusted odds ratio [OR], 2.1; 95% CI, 1.0-4.1; $P = .04$). There were no significant associations of migraine with progression of infra-tentorial hyperintensities: 21 participants (15%) in the migraine group and 1 of 57 participants (2%) in the control group showed progression (adjusted OR, 7.7; 95% CI, 1.0-59.5; $P = .05$) or new posterior circulation territory infarctlike lesions: 10 of 203 participants (5%) in the migraine group but none of 83 in the control group ($P = .07$). There was no association of number or frequency of migraine headaches with progression of lesions. There was no significant association of high vs nonhigh deep white matter hyperintensity load with change in cognitive scores (-3.7 in the migraine group vs 1.4 in the control group; 95% CI, -4.4 to 0.2; adjusted $P = .07$).

Conclusions.—In a community-based cohort followed up after 9 years, women with migraine had a higher incidence of deep white matter hyper-intensities but did not have significantly higher progression of other MRI-measured brain changes. There was no association of migraine with progression of any MRI-measured brain lesions in men.

▶ Migraine affects both children and adults. Although magnetic resonance imaging (MRI) data in children are scant in terms of structural damage caused by migraine, data are emerging in adults that suggest migraines are not innocent at all. There is an increasing body of evidence from cross-sectional, population-based studies suggesting that an MRI to measure white matter hyperintensities in the brain is more common in people with migraine compared with people who have no history of migraine. For example, 1 study has shown a 3.9 greater probability of white matter hyperintensities in migraine-affected adults in comparison with those without migraine.[1]

These authors reveal the results of a longitudinal population-based study from the Netherlands in which several hundred participants with migraine were compared with sex-matched control adults without migraine. The study determined the number and volume change of deep white matter hyperintensities, infratentorial hyperintensities, and posterior circulation infarct-like lesions over a period of 9 years in patients with migraine. Progression of deep white matter hyperintensities was found and was greatest in women with migraine without aura (odds ratio, 2.1). This progression of white matter abnormalities was not associated with the frequency of migraine episodes, duration of migraine, types of attacks, migraine therapy, or systemic hypertension. Fortunately, although there was progression of the MRI findings in the patient population study, the overall lesion burden in the brain was quite small and most likely clinically insignificant. Although other studies have suggested that such findings are associated with a higher incidence of stroke, mild cognitive impairment, and dementia, this study found no increased risk of clinically obvious stroke or a decline in fine motor skills or cognition as measured by memory, concentration, attention, executive function, psychomotor and processing speed, organization, fluid intelligence, and visual-spacial skills.

It is not known whether preventive migraine therapy reduces either progression of white matter lesions or the risk of stroke. At the same time it is not known whether the use of migraine medications such as triptans or ergots actually increased the risk of white matter hyperintensity.

This article is interesting but does not assist care providers in knowing what more to do or not do for patients who suffer from serious migraine. The study findings do imply that small white matter hyperintensities in most patients with migraine should not be a reason in and of themselves for alarm. It is possible, however, that certain subpopulations of patients with migraine and white matter hyperintensities may be at increased genetic risk for significant white matter disease and neurologic morbidity, including stroke, transient ischemic attacks, cognitive impairment, and other neurologic outcomes. As is true for adults, modifying other risk factors for vascular disease is important in children. This includes management of obesity, prevention of onset of smoking, management of hypertension and high cholesterol levels, and physical inactivity.

J. A. Stockman III, MD

Reference

1. Swartz RH, Kern RZ. Migraine is associated with magnetic resonance imaging white matter abnormalities: a meta-analysis. *Arch Neurol.* 2004;61:1366-1368.

Botulinum Toxin A for Prophylactic Treatment of Migraine and Tension Headaches in Adults: A Meta-Analysis
Jackson JL, Kuriyama A, Hayashino Y (Zablocki Veterans Affairs Med Ctr, Milwaukee, WI; Rakuwakai Otowa Hosp, Kyoto, Japan; Kyoto Univ Graduate School of Medicine and Public Health, Japan)
JAMA 307:1736-1745, 2012

Context.—Botulinum toxin A is US Food and Drug Administration approved for prophylactic treatment for chronic migraines.

Objective.—To assess botulinum toxin A for the prophylactic treatment of headaches in adults.

Data Sources.—A search of MEDLINE, EMBASE, bibliographies of published systematic reviews, and the Cochrane trial registries between 1966 and March 15, 2012. Inclusion and exclusion criteria of each study were reviewed. Headaches were categorized as episodic (<15 headaches per month) or chronic (≥15 headaches per month) migraine and episodic or chronic daily or tension headaches.

Study Selection.—Randomized controlled trials comparing botulinum toxin A with placebo or other interventions for headaches among adults.

Data Extraction.—Data were abstracted and quality assessed independently by 2 reviewers. Outcomes were pooled using a random-effects model.

Data Synthesis.—Pooled analyses suggested that botulinum toxin A was associated with fewer headaches per month among patients with chronic daily headaches (1115 patients, 2.06 headaches per month; 95% CI, −3.56 to −0.56; 3 studies) and among patients with chronic migraine headaches (n = 1508, −2.30 headaches per month; 95% CI, −3.66 to −0.94; 5 studies). There was no significant association between use of botulinum toxin A and reduction in the number of episodic migraine (n = 1838, 0.05 headaches per month; 95% CI, −0.26 to 0.36; 9 studies) or chronic tension-type headaches (n = 675, −1.43 headaches per month; 95% CI, −3.13 to 0.27; 7 studies). In single trials, botulinum toxin A was not associated with fewer migraine headaches per month vs valproate (standardized mean difference [SMD], −0.20; 95% CI, −0.91 to 0.31), topiramate (SMD, 0.20; 95% CI, −0.36 to 0.76), or amitriptyline (SMD, 0.29; 95% CI, −0.17 to 0.76). Botulinum toxin A was associated with fewer chronic tension-type headaches per month vs methylprednisolone injections (SMD, −2.5; 95% CI, −3.5 to −1.5). Compared with placebo, botulinum toxin A was associated with a greater frequency of blepharoptosis, skin tightness, paresthesias, neck stiffness, muscle weakness, and neck pain.

Conclusion.—Botulinum toxin A compared with placebo was associated with a small to modest benefit for chronic daily headaches and chronic migraines but was not associated with fewer episodic migraine or chronic tension-type headaches per month.

▶ Migraine headaches are common in adults and children. As many as 40% of adults have migraine headaches. It is also estimated that migraine headaches are responsible for $1 billion in medical costs and several-fold that amount in loss of productivity. There are many methods used to prophylactically manage migraine. Common measures include anticonvulsants, beta-blockers, calcium channel blockers, serotonin reuptake inhibitors, and tricyclic antidepressants. Botulinum toxin A injections were proposed several years ago as a headache treatment when it was observed that patients with chronic headaches receiving cosmetic botulinum injections experienced improvement in their headaches. In 2010, the Food and Drug Administration approved botulinum toxin A for prophylactic treatment of chronic migraine headaches. Several clinical trials have been undertaken to determine the effectiveness of this form of therapy. The results of these clinical trials have been mixed.

These authors performed a systematic review to assess the association of botulinum toxin A in reducing headache frequency as part of prophylactic treatment of migraine, tension, or chronic daily headaches in adults. They analyzed prior randomized studies examining botulinum A toxin with other interventions. The bottom line was that botulinum toxin A may be associated with improvement in the frequency of chronic migraine and chronic daily headaches, but no improvement in the frequency of episodic migraine, chronic tension-type headaches, or the episodic tension-type headaches was found. It should be noted that the response to botulinum toxin A was fairly modest. The reduction in number of headaches per month was from 19.5 to 17.2 for chronic migraine.

It is clear that botulinum toxin A is not associated with greater benefit than placebo in the prophylactic treatment recurrent tension headache. Some patients, however, will benefit from prophylaxis of chronic daily headaches and chronic migraine. Those receiving botulinum toxin A may experience more side effects than those receiving a placebo. Side effect may include eye lid droop, neck stiffness, and skin tightness.

If all else fails, one may wish to attempt a trial of botulinum toxin A in teenagers with chronic migraine. Beta-blockers are less expensive as a first therapy, however.

J. A. Stockman III, MD

Placebo-Controlled Phase 3 Study of Oral BG-12 for Relapsing Multiple Sclerosis
Gold R, for the DEFINE Study Investigators (St Josef-Hosp/Ruhr-Univ Bochum, Germany; et al)
N Engl J Med 367:1098-1107, 2012

Background.—BG-12 (dimethyl fumarate) was shown to have antiinflammatory and cytoprotective properties in preclinical experiments and to result in significant reductions in disease activity on magnetic resonance imaging (MRI) in a phase 2, placebo-controlled study involving patients with relapsing—remitting multiple sclerosis.

Methods.—We conducted a randomized, double-blind, placebo-controlled phase 3 study involving patients with relapsing—remitting multiple sclerosis. Patients were randomly assigned to receive oral BG-12 at a dose of 240 mg twice daily, BG-12 at a dose of 240 mg three times daily, or placebo. The primary end point was the proportion of patients who had a relapse by 2 years. Other end points included the annualized relapse rate, the time to confirmed progression of disability, and findings on MRI.

Results.—The estimated proportion of patients who had a relapse was significantly lower in the two BG-12 groups than in the placebo group (27% with BG-12 twice daily and 26% with BG-12 thrice daily vs. 46% with placebo, $P < 0.001$ for both comparisons). The annualized relapse rate at 2 years was 0.17 in the twice-daily BG-12 group and 0.19 in the thrice-daily BG-12 group, as compared with 0.36 in the placebo group, representing relative reductions of 53% and 48% with the two BG-12 regimens, respectively ($P < 0.001$ for the comparison of each BG-12 regimen with placebo). The estimated proportion of patients with confirmed progression of disability was 16% in the twice-daily BG-12 group, 18% in the thrice-daily BG-12 group, and 27% in the placebo group, with significant relative risk reductions of 38% with BG-12 twice daily ($P = 0.005$) and 34% with BG-12 thrice daily ($P = 0.01$). BG-12 also significantly reduced the number of gadolinium-enhancing lesions and of new or enlarging T_2-weighted hyperintense lesions ($P < 0.001$ for the comparison of each BG-12 regimen with placebo). Adverse events associated with BG-12 included flushing and gastrointestinal events, such as diarrhea, nausea, and upper abdominal pain, as well as decreased lymphocyte counts and elevated liver aminotransferase levels.

Conclusions.—In patients with relapsing remitting multiple sclerosis, both BG-12 regimens, as compared with placebo, significantly reduced the proportion of patients who had a relapse, the annualized relapse rate, the rate of disability progression, and the number of lesions on MRI. (Funded by Biogen Idec; DEFINE ClinicalTrials.gov number, NCT00420212.).

▶ This report and 1 other appeared in the same issue of the *New England Journal of Medicine*. Both studies tell us about a new medication, given orally, for treatment of multiple sclerosis. The medication has been used for psoriasis management for some time, as does its background. In a very curious incident of the "poison chair," hundreds of people in several European cities appeared at clinics with eczematous burns that had no apparent cause. The source was found to be dimethyl fumarate (fumarate), used as a fungicide and desiccant in the shipping of sofas. A Finnish physician uncovered the toxin by doggedly pursuing a local outbreak in Finland.[1] Fumarate and its esters have had a much better safety record as a medicinal than as an industrial agent. It was back in 1959 that a biochemist administered fumaric acid to himself to treat his psoriasis which he considered to be due to a deficiency of fumarate. A formulation of fumarate known as Fumaderm has been marketed for the treatment of psoriasis for the better part of 20 years. What is most interesting is the encounter between a German dermatologist and a neurologist over 2 patients with psoriasis whose multiple sclerosis stabilized after treatment with oral fumarate. The drug is known to have immunosuppressive and neuroprotectant properties. This encounter eventually led to the study abstracted.

All newly diagnosed patients with multiple sclerosis are now initially managed with medication therapy. The most longstanding of these medications is interferon, which has a quarter of a century history of experience. It reduces relapses by approximately one third, although it has not changed the ultimate overall course of patients with multiple sclerosis. There have been relatively few direct comparisons between oral and parenteral treatments. The interferons and a second parenteral compound, glatiramer acetate, have surpassed in terms of effectiveness in reducing relapses by some of the newly introduced orally administered drugs. None have quite attained the suppression of disease activity shown with monthly intravenous use of natalizumab, but the risk of progressive multifocal leukoencephalopathy (PML) has restricted the application of the latter agent. None of the oral agents—except for teriflunomide (the active metabolite of leflunomide that was approved for treatment of rheumatoid arthritis in 1998)—has had more than a few years of study for effectiveness and/or side effects.

Although the average age of onset of multiple sclerosis is in the late 20s, it can present in childhood. Significant disability tends to occur only after a decade or 2 from the time of diagnosis. Fumarate, as described in the report of Fox et al, will need to prove its efficacy and durability over many decades. Hopefully, along this journey there will be new drugs introduced. The risk of PML hangs heavily over the history of drug introduction as part of the management of multiple sclerosis, however.

Those involved with the care of individuals with multiple sclerosis now know at least 1 new drug has been added to the therapeutic armamentarium. The question that will need to be asked is whether it is reasonable to switch patients who are doing reasonably well on whatever current therapy they are on to these newer oral agents.

J. A. Stockman III, MD

Reference

1. Rantanen T. The cause of the Chinese sofa/chair dermatitis epidemic is likely to be contact allergy to dimethylfumarate, a novel potent contact sensitizer. *Br J Dermatol.* 2008;159:218-221.

Effectiveness of internet-based cognitive behavioural treatment for adolescents with chronic fatigue syndrome (FITNET): a randomised controlled trial

Nijhof SL, Bleijenberg G, Uiterwaal CSPM, et al (Univ Med Centre, Utrecht, Netherlands; Radboud Univ Nijmegen Med Centre, Netherlands)
Lancet 379:1412-1418, 2012

Background.—Chronic fatigue syndrome is characterised by persistent fatigue and severe disability. Cognitive behavioural therapy seems to be a promising treatment, but its availability is restricted. We developed Fatigue In Teenagers on the interNET (FITNET), the first dedicated internet-based therapeutic program for adolescents with this disorder, and compared its effectiveness with that of usual care.

Methods.—Adolescents aged 12–18 years with chronic fatigue syndrome were assigned to FITNET or usual care in a 1:1 ratio at one tertiary treatment centre in the Netherlands by use of a computer-generated blocked randomisation allocation schedule. The study was open label. Primary outcomes were school attendance, fatigue severity, and physical functioning, and were assessed at 6 months with computerised questionnaires. Analysis was by intention to treat. Thereafter, all patients were offered FITNET if needed. This trial is registered, number ISRCTN59878666.

Findings.—68 of 135 adolescents were assigned to FITNET and 67 to usual care, and 67 and 64, respectively, were analysed. FITNET was significantly more effective than was usual care for all dichotomised primary outcomes at 6 months—full school attendance (50 [75%] *vs* 10 [16%], relative risk 4·8, 95% CI 2·7—8·9; *p* < 0·0001), absence of severe fatigue (57 [85%] *vs* 17 [27%], 3·2, 2·1—4·9; *p* < 0·0001), and normal physical functioning (52 [78%] *vs* 13 [20%], 3·8, 2·3—6·3; *p* < 0·0001). No serious adverse events were reported.

Interpretation.—FITNET offers a readily accessible and highly effective treatment for adolescents with chronic fatigue syndrome. The results of this study justify implementation on a broader scale.

▶ These investigators report a trial of an effective, Internet-delivered treatment for adolescents with chronic fatigue syndrome, Fatigue In Teenagers on the InterNET (FITNET). The trial was based on data from a tertiary care center in the Netherlands. One hundred thirty five adolescents were recruited, with few eligible patients declining to participate and few dropouts from either treatment or control arm assessments. Usual care included individual and group delivered cognitive behavioral therapy or graded exercise therapy. Outcomes included assessment of school attendance, fatigue severity, and physical functioning. All 3 of these parameters improved more in patients given the new treatment using Internet-delivered behavioral therapy than in those given the alternative care when assessed at 6 months. For example, achievement of full school attendance was 5-fold greater; absence of severe fatigue was 3.2 fold greater and improvement in physical functioning was almost 4 times greater in those receiving the Internet-delivered treatment. This effect was sustained at 12 months. If one looks at the overall magnitude of the outcomes, the treatment effect was quite impressive, with 63% of participants recovering, almost 8 times as many as those who received usual care. This effect was much more than might be expected from information of previous trials of cognitive behavioral therapy in adolescents. It is known that adolescents tend to have a better outcome than adults with chronic fatigue syndrome, but even this would not account for the remarkable improvement seen with the new form of intervention therapy.

The logical question to ask is why there was such a good effect. In an editorial that accompanied this report, White and Chalder speculate on the reasons.[1] It is suspected that one of the reasons for the good effect was that the intervention was systemic, given to both patients and their parents. Second, the intervention was complex, involving both regular interactive e-mails and multiple multimodular educational and therapeutic components. Third, the therapeutic dose was huge—participants logged in on average 255 times to the program modules of cognitive behavioral therapy, e-mailed the therapist a mean of 90 times, and received 49 replies from the therapist. The results suggest that the dose of treatment is in fact a contributing factor in the response to cognitive behavioral therapy. Fourth, the response rate in the control group (usual care), which included 2 evidence-based treatments, was surprisingly poor, perhaps related to the participant's knowledge that they would be offered Internet-based treatment after 6 months. Last, the intervention was available when most needed or convenient. Internet-delivered treatments clearly appeal to adolescents.

The authors of this report do indicate that there are some difficulties with generalizability of the form of therapy described because only 30% of the world's population have Internet access (the percentage is higher in Europe, 80%, than in the United States, 58%). This disclaimer is not likely to persist at its current magnitude indefinitely, however. Also, it is necessary that parents of patients to be somewhat literate with no language barriers. The results of the trial cannot be generalized to adults who are not perhaps as Internet savvy as virtually all teens are, at least in the United States.

You can bet that a whole industry will now develop around Internet-delivered behavioral therapy for a variety of disorders, not just chronic fatigue syndrome. It would be wise to target teens in this regard because there is likely to be a greater receptivity, at least initially, to this modality of delivery.

J. A. Stockman III, MD

Reference

1. White PD, Chalder T. Chronic fatigue syndrome: treatment without a cause. *Lancet.* 2012;379:1372-1373.

Age and Gender Correlates of Pulling in Pediatric Trichotillomania

Panza KE, Pittenger C, Bloch MH (Child Study Ctr at Yale Univ, New Haven, CT)
J Am Acad Child Adolesc Psychiatry 52:241-249, 2013

Objective.—Our goals were to examine clinical characteristics and age and gender correlates in pediatric trichotillomania.

Method.—A total of 62 children (8–17 years of age) were recruited for a pediatric trichotillomania treatment trial and characterized using structured rating scales of symptoms of hairpulling and common comorbid conditions. We analyzed the association between qualitative and quantitative characteristics of pulling, comorbidities, and age and gender. We also examined the type of treatments these children previously received in the community.

Results.—We found lower rates of comorbid depression and anxiety disorders than have been reported in adult trichotillomania samples. Focused hairpulling significantly increased with age, whereas automatic pulling remained constant. Older children with hairpulling experienced more frequent urges and a decreased ability to refrain from pulling. Female participants reported greater distress and impairment associated with hairpulling, even though the severity of pulling did not differ from that of male participants.

Conclusion.—These results confirm several findings from the Children and Adolescent Trichotillomania Impact Project (CA-TIP). Our cross-sectional findings suggest there may be a developmental progress of symptoms in trichotillomania. Children appeared to develop more focused pulling, to become more aware of their urges, and to experience more frequent urges to pull, as they get older. Although these are important findings, they need to be confirmed in prospective longitudinal studies.

▶ If you look at Diagnostic and Statistical Manual of Mental Disorders IV (DSM-IV), you will see that trichotillomania (TTM) is classified as an impulse disorder that involves repetitive pulling of one's hair, which produces noticeable hair loss, distress, and impairment.[1] Somewhere between 1% and 3% of the population at some time during life exhibits this disorder, which tends to be more common in women and certainly is associated with significant physical, emotional, and functional impairment. Most cases begin in childhood. Unfortunately, there are no published, randomized, placebo-controlled trials of any pharmacologic agents for the treatment of pediatric TTM. Thus, unfortunately, our knowledge about the phenomenology and effective treatment of TTM is quite limited.

The pulling of one's hair seems to have a bimodal age of onset, and these ages occur in childhood. Very young children begin to pull before the age of 2 years, but this particular type of pulling is often limited and not associated with high degrees of psychopathology. In contrast, pulling with onset of late childhood/early adolescence (eg, 9 to 12 years) is more often chronic and, once present, often will continue without active intervention. Early-onset pulling is believed to be simply something similar to the common use of attachment objects, whereas later-onset pulling seems to occur in 2 patterns, which occur to a greater or lesser degree in most patients. Automatic pulling is habitual pulling that seems to be maintained by the sensory consequences of the behavior and often occurs out of the person's awareness. In contrast, focused pulling involves pulling that is done intentionally, often to decrease an unpleasant urge to pull or a negatively emotional experience (eg, stress, anxiety).

Although there is no known effective pharmacotherapy, there is mounting evidence that behavior therapy is effective for the treatment of TTM in adults and children. In most treatment outcome trials focusing on TTM in children, treatment has involved the core components of stimulus control and habit reversal. These procedures are designed to make pulling more difficult and to increase the patient's awareness of the behavior and give him or her something to do when he or she notices the pulling has begun or is about to begin. This particular intervention seems to work better in automatic pulling.

The report of Panza et al provides support for the notion that TTM must be understood against a developmental backdrop. The disorder and its response to treatment change across time, and researchers and clinicians should be aware of this when designing selective treatments for children with TTM.

With regard to drug therapy, although it has not been found to be effective, at least currently in children, a recent study looking at an N-acetylcysteine has found some effectiveness in adults.[2] Thus far, however, this agent has failed to produce improvements in clinical studies in children.

J. A. Stockman III, MD

References

1. American Psychiatric Association. *Diagnostic and Statistical Manual of Mental Disorders: DMS-IV—TR.* Washington, DC: American Psychiatric Association; 2000.
2. Grant JE, Odlaug BL, Kim SW. N-acetylcysteine, a glutamate modulator, in the treatment of trichotillomania: a double-blind, placebo-controlled study. *Arch Gen Psychiatry.* 2009;66:756-763.

Suicide mortality in India: a nationally representative survey

Patel V, for the Million Death Study Collaborators (The London School of Hygiene and Tropical Medicine, UK; et al)

Lancet 379:2343-2351, 2012

Background.—WHO estimates that about 170 000 deaths by suicide occur in India every year, but few epidemiological studies of suicide have been done in the country. We aimed to quantify suicide mortality in India in 2010.

Methods.—The Registrar General of India implemented a nationally representative mortality survey to determine the cause of deaths occurring between 2001 and 2003 in 1·1 million homes in 6671 small areas chosen randomly from all parts of India. As part of this survey, fieldworkers obtained information about cause of death and risk factors for suicide from close associates or relatives of the deceased individual. Two of 140 trained physicians were randomly allocated (stratified only by their ability to read the local language in which each survey was done) to independently and anonymously assign a cause to each death on the basis of electronic field reports. We then applied the age-specific and sex-specific proportion of suicide deaths in this survey to the 2010 UN estimates of absolute numbers of deaths in India to estimate the number of suicide deaths in India in 2010.

Findings.—About 3% of the surveyed deaths (2684 of 95 335) in individuals aged 15 years or older were due to suicide, corresponding to about 187 000 suicide deaths in India in 2010 at these ages (115 000 men and 72 000 women; age-standardised rates per 100 000 people aged 15 years or older of 26·3 for men and 17·5 for women). For suicide deaths at ages 15 years or older, 40% of suicide deaths in men (45 100 of 114 800) and 56% of suicide deaths in women (40 500 of 72 100) occurred at ages 15—29 years. A 15-year-old individual in India had a cumulative risk of about 1·3% of dying before the age of 80 years by suicide; men had a higher risk (1·7%) than did women (1·0%), with especially high risks in south India (3·5% in men and 1·8% in women). About half of suicide deaths were due to poisoning (mainly ingestions of pesticides).

Interpretation.—Suicide death rates in India are among the highest in the world. A large proportion of adult suicide deaths occur between the ages of 15 years and 29 years, especially in women. Public health interventions such as restrictions in access to pesticides might prevent many suicide deaths in India.

▶ The World Health Organization estimates that nearly 900 000 people worldwide die from suicide every year. This includes adolescents. This article from India is important as it provides insights into the global aspects of this problem and informs us about issues that we might not otherwise have been aware of that predispose individuals to commit suicide.

On the basis of world health estimates, India and China account for almost half of all global suicides. All low-income and middle-income countries combined account for about 85% of all suicides. This article, the first nationally representative study to estimate suicide rates in India, is an important contribution. The high estimated overall suicide rates in India of 18.6 per 100 000 boys and men and 12.7 per 100 000 girls and women, and the fact that suicide is the second most important cause of death in young adults age 15 to 29 years, parallel findings from China and confirm what has been suspected for decades: suicide is a major public health problem in low-income and middle-income countries that has not received the attention it deserves. The data from India also suggest that data collection in that country underestimates suicide in men by at least 25% and suicides in women by at least 36%. As better information about suicide in low-income and middle-income countries emerges, it is starting to challenge conventional beliefs about suicide that, up to the past decade or so, have been almost completely based on research from high-income countries, countries that account for only 15% of worldwide suicides. Studies from high-income countries typically show male-to-female suicide death rates of about 3 to 1, but we learn in India that the male-to-female suicide death ratio is about 1.5 to 1 at all ages and about the same in young adults aged 15 to 29 years. The main method of suicide in this article is poisoning, mostly from the use of organophosphate pesticides used in agriculture, as has been noted in other Asian countries. Also, suicide rates are significantly higher in rural India than they are in urban India, perhaps because of the higher availability of pesticides combined with poorer access to emergency medical care.

This article is the first study to provide national representative estimates and rates of suicide deaths in men and women in India. The findings show that suicide is an important cause of avoidable deaths in India, especially in young adults. Suicide rates for both sexes are higher in rural areas than they are in urban areas, and suicide rates vary substantially between the north and south of India. The southern states have nearly a 10 times greater age-standardized suicide rate than some of the northern states. Higher education and residency in southern India appears to be associated with an increased risk of suicide. The article also highlights that women who are widowed, divorced, or separated, compared with married women and men, have a much higher risk of suicide.

Death from suicide in India, a typical lower-income to middle-income country, occurs at about the same rate as deaths from HIV-AIDS and other typical disorders leading to death. However, unlike other causes of death, suicide attracts very little public health attention. At the same time, most Indians do not have community or other support services for the prevention of suicide and have restricted access to care for mental health illnesses. When one thinks about it, this is the exact same scenario in very low-income parts of rural United States.

Improving suicide prevention globally will require a greater understanding of why and how people decide to take their own lives in different settings. Suicide is a major public health problem that needs to be addressed sensitively by health professionals, legislators, and the media. In too many countries, India included, suicide is considered a criminal act, which only serves to put its underlying causes undercover.

J. A. Stockman III, MD

14 Newborn

Maternal deaths averted by contraceptive use: an analysis of 172 countries
Ahmed S, Li Q, Liu L, et al (Johns Hopkins Univ, Baltimore, MD)
Lancet 379:111 126, 2012

Background.—Family planning is one of the four pillars of the Safe Motherhood Initiative to reduce maternal death in developing countries. We aimed to estimate the effect of contraceptive use on maternal mortality and the expected reduction in maternal mortality if the unmet need for contraception were met, at country, regional, and world levels.

Method.—We extracted relevant data from the Maternal Mortality Estimation Inter-Agency Group (MMEIG) database, the UN World Contraceptive Use 2010 database, and the UN World Population Prospects 2010 database, and applied a counterfactual modelling approach (model I), replicating the MMEIG (WHO) maternal mortality estimation method, to estimate maternal deaths averted by contraceptive use in 172 countries. We used a second model (model II) to make the same estimate for 167 countries and to estimate the effect of satisfying unmet need for contraception. We did sensitivity analyses and compared agreement between the models.

Findings.—We estimate, using model I, that 342 203 women died of maternal causes in 2008, but that contraceptive use averted 272 040 (uncertainty interval 127 937—407 134) maternal deaths (44% reduction), so without contraceptive use, the number of maternal deaths would have been 1·8 times higher than the 2008 total. Satisfying unmet need for contraception could prevent another 104 000 maternal deaths per year (29% reduction).

Interpretation.—Numbers of unwanted pregnancies and unmet contraceptive need are still high in many developing countries. We provide evidence that use of contraception is a substantial and effective primary prevention strategy to reduce maternal mortality in developing countries.

► Whether or not one accepts contraceptives as a method for birth control based on religious or other beliefs, it is important to know about the effect of contraception from the medical outcome's point of view. The most substantial benefits of contraceptive use for the health and survival of women and children stem from reductions in the number of pregnancies, especially those that are greater than average risk to maternal, perinatal, and child survival. These risks are associated with pregnancies in the very young (< 18 years) and in the "old" (> 34 years), with maternal high parities, with short pregnancy intervals and with pregnancies that would have ended in unsafe abortion.

It has been estimated that an increase in contraceptive use of 10 percentage points reduces fertility by 0.6 births per woman, decreases the proportion of all births to women with 4 or more children by 5 percentage points, reduces births to women age 35 and older, and lowers birth intervals of less than two years by 3.5 percentage points.[1] It has been suggested that by preventing high-risk pregnancies, especially in women of high parities, and those that would have ended in unsafe abortion, increased contraceptive use has reduced the maternal mortality ratio—the risk of high maternal death per 100 000 live births—by about 26% in a little more than a decade. A further 30% of maternal deaths are said to be avoided by fulfillment of unmet needs for contraception. Most data suggest that throughout the world, the benefit of modern contraceptives to women's health outweigh the risks associated with their use. In many countries, this beneficial effect of contraception is largely the result of lengthening interpregnancy intervals. For example, in developing countries, the risk of prematurity and low birth weight doubles when conception occurs within 6 months of the previous birth. Children born within 2 years of an elder sibling are 60% more likely to die in infancy than those born more than 2 years after their sibling.

The report of Ahmed et al provides data from the Maternal Mortality Estimation Inter-Agency Group database, the United Nations' World Contraceptive Use 2010 database, and the United Nations' World Population Prospects 2010 database. From these databases, it was estimated in 2008 that 342 230 women died of natural causes, but that contraception use averted 272 040 maternal deaths, a full 44% reduction.

There does appear to be strong evidence that contraceptive use is a substantive and effective primary prevention strategy to reduce maternal mortality in developing countries. The findings from this report support increased access to contraception in countries with a low prevalence of contraceptive use, where gains in maternal mortality prevention stand to be the greatest. In such countries, reduction of unmet contraceptive need should be a major part of efforts to improve women's well-being.

While on the topic of newborn issues, there is good news coming from the US Centers for Disease Control about life expectancy in the US Hispanic population. Based on death rate data, a Hispanic newborn can expect to live for 80.6 years — a 2.5 year advantage in life expectancy over non-Hispanic whites and 7.7 years over non-Hispanic blacks.[2]

J. A. Stockman III, MD

References

1. Cleland J, Conde-Ajudelo A, Peterson H, Ross J, Tsui A. Contraception and health. *Lancet.* 2012;380:149-156.
2. Editorial comment. US life expectancy. *Lancet.* 2012;376.

Reproductive Technologies and the Risk of Birth Defects

Davies MJ, Moore VM, Willson KJ, et al (Robinson Inst, Adelaide, South Australia; et al)

N Engl J Med 366:1803-1813, 2012

Background.—The extent to which birth defects after infertility treatment may be explained by underlying parental factors is uncertain.

Methods.—We linked a census of treatment with assisted reproductive technology in South Australia to a registry of births and terminations with a gestation period of at least 20 weeks or a birth weight of at least 400 g and registries of birth defects (including cerebral palsy and terminations for defects at any gestational period). We compared risks of birth defects (diagnosed before a child's fifth birthday) among pregnancies in women who received treatment with assisted reproductive technology, spontaneous pregnancies (i.e., without assisted conception) in women who had a previous birth with assisted conception, pregnancies in women with a record of infertility but no treatment with assisted reproductive technology, and pregnancies in women with no record of infertility.

Results.—Of the 308,974 births, 6163 resulted from assisted conception. The unadjusted odds ratio for any birth defect in pregnancies involving assisted conception (513 defects, 8.3%) as compared with pregnancies not involving assisted conception (17,546 defects, 5.8%) was 1.47 (95% confidence interval [CI], 1.33 to 1.62); the multivariate-adjusted odds ratio was 1.28 (95% CI, 1.16 to 1.41). The corresponding odds ratios with in vitro fertilization (IVF) (165 birth defects, 7.2%) were 1.26 (95% CI, 1.07 to 1.48) and 1.07 (95% CI, 0.90 to 1.26), and the odds ratios with intracytoplasmic sperm injection (ICSI) (139 defects, 9.9%) were 1.77 (95% CI, 1.47 to 2.12) and 1.57 (95% CI, 1.30 to 1.90). A history of infertility, either with or without assisted conception, was also significantly associated with birth defects.

Conclusions.—The increased risk of birth defects associated with IVF was no longer significant after adjustment for parental factors. The risk of birth defects associated with ICSI remained increased after multivariate adjustment, although the possibility of residual confounding cannot be excluded. (Funded by the National Health and Medical Research Council and the Australian Research Council.)

▶ It has been known for some time that there is an association between intracytoplasmic sperm injection (ICSI) as part of in vitro fertilization (IVF) and an increased risk of birth defects. The association between the use of these techniques and birth defects appears to be stronger for single births than for multiple births. It is unclear, however, whether the excess of birth defects after IVF or ICSI may be attributed to patient characteristics related to infertility as opposed to the effects of the treatment itself and whether the risk is similar across all assisted reproductive technologies and related therapies.

These authors have attempted to sort this out by performing a population-wide cohort study examining births and pregnancies terminated because of birth defects. They assessed the risks of defects from pregnancy to a child's fifth birthday across a range of methods for treating infertility as compared with the risk associated with the pregnancy that was not assisted by reproductive technology (spontaneous pregnancy). Additionally, they assessed the risk of birth defects associated with spontaneous pregnancy among women with a previous birth with assisted contraception versus women with a documented history of infertility but no treatment at assisted reproductive technology clinics. The study was performed in Australia, where detailed records are kept at a national level. This allowed the investigators to draw very firm conclusions.

The data obtained as part of this article contained a total of 327 420 births and terminations of pregnancy. Births after any assisted contraception were associated with a significantly increased risk of birth defects (8.3%) compared with births to fertile women that did not involve assisted contraception. The risk of birth defects ran about 50% higher with assisted contraception. This increased risk occurred with both IVF and ICSI.

This observational study confirms previous findings of an increased risk of birth defects among births conceived with assisted reproductive technologies as compared with births from spontaneous conception. However, after multivariate adjustment, the association between IVF and the risk of any birth defect was no longer significant, whereas the increased risk of any birth defect associated with ICSI remained significant. When looked at in detail, the use of clomiphene citrate as a single agent used at home to increase fertility was associated with an increased risk of birth defects. This finding is consistent with prior studies. The risk of birth defects associated with other forms of minimal treatment (eg, timed intercourse, semen test, or low-dose hormonal stimulation) was not significantly different from the risk with spontaneous conception. There was a significant increased risk of birth defects associated with fresh embryo cycles but not with frozen embryo cycles. The risk of birth defects in fresh embryo cycles of IVF was also significantly lower than that in fresh embryo cycles of ICSI. The risk of a birth defect was increased among women with a history of infertility but no accompanying history of treatment with assisted reproductive technology. Significant associations between assisted contraception and birth defects were evident for single births but not multiple births.

The authors concluded that although the large majority of births resulting from assisted contraception are free of birth defects, treatment with assisted reproductive technology is associated with an increased risk of birth defects, including cerebral palsy, as compared with spontaneous conception. In the case of ICSI, but not IVF, the increased risk of birth defects persists after adjustment for maternal age and other risk factors. The authors could not rule out the possibility that other patient factors contribute to or explain the observed associations.

This is an important article for all pediatricians to read and understand because those in general practice are often called upon to provide counseling about the outcomes of pregnancy.

J. A. Stockman III, MD

Chromosomal Microarray versus Karyotyping for Prenatal Diagnosis

Wapner RJ, Martin CL, Levy B, et al (Columbia Univ Med Ctr, NY; Emory Univ School of Medicine, Atlanta, GA; et al)

N Engl J Med 367:2175-2184, 2012

Background.—Chromosomal microarray analysis has emerged as a primary diagnostic tool for the evaluation of developmental delay and structural malformations in children. We aimed to evaluate the accuracy, efficacy, and incremental yield of chromosomal microarray analysis as compared with karyotyping for routine prenatal diagnosis.

Methods.—Samples from women undergoing prenatal diagnosis at 29 centers were sent to a central karyotyping laboratory. Each sample was split in two; standard karyotyping was performed on one portion and the other was sent to one of four laboratories for chromosomal microarray.

Results.—We enrolled a total of 4406 women. Indications for prenatal diagnosis were advanced maternal age (46.6%), abnormal result on Down's syndrome screening (18.8%), structural anomalies on ultrasonography (25.2%), and other indications (9.4%). In 4340 (98.8%) of the fetal samples, microarray analysis was successful; 87.9% of samples could be used without tissue culture. Microarray analysis of the 4282 nonmosaic samples identified all the aneuploidies and unbalanced rearrangements identified on karyotyping but did not identify balanced translocations and fetal triploidy. In samples with a normal karyotype, microarray analysis revealed clinically relevant deletions or duplications in 6.0% with a structural anomaly and in 1.7% of those whose indications were advanced maternal age or positive screening results.

Conclusions.—In the context of prenatal diagnostic testing, chromosomal microarray analysis identified additional, clinically significant cytogenetic information as compared with karyotyping and was equally efficacious in identifying aneuploidies and unbalanced rearrangements but did not identify balanced translocations and triploidies. (Funded by the Eunice Kennedy Shriver National Institute of Child Health and Human Development and others; ClinicalTrials.gov number, NCT01279733.)

▶ A number of articles have appeared recently on the application of microarray technology in prenatal and reproductive genetics. These studies tell us about the complexity of such investigations, but also the power they offer along with some of the pitfalls of using the new genomic technology for clinical practice.

By way of background, chromosomal microarrays can detect almost all of the chromosomal imbalances detected with conventional cytogenetic analysis in addition to submicroscopic deletions and duplications termed copy-number variants. These variants are typically classified as benign, pathogenic, or of uncertain clinical significance. Chromosomal microarrays are recommended as the first-tier diagnostic test for the postnatal evaluation of patients with developmental delay or intellectual disability, autism spectrum disorders, or multiple congenital anomalies. Clinically significant findings have been reported in up to 15% of patients who have otherwise shown normal conventional karyotypes. In addition to providing higher resolution, the chromosomal microarray offers potential advantages over conventional karyotyping, such as automation (and therefore faster turnaround times) and elimination of the need to culture amniocytes or chorionic villi. Because microarray analysis does not require dividing cells, it is useful in cases of fetal death, when it is often not possible to culture cells. In pediatric practice, identifying a diagnosis is important to parents for many reasons, so the odds of finding a clinically significant abnormality on array may offset the downside of finding a copy-number variant of little or uncertain clinical significance. During pregnancy, the detection of a copy-number variant of uncertain clinical significance may cause considerable stress and anxiety for parents who may then consider termination of the pregnancy. This article helps us understand how to implement microarray analysis in clinical practice.

These authors compare chromosomal microarray with standard karyotyping in 4406 women undergoing prenatal diagnosis. Microarray analysis identified all the common autosomal and sex-chromosome abnormalities and the unbalanced rearrangements identified on standard karyotyping. Microdeletions or duplications of clinical significance were found in 2.5% of fetal samples with normal karyotypes, including 6% of cases in which fetal anomalies were detected on ultrasonography. There were 94 copy-numbered variants of uncertain clinical significance. Some 65% of the latter findings were deemed to be of sufficient clinical relevance to be reported to the participant in the study. With this updated information, the pathogenicity of 1.5% of copy-numbered variants detected on microarray analysis remained uncertain.

These authors tell us that they are still in the process of gauging the extent of incremental information that should be sought in the context of prenatal testing and how that information should be introduced into clinical care. Lessons learned from microarray analysis will be helpful when whole-genome sequencing of the fetus, perhaps with the use of maternal blood samples, becomes clinically available and should help to ensure the sensible application of new technology. Without question, chromosomal microarray analysis will identify additional, clinically significant cytogenetic information as compared with karyotyping and is equally efficacious in identifying other types of chromosomal abnormalities.

J. A. Stockman III, MD

Candidate gene linkage approach to identify DNA variants that predispose to preterm birth
Bream ENA, Leppellere CR, Cooper ME, et al (Univ of Iowa; Univ of Pittsburgh, PA; et al)
Pediatr Res 73:135-141, 2013

Background.—The aim of this study was to identify genetic variants contributing to preterm birth (PTB) using a linkage candidate gene approach.

Methods.—We studied 99 single-nucleotide polymorphisms (SNPs) for 33 genes in 257 families with PTBs segregating. Nonparametric and parametric analyses were used. Premature infants and mothers of premature infants were defined as affected cases in independent analyses.

Results.—Analyses with the infant as the case identified two genes with evidence of linkage: *CRHR1* ($P = 0.0012$) and *CYP2E1* ($P = 0.0011$). Analyses with the mother as the case identified four genes with evidence of linkage: *ENPP1* ($P = 0.003$), *IGFBP3* ($P = 0.006$), *DHCR7* ($P = 0.009$), and *TRAF2* ($P = 0.01$). DNA sequence analysis of the coding exons and splice sites for *CRHR1* and *TRAF2* identified no new likely etiologic variants.

Conclusion.—These findings suggest the involvement of six genes acting through the infant and/or the mother in the etiology of PTB.

▶ Anything we can learn that might diminish the probability of preterm birth is welcomed these days. Preterm birth remains a major public health issue in the United States and one of the reasons why we are not leading the world in neonatal survivorship. Preterm birth remains associated with substantial rates of morbidities, including chronic lung disease, patent ductus arteriosus, retinopathy of prematurity, intracranial hemorrhage, and cerebral palsy, particularly in extremely preterm infants. Most (70% or more) of preterm births are spontaneous and without known etiology. There are some clues, however, for this unknown etiology group. One substantial risk for preterm birth is genetic predisposition. For example, an infant has an increased risk of being born premature if the mother was born premature, if a maternal aunt had a premature infant, and especially if the mother had a prior preterm birth. Twin studies suggest that the hereditary aspect of preterm birth ranges from 15% to 40% of affected pregnancies. Other additional maternal factors resulting in spontaneous preterm birth include low socioeconomic status, black race, younger age, intrauterine infection, inflammation, low prepregnancy weight, low cholesterol levels, and substance abuse. Certain medical conditions such as preeclampsia or fetal distress of course can lead to induction of labor or cesarean delivery earlier in pregnancy than hoped for. If there are significant genetic factors related to preterm birth, most of these come from the mother's side rather than the father's.

These authors discuss one of a variety of approaches to identifying genes associated with a complex trait such as preterm birthing. They score the "candidate gene approach," which has the advantage of the known biology associated with labor and delivery, whereas a genome-wide approach implicates other physiologic pathways. There are other strong arguments for pursuing candidate gene studies and preterm birth because such studies have the ability to detect rare, high-risk variants and could identify causal genes as well.

These authors studied over 250 extended families of infants born prematurely, assaying almost 100 single-nucleotide polymorphisms for several dozen genes thought to segregate in families with preterm deliveries. Their findings suggest involvement of a very few specific genes that might play a role in preterm births. One gene in particular, *CRHR1*, looks particularly promising. Overall, the findings suggest the involvement of perhaps 6 genes acting through the infant or mother in the etiology of preterm births.

Stay tuned for further information in this regard. Obviously the occurrence of a preterm birth is a complex multifactorial issue. We will likely find out soon how much of the problem is related to our genes.

J. A. Stockman III, MD

Characteristics and outcome of brachial plexus birth palsy in neonates

Lindqvist PG, Erichs K, Molnar C, et al (Karolinska Univ Hosp, Huddinge, Stockholm, Sweden; Skåne Univ Hosp, Malmö, Sweden; Kalmar Hosp, Sweden; et al)
Acta Paediatr 101:579-582, 2012

Aim.—To relate pregnancy characteristics to extent and reversibility of brachial plexus birth palsy (BPBP) in neonates.

Methods.—Retrospective case–control study: newborns with a registered diagnosis of BPBP (n = 168) 1990–2005 were compared to data from a randomly selected control group (n = 1000). Characteristics were related to the level of injury, reversibility and outcome.

Results.—Among 51 841 newborns, 168 cases with BPBP were found (incidence 3.2/1000 newborns/year). Extent and reversibility of lesion did not differ with respect to characteristics of mothers, foetuses or deliveries. Children with C5–C6 and C5–C6–C7 injuries had complete recovery in 86% and 38%, respectively. Global injuries (C5-Th1) always had permanent disability. Accelerators (foetal weight gain > 35 g/day after 32 weeks of gestation) and foetuses with estimated weight deviation $\geq$ +22% at 32 weeks were at seven- and ninefold increased risk of BPBP. Parous women were at doubled risk as compared to nulliparous women.

Conclusion.—Maternal and foetal characteristics influence risk of BPBP, but not the extent of injury or reversibility of injury. Because of the high risk of permanent disability and modest risk of low Apgar or pH among newborns with BPBP, the recommendation of prompt delivery may need to be re-evaluated.

▶ The main cause of brachial plexus birth palsy is strain to the brachial plexus, thought to occur during the downward traction of the fetal head during delivery. The problem has also been reported to occur in utero, but that is probably extremely rare. It is not isolated to vaginal delivery alone; it has also been reported as a complication of cesarean section and it can happen during breech delivery. The clinical presentation of brachial plexus palsy is the result of damage to 2 or several of the spinal nerve roots, C5-T1. If the injury involves C5-6, the presentation is usually shoulder dysfunction and impaired elbow flexion. If it also involves C7, there will be impaired wrist, finger, and thumb extension. Injury can involve the entire brachial plexus (C5-T1), producing a global paralysis of the arm, with or without Horner syndrome. Isolated C8-T1 is extremely rare. Recovery depends on the localization of the injury. A C5-6 (C7) injury may resolve in 80% to 92% of cases, while a global lesion has a recovery of only 40%.

Risk factors for brachial plexus palsy vary. It is certainly closely related to fetal size. The larger the baby, the greater the risk. Shoulder dystocia, diabetes mellitus, the need of instrumented vaginal delivery, time required for vacuum extraction, external fundal pressure, and increased maternal body mass index are additional risk factors. The largest study of deliveries with difficulties showed that almost all brachial plexus palsies were observed in deliveries in which there was difficulty relieving the shoulders.[1]

These authors designed a study to provide additional information on risk factors as well as the outcomes of infants affected with a brachial plexus palsy. Their study was undertaken in Sweden where information was culled from the medical records of a large university hospital in Malmö. The records covered a 15-year period from 1990 through 2005. A total of 51 968 newborn records were reviewed. The incidence of this problem was found to be 3.2 of 1000 newborns per year. Of the 168 palsies, 36 were also diagnosed as having shoulder dystocia. A careful analysis revealed a number of risk factors for the development of a brachial plexus palsy. These risk factors did not differ with the extent of injury (ie, C5-6 or injuries including C7) or if the palsy ultimately was reversible. Large for gestational age infants were at a 9-fold increased risk for the development of this complication. Newborns with brachial plexus palsy were characterized by increased growth in late pregnancy, which made the predictive use of ultrasound at 32 weeks (routine in Sweden) problematic in alerting obstetricians that there may be a problem. Women who had prior pregnancies, as compared with nulliparous women, were found to be at double the risk of having a child with a brachial plexus palsy. Presumably this is because of the greater incidence of having fetuses that are large for gestational age. Data from the report showed that 86% of palsies that involved only C5-6 resolved on their own. The majority (62%) of injuries also involving C7 did not have complete recovery. In terms of other risk factors, the more force put into the downward traction of the fetal head at delivery, the higher the risk of palsy (a 0.2 of 1000 risk for low strength up to a 5% risk of injury at 80% or more of conceivable force).

The most important finding in this article is the observation that fetuses that grow disproportionately fast in the last trimester are at the greatest risk for the development of brachial plexus palsy. It is hard to say how this observation can be translated into different obstetrical care, but at least obstetricians and pediatricians are forewarned of the problem.

J. A. Stockman III, MD

Reference

1. Mollberg M, Wennergren M, Bager B, Ladfors L, Hagberg H. Obstetric brachial plexus palsy: a prospective study on risk factors related to manual assistance during the second stage of labor. *Acta Obstet Gynecol Scand.* 2007;86:198-204.

Neonatal Abstinence Syndrome and Associated Health Care Expenditures: United States, 2000-2009
Patrick SW, Schumacher RE, Benneyworth BD, et al (Univ of Michigan Health System, Ann Arbor; et al)
JAMA 307:1934-1940, 2012

Context.—Neonatal abstinence syndrome (NAS) is a postnatal drug withdrawal syndrome primarily caused by maternal opiate use. No national estimates are available for the incidence of maternal opiate use at the time of delivery or NAS.

Objectives.—To determine the national incidence of NAS and antepartum maternal opiate use and to characterize trends in national health care expenditures associated with NAS between 2000 and 2009.

Design, Setting, and Patients.—A retrospective, serial, cross-sectional analysis of a nationally representative sample of newborns with NAS. The Kids' Inpatient Database (KID) was used to identify newborns with NAS by *International Classification of Diseases, Ninth Revision, Clinical Modification (ICD-9-CM)* code. The Nationwide Inpatient Sample (NIS) was used to identify mothers using diagnosis related groups for vaginal and cesarean deliveries. Clinical conditions were identified using *ICD-9-CM* diagnosis codes. NAS and maternal opiate use were described as an annual frequency per 1000 hospital births. Missing hospital charges (< 5% of cases) were estimated using multiple imputation. Trends in health care utilization outcomes over time were evaluated using variance-weighted regression. All hospital charges were adjusted for inflation to 2009 US dollars.

Main Outcome Measures.—Incidence of NAS and maternal opiate use, and related hospital charges.

Results.—The separate years (2000, 2003, 2006, and 2009) of national discharge data included 2920 to 9674 unweighted discharges with NAS and 987 to 4563 unweighted discharges for mothers diagnosed with antepartum opiate use, within data sets including 784 191 to 1.1 million discharges for children (KID) and 816 554 to 879 910 discharges for all ages of delivering mothers (NIS). Between 2000 and 2009, the incidence of NAS among newborns increased from 1.20 (95% CI, 1.04-1.37) to 3.39 (95% CI, 3.12-3.67) per 1000 hospital births per year (P for trend < .001). Antepartum maternal opiate use also increased from 1.19 (95% CI, 1.01-1.35) to 5.63 (95% CI, 4.40-6.71) per 1000 hospital births per year (P for trend < .001). In 2009, newborns with NAS were more likely than all other hospital births to have low birthweight (19.1%; SE, 0.5%; vs 7.0%; SE, 0.2%), have respiratory complications (30.9%; SE, 0.7%; vs 8.9%; SE, 0.1%), and be covered by Medicaid (78.1%; SE, 0.8%; vs 45.5%; SE, 0.7%; all P < .001). Mean hospital charges for discharges with NAS increased from $39 400 (95% CI, $33 400-$45 400) in 2000 to $53 400 (95% CI, $49 000-$57 700) in 2009 (P for trend < .001). By 2009, 77.6% of charges for NAS were attributed to state Medicaid programs.

Conclusion.—Between 2000 and 2009, a substantial increase in the incidence of NAS and maternal opiate use in the United States was observed, as well as hospital charges related to NAS.

▶ Neonatal abstinence syndrome (NAS) is a drug withdrawal syndrome. This syndrome most commonly occurs in the context of maternal antepartum opiate use, although other drugs have also been implicated. Such illicit drug use, particularly opioid dependence during pregnancy, is also significantly associated with increased risk of adverse neonatal outcomes, such as low birth weight and high mortality. NAS is characterized by a wide array of signs and symptoms, including irritability, hypertonia, tremors, feeding intolerance, emesis, watery stools, seizures, and respiratory distress.

These authors demonstrate that the increase in NAS (from an incidence of 1.2 per 1000 hospital births per year in 2000 to 3.39 per 1000 hospital births per year in 2009) has created a health care problem primarily for state Medicaid budgets. In a number of states, methadone treatment programs have had to expand rapidly. The cost burden to many states has caused them to begin to cut back on services. This poses a crisis of care for affected fetuses and newborns. These investigators also observed that over the past decade there has been no improvement in NAS treatment efficacy as measured by hospital length of stay for newborns. Some 60% to 80% of infants exposed in utero to opiates will develop NAS and require prolonged hospitalization, averaging 16 days. As part of the management of NAS, most neonatologists use oral opiate medication such as methadone or morphine and, in difficult cases a second line nonopiate drug containing gamma-aminobutyric acid (eg, phenobarbital), benzodiazepine (eg, clonazepam), or an antiadrenergic (eg, clonidine). Neonatal withdrawal status is monitored every few hours after birth by nursing personnel in most centers using the Finnegan scoring system, a clinical measure that rates sleep, movement, and feeding difficulty, as well as signs of opiate withdrawal similar to those established for withdrawing adults, such as yawning, tremors, and watery stools. Currently, this is the best method of diagnosing NAS, evaluating severity, and titrating drug dosage changes during weaning of neuropharmacologic agents. Everyone agrees that these approaches are less than adequate.

These authors tell us that future directions in NAS research must address the need for clinical trials of new medications to establish optimal protocols for maternal opiate dependence, with particular focus on methadone treatment induction of the mother early in pregnancy, maternal adherence to treatment, ancillary alcohol use monitoring, and psychiatric care. Postnatally, early identification and aggressive opiate replacement in infants with early signs of NAS may help decrease severity and hospital length of stay. This article and other studies indicate that breastfeeding may reduce treatment and length of stay in opiate-exposed infants. Better management of opiate dependency during pregnancy will also be of help.

J. A. Stockman III, MD

Association Between Hospital Recognition for Nursing Excellence and Outcomes of Very Low-Birth-Weight Infants
Lake ET, Staiger D, Horbar J, et al (Univ of Pennsylvania, Philadelphia; Dartmouth College, Hanover, NH; Univ of Vermont and Vermont Oxford Network, Burlington; et al)
JAMA 307:1709-1716, 2012

Context.—Infants born at very low birth weight (VLBW) require high levels of nursing intensity. The role of nursing in outcomes for these infants in the United States is not known.

Objective.—To examine the relationships between hospital recognition for nursing excellence (RNE) and VLBW infant outcomes.

Design, Setting, and Patients.—Cohort study of 72 235 inborn VLBW infants weighing 501 to 1500 g born in 558 Vermont Oxford Network hospital neonatal intensive care units between January 1, 2007, and December 31, 2008. Hospital RNE was determined from the American Nurses Credentialing Center. The RNE designation is awarded when nursing care achieves exemplary practice or leadership in 5 areas.

Main Outcome Measures.—Seven-day, 28-day, and hospital stay mortality; nosocomial infection, defined as an infection in blood or cerebrospinal fluid culture occurring more than 3 days after birth; and severe (grade 3 or 4) intraventricular hemorrhage.

Results.—Overall, the outcome rates were as follows: for 7-day mortality, 7.3% (5258/71 955); 28-day mortality, 10.4% (7450/71 953); hospital stay mortality, 12.9% (9278/71 936); severe intraventricular hemorrhage, 7.6% (4842/63 525); and infection, 17.9% (11 915/66 496). The 7-day mortality was 7.0% in RNE hospitals and 7.4% in non-RNE hospitals (adjusted odds ratio [OR], 0.87; 95% CI, 0.76-0.99; $P = .04$). The 28-day mortality was 10.0% in RNE hospitals and 10.5% in non-RNE hospitals (adjusted OR, 0.90; 95% CI, 0.80-1.01; $P = .08$). Hospital stay mortality was 12.4% in RNE hospitals and 13.1% in non-RNE hospitals (adjusted OR, 0.90; 95% CI, 0.81-1.01; $P = .06$). Severe intraventricular hemorrhage was 7.2% in RNE hospitals and 7.8% in non-RNE hospitals (adjusted OR, 0.88; 95% CI, 0.77-1.00; $P = .045$). Infection was 16.7% in RNE hospitals and 18.3% in non-RNE hospitals (adjusted OR, 0.86; 95% CI, 0.75-0.99; $P = .04$). Compared with RNE hospitals, the adjusted absolute decrease in risk of outcomes in RNE hospitals ranged from 0.9% to 2.1%. All 5 outcomes were jointly significant ($P < .001$). The mean effect across all 5 outcomes was OR, 0.88 (95% CI, 0.83-0.94; $P < .001$). In a subgroup of 68 253 infants with gestational age of 24 weeks or older, the ORs for RNE for all 3 mortality outcomes and infection were statistically significant.

Conclusion.—Among VLBW infants born in RNE hospitals compared with non-RNE hospitals, there was a significantly lower risk-adjusted rate of 7-day mortality, nosocomial infection, and severe intraventricular hemorrhage but not of 28-day mortality or hospital stay mortality.

▶ Everyone knows that preterm infants and those otherwise with very low birth weight, if born at an institution with a level III neonatal intensive care unit (NICU), will do better than those born at lower-level facilities. What is not known, however, is what the specific components are of the quality of care provided within these NICUs that determine the improved survival rate. This is what these authors have examined in detail. These investigators studied a 2-year cohort (2007 to 2008) of more than 72 000 very low birth weight (< 1500 g) infants born in 558 hospitals in the Vermont Oxford Network, comparing hospitals that have earned the American Nurses Credentialing Center Recognition for Nursing Excellence (RNE) with non-RNE hospitals within the network. After adjusting for patient, neonatal intensive care unit, and hospital characteristics, the authors found that RNE hospitals, compared with non-RNE hospitals, had lower percentages of mortality within 7 days after birth (7.0% vs 7.4%) and nosocomial infections more than 3 days after birth (16.7% vs 18.3%) among very low birth weight infants. The odds of mortality within 7 days of birth (odds ratio 0.87) and of nosocomial infection (odds ratio 0.86) were slightly but statistically significantly lower in RNE versus non-RNE hospitals. Nonsignificant differences in the odds of 28-day mortality (10.0% vs 10.5%; odds ratio 0.90), predischarge mortality (12.4% vs 13.1%; odds ratio 0.9), and severe intraventricular hemorrhage (7.2% vs 7.8%; odds ratio 0.88) were found between RNE and non-RNE hospitals.

Interestingly, although the findings from this article are important for all of us to know, the benefits of being born in an RNE hospital did not appear as large as might be expected. In an editorial that accompanied this article by Barfield,[1] it was noted that this may be because all hospitals in this study, both RNE and non-RNE, voluntarily participated in quality improvement activities through the Vermont Oxford Network, a collaborative of hospitals with NICUs that focus on improving the quality of care to newborns, particularly very low birth weight infants. Non-RNE hospitals that participate in the network may have high quality standards within their NICUs, but do not meet hospital-wide provision for RNE, thus potentially reducing the independent effect of better neonatal intensive care.

The authors of this article suggest that the components of hospital RNE, including exemplary professional practice, structural empowerment, new knowledge, transformational leadership, and empirical outcomes, help these hospitals to achieve high-quality care and decreased infant mortality and severe morbidity. It is proposed that these principles may not only make better nurses, but also better physicians, respiratory therapists, laboratory technicians, social workers, and hospital executives. Recognition, therefore, for nursing excellence status may serve as a proxy for a hospital's commitment for improving quality of care and providing available resources for this purpose.

For more on this topic of the association between hospital recognition and outcomes of low birth weight infants, see the editorial of Barfield,[1] who notes that to date, the discourse on perinatal regionalization has been focused mostly on quantity, not quality. In fact there appears to be an inverse relationship between the number of intensive care units and the quality of care they provide. For example, the number of NICUs and neonatologists throughout the United States continues to increase with little correlation to the numbers of very low birth weight infants. Also, a study of all 50 states and the District of Columbia to identify state certificate of need legislation (a mechanism that regulates the construction and expansion of NICU facilities) found a strong inverse association between certificate of need programs and the number of facilities. Specifically, noncertificate of need states are associated with more NICU facilities by a factor of 2-fold as well as more neonatal intensive care beds, also by a factor of 2-fold. At the same time, noncertificate of need states appear to have higher infant mortality for all birth weight groups. The editorial also notes that there seems to be little more that can be done in the very first day of life to reduce neonatal mortality, and therefore, until a way is found to prevent prematurity and low birth weight, we will continue to push against the tide of problems created for these tiny infants.

J. A. Stockman III, MD

Reference

1. Barfield WD. Improving systems in perinatal care: quality, not quantity. *JAMA.* 2012;307:1750-1751.

Follow-up of Neonates With Total Serum Bilirubin Levels ≥25 mg/dL: A Danish Population-Based Study

Vandborg PK, Hansen BM, Greisen G, et al (Aarhus Univ Hosp, Aalborg, Denmark; Copenhagen Univ Hosp, Denmark)
Pediatrics 130:61-66, 2012

Objective.—To study if severe hyperbilirubinemia in infants with no or minor neurologic symptoms in the neonatal period affects children's development at the age of 1 to 5 years.

Methods.—Controlled descriptive follow-up study of a national cohort of Danish children. The exposed group consisted of all live-born infants in Denmark from 2004 to 2007 with a gestational age ≥35 weeks and severe hyperbilirubinemia in the neonatal period, defined as at least 1 measure of total serum bilirubin level ≥25 mg/dL during the first 3 weeks of life. The exposed group of 206 children was matched with a control group of 208 children. The Ages and Stages Questionnaire (ASQ), a method of evaluating the child's development, was filled in by parents. Main outcome measure was effect size of ASQ total score. Statistical analyses comprised a matched analysis of 102 pairs and a nonmatched regression analysis of all participants.

Results.—The response rate was 79% ($n = 162$ of 206) in the study group and 70% ($n = 146$ of 208) in the control group. Neither the matched nor the nonmatched analysis showed any statistically significant differences between the groups; the effect size of the total score was 0.04 (−0.24 to 0.32) and −0.04 (−0.26 to 0.19), respectively.

Conclusions.—Using the parent-completed ASQ, we found no evidence of developmental delay in children aged between 1 and 5 years with severe neonatal hyperbilirubinemia compared with a matched control group.

▶ This article emanates from Denmark. It reminds us that acute bilirubin encephalopathy can be divided into 3 phases: early, intermediate, and advanced. The early phase is characterized by lethargy, hypotonia, and decreased feeding; the intermediate phase is characterized by alternating tonus, irritability, high-pitched cry, retrocollis, and opisthotonus; and the advanced phase is characterized by sun setting, seizures, coma, and eventually death. What has remained controversial is whether infants with severe or extreme hyperbilirubinemia presenting with minor or no neurologic symptoms in the neonatal period might develop more subtle brain injury, causing developmental problems later.

These authors designed a study to assess the developmental status of term and late preterm infants with severe and extreme neonatal hyperbilirubinemia (total serum bilirubin level greater than 25 mg/dL with no symptoms or advanced bilirubin encephalopathy in the neonatal period) compared with a matched control group. They were able to examine data for more than one-quarter of a million live-born infants during a study period from January 1, 2004, through December 31, 2007, in Denmark. In that country, the Danish National Patient Registry collates information on a wide variety of clinical diagnoses. During the study period, 258 infants with gestational age greater than 35 weeks with a total serum bilirubin level greater than 25 mg/dL were identified, equivalent to an incidence of 103 of 100 000 newborns. In this group, the median total serum bilirubin level was 26 mg/dL and the median time to the peak level was 4 days. The children included in the analysis had either no neurologic symptoms or only early acute bilirubin encephalopathy. The authors found no evidence of a general effect on the development in children exposed to severe and extreme hyperbilirubin levels in comparison with a control group. The findings were based on parent completion of the Ages and Stages Questionnaire, a method of evaluating a child's development

If the data from this report hold up, clinicians can now inform parents of newborns who develop bilirubin levels in excess of 25 mg/dL that if their infant has no clinical symptomatology in the neonatal period, chances are extremely good that their overall development later in infancy and childhood will be normal. This is a very important finding.

J. A. Stockman III, MD

Glucose-6-Phosphate Dehydrogenase Deficiency and Borderline Deficiency: Association with Neonatal Hyperbilirubinemia
Riskin A, Gery N, Kugelman A, et al (Technion-Israel Inst of Technology, Haifa)
J Pediatr 161:191-196, 2012

Objective.—To characterize the occurrence of glucose-6-phosphate dehydrogenase (G6PD) deficiency and its association with neonatal hyperbilirubinemia.

Study Design.—This study involved an evaluation of G6PD data for 2656 newborns from a universal newborn screening program.

Results.—Mean G6PD activity was 14.2 ± 3.3 U/g Hb. Some 2.71% of the newborns were G6PD-deficient, and 1.77% had borderline G6PD activity, with male and female predominance, respectively. G6PD deficiency was more prevalent in newborns of Sephardic Jew and Muslim Arab backgrounds. The infants with G6PD deficiency had higher bilirubin levels at the time of discharge from the nursery. Infants with low and borderline G6PD activity were more likely to require phototherapy (22.2% and 25.5%, respectively, vs 7.6% of infants with normal G6PD activity; $P < .005$) and to have more referrals for exacerbation of jaundice (15.3% and 14.9%, respectively, vs 6.1%; $P < .005$). Mean G6PD activity was higher in preterm infants born at 27-34 weeks gestational age compared with those born later (16.3 ± 1.8 U/g Hb vs 14.8 ± 2.0 U/g Hb). Based on sex distribution and theoretical genetic calculations for the rate of heterozygous females, we propose that the range of borderline G6PD activity should be 2-10 U/g Hb rather than the currently accepted range of 2-7 U/g Hb.

Conclusions.—There is association between G6PD deficiency and significant neonatal hyperbilirubinemia. Increased risk is also associated with borderline G6PD activity. The suggested new range for borderline G6PD activity should enhance the identification of females at risk. G6PD activity is higher in preterm infants (Fig 1).

▶ There is not a primary care physician in practice who is not familiar with the various causes of neonatal hyperbilirubinemia. In its most simplistic form, elevated bilirubin levels in the newborn are the result of an imbalance between the production and conjugation of bilirubin. The risk for development of high bilirubin levels involves a delicate balance between the rate of hemolysis and the rate of conjugation of bilirubin.

These authors recognized that glucose-6-phosphate dehydrogenase (G6PD) deficiency is an important cause of severe neonatal hyperbilirubinemia, which can lead to the development of kernicterus. They evaluated G6PD levels in newborns with a variety of demographic characteristics including, but not limited to, race, ethnicity, and sex in an attempt to determine what level of G6PD activity might be associated with hyperbilirubinemia in both preterm and term infants. More than 2500 newborns were studied. Correlations were made between bilirubin levels and G6PD levels: 2.71% of the newborns were found to be G6PD deficient, and 1.77% had borderline G6PD activity. Because the study was performed in Israel, differences in G6PD activity could be studied among various subgroups of both Jewish newborns and Muslim Arab newborns. Fig 1 shows the distribution of G6PD activities by sex and documents the differences between male and female infants. G6PD deficiency (G6PD < 2.0 U/gHb) was most

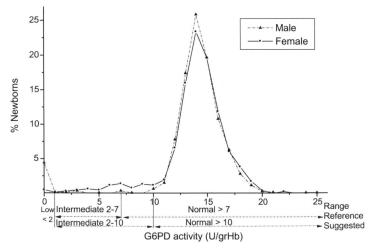

FIGURE 1.—Distribution of G6PD activities by sex. The proportion of females:males in the intermediate G6PD using the reference range (2.00-6.99 U/g Hb) was 4.87:1.00. This proportion increased to 6.00:1.00 using the suggested intermediate range (2.00-9.99 U/g Hb). This is because the proportion of females:males in the added G6PD range (7.00-9.99 U/g Hb) was 7.50:1.00. (Reprinted Journal Pediatrics. Riskin A, Gery N, Kugelman A, et al. Glucose-6-phosphate dehydrogenase deficiency and borderline deficiency: association with neonatal hyperbilirubinemia. *J Pediatr.* 2012;161:191-196, Copyright 2012, with permission from Elsevier.)

prevalent in males born to mothers of Sephardic Jew and Muslim Arab origin (10.7% and 6.2%, respectively), compared with 1.0% in Ashkenazi Jews, 10.6% in Christian Arabs, and 0% in Ethiopian Jews and Druze Arabs.

The *G6PD* gene, of course, is X linked. Females, as opposed to males, can be either homozygous, with both *G6PD* genes either normal or deficient or heterozygous with only 1 mutant gene. In the latter case, based on the Lyon hypothesis of X inactivation, we would expect 2 populations of red blood cells—1 in which the normal X was inactivated and 1 in which the mutant X was inactivated. In this report, had inactivation occurred, 50% of the red blood cells would have had normal G6PD activity and the total G6PD level would have been in the intermediate range. However, inactivation is not always random and some clones might be preferred over others, resulting in 3 possible phenotypes for heterozygous females: normal, intermediate, and low G6PD activity. On average, up to 10% of heterozygous females have normal G6PD activity, 10% have low activity, and 80% have intermediate or borderline activity. Thus, even female infants can develop hyperbilirubinemia on the basis of variations in G6PD activity.

It should be recognized that G6PD activity is normally higher in newborns than in older children and adults, mainly because of the large number of immature red blood cells and reticulocytes, which are known to have greater G6PD activity in normal newborns, compared with the more mature cells of older infants and children. Even higher levels of G6PD activity are known to be associated with being born preterm. The higher G6PD activity seen in preterm infants raises the question of whether the ranges of values indicating deficient and borderline G6PD activity should be raised accordingly. Such a change might have implications, especially in defining those at risk for significant neonatal hyperbilirubinemia. If we make such an adjustment, the prevalence of borderline or deficient G6PD activity as reported in this article would have actually been higher in preterm infants than in term infants.

If there is a bottom line to this study, it is that there is an increased risk of hyperbilirubinemia associated with borderline G6PD activities, and we should consider a new range for borderline G6PD activities based on the data from this article, particularly in female babies. It should be noted that another article that appeared recently from Israel also showed that accurate identification of G6PD-deficient states could be made despite the high normal neonatal G6PD values observed at this young age.[1]

J. A. Stockman III, MD

Reference

1. Algur N, Avraham I, Hammerman C, Kaplan M. Quantitative neonatal glucose-6-phosphate dehydrogenase screening: distribution, reference values, and classification by phenotype. *J Pediatr.* 2012;161:197-200.

Clinical Sepsis in Neonates and Young Infants, United States, 1988-2006

Lukacs SL, Schrag SJ (Ctrs for Disease Control and Prevention, Hyattsville, MD; Ctrs for Disease Control and Prevention, Atlanta, GA)
J Pediatr 160:960-965.e1, 2012

Objective.—To describe the burden and characteristics of clinical neonatal sepsis in the United States and evaluate incidence rates after the issuance of intrapartum antibiotic prophylaxis (IAP) guidelines.

Study Design.—This is a cross-sectional study of hospitalizations of infants aged <3 months diagnosed with sepsis from the 1988-2006 National Hospital Discharge Survey. The National Hospital Discharge Survey collects data annually on inpatient discharges from a national probability sample of approximately 500 short-stay hospitals. We examined sepsis hospitalizations, defined by *International Classification of Diseases, Ninth Revision, Clinical Modification* codes, and compared sepsis hospitalization rates for 2 time periods after the issuance of IAP guidelines (1996-2001 and 2002-2006) with 1988-1995 using national natality data as the population denominator. We used Joinpoint (Surveillance Research Program, National Cancer Institute, Bethesda, Maryland) regression to assess the average annual percent change (AAPC) in rates.

Results.—Between 1988 and 2006, there were more than 2.5 million sepsis-related hospitalizations in infants aged <3 months (112 000-146 000 annually). In 2006, the sepsis hospitalization rate was 30.8/1000 births. The rate was more than 3 times higher in preterm infants compared with term infants (85.4/1000 preterm births vs 23.1/1000 term births). The AAPC in sepsis hospitalization rate was -3.6% (95% CI, -2.1% to 5.1%) for term infants during 1996-2002 and did not change significantly after issuance of the revised 2002 guidelines. For preterm infants, the AAPC was -1.2% (95% CI, -2.2% to 0.1%) annually from 1988 to 2006.

Conclusion.—Clinical neonatal sepsis declined in the post-IAP era, mirroring trends observed in group B streptococcal early-onset neonatal sepsis surveillance. Preterm infants were affected disproportionately and exhibited a modest but steady decline in sepsis hospitalization rate.

▶ All of us know there have been changes over time in the organisms that cause clinical sepsis in neonates and young infants. Unfortunately, in most infants treated for sepsis, a pathogen is not isolated and a diagnosis is based on a combination of clinical signs and other laboratory testing. Recent trends in clinical sepsis (physician-diagnosed sepsis lacking culture confirmation) have not been described and might not mirror the trends observed for proven invasive sepsis. Indeed, trends in clinical sepsis likely have changed over the past 20 or more years as a result of changes in clinical practice. For example, guidelines recommending intrapartum antibiotic prophylaxis (IAP) to prevent group B streptococcus (GBS) and neonatal sepsis were issued in the mid-1990s and were revised in 2002. There has been a greater than 80% decline in the incidence of culture-confirmed early-onset GBS infections over a 15-year period, with the most dramatic decline occurring between 1996 and 1999. Of some concern is the fact that with the widespread use of IAP, there may now be a potential increase in false-negative neonatal blood cultures, resulting from intrapartum antibiotic exposure, and in neonatal sepsis caused by pathogens other than GBS.

These authors provide further insights into the current neonatal sepsis burden and recent incidence trends by examining sepsis-associated hospitalizations in young infants in the United States between 1988 and 2006, utilizing data from the National Center for Health Statistics National Hospital Discharge Survey, a representative survey of discharges from the nation's nonfederal, short-stay hospitals. Data from this article show that between 1988 and 2006, there were an estimated 2.5 million sepsis hospitalizations in newborns and infants under 3 months of age, one-third of which were preterm infants. Nearly 60% of the sepsis hospitalizations for term infants were in the early-onset group. Among the 12% of sepsis hospitalizations that had a proven pathogen, 38% were due to *Streptococcus* spp (9% identified as GBS), 26% due to *Staphylococcus* spp, and 31% due to gram-negative bacteria (23% *Escherichia coli*). Hospitalizations for neonatal sepsis for term infants decreased by approximately 4% annually immediately after the issuance of the initial IAP guidelines to prevent GBS sepsis. No further decline was observed after issuance of the revised IAP guidelines. The stabilization of sepsis rates and the lack of decline in the second post-IAP time period are not surprising, given the smaller predicted impact of the 2002 recommendations on invasive GBS disease (a 32% further decline in incidence, from 0.5 to 0.3 cases per 1000 live births) compared with the impact of the 1996 guidelines.

Unfortunately, there is no national surveillance system for clinical sepsis syndromes in young infants. This article, however, should suffice for this purpose. Clearly the IAP recommendations have made a major impact on the prevalence of sepsis in the United States.

J. A. Stockman III, MD

Respiratory Function in Healthy Late Preterm Infants Delivered at 33-36 Weeks of Gestation

McEvoy C, Venigalla S, Schilling D, et al (Oregon Health and Science Univ, Portland)
J Pediatr 162:464-469, 2013

Objective.—To compare pulmonary function testing including respiratory compliance (Crs) and time to peak tidal expiratory flow to expiratory time (TPTEF:TE) at term corrected age in healthy infants born at 33-36 weeks of gestation versus healthy infants delivered at term.

Study Design.—We performed a prospective cohort study of late preterm infants born at 33-36 weeks without clinical respiratory disease (<12 hours of >0.21 fraction of inspired oxygen) and studied at term corrected age. The comparison group was term infants matched for race and sex to the preterm infants and studied within 72 hours of delivery. Crs was measured with the single breath occlusion technique. A minimum of 50 flow-volume loops were collected to estimate TPTEF:TE.

Results.—Late preterm infants (n = 31; mean gestational age 34.1 weeks, birth weight 2150 g) and 31 term infants were studied at term corrected age. The late preterm infants had decreased Crs (1.14 vs 1.32 mL/cm H_2O/kg; $P < .02$) and decreased TPTEF:TE (0.308 vs 0.423; $P < .01$) when compared with the term infants. Late preterm infants also had an increased respiratory resistance (0.064 vs 0.043 cm H_2O/mL/s; $P < .01$).

Conclusions.—Healthy late preterm infants (33-36 weeks of gestation) studied at term corrected age have altered pulmonary function when compared with healthy term infants.

▶ It is well known that preterm birth and the complications related to early delivery can affect long-term pulmonary function. Alveolarization in the human lung occurs in the third trimester of gestation and, therefore, preterm delivery, without any clinical signs of respiratory distress, can affect lung structure and development. Changes in bronchial muscle, collagen, and elastin have been reported in preterm infants later in life. Studies examining premature infants clearly have demonstrated altered airway and alveolar development in the first decade of life.[1]

These authors designed a study to evaluate respiratory function in an otherwise healthy group of late preterm infants born in Portland, Oregon. Using sophisticated pulmonary function testing assessment instruments, studies were undertaken at 40 weeks' postmenstrual age for both a late preterm and a term control group. The most striking finding in this article was a 33% higher respiratory resistance in the preterm group at comparable weights. Unfortunately, there were no follow-up data, so it is not possible to speculate on whether the observed changes would have long-lasting structural and functional impact later in life.

In an editorial that accompanied this report, Martin et al[2] remind us there is no doubt that very low birth weight infants are at greater risk of later wheezing disorders, and this is aggravated by the presence of bronchopulmonary dysplasia (BPD). Even healthy late preterm infants now have been shown to have significantly decreased passive resistance compliances and respiratory flow ratios compared with term infants matched for race and sex, setting such infants up for all sorts of problems, including wheezing disorders, later in infancy and childhood. The results of this study suggest that preterm infants may have delayed or abnormal pulmonary development compared with term infants and, thus, may be at greater risk for later pulmonary difficulties.

J. A. Stockman III, MD

References

1. Hoo AF, Dezateux C, Henschen M, Costeloe K, Stocks J. Development of airway function in infancy after preterm delivery. *J Pediatr.* 2002;141:652-658.
2. Martin RJ, Prakash YS, Hibbs AM. Why do former preterm infants wheeze? *J Pediatr.* 2013;162:443-444.

Childhood Outcomes after Hypothermia for Neonatal Encephalopathy

Shankaran S, for the Eunice Kennedy Shriver NICHD Neonatal Research Network (Wayne State Univ, Detroit, MI; et al)

N Engl J Med 366:2085-2092, 2012

Background.—We previously reported early results of a randomized trial of whole-body hypothermia for neonatal hypoxic—ischemic encephalopathy showing a significant reduction in the rate of death or moderate or severe disability at 18 to 22 months of age. Long-term outcomes are now available.

Methods.—In the original trial, we assigned infants with moderate or severe encephalopathy to usual care (the control group) or whole-body cooling to an esophageal temperature of 33.5°C for 72 hours, followed by slow rewarming (the hypothermia group). We evaluated cognitive, attention and executive, and visuospatial function; neurologic outcomes; and physical and psychosocial health among participants at 6 to 7 years of age. The primary outcome of the present analyses was death or an IQ score below 70.

Results.—Of the 208 trial participants, primary outcome data were available for 190. Of the 97 children in the hypothermia group and the 93 children in the control group, death or an IQ score below 70 occurred in 46 (47%) and 58 (62%), respectively ($P = 0.06$); death occurred in 27 (28%) and 41 (44%) ($P = 0.04$); and death or severe disability occurred in 38 (41%) and 53 (60%) ($P = 0.03$). Other outcome data were available for the 122 surviving children, 70 in the hypothermia group and 52 in the control group. Moderate or severe disability occurred in 24 of 69 children (35%) and 19 of 50 children (38%), respectively ($P = 0.87$). Attention—executive dysfunction occurred in 4% and 13%, respectively, of children receiving hypothermia and those receiving usual care ($P = 0.19$), and visuospatial dysfunction occurred in 4% and 3% ($P = 0.80$).

Conclusions.—The rate of the combined end point of death or an IQ score of less than 70 at 6 to 7 years of age was lower among children undergoing whole-body hypothermia than among those undergoing usual care, but the differences were not significant. However, hypothermia resulted in lower death rates and did not increase rates of severe disability among survivors. (Funded by the National Institutes of Health and the Eunice Kennedy Shriver NICHD Neonatal Research Network; ClinicalTrials.gov number, NCT00005772.)

▶ The authors of this article have previously studied the effects of hypothermia as part of the management of neonatal encephalopathy. They showed that hypothermia to 33°C to 34°C for 72 hours, when initiated within 6 hours after birth among infants of more than 35 weeks gestation with hypoxic-ischemic encephalopathy, would reduce the risk of death or disability and increase the rate of survival free of disability at 18 to 24 months of age. In their earlier report of a randomized, controlled trial of whole-body hypothermia for neonatal hypoxic-ischemic encephalopathy, the rate of death or moderate to severe disability at 18 to 22 months was 62% in the control group versus 44% in the hypothermia group, with mortality of 37% and 24%, respectively.[1] As compared with the control group, there was no significant increase in major disability among survivors in the hypothermia group; the rates of moderate or severe cerebral palsy grew 30% in the control group versus 19% in the hypothermia group, with corresponding rates of blindness of 14% versus 7% and hearing impairment of 6% versus 4%. However, longer-term data have not been available previously to assess whether the benefits of hypothermia for neonatal hypoxic-ischemic encephalopathy persist after 2 years of age.

In order to fill in some of the gaps in our understanding of the long-term effects of hypothermia, these authors designed this study to assess rates of death, cognitive impairment, and other neurodevelopmental and behavioral outcomes associated with whole-body hypothermia at 6 to 7 years of age, at which time outcomes of neonatal intervention are believed to be much more definitive. Newborns were recruited between July 2000 and May 2003 and were eligible if they had either moderate or severe encephalopathy within 6 hours after birth, with severe acidosis or resuscitation at birth and after an acute perinatal event. Infants were randomly assigned to undergo either whole-body hypothermia at 33.5°C for 72 hours or to usual care. All surviving children were then evaluated at 6 to 7 years of age. IQ scores were measured with the use of the Wechsler Preschool and Primary Scale of Intelligence III in the 96 children under 7 years 3 months of age, and the Wechsler Intelligent Scale for Children IV was used for older children. These tests assess verbal comprehension, perceptual organization, and processing speed, yielding verbal and performance IQ scores that are combined to give a full-scale IQ score with a mean score of 100 ± 15 being normal. Higher cognitive function including attention and executive function and visuospatial processing were evaluated by means of the Developmental Neuropsychological Assessment, on which a score of 100 ± 15 is normal.

In this study, when assessing children at 6 to 7 years of age, the difference in rates of composite outcomes of death or IQ score below 70 between the hypothermia and the usual care groups did not achieve statistical significance; however, the previous finding of reduced mortality with hypothermia was maintained, with no appreciable increase in the risk of neurodevelopmental deficients among survivors. These results are reassuring since hypothermia is being used extensively around the world and currently is recommended by health policymakers. The 2010 American Heart Association guidelines for pulmonary resuscitation state that during the postresuscitation period in neonates who are 36 weeks' gestational age or older with progressing moderate to severe encephalopathy, hypothermia should be offered in the context of clearly defined protocols similar to those used in published clinical trials. This study found a nonsignificant decrease (from 29% to 20%) in the rate of moderate or severe cerebral palsy in the hypothermia group compared with the control group. The authors did not find a decrease in the risk of abnormalities in motor function among the nondisabled children in the hypothermia group as compared with those in the control group.

It should be noted that the significant difference in the rate of the primary outcome between the hypothermia group and the control group seen in the authors' earlier report at 18 to 22 months of age and the borderline significant difference in the rate of this outcome at 6 to 7 years of age in the current report are largely driven by deaths, mainly occurring within the first 18 months of life. A concern with any therapy that reduces mortality among infants at high risk of death and disability is the possibility of an increase in the number of children who survive with disabilities. As reported here, there is no evidence of increased risk of IQ score below 70, severe disability, or cerebral palsy at 6 to 7 years of age among surviving children treated with hypothermia. Thus, our nurseries will likely continue to follow existing recommendations regarding the institution of hypothermia as part of the management of neonatal encephalopathy.

J. A. Stockman III, MD

Reference

1. Shankaran S, Laptook AR, Ehrenkranz RA, et al. Whole-body hypothermia for neonates with hypoxic-ischemic encephalopathy. *N Engl J Med.* 2005;353: 1575-1584.

15 Nutrition and Metabolism

Effects of Promoting Longer-term and Exclusive Breastfeeding on Adiposity and Insulin-like Growth Factor-I at Age 11.5 Years: A Randomized Trial

Martin RM, Patel R, Kramer MS, et al (Univ of Bristol, England, UK; McGill Univ Faculty of Medicine, Montréal, Québec, Canada; et al)

JAMA 309:1005-1013, 2013

Importance.—Evidence that longer-term and exclusive breastfeeding reduces child obesity risk is based on observational studies that are prone to confounding.

Objective.—To investigate effects of an intervention to promote increased duration and exclusivity of breastfeeding on child adiposity and circulating insulin-like growth factor (IGF)-I, which regulates growth.

Design, Setting, and Participants.—Cluster-randomized controlled trial in 31 Belarusian maternity hospitals and their affiliated clinics, randomized into 1 of 2 groups: breastfeeding promotion intervention (n = 16) or usual practices (n = 15). Participants were 17 046 breastfeeding mother-infant pairs enrolled in 1996 and 1997, of whom 13 879 (81.4%) were followed up between January 2008 and December 2010 at a median age of 11.5 years.

Intervention.—Breastfeeding promotion intervention modeled on the WHO/UNICEF Baby-Friendly Hospital Initiative (World Health Organization/United Nations Children's Fund).

Main Outcome Measures.—Body mass index (BMI), fat and fat-free mass indices (FMI and FFMI), percent body fat, waist circumference, triceps and subscapular skinfold thicknesses, overweight and obesity, and whole-blood IGF-I. Primary analysis was based on modified intention-to-treat (without imputation), accounting for clustering within hospitals and clinics.

Results.—The experimental intervention substantially increased breastfeeding duration and exclusivity when compared with the control (43% vs 6% exclusively breast-fed at 3 months and 7.9% vs 0.6% at 6 months). Cluster-adjusted mean differences in outcomes at 11.5 years of age between experimental vs control groups were: 0.19 (95% CI, −0.09 to 0.46) for BMI; 0.12 (−0.03 to 0.28) for FMI; 0.04 (−0.11 to 0.18) for FFMI; 0.47% (−0.11% to 1.05%) for percent body fat; 0.30 cm (−1.41 to 2.01) for waist circumference; −0.07 mm (−1.71 to 1.57) for triceps and −0.02 mm (−0.79 to 0.75) for subscapular skinfold thicknesses; and

−0.02 standard deviations (−0.12 to 0.08) for IGF-I. The cluster-adjusted odds ratio for overweight/obesity (BMI ≥85th vs <85th percentile) was 1.18 (95% CI, 1.01 to 1.39) and for obesity (BMI ≥95th vs <85th percentile) was 1.17 (95% CI, 0.97 to 1.41).

Conclusions and Relevance.—Among healthy term infants in Belarus, an intervention that succeeded in improving the duration and exclusivity of breastfeeding did not prevent overweight or obesity, nor did it affect IGF-I levels at age 11.5 years. Breastfeeding has many advantages but population strategies to increase the duration and exclusivity of breastfeeding are unlikely to curb the obesity epidemic.

Trial Registration.—isrctn.org: ISRCTN37687716; and clinicaltrials. gov: NCT01561612.

▶ It has been thought for ages that greater duration and exclusive breastfeeding is associated with greater lean body mass and is positively associated with stature and later-life serum insulinlike growth factor (IGF)-I, a known regulator of childhood linear growth and body composition. The report of Martin et al provides us information from the Promotion of Breastfeeding Intervention Trial (PROBIT). The current PROBIT study (PROBIT III) provides experimental evidence on whether beneficial effects of increased duration and exclusivity of breastfeeding on growth develop later in childhood, based on direct measurements by bioimpedance of body fat and lean mass and on circulating IGF-I. The original PROBIT study began in the 1990s and included a follow-up study of more than 17 000 children. PROBIT III takes off where earlier studies end by actually directly measuring adiposity in an objective manner with bioimpedance technology.

The results from this large cluster-randomized trial indicate that the experimental intervention to promote increased duration and exclusivity of breastfeeding does not reduce continuous measures of adiposity nor reduce the prevalence of overweight or obesity in children age 11.5 years, despite causing large increases in the duration and exclusivity of breastfeeding. These results are similar to data from the PROBIT II study that looked at this phenomenon at 6.5 years of age. The findings also are consistent with evidence provided by other investigators attempting to systematically assess unbiased and unconfounded associations of breastfeeding on adiposity.

Among healthy-term infants, at least in Belarus, the intervention provided by PROBIT III to improve the duration and exclusivity of infant breastfeeding did not prevent overweight or obesity, nor did it affect IGF-I levels among children entering adolescence. This is not to say that breastfeeding does not have many health advantages that are otherwise seen in the PROBIT trials with respect to gastrointestinal infections, the prevalence of atopic eczema in infancy, and improved cognitive development when measured at 6.5 years. The bottom line is that breastfeeding cannot be expected to stem the current epidemic of obesity, which requires much more in the way of public health efforts to promote better eating habits and the endorsement of physical activity in children.

This commentary on dealing with a nutrition topic ends on a culinary observation that might be of interest to readers who enjoy the art of food preparation. A common endeavor in the kitchen is the reduction of liquids into a more concentrated form. The traditional method to accomplish this is to heat slowly, allowing moisture in a brew to boil off. The rub with this is that while it makes the room smell good, it does so at the cost of a duller sauce. A lengthy sit on the burner also chemically alters many of the compounds that remain in a sauce, so they no longer taste or smell fresh. Scientists have now figured out how to address this ... Mario Malto, take note. The new technique is called vacuum reduction. This uses a vacuum reduction methodology rather than high heat to accelerate evaporation of liquid materials. First, pour the cooking liquid into a Pyrex flask that has a side port connected to a vacuum pump; second, stopper the flask; and third, put on a hot plate and gently warm the liquid to be reduced. The pump reduces the air pressure and thus the boiling point of the liquid, allowing evaporation to occur not only fast but at remarkably low temperatures producing a perfect sauce reduction with little or no alterations in quality.[1]

BAM: cooking that sucks.

J. A. Stockman III, MD

Reference

1. Gibbs WW, Myhrvold N. Cooking that sucks. *Scientific American*. 2012;5:21.

Effects of Freezing on the Bactericidal Activity of Human Milk
Takci S, Gulmez D, Yigit S, et al (Hacettepe Univ Ihsan Dogramaci Children's Hosp, Ankara, Turkey; Hacettepe Univ School of Medicine, Ankara, Turkey)
J Pediatr Gastroenterol Nutr 55.146-149, 2012

Objectives.—Storage of human milk by freezing has been recommended for long-term storage. The present study analyzed the bactericidal activity of human milk on *Escherichia coli* and *Pseudomonas aeruginosa* and determined the changes in bactericidal activity following freezing at −20°C and −80°C for 1 month and 3 months.

Methods.—Forty-eight milk samples were collected from 48 lactating mothers. Each sample was divided into 10 aliquots. Two of the samples were processed immediately and the others were stored at both −20°C and −80°C until analysis after 1 month and 3 months of freezing.

Results.—All of the fresh milk samples showed bactericidal activity against *E coli* and *P aeruginosa*. Freezing at −20°C for 1 month did not cause statistically significant alteration in bactericidal activity ($P > 0.017$), whereas storage for 3 months lowered the degree of bactericidal activity significantly ($P < 0.017$) against *E coli*. Bactericidal activity was protected when the samples were stored at −80°C. There was no statistically significant difference in the bactericidal activity of human milk against *E coli* between freezing at −20°C and −80°C for 1 month ($P > 0.017$); however, when milk was stored for 3 months, −80°C was significantly more protective ($P < 0.017$). Freezing at −20°C and −80°C for 1 month and 3 months did not cause any significant change in bactericidal activity against *P aeruginosa* ($P > 0.05$).

Conclusions.—Storage by freezing at −80°C is more appropriate to keep bactericidal capacity of stored human milk > 1 month if affordable and available, especially in intensive care settings.

▶ No one would argue that when it comes to infant feeding, cow milk is for cows and breast milk is for infants. It has been clearly demonstrated that breast milk-fed infants, particularly in neonatal units, have less necrotizing enterocolitis and sepsis. This action of human milk is extremely important for premature and ill infants who are exposed to abundant pathogenic organisms during their stays in neonatal intensive care units. Human milk provides such infants with large numbers of antimicrobial substances while exerting bacteriostatic and bacteriocidal action. Breast milk can be supplied for infants by their own mothers or by donor milk that is available from breast milk banks. There is no doubt that mothers' own milk is the first choice for preterm and other high-risk infants, but in many cases donor milk must be used when mothers' own milk is not available in sufficient quantity. When it comes to some small preterm infants, many cannot receive feedings at all or only receive extremely small amounts of breast milk even though mother's milk is available. In this situation, the common practice is to store mother's milk for the future. The storage of human milk is generally advisable by refrigeration for 5 to 8 days; however, for long storage periods, freezing is recommended. The common existing freezing temperature for storage is −28°C. Freezing of milk at −70°C or −80°C is not a common storage practice except for laboratory purposes.

The aim of the report of Takci et al was to analyze the bacteriocidal activity of human milk on different pathogenic organisms and to determine the changes in bacteriocidal activity following freezing at −20°C and −80°C for 1 month and 3 months. Bacteriocidal activity against *Escherichia coli* and *Pseudomonas aeruginosa* was examined. The data from this result showed that freezing at −20°C for 1 month did not cause statistically significant alterations in the bacteriocidal activity of the human milk, whereas storage for 3 months lowered the degree of bacteriocidal activity significantly. Bacteriocidal activity was protected to a significant degree for longer periods when samples were stored at −80°C.

The data from this report suggest that milk can be stored safely for an unlimited period or at least for more than 12 months at −70°C to −80°C. This is likely true also for colostrum as well as more mature breast milk itself. The authors of this report conclude that storage by freezing at −80°C is more appropriate to keep the bacteriocidal activity of stored milk if the freezing methodology is affordable and available.

J. A. Stockman III, MD

Maternal Exercise and Growth in Breastfed Infants: A Meta-analysis of Randomized Controlled Trials

Daley AJ, Thomas A, Cooper H, et al (Univ of Birmingham, UK)
Pediatrics 130:108-114, 2012

Background and Objectives.—Studies have revealed that women who breastfeed their infants may be reluctant to exercise due to concerns that to do so would adversely affect their breast milk and consequently the growth of their infants. In this review, we seek to systematically review and statistically synthesize evidence from randomized controlled trials (RCTs) that have assessed the effects of maternal exercise on breastfed infant growth (weight gain and gain in length).

Methods.—Searches of the following electronic bibliographic databases were performed to identify RCTs: Cochrane Library (CENTRAL), Medline/PubMed, Embase, Cumulative Index to Nursing and Allied Health Literature, and SPORT Discus. RCTs that compared any type of exercise intervention with other treatments or no treatment in women exclusively or predominately breastfeeding were eligible for inclusion, as were trials involving exercise as a cointervention. Two authors extracted data from studies independently.

Results.—Four RCTs (5 comparisons) were included in the meta-analysis of infant weight gain that incorporated 170 participants. In breastfed infants, maternal exercise did not significantly affect infant weight gain (difference in mean weight gain $= 18.6$ g [95% confidence interval: -113.52 to 150.80, $P = .73$]). Only 1 trial assessed infant gain in length; no difference between the exercise and control groups was reported. Trials were classified as moderate or good methodological quality (moderate risk of bias).

Conclusions.—It appears that mothers can exercise and breastfeed without detriment to the growth of their infants, but this is based on limited evidence, and more research is required before this finding is confirmed.

▶ There is a great deal written about the relationship between maternal exercise and its effects on breastfeeding. Unfortunately, the literature has not provided a clear message to either care providers or mothers in this regard. Early experimental studies done immediately before or after exercise have suggested that lactic acid concentration in breast milk rises significantly with exercise, and that this might negatively affect infant milk acceptance based on taste changes in the breast milk. Studies on dairy cows have suggested that short bouts of aerobic exercise in these animals will result in negative effects by draining the body of fluid and energy, causing a substantial energy deficit in a lactating cow and resulting in reduced milk volume after exercise. Studies in humans, however, suggest that the effects of lactic acid on taste primarily occur only with maximal exercise, and that this would not be the typical case with a routine exercise session for most women. The counter to all this is that aerobic exercise could have several benefits for breastfeeding, serving to protect lactation when energy deficiency occurs because prolactin (an important hormone implicated in the maintenance of lactation) increases in response to short bouts of aerobic exercise.

These authors have accepted the challenge of sifting through all the literature, systematically reviewing the evidence from randomized controlled trials that have attempted to assess the effects of maternal exercise on breastfed infant growth (weight gain and gain in length). The authors intended to produce evidence regarding whether mothers can exercise and breastfeed without detriment to the growth of their infants. A secondary aim of the review was to evaluate the effects of exercise on infant length and maternal weight loss. The study was designed to help clinicians answer a frequently asked question by mothers: "Can I exercise and breastfeed my baby?"

This article does provide evidence that participation in exercise while breast-feeding does not adversely affect infant weight gain. However, although these findings might appear initially encouraging, consideration should be given to the fact that only 4 small trials turned out to be eligible for inclusion in this meta-analysis. There were insufficient data to make any conclusions regarding infant gain in length, but the 1 study that assessed this indicated no detrimental effects. Thus the findings from this report should be considered in light of the potential limitations and strengths of the methods and analyses used in the review. The bottom line, however, was that the authors found that breastfed infants whose mothers exercised did not gain less weight than infants of seden-tary mothers. Although these findings are encouraging and suggest exercise and breastfeeding are compatible, this analysis is based on data only from 170 breast-feeding women, and therefore a large high-quality trial needs to be undertaken to substantiate these findings. The authors of this article suggest that such a trial should include data on infant body length, breastfeeding frequency and duration, infant fussiness, milk volume, and milk composition. Is there a group of investigators out there willing to undertake such a trial?

J. A. Stockman III, MD

Timing of the Introduction of Complementary Foods in Infancy: A Randomized Controlled Trial

Jonsdottir OH, Thorsdottir I, Hibberd PL, et al (Univ of Iceland, Reykjavik; Massachusetts General Hosp for Children, Boston; et al)
Pediatrics 130:1038-1045, 2012

Objective.—To increase knowledge on iron status and growth during the first 6 months of life. We hypothesized that iron status would be better in infants who received complementary foods in addition to breast milk compared with those exclusively breastfed.

Methods.—One hundred nineteen healthy term (≥37 weeks) singleton infants were randomly assigned to receive either complementary foods in addition to breast milk from age 4 months (CF) or to exclusive breastfeeding for 6 months (EBF). Dietary data were collected by 3-day weighed food records, and data on iron status and growth were also collected.

Results.—One hundred infants (84%) completed the trial. Infants in the CF group had higher mean serum ferritin levels at 6 months ($P = .02$), which remained significant when adjusted for baseline characteristics. No difference was seen between groups in iron deficiency anemia, iron deficiency, or iron depletion. The average daily energy intake from complementary foods of 5-month-olds in the CF group was 36.8 kJ per kg body weight. Infants in both groups grew at the same rate between 4 and 6 months of age.

Conclusions.—In a high-income country, adding a small amount of complementary food in addition to breast milk to infants' diets from 4 months of age does not affect growth rate between 4 and 6 months, but has a small and positive effect on iron status at 6 months. The biological importance of this finding remains to be determined.

▶ Before 2001, the World Health Organization (WHO) recommended exclusive breastfeeding for the first 4 to 6 months of life. In 2001, the WHO Expert Consultation on Optimal Duration of Exclusive Breastfeeding changed this recommendation of exclusive breastfeeding to the first 6 months of life. The reason for this was to provide optimal nutrition to young infants in low resource countries where available water and complementary foods that were nutritionally adequate were not available or were contaminated. On the other hand, in high-income countries, the evidence for recommending 6 months of exclusive breastfeeding has remained less clear. Parents have been left confused about when to introduce complementary foods in addition to breastfeeding. Jonsdottir et al have examined this issue of optimal duration of exclusive breastfeeding by conducting a randomized, controlled trial comparing iron status and the growth of infants randomly assigned to 4 months versus 6 months of exclusive breastfeeding before introduction of complementary foods. The study was performed in Iceland.

In this study, eligible infant—mother pairs were randomly assigned to receive complementary foods from 4 months in addition to breast milk or to continue being exclusively breastfed to 6 months of age. Vitamin D supplements were recommended in both groups. Measurements were made of iron status along with regular measurements of each infant's weight, length, and head circumference, all measured at birth, 6 weeks, 3 months, 4 months, 5 months, and 6 months of age.

The results of this study were consistent with the earlier observations made by the WHO regarding the optimal duration of exclusive breastfeeding. There was no reduction found in growth in children exclusively breastfed for 4 months versus those breastfed for 6 months of life. Iron stores were higher at 6 months in those who had complementary foods introduced at 4 months of age, but both those exclusively breastfed for 4 months and 6 months did have adequate stores as measured by serum iron levels. There was no difference in the prevalence of iron deficiency with or without anemia. It is presumed that the higher serum ferritin levels reflected greater sourcing of iron from the complementary foods these infants were fed. It should be noted that the amount of complementary foods consumed from age 4 months by infants in this study was small and did not affect the growth of these infants compared with those exclusively breastfed.

Thus, at least on the short haul, it seems that there is no demonstrable down-side with respect to iron status to the introduction of complementary foods at 4 months of age as long as breastfeeding is continued past that time.

J. A. Stockman III, MD

Taste Perception and Food Choices

Negri R, Di Feola M, Di Domenico S, et al (Univ of Naples "Federico II," Italy; et al)

J Pediatr Gastroenterol Nutr 54:624-629, 2012

Objectives.—The extent to which variation in taste perception influences food preferences is, to date, controversial. Bitterness in food triggers an innate aversion that is responsible for dietary restriction in children. We investigated the association among genetic variations in bitter receptor TAS2R38 and food choices in healthy children in the Mediterranean area, to develop appropriate tools to evaluate the relation among genetic predis-position, dietary habits, and feeding disorders. The aims of the study were to get a first baseline picture of taste sensitivity in healthy adults and their chil-dren and to explore taste sensitivity in a preliminary sample of obese children and in samples affected by functional gastrointestinal diseases.

Methods.—Individuals (98 children, 87 parents, 120 adults) were re-cruited from the general population in southern Italy. Bitterness sensitivity was assessed by means of a suprathreshold method with 6-propyl-2-thiouracil. Genomic DNA from saliva was used to genotype individuals for 3 polymorphisms of TAS2R38 receptor, A49P, A262V, and V296I. Food intake was assessed by a food frequency questionnaire.

Results.—Children's taste sensation differed from that of adults: we observed a higher frequency of supertasters among children even in the mother–child dyads with the same diplotypes. Among adults, supertaster status was related with proline-alanine-valine (taster allele) homozygous haplotype, whereas supertaster children were mainly heterozygous. Regarding the food choices, we found that a higher percentage of taster chil-dren avoided bitter vegetables or greens altogether compared with taster adults. Taster status was also associated with body mass index in boys.

Conclusions.—Greater sensitivity to 6-propyl-2-thiouracil predicts lower preferences for vegetables in children, showing an appreciable effect of the genetic predisposition on food choices. None of the obese boys was a supertaster.

▶ This is an absolutely fascinating article that tells us a great deal of how the taste of certain foods is perceived by some and not by others and how taste perception has evolved within different societies. We learn that good (pleasant) taste, such as sweet and umami (the savory taste of some L-amino acids), elicited by energetic compounds such as carbohydrates and proteins, trigger attraction toward nutri-tive food as man has evolved over many millennia. Bad (unpleasant) taste, such as bitter and sour, evolved to detect potentially lethal compounds such as plant secondary metabolites or microbial toxins. Salty taste, developed to ensure ion and water homeostasis when life moved from sea to land, can be good or bad depending on the concentration of sodium and on the psychological context. Ancestral feeding behavior has been retained by contemporary humans, although food choices do not pertain to life or death. Nevertheless, taste is still a critical determinant of food selection, especially in children. As a legacy of the prehistoric age, neophobia, the fear of the new and unknown, in this case, food, restrains the dietary habit of infants and is related to feeding behavioral disorders.

What we learn from this article relates to new information about taste sensors and how they are controlled by certain genes we inherit. Taste sensors are specific receptors located in the taste buds of the gustatory papillae on the tongue and soft palate. Sweet and bitter tastants are recognized by protein receptors encoded by certain taste receptor gene families such as *TAS1R* and *TAS2R*. Salty and sour compounds are detected by ion channels. Based on genetics, some individuals are hypersensitive, particularly to bitter taste, but also to the wide behavior spectrum of other foods. Hypersensitive individuals tend to have a more restricted diet, compared with sensitive or insensitive taste individuals. These issues are of paramount importance to children after weaning, as this is the time when many children gradually develop erratic food acceptance, often generating anxiety in mothers.

These authors have undertaken research looking at the relationship between the genotype of an individual and his or her taste phenotype in an attempt to correlate bitter taste sensitivity in mothers as well as their children. They also looked at whether bitter taste sensitivity differed in obese children. The data from the report show that children's taste sensation does differ from that of adults. Children have a much greater likelihood of having "super tasters" in their population, that is, children who are much more sensitive to certain tastes, including bitter taste. Regarding food choices, those with higher percentages of taste stimulation tended to avoid bitter vegetables or greens altogether compared with less taste-sensitive children. Obese children appear to have a diminished sensitivity to bitter substances. Increased sensitivity to bitterness was shown to be associated with infant and child neophobia and presumably is responsible for a child's rejection of new, unfamiliar foods. This results in a diet particularly poor in food variety. The mode of inheritance for this phenomenon is described in some detail in this article.

This article, which emanates from Naples, Italy, should be read by every pediatrician. We all too frequently hear complaints from mothers that their youngster will not try new foods. Why some kids will eat everything and others are picky eaters is based on a complex interaction between one's genes as inherited from both parents and the foods they are presented with.

This commentary closes with an interesting tidbit having to do with one particular form of nutrition: the cheeseburger. Have you ever wondered why the cheeseburger did not become a popular food item until sometime early in the last century. One-hundred years ago you could not make a cheeseburger as we know it even if you knew how to. Tomatoes were in season only in the late summer. Lettuce was available in spring and fall. Large mammals were slaughtered usually in early winter after a grazing period earlier in the year. Thus, the process of making a hamburger would take nearly a year and would necessitate omitting some core ingredients. The fact we now can eat cheeseburgers to our hearts delight (or its demise) is a shining, albeit greasy, example of all that is both right and wrong with our modern food economy. Thanks to fertilizers, genetically modified crops, concentrated farming operations and global overnight shipping, much of the world was lifted out of starvation because food could be finally grown in sufficient quantities with decreasing labor inputs.[1] At the same time, such technologies contribute to a variety of environmental issues from deforestation and nitrogen loading of water sources to excessive quantities of water being utilized for growing crops, leading to massive shortages of this life sustaining liquid. This situation is not likely to get better since projected world food supply needs are expected to double over the next 40 years.

J. A. Stockman III, MD

Reference

1. Wogan D. The impracticality of the cheeseburger. *Scientific American.* 2012;2:2.

Evaluating iron status and the risk of anemia in young infants using erythrocyte parameters
Torsvik IK, Markestad T, Ueland PM, et al (Haukeland Univ Hosp, Bergen, Norway)
Pediatr Res 73:214-220, 2013

Background.—Correct evaluation of iron status is important in young infants because both iron deficiency and excess may have negative effects on development, growth, and morbidity.

Methods.—We evaluated iron status using erythrocyte parameters, including reticulocyte hemoglobin content (CHr) in infants with birth weight <3,000 g ($n = 80$). Blood samples and infant characteristics were recorded at 6 wk and at 4 and 6 months. Infants with a birth weight ≤2,500 g ($n = 36$) were recommended for iron supplementation.

Results.—Despite a significantly poorer status at 6 wk, iron-supplemented infants had significantly higher hemoglobin level (Hb): 12.2 (SD = 0.8) g/dl and CHr: 28.3 (SD = 1.4) pg at 6 mo, as compared with nonsupplemented infants, Hb: 11.7 (SD = 1.0) g/dl, $P = 0.02$ and CHr: 26.5 (SD = 2.5) pg, $P < 0.001$. Prolonged exclusive breastfeeding, high weight gain, and male gender were the predisposing factors for a low iron status at 6 mo. A CHr cutoff level of 26.9 pg at 4 mo proved to be a sensitive predictor for anemia at 6 mo.

Conclusion.—Signs of an iron-restricted erythropoiesis were observed in nonsupplemented infants (birth weight 2,501–3,000 g), and CHr was a useful tool for evaluating iron status. The need for iron supplementation in certain infant risk populations should be further evaluated.

▶ This is another article documenting how useful reticulocyte hemoglobin content (CHr) is in the detection of iron deficiency in young infants. In this study, investigators used a variety of red cell parameters to evaluate iron status and the risk of subsequent development of anemia as defined by hemoglobin less than 11 g/dL in iron-supplemented infants with low birth weight and nonsupplemented infants with a birth weight between 2500 and 3000 g. Correlations were then made with infant nutritional status, weight gain, and gender during the first 6 months of life. Studies included hemoglobin, mean corpuscular volume, number of red blood cells, red cell distribution width, and percentage of hypochromic erythrocytes as well as CHr parameters.

This study documented that CHr is a real-time iron parameter reflecting bone marrow iron availability for hemoglobin production during the preceding 48 hours in comparison with other red cell parameters that reflect mean values based on an erythrocyte lifespan of 120 days. Rapid changes in erythrocyte and common iron markers, such as ferritin and soluble transfer and receptor, during the first months of life make these parameters less useful in infants. By comparison, CHr is considered a reliable iron marker during this period based on prior studies. The investigators found that using a CHr cutoff of 26.9 pg at 4 months of age had the best sensitivity and specificity for predicting anemia (hemoglobin < 11 g/dL at 6 months of age). However, it should be noted that anemia is a late sign of iron deficiency, and the optimal CHr cutoff level for predicting iron deficiency in infants may be higher. A CHr threshold of less than 27.5 pg has been found to have a good sensitivity and specificity for detecting iron deficiency before the onset of anemia in infants aged 9 to 12 months [1]

The authors conclude that erythrocyte parameters are useful for identifying infants with low iron status even during the first 6 months of life. The study did find iron restricted erythropoiesis from 6 weeks to 6 months in nonsupplemented infants with birth weights 2500 to 3000 g. Exclusive breastfeeding, rapid weight gain, and male sex tended to be predisposing factors for low iron status.

J. A. Stockman III, MD

Reference

1. Ullrich C, Wu A, Armsby C, et al. Screening healthy infants for iron deficiency using reticulocyte hemoglobin content. *JAMA.* 2005;294:924-930.

Iron Deficiency in Infancy is Associated with Altered Neural Correlates of Recognition Memory at 10 Years

Congdon EL, Westerlund A, Algarin CR, et al (Children's Hosp Boston, MA; Univ of Chile, Santiago, Chile; et al)
J Pediatr 160:1027-1033, 2012

Objective.—To determine the long-term effects of iron deficiency on the neural correlates of recognition memory.

Study Design.—Non-anemic control participants (n = 93) and 116 otherwise healthy formerly iron-deficient anemic Chilean children were selected from a larger longitudinal study. Participants were identified at 6, 12, or 18 months as iron-deficient anemic or non-anemic and subsequently received oral iron treatment. This follow-up was conducted when participants were 10 years old. Behavioral measures and event-related potentials from 28 scalp electrodes were measured during an new/old word recognition memory task.

Results.—The new/old effect of the FN400 amplitude, in which new words are associated with greater amplitude than old words, was present within the control group only. The control group also showed faster FN400 latency than the formerly iron-deficient anemic group and larger mean amplitude for the P300 component.

Conclusions.—Although overall behavioral accuracy is comparable in groups, the results show that group differences in cognitive function have not been resolved 10 years after iron treatment. Long-lasting changes in myelination and energy metabolism, perhaps especially in the hippo-campus, may account for these long-term effects on an important aspect of human cognitive development.

▶ There are numerous studies reported in the literature over the past 30 years strongly suggesting that iron deficiency and iron deficiency anemia, presenting early in life, can result in long-term as well as short-term neurocognitive and behavioral disturbances. Early-onset iron deficiency, for example, neurochemi-cally alters the function of neurotransmitters. Neurotransmitters affect a variety of cognitive and behavioral tasks and can produce changes in startle responses, auditory evoke potentials, and motor function in infants. Iron deficiency can negatively affect the ability of the brain to generate and use metabolic energy, believed to be the result of alterations in the metabolism of cytochrome oxidase in the brain.

Congdon et al have attempted to study the effects of iron deficiency that occurs in utero and in early postnatal life as it affects brain development. This study involved a population of Chilean school-age children identified as having iron deficiency anemia at 6, 12, and 18 months of age who were then treated for the iron deficiency and were compared with control subjects. After treatment, all chil-dren reached normal iron status, and at 4 years of age, analyses were performed of auditory brain stem responses and visual evoked potentials. The study shows that formerly iron-deficient anemic children had persistent variation in auditory and visual systems in comparison to control subjects. These findings suggest that early iron deficiency anemia, despite treatment, has persistent abnormalities in brain neurotransmission—at least at 4 years of age. With follow-up at age 10, the study results also show that there are group differences in cognitive function not resolved over the first decade of life after adequate iron treatment. If there is any single conclusion from this report, it is that nutrient deficiencies occurring during periods of rapid cognitive development can cause long-lasting changes in the brain.

This commentary closes with an observation having to do with Dr Leila Daughtry Denmark, a pediatrician who very early in her career recognized the association between iron deficiency and cow's milk ingestion, telling her patients that if cows grew strong by not drinking any milk after they were weaned, why shouldn't humans learn from that experience? Interestingly, many years later, Dr Frank Oski wrote a book on this topic called: "Don't Drink Your Milk." What is unique about Denmark is she practiced pediatrics until she was 103 years old, passing away only at the age of 114 on April 1, 2012. The only reason she quit practice, according to her daughter, was that her eyesight was getting poor and she did not wish to make any mistakes. When she retired, Denmark was the oldest practicing physician in the United States, and before her death, the Gerontology Research Group, which verifies claims of extreme old age, reported her as the fourth oldest person in the world. She was turned down for admission to the medical school at Emory (which remained all male and all white until 1953), but was accepted by the Medical College of Georgia in Augusta, the only woman in a class of 52, at age 26. Her husband, John Eustace Denmark, was later vice president of the US Federal Reserve Bank of Atlanta. She did part of her residency at the Children's Hospital of Philadelphia. Her practice was undertaken out of her home. She never had a receptionist or nurse and did not require appointments. In her earlier years, her fee for a routine office visit was $4.00 and by the time she retired it had risen only to $10.00. In addition to her pet peeve about cow's milk, she was opposed to children using pacifiers and consuming sugar, including in fruit juices—a pioneer way ahead of her time in this regard. It should be noted that in 2000, the university that denied her admission, Emory, gave her an honorary degree. She received a standing ovation. William Chace, Emory's president from 1994 to 2003, recalled only 2 similar outpourings of emotion at graduation ceremonies during his tenure: one for the Dalai Lama and the other for the African-American baseball legend Hank Aaron.

To read more about Dr Leila Denmark, see the remarkable story of her life summarized in the *British Medical Journal*.[1]

J. A. Stockman III, MD

Reference

1. Obituary Leila Denmark. *BMJ*. 2012;344:e3361.

Post-Term Birth is Associated with Greater Risk of Obesity in Adolescent Males

Beltrand J, Soboleva TK, Shorten PR, et al (Univ of Auckland, New Zealand; et al)
J Pediatr 160:769-773, 2012

Objective.—To test the hypothesise that post-term birth (>42 weeks gestation) adversely affects longitudinal growth and weight gain throughout childhood.

Study Design.—A total of 525 children (including 17 boys and 20 girls born post-term) were followed from birth to age 16 years. Weight and height were recorded prospectively throughout childhood, and respective velocities from birth to end of puberty were calculated using a mathematical model.

Results.—At birth, post-term girls were slimmer than term girls (ponderal index, 27.7 ± 2.6 kg/m^3 vs 26.3 ± 2.8 kg/m^3; $P < .05$). At age 16 years, post-term boys were 11.8 kg heavier than term subjects (body mass index

[BMI], 25.4 ± 5.5 kg/m² vs 21.7 ± 3.1 kg/m²; $P < .01$). The rate of obesity was 29% in post-term boys and 7% in term boys ($P < .01$), and the combined rate of overweight and obesity was 47% in post-term boys and 13% in term boys ($P < .01$). Weight velocity, but not height velocity, was higher in post-term boys at age 1.5-7 years ($P < .05$) and again at age 11.5-16 years ($P < .05$). BMI was higher in post-term boys at age 3 years, with the difference increasing thereafter. BMI and growth were similar in post-term and term girls.

Conclusion.—In this post-term birth cohort, boys, but not girls, demonstrated accelerated weight gain during childhood, leading to greater risk of obesity in adolescence.

▶ A great deal has been written about the effects of being small at birth. Small at birth is associated with a variety of adult diseases, including type 2 diabetes, ischemic heart disease, and obesity. Preterm infants are more prone to insulin resistance. Rapid weight gain during infancy and childhood in low-birth-weight and preterm infants is a risk factor for obesity and insulin resistance as well as for adult metabolic and cardiovascular disease. On the other hand, being born post-term (> 42 weeks of gestation) has not been known to be associated with long-term sequelae, even though it can result in greater perinatal mortality and morbidity. Beltrand et al now tell us the impact of postterm birth on weight gain throughout childhood and adolescence and its effects on the likelihood obesity in adolescence.

Beltrand et al undertook a study in Sweden of infants born between 1980 and 1986, comparing those born at term (37 to 42 weeks of gestation) with those born postterm (> 42 weeks of gestation). Children were measured between 3 and 5 times a year from birth through 3 years of age and then yearly until the end of the study. The final measurements of weight were made between 16 and 17 years of age. Values of height velocity, weight velocity, weight, height, and body mass index (BMI) were calculated at each of these visits. A total of 250 boys and 275 girls met the criteria for inclusion in the study. There were clear differences in weight gain patterns between postterm boys and girls. Postterm boys had 2 periods of rapid weight gain, at age 1.5 to 7.0 years and 11.5 to 16 years. Weight gain and height were similar in postterm and term boys as soon as 1.5 and 9 weeks of age, respectively, but subsequent weight velocity changes resulted in a divergent set of mean weight curves. The rapid weight gain in post-term boys was associated with higher BMI as early as 3 years. Conversely, there were no differences in weight gain throughout childhood between postterm and term girls.

Height velocity throughout childhood did not differ between postterm boys and girls and their term counterparts. However, pubertal growth spurt began at an earlier age in postterm boys than in term boys (12.5 ± 2 years vs 13.5 ± 1.4 years). At 16 years of age, the postterm and term groups were of similar height, but postterm boys were approximately 11.8 kg heavier and had a 3.7 kg/m² greater BMI than term boys. The rate of obesity (BMI > 95th percentile for age) was 29% in postterm boys and 7% in term boys. The BMI differences were even more marked than the prevalence of obese and overweight (BMI > 85th percentile for age) boys were combined, with rates of 47% in preterm boys and 13% in term boys. In contrast, weight, height, and BMI were similar in term girls and postterm girls.

The results of this study are quite astounding. Almost half of postterm boys are overweight or obese at 16 years of age. It is likely that this population will develop even greater levels of obesity during adulthood and, therefore, be at excess risk for obesity-related diseases such as type 2 diabetes mellitus, hypertension, and dyslipidemia. Why girls are spared these problems is not known. This report is worth reading in detail because it attempts to apply some explanation to the findings about why postterm boys get into trouble with their weight during childhood.

Those providing care to children should pay great attention to postterm male infants. They are much more likely than their counterparts of the opposite sex or infants born at term to have obesity, insulin resistance, and metabolic syndrome later in life. Whether these problems can be prevented remains to be seen.

J. A. Stockman III, MD

Sugar-Sweetened Beverages and Genetic Risk of Obesity

Qi Q, Chu AY, Kang JH, et al (Harvard School of Public Health, Boston, MA; Brigham and Women's Hosp and Harvard Med School, Boston, MA)
N Engl J Med 367:1387-1396, 2012

Background.—Temporal increases in the consumption of sugar-sweetened beverages have paralleled the rise in obesity prevalence, but whether the intake of such beverages interacts with the genetic predisposition to adiposity is unknown.

Methods.—We analyzed the interaction between genetic predisposition and the intake of sugar-sweetened beverages in relation to body-mass index (BMI; the weight in kilograms divided by the square of the height in meters) and obesity risk in 6934 women from the Nurses' Health Study (NHS) and in 4423 men from the Health Professionals Follow-up Study (HPFS) and also in a replication cohort of 21 740 women from the Women's Genome Health Study (WGHS). The genetic-predisposition score was calculated on the basis of 32 BMI-associated loci. The intake of sugar-sweetened beverages was examined prospectively in relation to BMI.

Results.—In the NHS and HPFS cohorts, the genetic association with BMI was stronger among participants with higher intake of sugar-sweetened beverages than among those with lower intake. In the combined cohorts, the increases in BMI per increment of 10 risk alleles were 1.00 for an intake of less than one serving per month, 1.12 for one to four servings per month, 1.38 for two to six servings per week, and 1.78 for one or more servings per day ($P < 0.001$ for interaction). For the same categories of intake, the relative risks of incident obesity per increment of 10 risk alleles were 1.19 (95% confidence interval [CI], 0.90 to 1.59), 1.67 (95% CI, 1.28 to 2.16), 1.58 (95% CI, 1.01 to 2.47), and 5.06 (95% CI, 1.66 to 15.5) ($P = 0.02$ for interaction). In the WGHS cohort, the increases in BMI per increment of 10 risk alleles were 1.39, 1.64, 1.90, and 2.53 across the four categories of intake ($P = 0.001$ for interaction); the relative risks for incident obesity were 1.40 (95% CI, 1.19 to 1.64), 1.50 (95% CI, 1.16 to 1.93), 1.54 (95% CI, 1.21 to 1.94), and 3.16 (95% CI, 2.03 to 4.92), respectively ($P = 0.007$ for interaction).

Conclusions.—The genetic association with adiposity appeared to be more pronounced with greater intake of sugar-sweetened beverages. (Funded by the National Institutes of Health and others.)

▶ This is the first of 3 reports in a series dealing with the relationship between sugar-sweetened beverages and the consequences on children's health and well being. The report of Qi et al reminds us that there is a temporal increase described in the consumption of sugar-sweetened beverages and an increase in obesity prevalence in the United States. Studied was the issue of whether the intake of such beverages actually increases the rate of obesity based on a subpopulation of patients with a genetic predisposition to adiposity. The authors of this report note that during the last 30 years, the consumption of sugar-sweetened beverages has increased almost logarithmically and that there is compelling evidence to support a positive link between the consumption of sugar-sweetened beverages and a risk of obesity. The intake of sugar-sweetened beverages and its increased use directly parallels the increasing prevalence of obesity since the late 1970s.

To test the hypothesis that a high intake of sugar-sweetened beverages would influence the association between genetic predisposition and adiposity, the authors used a longitudinal database to examine the interaction between the intake of sugar-sweetened beverages and a genetic-predisposition score, calculated on the basis of 32 genetic loci that have an established association with body mass index (BMI).

In 2 prospective cohorts of women and men in the United States, the investigators found that a greater consumption of sugar-sweetened beverages was associated with a more pronounced genetic predisposition to an elevated BMI and an increased risk of obesity. Specifically, the combined genetic effects on BMI and obesity risk among individuals consuming one or more servings of sugar-sweetened beverages per day were approximately twice as large as those among people consuming less than one serving per month. These data suggest that people with a greater genetic predisposition to obesity appear to be much more susceptible to the deleterious effects of sugar-sweetened beverages on BMI. In the current analysis, the investigators calculated a genetic-predisposition score that was composed of multiple genetic variants, which has become the preferred method in analyses of gene-environment interactions.

The authors of this report speculate that the intake of sugar-sweetened beverages contributes to obesity through several potential mechanisms, including a high caloric content with low satiety and incomplete compensation for these liquid calories, resulting in an increased total energy intake. In addition, because of the large amounts of rapidly absorbable carbohydrates in sugar-sweetened beverages, greater consumption may increase the risk of insulin resistance, β-cell dysfunction, inflammation, visceral adiposity, and other metabolic disorders.

It is not clear, however, whether these factors linking the intake of sugar-sweetened beverages to obesity modify the genetic effect, accounting for the observed interactions. Nonetheless, the data do provide consistent evidence from several separate cohorts that greater consumption of sugar-sweetened beverages is associated with a more pronounced genetic predisposition to an elevated BMI and obesity risk among men and women. Needless to say that although this study did not include children, it seems likely that the same effects would be seen, given that calories are calories and genes are genes at any age. The reports that follow[1,2] show that a reduction in the consumption of sugar-sweetened beverages and a replacement of sugar-sweetened beverages with noncaloric sweetened beverages will reduce weight gain in children. Although further evidence is warranted, data do support a causal relationship between the consumption of sugar-sweetened beverages, weight gain, and the risk of obesity in younger individuals.

J. A. Stockman III, MD

References

1. Ebbeling CB, Feldman HA, Chomitz VR, et al. A randomized trial of sugar-sweetened beverages and adolescent body weight. *N Engl J Med.* 2012;367:1407-1416.
2. de Ruyter JC, Olthof MR, Seidell JC, et al. A trial of sugar-free or sugar-sweetened beverages and body weight in children. *N Engl J Med.* 2012;367:1397-1406.

A Randomized Trial of Sugar-Sweetened Beverages and Adolescent Body Weight

Ebbeling CB, Feldman HA, Chomitz VR, et al (Boston Children's Hosp, MA; Inst for Community Health, Cambridge, MA; et al)
N Engl J Med 367:1407-1416, 2012

Background.—Consumption of sugar-sweetened beverages may cause excessive weight gain. We aimed to assess the effect on weight gain of an intervention that included the provision of noncaloric beverages at home for overweight and obese adolescents.

Methods.—We randomly assigned 224 overweight and obese adolescents who regularly consumed sugar-sweetened beverages to experimental and control groups. The experimental group received a 1-year intervention designed to decrease consumption of sugar-sweetened beverages, with follow-up for an additional year without intervention. We hypothesized that the experimental group would gain weight at a slower rate than the control group.

Results.—Retention rates were 97% at 1 year and 93% at 2 years. Reported consumption of sugar-sweetened beverages was similar at baseline in the experimental and control groups (1.7 servings per day), declined to nearly 0 in the experimental group at 1 year, and remained lower in the experimental group than in the control group at 2 years. The primary outcome, the change in mean body-mass index (BMI, the weight in kilograms divided by the square of the height in meters) at 2 years, did not differ significantly between the two groups (change in experimental group minus change in control group, -0.3; $P = 0.46$). At 1 year, however, there were significant between-group differences for changes in BMI (-0.57, $P = 0.045$) and weight (-1.9 kg, $P = 0.04$). We found evidence of effect modification according to ethnic group at 1 year ($P = 0.04$) and 2 years ($P = 0.01$). In a prespecified analysis according to ethnic group, among Hispanic participants (27 in the experimental group and 19 in the control group), there was a significant between-group difference in the change in BMI at 1 year (-1.79, $P = 0.007$) and 2 years (-2.35, $P = 0.01$), but not among non-Hispanic participants ($P > 0.35$ at years 1 and 2). The change in body fat as a percentage of total weight did not differ significantly between groups at 2 years (-0.5%, $P = 0.40$). There were no adverse events related to study participation.

Conclusions.—Among overweight and obese adolescents, the increase in BMI was smaller in the experimental group than in the control group after a 1-year intervention designed to reduce consumption of sugar-sweetened beverages, but not at the 2-year follow-up (the prespecified primary outcome). (Funded by the National Institute of Diabetes and Digestive and Kidney Diseases and others; ClinicalTrials.gov number, NCT00381160.)

▶ Sugar intake from sugar-sweetened beverages, which are the highest single caloric food source in the United States, approximates 15% of the daily caloric intake in several population groups. Adolescent boys in the United States consume an average of 357 kcal of such beverages per day. All other calories in and out being equal, this can equate to 1 pound of weight gained per week if these drinks are on top of a normal caloric balance. Such sugar-sweetened beverages are nutrient poor and often associated with consumption of salty foods and fast foods. There is an emerging set of data showing an association between the increased consumption of sugar-sweetened beverages and several chronic diseases, such as type 2 diabetes, hypertension, and coronary heart disease. A widely proposed explanation for the association is that caloric beverages elicit weak satiety and compensatory dietary responses, although the evidence supporting this hypothesis has not been conclusively documented. Another possible explanation is the content of high fructose corn syrup, a key ingredient in most sugar-sweetened beverages. Numerous studies have found that dietary fructose promotes hepatic lipogenesis and the development of insulin resistance, fueling the development of fatty liver and type 2 diabetes.

The report of Ebbeling et al and the one of de Ruyter et al that follows describe the effects of interventions to reduce consumption of sugar-sweetened beverages on weight gain in normal-weight children and overweight and obese adolescents. The study by de Ruyter et al represents a double-blind design that includes a large sample of normal weight school children from 4 years, 10 months to 11 years, 11 months of age using measurements of sucralose in urine as an additional compliance marker. The results clearly suggest that replacement of sugar-containing beverages containing 104 kcal with a sugar-free beverage significantly reduces weight gain and fat accumulation in normal-weight children. The study of Ebbeling et al randomly assigned 224 overweight and obese adolescents who regularly consume sugar-sweetened beverages to experimental and control groups. The experimental group received a 1-year intervention consisting of home delivery of noncaloric beverages. This intervention was designed to decrease the consumption of sugar-sweetened beverages, with a follow-up for an additional year. The difference in the primary outcome from this study, the change in body mass index (BMI) at 2 years between the experimental and control groups, was not significant, but at 1 year, significant changes in BMI were observed, particularly among Hispanic participants. These changes were modest, occurring mainly in very small numbers of obese Hispanic adolescents, and they were not sustained at 2 years. Nonetheless, this report, the one of de Ruyter et al, and as the study of Qi et al do provide a strong impetus to develop recommendations and policy decisions to limit consumption of sugar-sweetened beverages, especially those served at low cost and in excessive proportions to attempt to reverse the increase in childhood obesity. These interventions, if successful, could prevent the development of type 2 diabetes in a large number of individuals starting at an early age.

This report, the preceding one, and the one that follows suggest that calories from sugar-sweetened beverages do matter and that policy makers should take the results of these studies into account. Clearly, policy makers in New York City have done so, and we are beginning to see a spread across the country of dialogue about the long term risks of continuing to allow no regulation of sugar-sweetened beverages. America has been a free society, but the societal cost to our health care system demand at least a reasonable debate on the subject of regulatory influences on the foods we consume.

J. A. Stockman III, MD

A Trial of Sugar-free or Sugar-Sweetened Beverages and Body Weight in Children

de Ruyter JC, Olthof MR, Seidell JC, et al (VU Univ Amsterdam, the Netherlands)
N Engl J Med 367:1397-1406, 2012

Background.—The consumption of beverages that contain sugar is associated with overweight, possibly because liquid sugars do not lead to a sense of satiety, so the consumption of other foods is not reduced. However, data are lacking to show that the replacement of sugar-containing beverages with noncaloric beverages diminishes weight gain.

Methods.—We conducted an 18-month trial involving 641 primarily normal-weight children from 4 years 10 months to 11 years 11 months of age. Participants were randomly assigned to receive 250 ml (8 oz) per day of a sugar-free, artificially sweetened beverage (sugar-free group) or a similar sugar-containing beverage that provided 104 kcal (sugar group). Beverages were distributed through schools. At 18 months, 26% of the children had stopped consuming the beverages; the data from children who did not complete the study were imputed.

Results.—The z score for the body-mass index (BMI, the weight in kilograms divided by the square of the height in meters) increased on average by

0.02 SD units in the sugar-free group and by 0.15 SD units in the sugar group; the 95% confidence interval (CI) of the difference was -0.21 to -0.05. Weight increased by 6.35 kg in the sugar-free group as compared with 7.37 kg in the sugar group (95% CI for the difference, -1.54 to -0.48). The skinfold-thickness measurements, waist-to-height ratio, and fat mass also increased significantly less in the sugar-free group. Adverse events were minor. When we combined measurements at 18 months in 136 children who had discontinued the study with those in 477 children who completed the study, the BMI z score increased by 0.06 SD units in the sugar-free group and by 0.12 SD units in the sugar group ($P = 0.06$).

Conclusions.—Masked replacement of sugar-containing beverages with noncaloric beverages reduced weight gain and fat accumulation in normal-weight children. (Funded by the Netherlands Organization for Health Research and Development and others; DRINK ClinicalTrials.gov number, NCT00893529.)

▶ This report and the preceding 2 reports tell a potent story about the interrelationship between sugar-sweetened beverages and weight gain in the US population. Reviewing the strength of the data from these reports and others that preceded them, the issue that has arisen recently is whether government has any role or legal authority to regulate food-industry processes. One such measure introduced recently is the proposal by the New York City Department of Health supported by Mayor Michael Bloomberg to prohibit sugar-sweetened beverages from being sold in containers larger than 16 ounces in restaurants, movie theaters, and mobile food vendors, all venues in which the health department does appear to have jurisdiction. Needless to say, many came out of the woodwork to oppose the plans of the New York City Department of Health, suggesting that such policy is a slippery slope to regulate supermarkets and children's access to certain foods and the potential banning of other harmful products such as caffeinated drinks.

In an editorial that appeared in the *New England Journal of Medicine*, the Commissioner of the Department of Health of the city of New York, Dr Thomas Farley, noted that if harmful chemicals in schools were causing our children to get sick, people would demand government regulation to protect them and, thus, it is difficult to argue against a government response to an epidemic of obesity that kills more than 100 000 persons a year in the United States and does have an environmental origin.[1] He also notes that federal, state, and local governments already regulate the food system, from farm to retail, in many ways and for many purposes, ranging from support of agriculture to prevention of food-borne illness. The issue then is not whether we should regulate food, but rather whether we should update food regulations to address the epidemic of obesity related to the intake of sugar-sweetened beverages. A number of public health professional proposals have already been introduced to reduce the consumption of sugary drinks. Besides restrictions on sales in schools, proposals include volume-based excise taxes, which encourage customers to switch to zero-calorie beverages or to choose smaller portion sizes; a prohibition on the use of Supplemental Nutrition Assistance Program benefits to purchase such drinks, which would remove an inappropriate government subsidy; and an upper limit on portion size in restaurants, which encourages moderation.

In a second editorial, one that followed Dr Farley's commentary, there was a contrarian view presented by Just and Wansink.[2] These authors suggest that we have gone down the regulatory pathway numerous times before with more evidence than there is to support the case of sugar-sweetened beverage reduction and with fewer potential costs in terms of individual freedoms, and still we have failed to change behavior. These authors remind us that prohibition was intended to wipe out the ills of alcohol, but it could not withstand the violent backlash, subversion, and illegal consequences that quickly followed. The authors also suggest that consumption of other choices will not remain constant if one tinkers with what is available to eat or drink, in the language of economists, "certeris paribus" (with all other things constant) does not hold. These authors published a study commonly called *Coke to Coors*, showing that taxing soft drinks in Utica, New York, led beer-buying households to increase their purchases of beer.[3] It is suggested that if soft drinks are not available, children may very well drink high caloric fruit juice or eat more cookies and candy. These same authors remind us of a quotation of Ben Franklin, who poetically said, "A man convinced against his will is of the same opinion still." You can rob a man of something less healthful to him, and he will likely find something to quickly fill the void just as bad, or so say these contrarians.

Whether you are a supporter of the regulation of sugar-sweetened beverages or one who abhors the loss of personal freedoms that can come with regulatory oversight, it is generally agreed that the use of simple behavioral modification techniques should be put into place, such as making soft drinks less visible and less convenient, while still allowing both children and adults to have choices. It has been suggested that there are opportunities to work with the soft drink companies to find ways to encourage better consumer habits without creating a potential backlash (eg, healthy habit loyalty cards for zero-calorie beverages). Such behavioral approaches have been successful in guiding children to eat more fruits and vegetables by simply making them more visible and attractive, by associating them with exciting names such as "X-ray-Vision" carrots or by associating them with well-known fictional characters such as Elmo or Batman.

For more on the role of government in preventing excess calorie consumption and the example of New York City, see the additional commentary by Dr Farley that appeared in *JAMA*.[4] Data recently published in the *Annals of Internal Medicine* show that New York's bold legislation in terms of regulation of trans fats seems to have worked in terms of improving the diet of the average New Yorker.[5] Lunches at fast food chains improved in terms of nutritional content in high-income and low-income neighborhoods. Unfortunately, both children and adults here in the United States still eat too much, and there is a danger that labeling fast foods as zero trans fats could encourage them to eat even more if such foods are thought to be healthful; they still have calories. These adverse consequences have been dubbed a *health halo*.

J. A. Stockman III, MD

References

1. Farley T. Support regulation of sugar-sweetened beverages. *N Engl J Med.* 2012; 367:1464-1465.
2. Just DR, Wansink B. Do not support regulation of sugar-sweetened beverages. *N Engl J Med.* 2012;367:465-466.
3. Wansink B, Hanks D, Just DR, et al. From coke to coors: a field study of a sugar-sweetened beverage tax and its unintended consequences. Socia Scine Research Network. 2012. http://www.ssrn.com/abstract-2079840. Accessed February 26, 2013.
4. Farley TA. The role of government in preventing excess calorie consumption: the example of New York City. *JAMA.* 2012;308:1093-1094.
5. Angell SY, Cobb LK, Curtis CJ, et al. Change in trans fatty acid content of fast-food purchases associated with New York City's restaurant regulation: a pre—post study. *Ann Intern Med.* 2012;157:81-86.

Potential nutritional and economic effects of replacing juice with fruit in the diets of children in the United States
Monsiváis P, Rehm CD (Univ of Washington, Seattle)
Arch Pediatr Adolesc Med 166:459-464, 2012

Objective.—To estimate the nutritional and economic effects of substituting whole fruit for juice in the diets of children in the United States.

Design.—Secondary analyses using the 2001-2004 National Health and Nutrition Examination Survey and a national food prices database. Energy intakes, nutrient intakes, and diet costs were estimated before and after fruit juices were completely replaced with fruit in 3 models that emphasized fruits that were fresh, inexpensive, and widely consumed and in a fourth model that partially replaced juice with fruit, capping juice at recommended levels.

Setting.—A nationwide, representative sample of children in the United States.

Participants.—A total of 7023 children aged 3 to 18 years.

Main Exposures.—Systematic complete or partial replacement of juice with fruit.

Main Outcome Measures.—Difference in energy intakes, nutrient intakes, and diet costs between observed and modeled diets.

Results.—For children who consumed juice, replacement of all juice servings with fresh, whole fruit led to a projected reduction in dietary energy of 233 kJ/d (-2.6% difference [95% CI, -5.1% to -0.1%]), an increase in fiber of 4.3 g/d (31.1% difference [95% CI, 26.4%-35.9%]), and an increase in diet cost of \$0.54/d (13.3% difference [95% CI, 8.8%-17.8%]).

Conclusions.—Substitution of juice with fresh fruit has the potential to reduce energy intake and improve the adequacy of fiber intake in children's diets. This would likely increase costs for schools, childcare providers, and families. These cost effects could be minimized by selecting processed fruits, but fewer nutritional gains would be achieved.

▶ This is an interesting report. There has been a literal stampede away from the use of 100% fruit juice as a substantial part of the total fruit intake of children.

Fruit juices have energy densities similar to sugar-sweetened beverages and could contribute to excess energy intake, obesity, and weight gain, although the evidence linking fruit juices with obesity has been mixed. The American Academy of Pediatrics and the Institute of Medicine in its recommendations for improving school meals have supported prioritizing whole fruit over fruit juices. The 2010 Dietary Guidelines have recommended that no more than half of total fruit servings be in the form of fruit juice, based on the suggestions that whole fruits confer greater health benefits.[1]

Unfortunately, there has been little information about the potential nutritional effects of substituting fruit for fruit juices in the diets of children. It is possible that there is an unintended consequence that such substitutions might drive up food costs given that fruit juices are usually more affordable than fresh fruits. The complete substitution of whole fruit for juice has the potential to substantially improve the nutrient intakes of children while at the same time increasing cost for schools, childcare providers, and families.

Monsivais et al used data from the National Health and Nutrition Examination Survey to assess what would actually happen if all fruit juice servings given to children were replaced with fresh whole fruits. Their findings were consistent with previous analyses commissioned by the Dietary Guidelines Advisory Committee showing that replacing fruit juices with fruit reduces the content of energy while increasing intakes of dietary fiber. It was calculated that such a maneuver would result in a reduction in energy intake of 56 kcal per day. Such a reduction, if sustained, would translate into a reduction in body weight of more than 2.3 kg per year, assuming no compensatory increases in energy intake from other sources. The latter assumption is probably reasonable given the greater satiety effects of fresh fruit compared with fruit juices. It should be noted that replacement of fruit juices with fresh fruit will have the unintended consequence of reducing potassium and vitamin C intake, although there are many other sources for both of these nutrients in the average diet. Replacing fruit juices with fresh fruit also led to higher costs, on average $0.54 per day.

The authors of this report conclude that complete replacement of fruit juice with a variety of whole, fresh fruits has the potential to reduce the dietary energy intake of youngsters and to increase the intake of dietary fiber. These benefits do come at the cost of lower intakes of some vitamins and minerals and higher food costs. We should be grateful to these investigators for providing us with some concrete data about the pros and cons of replacing fruit juices with fresh fruits. In a perfect world, it is clear that fruits picked freshly off the vine or tree are the way to go.

J. A. Stockman III, MD

Reference

1. US Department of Health and Human Services. Report of the dietary guidelines advisory committee on the dietary guidelines for Americans, 2010. US Department of Health and Human Services. http://www.cnpp.usda.gov/dgas2010-policydocument.htm. Accessed September 7, 2012.

Change in Trans Fatty Acid Content of Fast-Food Purchases Associated With New York City's Restaurant Regulation: A Pre–Post Study

Angell SY, Cobb LK, Curtis CJ, et al (New York City Dept of Health and Mental Hygiene)

Ann Intern Med 157:81-86, 2012

Background.—Dietary trans fat increases risk for coronary heart disease. In 2006, New York City (NYC) passed the first regulation in the United States restricting trans fat use in restaurants.

Objective.—To assess the effect of the NYC regulation on the trans and saturated fat content of fast-food purchases.

Design.—Cross-sectional study that included purchase receipts matched to available nutritional information and brief surveys of adult lunchtime restaurant customers conducted in 2007 and 2009, before and after implementation of the regulation.

Setting.—168 randomly selected NYC restaurant locations of 11 fast-food chains.

Participants.—Adult restaurant customers interviewed in 2007 and 2009.

Measurements.—Change in mean grams of trans fat, saturated fat, trans plus saturated fat, and trans fat per 1000 kcal per purchase, overall and by chain type.

Results.—The final sample included 6969 purchases in 2007 and 7885 purchases in 2009. Overall, mean trans fat per purchase decreased by 2.4 g (95% CI, −2.8 to −2.0 g; $P < 0.001$), whereas saturated fat showed a slight increase of 0.55 g (CI, 0.1 to 1.0 g; $P = 0.011$). Mean trans plus saturated fat content decreased by 1.9 g overall (CI, −2.5 to −1.2 g; $P < 0.001$). Mean trans fat per 1000 kcal decreased by 2.7 g per 1000 kcal (CI, −3.1 to −2.3 g per 1000 kcal; $P < 0.001$). Purchases with zero grams of trans fat increased from 32% to 59%. In a multivariate analysis, the poverty rate of the neighborhood in which the restaurant was located was not associated with changes.

Limitation.—Fast-food restaurants that were included may not be representative of all NYC restaurants.

Conclusion.—The introduction of a local restaurant regulation was associated with a substantial and statistically significant decrease in the trans fat content of purchases at fast-food chains, without a commensurate increase in saturated fat. Restaurant patrons from high- and low-poverty neighborhoods benefited equally. However, federal regulation will be necessary to fully eliminate population exposure to industrial trans fat sources.

▶ Because of the increased risk for cardiovascular disease conferred by trans fat intake and because industrial sources of trans fat can be replaced with more healthful alternatives, many countries and localities have recently introduced policies that decrease trans fat intake by prompting its removal from the food supply. In 2003, Denmark became the first country to introduce regulatory limits on trans fat content of foods sold everywhere. It was in 2005 and 2006 that the Canada and United States, respectively, introduced nutritional labeling of trans fat content on packaged foods. New York City in 2006 became the first locality in the United States to pass a regulatory restriction on the use of partially hydrogenated vegetable oil, targeting the restaurant environment throughout the city. One would expect that targeting restaurants would have some significant impact because more than one-third of daily calorie intake in the United States is from food prepared away from the home. This New York City regulation was phased in starting in July 2007 and became fully in effect by the following summer. The New York regulation restricts all food service establishments, including both chain and nonchain restaurants, from using, storing, or serving goods that contains partially hydrogenated vegetable oil that has 0.5 g or more trans fat per serving. Similar trans fat restrictions for restaurants since that time have been adopted by well over a dozen local and state jurisdictions.

So have the regulations reduced exposure to trans fat? Since the introduction of trans fat labeling in Canada and food restrictions in Denmark, many studies of changes in total trans fat, saturated fat, or trans fat content in packaged foods have shown generally favorable results. In New York City, statistically significant decreases in trans fat and trans fat plus saturated fat content in French fries were found in chain restaurants after full implementation of the restaurant restrictions (97.9% and 54.2% decreases, respectively).[1]

These authors evaluated the effect of New York City's restaurant trans fat regulation as reflected by food purchases using a unique survey dataset of customers of lunchtime chain restaurants fielded before and after full implementation of the trans fat regulation. The dataset obtained was initially collected to assess New York City's calorie-labeling regulation, but it included information on nutrients in addition to calories. The study was designed to assess trans fat and trans fat plus saturated fat content of lunchtime purchases with a hypothesis that there would be a decrease after the New York City regulation that restricted the use of trans fat in restaurants was implemented. They looked at the period between 2007 and 2009 and found that between these years, there was a substantial decrease in the amount of trans fat purchased per meal, without a commensurate increase in saturated fat. The results did not differ according to the poverty rate of the neighborhood in which the restaurant was located.

This study clearly suggests that reductions in the trans fat content of restaurant purchases can be achieved without an offsetting increase in saturated fat through regulation of the restaurant food environment. The study provides objective findings that warrant consideration of federal action that would carry the New York experience throughout the United States as a whole. Although the latter would be a neat trick on the part of the federal government, the US population's outlook has changed in recent years so it might find such regulation acceptable. Full elimination of exposure to the industrially produced form of harmful trans fats and the unnecessary addition of such fats to our food supply, found in partially hydrogenated oils, will require federal action, as these authors point out.

J. A. Stockman III, MD

Reference

1. Angell SY, Silver LD, Goldstein GP. Cholesterol control beyond the clinic: New York City's trans fat restriction. *Ann Intern Med.* 2009;151:129-134.

Occurrence and Timing of Childhood Overweight and Mortality: Findings from the Third Harvard Growth Study

Must A, Phillips SM, Naumova EN (Tufts Univ School of Medicine, Boston, MA)
J Pediatr 160:743-750, 2012

Objective.—To assess the mortality experience of participants in the Third Harvard Growth Study (1922-1935) who provided ≥8 years of growth data.

Study Design.—A total of 1877 participants provided an average of 10.5 body mass index measurements between age 6 and 18 years. Based on these measurements, the participants were classified as ever overweight or ever >85th percentile for height in childhood. Age at peak height velocity was used to indicate timing of overweight relative to puberty. Relative risks of all-cause and cause-specific mortality according to measures of childhood growth were estimated using Cox proportional hazards survival analysis.

Results.—For women, ever being overweight in childhood increased the risks of all-cause and breast cancer death; the risk of death from ischemic heart disease was increased in men. Men with a first incidence of overweight before puberty were significantly more likely to die from ischemic heart disease; women in the same category were more likely to die from all causes and from breast cancer.

Conclusion.—We find evidence of long-term effects of having ever been overweight, with some evidence that incidence before puberty influences the pattern of risk.

▶ The Third Harvard Growth Study is a longitudinal study of the physical and mental growth of more than 3000 school children conducted between 1922 and 1935 by the Harvard School of Education. The study subjects were first- and second-grade public school children from 3 middle-class cities north of Boston who were enrolled in 1922 and 1923. The subjects were measured annually until they graduated from or left high school. In 1968, when the cohort had reached the mean age of 51.7 years, 45% of the original cohort was able to be successfully contacted by mail for a midlife follow-up study. A second follow-up was conducted in 1988. As of December 31, 1999, 61% of the study subjects were deceased, and 25% were alive. For the remaining 13.9%, only partial follow-up data were able to be obtained. For the entire cohort, the mean age on December 31, 1999, would have been 83.7 ± 1.0 years had all subjects still been alive.

The investigators looking at data from the Harvard study were able to examine the vital status of each subject by looking at information from the Social Security Death Index, the Massachusetts Registry of Vital Records and Statistics, and the National Death Index Plus System. Data from all these sources allowed the investigators to make correlations between the occurrence and timing of child-hood overweight and obesity and its impact or relationship to adult mortality.

Data from this report documented an association between being overweight in adolescence and increased risk of all-cause mortality and coronary heart disease, specifically in men, but not in women. Findings from this study of largely white individuals living in the northeast support the concept that childhood weight gain status does have an effect on disease outcome but do not suggest that the adolescent period in and of itself is of particular significance. Being overweight before puberty increased the risk of mortality in men and the risks of all-cause and breast cancer mortality among women. It is well known that current body mass index (BMI) is a risk factor for death from breast cancer, but few prior studies have examined BMI in childhood in relationship to this risk of breast cancer later in life.

The Harvard study should be taken seriously. The lengthy follow-up period of an accumulated total of 129 686 person-years makes for powerful statistical analysis and firm conclusions. Particularly at risk are men with a first incidence of being overweight before puberty.

J. A. Stockman III, MD

Exercise Dose and Diabetes Risk in Overweight and Obese Children. A Randomized Controlled Trial

Davis CL, Pollock NK, Waller JL, et al (Med College of Georgia, Augusta; et al)
JAMA 308:1103-1112, 2012

Context.—Pediatric studies have shown that aerobic exercise reduces metabolic risk, but dose-response information is not available.

Objectives.—To test the effect of different doses of aerobic training on insulin resistance, fatness, visceral fat, and fitness in overweight, sedentary children and to test moderation by sex and race.

Design, Setting, and Participants.—Randomized controlled efficacy trial conducted from 2003 through 2007 in which 222 overweight or obese sedentary children (mean age, 9.4 years; 42% male; 58% black) were recruited from 15 public schools in the Augusta, Georgia, area.

Intervention.—Children were randomly assigned to low-dose (20 min/d; n = 71) or high-dose (40 min/d; n = 73) aerobic training (5 d/wk; mean duration, 13 [SD, 1.6] weeks) or a control condition (usual physical activity; n = 78).

Main Outcome Measures.—The prespecified primary outcomes were postintervention type 2 diabetes risk assessed by insulin area under the curve (AUC) from an oral glucose tolerance test, aerobic fitness (peak oxygen consumption [$\dot{V}O_2$]), percent body fat via dual-energy x-ray absorptiometry, and visceral fat via magnetic resonance, analyzed by intention to treat.

Results.—The study had 94% retention (n = 209). Most children (85%) were obese. At baseline, mean body mass index was 26 (SD, 4.4). Reductions in insulin AUC were larger in the high-dose group (adjusted mean difference, −3.56 [95% CI, −6.26 to −0.85] × 10^3 µU/mL; $P =.01$) and the low-dose group (adjusted mean difference, −2.96 [95% CI, −5.69 to −0.22] × 10^3 µU/mL; $P =.03$) than the control group. Dose-response trends were also observed for body fat (adjusted mean difference, −1.4% [95% CI, −2.2% to −0.7%]; $P <.001$ and −0.8% [95% CI, −1.6% to −0.07%];

$P = .03$) and visceral fat (adjusted mean difference, -3.9 cm^3 [95% CI, -6.0 to -1.7 cm^3]; $P < .001$ and -2.8 cm^3 [95% CI, -4.9 to -0.6 cm^3]; $P = .01$) in the high- and low-dose vs control groups, respectively. Effects in the high- and low-dose groups vs control were similar for fitness (adjusted mean difference in peak VO_2, 2.4 [95% CI, 0.4–4.5] mL/kg/min; $P = .02$ and 2.4 [95% CI, 0.3–4.5] mL/kg/min; $P = .03$, respectively). High- vs low-dose group effects were similar for these outcomes. There was no moderation by sex or race.

Conclusion.—In this trial, after 13 weeks, 20 or 40 min/d of aerobic training improved fitness and demonstrated dose-response benefits for insulin resistance and general and visceral adiposity in sedentary overweight or obese children, regardless of sex or race.

Trial Registration.—clinicaltrials.gov Identifier: NCT00108901.

▶ It is known that diet and exercise can reduce the probability of the development of diabetes and prediabetes among adults. The Diabetes Prevention Program documented this.[1] Studies performed in children have shown a downward risk in the development of metabolic abnormalities through exercise, but little has been done to calculate exactly what dose of exercise is necessary to achieve beneficial ends, particularly with respect to weight control and the risk of diabetes.

The report of Davis et al examines the dose-response effect of a training program on insulin resistance, total body fat, abdominal fat, and aerobic fitness in overweight children. Children were recruited from a variety of elementary schools to participate in the study. The children were randomized to low-dose or high-dose aerobic training for 5 days a week for 3 months. These were overweight or obese sedentary children whose average age was 9.4 years. A control population was also studied. The emphasis during the exercise, which was done in a gymnasium, was on intensity, enjoyment, and safety, not competition or skill enhancement. Activities were selected based on the ease of comprehension, fun, and eliciting intermittent vigorous movement. They included running games, jumping rope, and modified basketball and soccer. Outcomes looked at included insulin resistance, fatness, visceral fat, and aerobic fitness. Fasting glucose levels were a secondary outcome. A secondary aim of the study tested moderation of group effects by race and sex to determine the generalizability of the results. Measurements were made at baseline and repeated at 13 weeks of participation in the study. Of the obese and overweight children entering the study, 28% had prediabetes.

The results of this study were quite extraordinary. The trial had exceptional adherence and retention. A daily aerobic exercise intervention with duration of 13 weeks and no dietary restrictions showed dose-response benefits as assessed by insulin response to an oral glucose tolerance test and fasting insulin. The high-dose exercise intervention demonstrated significant benefit in many areas of pancreatic beta cell function. No intervention effects were detected on fasting glucose levels. No difference in efficacy was observed between boys and girls, black and white children, or children with prediabetes versus normoglycemic children. Reductions in insulin resistance were greatest in the high-dose group. Exercise dose trends were also observed for body fat and visceral fat.

This study clearly showed that 20 minutes or 40 minutes a day of aerobic training will improve fitness and will produce benefits for those destined to develop diabetes. The more exercise the better, although even a small amount does afford some benefit.

J. A. Stockman III, MD

Reference

1. Knowler WC, Barrett-Connor E, Fowler SE, et al; Diabetes prevention program research group. Reduction in the incidence of type 2 diabetes with lifestyle intervention or metformin. N Engl J Med. 2002;346:393-403.

Role of Carbohydrate Modification in Weight Management among Obese Children. A Randomized Clinical Trial

Kirk S, Brehm B, Saelens BE, et al (Cincinnati Children's Hosp Med Ctr, OH; Univ of Cincinnati, OH; Seattle Children's Res Inst, WA; et al)
J Pediatr 161:320-327.e1, 2012

Objective.—To compare the effectiveness and safety of carbohydrate (CHO)-modified diets with a standard portion-controlled (PC) diet in obese children.

Study Design.—Obese children (n = 102) aged 7-12 years were randomly assigned to a 3-month intervention of a low-CHO (LC), reduced glycemic load (RGL), or standard PC diet, along with weekly dietary counseling and biweekly group exercise. Anthropometry, dietary adherence, and clinical measures were evaluated at baseline and 3, 6, and 12 months. Analyses applied intention-to-treat longitudinal mixed models.

Results.—Eighty-five children (83%) completed the 12-month assessment. Daily caloric intake decreased from baseline to all time points for all diet groups (P < .0001), although LC diet adherence was persistently lower (P < .0002). At 3 months, body mass index z score was lower in all diet groups (LC, −0.27 ± 0.04; RGL, −0.20 ± 0.04; PC, −0.21 ± 0.04; P < .0001) and was maintained at 6 months, with similar results for waist circumference and percent body fat. At 12 months, participants in all diet groups had lower body mass index z scores than at baseline (LC, −0.21 ± 0.04; RGL, −0.28 ± 0.04; PC, −0.31 ± 0.04; P < .0001), and lower percent body fat, but no reductions in waist circumference were maintained. All diets demonstrated some improved clinical measures.

Conclusion.—Diets with modified CHO intake were as effective as a PC diet for weight management in obese children. However, the lower adherence to the LC diet suggests that this regimen is more difficult for children to follow, particularly in the long term.

▶ There has been a lot written about low-carbohydrate diets to help manage obesity. Recently, dietary interventions that modified the type or amount of carbohydrate intake have shown some promise for weight management. Low-carbohydrate diets limit carbohydrate intake to no more than 60 g/day, whereas reduced glycemic load diets restrict the intake of rapidly absorbed carbohydrates. Such diets have improved weight status in both adults and adolescents. Small studies have also suggested that low-carbohydrate diets might be of benefit to younger children as well, but no randomized control trials have investigated the acceptability, safety, and effectiveness of these approaches in younger children. Kirk et al have designed a randomized clinical trial to compare the safety and efficacy of low-carbohydrate and reduced glycemic load diets with a standard dietary intervention for the management of obesity in younger children. Their theory was that carbohydrate-modified diets would have greater beneficial effects on weight status and other metabolic parameters than a standard portion-controlled diet. A total of 102 obese children ages 7 to 12 years were randomly assigned to a 3-month intervention of a low-carbohydrate, reduced glycemic load, or standard calorie reduction diet. All these youngsters received dietary counseling and were instructed about the use of exercise. All 3 groups experienced a reduction in body mass index over a 3-month period. The weight reduction was maintained for the 6 months of observation. Percent age of body fat was reduced along with waist circumference. Although all 3 approaches produced the desired weight reduction, it was clear that a low-carbohydrate diet was much more difficult to implement based on acceptance by this age group of children. The results also do not support the hypothesis that carbohydrate-modified diets would be more effective in improving weight status than a standard caloric reduction diet in obese children. Each of the diets did lead to improvement in some of the clinical measures evaluated, but there was variability among the groups. The low-carbohydrate diet had significant improvement in high-density lipoprotein cholesterol and triglyceride levels, and the caloric reduction diet and reduced glycemic load groups had relatively lower fasting insulin and glucose levels. The degree to which the 3 study diets macronutrient compositions contributed to these variable outcomes is not clear. Nonetheless, none of the diets appears to have any systematic adverse effects on the prevalence of cardiovascular risk factors and in this regard the authors considered any 1 of the 3 diets as safe.

Whether a reduced-carbohydrate diet can be considered safe if used in the long haul is a far different question that needs to be looked at. There are serious reservations about such diets when used in adults and certainly in children. See the report and commentary with follow-up on this topic.[1]

J. A. Stockman III, MD

Reference

1. Lagiou P, Sandin S, Lof M, Trichopoulos D, Adami HO, Weiderpass E. Low carbohydrate-high protein diet and incidence of cardiovascular diseases in Swedish women: prospective cohort study. *BMJ.* 2012;344:e4026.

Low carbohydrate-high protein diet and incidence of cardiovascular diseases in Swedish women: prospective cohort study

Lagiou P, Sandin S, Lof M, et al (Univ of Athens Med School, Greece; Karolinska Institutet, Stockholm, Sweden; et al)
BMJ 344:e4026, 2012

Objective.—To study the long term consequences of low carbohydrate diets, generally characterised by concomitant increases in protein intake, on cardiovascular health.

Design.—Prospective cohort study.

Setting.—Uppsala, Sweden.

Participants.—From a random population sample, 43 396 Swedish women, aged 30-49 years at baseline, completed an extensive dietary questionnaire and were followed-up for an average of 15.7 years.

Main Outcome Measures.—Association of incident cardiovascular diseases (ascertained by linkage with nationwide registries), overall and by diagnostic category, with decreasing carbohydrate intake (in tenths), increasing protein intake (in tenths), and an additive combination of these variables (low carbohydrate-high protein score, from 2 to 20), adjusted for intake of energy, intake of saturated and unsaturated fat, and several non-dietary variables.

Results.—A one tenth decrease in carbohydrate intake or increase in protein intake or a 2 unit increase in the low carbohydrate-high protein score were all statistically significantly associated with increasing incidence of cardiovascular disease overall (n = 1270)—incidence rate ratio estimates 1.04 (95% confidence interval 1.00 to 1.08), 1.04 (1.02 to 1.06), and 1.05 (1.02 to 1.08). No heterogeneity existed in the association of any of these scores with the five studied cardiovascular outcomes: ischaemic heart disease (n = 703), ischaemic stroke (n = 294), haemorrhagic stroke (n = 70), subarachnoid haemorrhage (n = 121), and peripheral arterial disease (n = 82).

Conclusions.—Low carbohydrate-high protein diets, used on a regular basis and without consideration of the nature of carbohydrates or the source of proteins, are associated with increased risk of cardiovascular disease.

▶ The preceding report of Kirk et al examined the role of carbohydrate modification weight management among obese children. It concluded that low carbohydrate diets were about equally effective to straightforward caloric reduced diets and reduced glycemic load diets in managing obesity in pediatric age patients 7 to 12 years of age.[1] The authors considered all 3 diets equally safe. Unfortunately, the long-term consequences of a low-carbohydrate diet when used in children were not able to be examined to document safety. The report of Lagiou, while not undertaken in children, does provide data leading to serious reservations about the consequences of low-carbohydrate/high-protein diet and the incidence of cardiovascular diseases in young Swedish women.

Low-carbohydrate/high-protein diets and their combinations (such as the Atkins diet) have become popular worldwide and are frequently adopted for weight control. These diets have been suggested to have health benefits over low-fat diets, mainly on the basis of results from short-term intervention studies. These benefits include reductions in triglyceride levels, glycated hemoglobin and insulin concentrations, and systolic blood pressure. These have resulted in improvements and conditions such as type 2 diabetes and nonalcoholic steatohepatitis. There are data, however, to indicate that adherence to such diets might be associated with higher mortality from cardiovascular diseases.

This report investigated the association between adherence to low-carbohydrate/high-protein diets and the incidence of cardiovascular disease in a prospective cohort of 43 396 Swedish women followed up with for an average of 15.7 years. The investigators looked for a diagnosis of cardiovascular disease, including ischemic heart disease, ischemic or hemorrhagic stroke, subarachnoid hemorrhage, or peripheral artery disease. Adherence to a diet low in carbohydrate and high in protein was consistently associated with a higher incidence of cardiovascular disease in a dose-response manner independently of other risk factors. Specifically, women had a 5% higher incidence of cardiovascular disease for each tenth of an increase in the low-carbohydrate/high-protein score that was used in this study yielding a 62% higher incidence among women in the highest categories of low-carbohydrate/high-protein diet compared with the lowest. It is suggested that when one lowers carbohydrate in the diet significantly, one must be taking in a much higher percentage of the diet as protein, otherwise it is simply pure fat that you are eating. A high-protein diet may indicate higher intake of red and processed meats and therefore a higher intake of iron, cholesterol, and saturated fat. As a consequence, one may not be eating a more healthy diet just because one is eating a low-carbohydrate diet. Long-term adherence to low-carbohydrate/high-protein diets necessarily should require careful food choices, such as increased consumption of proteins from vegetables, and cautious monitoring of saturated versus unsaturated fat intake to avoid unfavorable eating patterns.

Despite the popularity of low-carbohydrate/high-protein diets, we should be careful about advising their use for long-term control of body weight. Maybe they are best used for getting down to the preferred weight followed by careful use of a balanced diet that is appropriate in terms of overall caloric content. The long-term news about low-carbohydrate/high-protein diets is not good. Pay attention to these studies as they evolve in the future.

J. A. Stockman III, MD

Reference

1. Kirk S, Brehm B, Saelens BE, et al. Role of carbohydrate modification in weight management among obese children: a randomized clinical trial. *J Pediatr.* 2012; 161:320-327.

Prevalence of Hypovitaminosis D Among Children With Upper Extremity Fractures

James JR, Massey PA, Hollister AM, et al (Louisiana State Univ Health Sciences Ctr, Shreveport)
J Pediatr Orthop 33:159-162, 2013

Background.—Recent publications show a high rate of hypovitaminosis D among children in general as well as among children with fractures. 25-hydroxyvitamin D levels were analyzed from hospital records to determine the prevalence of hypovitaminosis D, with the goal of using that information in fracture management and nutritional counseling.

Methods.—We retrospectively reviewed the records of 213 children with upper extremity fractures that were treated during a 14-month period. For 181 of those patients, the 25-hydroxyvitamin D level was measured at the time of emergency department presentation or at the first clinic appointment within 2 weeks after the initial presentation. The following information was collected from the charts: fracture mechanism (high or low energy), age, sex, race, and body mass index. Vitamin D levels were categorized as normal ($\geq$32 ng/mL), insufficient (20 to 32 ng/mL), or deficient (<20 ng/mL). The levels were analyzed with respect to fracture pattern and race.

Results.—Of the 181 patients, 24% had deficient vitamin D levels, 41% had insufficient levels, and 35% had normal levels. There was no significant correlation with vitamin D level and mechanism of injury. African American children were more likely to have insufficient or deficient levels of vitamin D.

Conclusions.—Hypovitaminosis D is common among children with upper extremity fractures. Further investigation is warranted on the use of the 25-hydroxyvitamin D level as a screening tool to predict risk of fracture and to design proper nutritional programs for children with fractures.

Level of Evidence.—Retrospective chart review; Level III evidence.

▶ It is generally believed that we are experiencing a worldwide epidemic of low vitamin D levels, and that this is occurring in virtually every population that has been looked at. This article reminds us that a study from Boston found 51% of blacks and 17% of Hispanics were determined to be vitamin D deficient.[1] In Northern Ireland, 36% of a representative sample of adolescents were found to be vitamin D deficient.[2] A wintertime prevalence study in Beijing showed that 89.2% of young Chinese girls were vitamin D deficient.[3] The consequences of vitamin D deficiency include a number of different bone diseases, muscle weakness, and increase in risk of certain forms of cancer, multiple sclerosis, hypertension, and diabetes mellitus. The risk for respiratory tract infections is greater in children with vitamin D deficiency and, of course, vitamin D deficiency can lead to rickets in children and to osteomalacia and osteoporosis in adults.

What has not been looked at carefully is whether those presenting with an acute fracture in childhood might be at greater risk for having vitamin D deficiency as a potential contributor to fracture onset. This is what this article is about. A total of 213 children with upper extremity fractures had vitamin D levels drawn. These fractures include 25 of the humerus, 90 of the radius or ulna, 61 metacarpal or phalanx fractures, and 3 carpal fractures. Vitamin D levels were deficient in 24% of youngsters with fractures, insufficient in 41%, and sufficient in 35%. The study defined vitamin D deficiency as a 25-hydroxy vitamin D concentration less than 20 ng/mL, insufficiency as 20 to 32 ng/mL, and sufficiency as greater than 32 ng/mL based on previously published literature.

We now recognize that normal vitamin D levels are important in many critical biological processes, including the functioning of the immune system, glucose metabolism, the prevention of muscle weakness, more than a dozen different types of cancers, multiple sclerosis, hypertension, and diabetes.[4] The media have caught on to this rapid evolution of understanding about the role of vitamin D. Vitamin D sales have surged from $40 million in 2001 to over $425 million in the past few years.[5] It is pretty clear that vitamin D is no longer just a "bone vitamin." Nonetheless, the data from this study remind us that those who are vitamin D deficient or insufficient do run a higher than expected risk of the development of fractures. Although only upper extremity fractures were noted in this article, presumably other types of fractures would have an increased probability of occurring in these deficiency states as well. It might be worthwhile the next time you see a child with a fracture to take a careful history about the likelihood of vitamin D deficiency or insufficiency.

This is the last commentary in the Nutrition and Metabolism chapter, so we will close with a quiz having to do with how metabolism issues led to the defeat of the French at the village of Agincourt by an English army far inferior in numbers under the command of the 27-year-old King Henry V, this on August 13, 1415. The question is, if you were to wear typical armor of the 15th century, what would it weigh and how would it affect your metabolic rate? Standard armor of the 15th century weighed up to approximately 50 kg and was spread head to toe. Researchers recently used volunteers to assess the effects of wearing such armor on metabolic rates. The researchers found that the suits of armor more than doubled the volunteers' metabolic rates.[6] O2 consumption was monitored while the volunteers exercised on a treadmill. Part of the added metabolism requirement was based on difficult ambulation as a consequence of the armor being so heavy about the legs since the same amount of weight if worn as a backpack would only increase metabolic rates by 70%. The French army wearing the 50kg of armor and numbering 30,000 had to slog 300 yards across a wet sloppy field while under the fire of arrows launched by just 7,000 armorless Brits. Proof positive that everything, even history, depends on having a favorable metabolism!

J. A. Stockman III, MD

References

1. Gordon C, DePeter DC, Feldman H, Grace E, Emans SJ. Prevalence of vitamin D deficiency among healthy adolescents. *Arch Pediatr Adolesc Med.* 2004;158: 531-537.
2. Hill TR, Cotter AA, Mitchell S, et al. Vitamin D status and its determinants in adolescents from the North Ireland Young Hearts 2000 cohort. *Br J Nutr.* 2008; 99:1061-1067.

3. Foo LH, Zhang Q, Zhu K, et al. Relationship between vitamin D status, body composition and physical exercise of adolescent girls in Beijing. *Osteoporos Int.* 2009;20:417-425.
4. Holick MF. Vitamin D deficiency. *N Engl J Med.* 2007;357:266-281.
5. Maxmen A. Nutrition advice: the vitamin D-lemma. *Nature.* 2011;475:23-25.
6. Mayer M. The trouble with armor. *Scientific American.* 2011;11:25.

16 Oncology

Peripheral-Blood Stem Cells versus Bone Marrow from Unrelated Donors

Anasetti C, for the Blood and Marrow Transplant Clinical Trials Network (H. Lee Moffitt Cancer Ctr and Res Inst; et al)
N Engl J Med 367:1487-1496, 2012

Background.—Randomized trials have shown that the transplantation of filgrastim-mobilized peripheral-blood stem cells from HLA-identical siblings accelerates engraftment but increases the risks of acute and chronic graft-versus-host disease (GVHD), as compared with the transplantation of bone marrow. Some studies have also shown that peripheral-blood stem cells are associated with a decreased rate of relapse and improved survival among recipients with high-risk leukemia.

Methods.—We conducted a phase 3, multicenter, randomized trial of transplantation of peripheral-blood stem cells versus bone marrow from unrelated donors to compare 2-year survival probabilities with the use of an intention-to-treat analysis. Between March 2004 and September 2009, we enrolled 551 patients at 48 centers. Patients were randomly assigned in a 1:1 ratio to peripheral-blood stem-cell or bone marrow transplantation, stratified according to transplantation center and disease risk. The median follow-up of surviving patients was 36 months (interquartile range, 30 to 37).

Results.—The overall survival rate at 2 years in the peripheral-blood group was 51% (95% confidence interval [CI], 45 to 57), as compared with 46% (95% CI, 40 to 52) in the bone marrow group ($P = 0.29$), with an absolute difference of 5 percentage points (95% CI, -3 to 14). The overall incidence of graft failure in the peripheral-blood group was 3% (95% CI, 1 to 5), versus 9% (95% CI, 6 to 13) in the bone marrow group ($P = 0.002$). The incidence of chronic GVHD at 2 years in the peripheral-blood group was 53% (95% CI, 45 to 61), as compared with 41% (95% CI, 34 to 48) in the bone marrow group ($P = 0.01$). There were no significant between-group differences in the incidence of acute GVHD or relapse.

Conclusions.—We did not detect significant survival differences between peripheral-blood stem-cell and bone marrow transplantation from unrelated donors. Exploratory analyses of secondary end points indicated that peripheral-blood stem cells may reduce the risk of graft failure, whereas bone marrow may reduce the risk of chronic GVHD. (Funded by the

National Heart, Lung, and Blood Institute—National Cancer Institute and others; ClinicalTrials.gov number, NCT00075816.)

▶ It has been 35 years since the first successful unrelated-donor transplantation was performed for a patient with leukemia. In 1979, the father of a 10-year-old girl with acute lymphocytic leukemia in need of a bone marrow transplant contacted the Fred Hutchinson Cancer Research Center in Seattle to ask whether they might have in their files a donor who could be matched against their daughter. There was no family member who was an HLA match. Luckily, a research technician in the research center in Seattle did have the same HLA type as the young girl, and a successful transplant was performed. Over the intervening years, registries for HLA typing of unrelated potential donors were established in Europe, North and South America, and Asia. There are more than 20 million potential unrelated donors now typed and listed in these registries. As recently as 2011, between 5000 and 6000 unrelated donor transplantations were performed here in the United States, actually more than the number of matched related-donor transplantations.

Early on, the donor stem cells came from donor bone marrow. Once it was discovered that hematopoietic growth factors, such as granulocyte colony-stimulating factor, could mobilize high numbers of stem cells into the blood where they can be easily harvested by apheresis, clinical trials of their use for autologous transplantation were conducted successfully for many patients without hematologic malignancies. This then quickly led to the use of matched sibling donor transplantation using peripheral blood stem cells as the source of transplanted materials. Randomized trials show that transplantation with peripheral-blood stem cells results in a much more rapid engraftment, a trend toward an increased risk of graft versus host disease, and improved overall survival of high-risk patients, despite the increased risks of graft versus host disease. With the advent of good solid results in this regard, peripheral blood stem cells became the preferred source for match-sibling transplants and, despite a lack of randomized trials, have become the norm for unrelated-donor transplants as well, accounting for 76% of all transplants this past half decade.

These authors have performed the first randomized trial comparing bone marrow with peripheral blood for unrelated-donor transplantation. Although they found no significant differences in survival, peripheral blood stem cells were associated with significantly faster engraftment, reduced risk of graft failure, and a significant increase in the risk of chronic graft versus host disease.

These data from this study suggest that, given the risk of chronic graft versus host disease, instead of being the default choice for most unrelated-donor transplants, mobilized peripheral blood stem cells should be used only in the minority of patients for whom the benefits outweigh the risks. This would include patients in need of rapid engraftment, such as those with life-threatening infections, and patients at high risk for graft rejection, including those undergoing reduced-intensity conditioning without prior exposure to intensive chemotherapy. However, for the majority of unrelated donor transplantations performed after the patient has undergone a standard, high-dose preparative regimen, bone marrow should be used, since survival is equivalent to the 2 transplant sources, but the incidence of chronic graft versus host disease, which can be a debilitating complication, is significantly lower with bone marrow.

In an editorial that accompanied this report, Appelbaum[1] notes that, although this study should change our practices, it is not clear whether it really will. The benefits of peripheral blood are seen early, under the watchful eye of the transplantation physician, whereas the deleterious effects occur late, often after the patient has left the transplant center. Appelbaum also notes that with more than 20 million potential donors registered, matched unrelated donors as a source of bone marrow or peripheral blood stem cells can be found, but only for most whites, because greater HLA polymorphisms and underrepresentation in the registry exist for most blacks, Hispanics, Asians, and Native Americans.

J. A. Stockman III, MD

Reference

1. Appelbaum FR. Pursuing the goal of a donor for everyone in need. *N Engl J Med.* 2012;367:1555-1556.

KI, WU, and Merkel Cell Polyomavirus DNA was not Detected in Guthrie Cards of Children who Later Developed Acute Lymphoblastic Leukemia
Gustafsson B, Honkaniemi E, Goh S, et al (Karolinska Univ Hosp Huddinge, Stockholm, Sweden; Karolinska Institutet, Stockholm, Sweden; et al)
J Pediatr Hematol Oncol 34:364-367, 2012

Background.—Neonatal dried blood spots (Guthrie cards) have been used to demonstrate a prenatal origin of clonal leukemia-specific genetic aberrations in several subgroups of childhood acute lymphoblastic leukemia (ALL). One hypothesis suggests that an infectious agent could initiate genetic transformation already in utero. In search for a possible viral agent, Guthrie cards were analyzed for the presence of 3 newly discovered polyomavirus Karolinska Institutet polymavirus (KIPyV), Washington University polyomavirus (WUPyV), and Merkel cell polyomavirus (MCPyV).

Methods.—Guthrie cards from 50 children who later developed ALL and 100 matched controls were collected and analyzed by standard or real-time polymerase chain reaction for the presence of the VP1 region of KIPyV, WUPyV, and MCPyV, and the LT region for MCPyV.

Results and Conclusions.—DNA from KIPyV, WUPyV, and MCPyV was not detected in neonatal blood samples from children with ALL or controls. Prenatal infections with these viruses are not likely to be etiological drivers for childhood leukemogenesis.

▶ Not all reports have to have the outcomes that the investigators desire. Some studies are just worth undertaking to find out the answers to important questions. The background to the study undertaken by Gustafsson et al is quite fascinating. Acute lymphoblastic leukemia remains the most frequently diagnosed childhood malignancy. Its etiology remains unknown except in those few who get it as a result of a proclivity to the development of this malignancy that occurs with inherited immunodeficiency syndromes and exposure to ionizing radiation or chemotherapeutic agents. One hypothesis has been that leukemia develops in 2 steps—a prenatal infection, which then would initiate a genetic transformation. It has been proposed that a human polyomavirus could cross the placenta and infect the fetus without causing fetal abnormalities but would induce genomic instability, with specific effects on B lymphocytes. The first 2 human polyomaviruses were described in 1971. In humans, these viruses produce a mild respiratory illness or no symptom at all in otherwise immunocompetent individuals. Once infected, the virus remains latent in the epithelial cells of the urinary tract. Reactivation of polyomavirus can occur during periods of immunosuppression. In recent years, a number of new polyomaviruses have been detected in humans. The seroprevalences for these viruses is high in children, and it is unclear whether most of these viruses produce any symptoms at all, but they can be transferred from mothers to fetuses. Polyomaviruses as a group are potentially oncogenic, and some have been shown to be strongly associated with cancers in humans.

The authors of this report from the Karolinska Institute in Stockholm, Sweden, have examined the Guthrie cards using neonatal blood spots on filter paper to not only screen for metabolic diseases, but also to detect whether viral DNA could be found in the blood of newborns, including those subsequently diagnosed with acute lymphocytic leukemia. No polyomaviruses were able to be detected in Guthrie cards either in children who later developed acute lymphocytic leukemia or from normal control children despite the use of very sensitive technology to detect the respective viruses.

Although the findings from this report did not show any association between polyomaviruses and the development of leukemic clones prenatally, these pathogens still remain candidates for a role in the etiology of leukemia during the second hit, which occurs postnatally. Nonetheless, such infections do not seem to play a major role in the first event of childhood acute lymphoblastic leukemia.

J. A. Stockman III, MD

Zebrafish screen identifies novel compound with selective toxicity against leukemia
Ridges S, Heaton WL, Joshi D, et al (Univ of Utah, Salt Lake City; et al)
Blood 119:5621-5631, 2012

To detect targeted antileukemia agents we have designed a novel, high-content in vivo screen using genetically engineered, T-cell reporting zebrafish. We exploited the developmental similarities between normal and malignant T lymphoblasts to screen a small molecule library for activity against immature T cells with a simple visual readout in zebrafish larvae. After screening 26 400 molecules, we identified Lenaldekar (LDK), a compound that eliminates immature T cells in developing zebrafish without affecting the cell cycle in other cell types. LDK is well tolerated in vertebrates and induces long-term remission in adult zebrafish with cMYC-induced T-cell acute lymphoblastic leukemia (T-ALL). LDK causes dephosphorylation of members of the PI3 kinase/AKT/mTOR pathway and delays sensitive cells in late mitosis. Among human cancers, LDK selectively affects survival of hematopoietic malignancy lines and primary leukemias, including therapy-refractory B-ALL and chronic myelogenous leukemia samples, and inhibits growth of human T-ALL xenografts. This work demonstrates the utility of our method using zebrafish for antineoplastic candidate drug identification and suggests a new approach for targeted leukemia therapy. Although our efforts focused on leukemia therapy, this screening approach has broad implications as it can be translated to other cancer types involving malignant degeneration of developmentally arrested cells.

▶ This is a fascinating report that links the zebrafish to a whole variety of childhood malignancies. The yearly incidence in the United States for all leukemia types including acute lymphoblastic leukemia (ALL), acute myeloid leukemia, and chronic myelogenous leukemia is estimated at more than 40 000 men and women in 2010, resulting in a death rate of 50% once an individual is diagnosed. With respect to children, more than 2000 cases of ALL are diagnosed in children every year, making it the most common childhood cancer. T-cell ALL (T-ALL) represents approximately 15% and 25% of pediatric and adult ALL cases, respectively. Although leukemia treatment has become increasingly effective over the past 50 years or so, overall mortality from ALL is still 20% for children and more than 40% for adults. T-ALL has been more difficult to treat than B-cell ALL.

A good bit of the research that is being undertaken these days in the management of these diseases is devoted to identifying patients at various levels of risk on the basis of molecular markers and the development of targeted therapies to limit side effects. The development of targeted cancer therapies typically requires knowledge of the molecular target itself. In the absence thereof, an alternative approach may be use of a robust methodology designed to screen large numbers of compounds for specific effects against the malignant cell type in question. This is where the zebrafish comes into play. Zebrafish and humans show striking similarities in hematopoietic development. Zebrafish demonstrate all human adult blood lineages, including T and B lymphocytes. For these reasons, it is conceivable that drugs that show hematopoietic effects in zebrafish might have similar effects on human cells. A pharmacologic screen for drugs that could cause alterations in hematopoietic stem cells during embryonic periods has already shown that prostaglandins can expand the pool of hematopoietic stem cells.

These authors have reasoned that because T-ALL generally involves immature blasts, looking for compounds that prevent T-cell maturation during embryonic development in zebrafish might identify compounds that would have similar effects on immature blasts found in T-ALL. They took advantage of a transgenic zebrafish line to determine whether various agents had the capacity to block T-cell development, which can be readily visualized by fluorescence in certain types of zebrafish. Their methodology allowed surveys of tens of thousands of small molecules and showed that a particular compound with a previously unappreciated biologic activity, which they termed Lenaldekar, specifically ablates immature T cells. There is a zebrafish T-ALL model that carries a human *cMYC* oncogene. Remarkably, although all untreated affected zebrafish will succumb to their cancer by 40 days, those treated with Lenaldekar remain in remission many months after an initial 14-day treatment course.

Although this article may seem a bit obscure, the data presented demonstrate how effectively investigators are now exploring new cancer therapies using, in this case, the zebrafish. Previously it has been shown that human oncogenes cause malignancy in zebrafish, that novel oncogenes can be discovered by mutagenesis, and that human cancer therapies can be effective in fish. These authors have now shown that novel human anticancer therapeutics can be discovered using small molecule screening methodologies in zebrafish. It is now time for cancer researchers to go all out fish farming for new cancer therapies.

J. A. Stockman III, MD

Outcomes after Induction Failure in Childhood Acute Lymphoblastic Leukemia

Schrappe M, Hunger SP, Pui C-H, et al (Christian-Albrechts-Univ, Kiel, Germany; Univ of Colorado Cancer Ctr and Children's Hosp Colorado, Aurora; St. Jude Children's Res Hosp and Univ of Tennessee Health Science Ctr, Memphis; et al)
N Engl J Med 366:1371-1381, 2012

Background.—Failure of remission-induction therapy is a rare but highly adverse event in children and adolescents with acute lymphoblastic leukemia (ALL).

Methods.—We identified induction failure, defined by the persistence of leukemic blasts in blood, bone marrow, or any extramedullary site after 4 to 6 weeks of remission-induction therapy, in 1041 of 44,017 patients (2.4%) 0 to 18 years of age with newly diagnosed ALL who were treated by a total of 14 cooperative study groups between 1985 and 2000. We analyzed the relationships among disease characteristics, treatments administered, and outcomes in these patients.

Results.—Patients with induction failure frequently presented with high-risk features, including older age, high leukocyte count, leukemia with a T-cell phenotype, the Philadelphia chromosome, and 11q23 rearrangement. With a median follow-up period of 8.3 years (range, 1.5 to 22.1), the 10-year survival rate ($\pm$SE) was estimated at only $32\pm1\%$. An age of 10 years or older, T-cell leukemia, the presence of an 11q23 rearrangement, and 25% or more blasts in the bone marrow at the end of induction therapy were associated with a particularly poor outcome. High hyperdiploidy (a modal chromosome number >50) and an age of 1 to 5 years were associated with a favorable outcome in patients with precursor B-cell leukemia. Allogeneic stem-cell transplantation from matched, related donors was associated with improved outcomes in T-cell leukemia. Children younger than 6 years of age with precursor B-cell leukemia and no adverse genetic features had a 10-year survival rate of $72\pm5\%$ when treated with chemotherapy only.

Conclusions.—Pediatric ALL with induction failure is highly heterogeneous. Patients who have T-cell leukemia appear to have a better outcome with allogeneic stem-cell transplantation than with chemotherapy, whereas patients who have precursor B-cell leukemia without other adverse features appear to have a better outcome with chemotherapy. (Funded by Deutsche Krebshilfe and others.)

▶ When I was a house officer, only about half of the children with acute lympho-blastic leukemia (ALL) survived to 5 years, and many of these patients were not truly cured. Now, approximately 80% of children with ALL are cured. It has been estimated that with current therapies this percentage is likely to rise to nearly 90%. Unfortunately, there is a subset of newly diagnosed children with ALL who will not respond well. In some groups the long-term survival is well under 50%.

These authors report on an observational analysis of 1041 patients with induc-tion failure who were treated between 1985 and 2000. This study provides extraordinarily useful information in identifying which clinical and biological features of ALL at diagnosis indicate a poorer prognosis right from the start of therapy. Poor risk features included T-cell disease, male sex, older age, hyperleu-kocytosis, Philadelphia chromosome positivity, and *MLL* rearrangements. The data from these studies highlight the complex interrelation between disease biology and early treatment response. Inferior initial responses to therapy portend different outcomes within unique biologic subgroups. Even if there is a poor prognostic outcome based on induction failure, certain other features might still allow a better outcome. For example, in a child who has failed induction, favorable-risk factors include high hyperdiploidy at young age along with precursor B-cell ALL in children younger than 6 years of age.

There is one other additional important finding from this article. Currently the standard of care for poor prognosis ALL is early transplantation. Data from this study seem to document no benefit of allogeneic transplantation in a specific subset of poor prognosis patients, specifically patients younger than 6 years of age who have precursor B-cell ALL and induction failure and no high-risk genetic features. Although we have come a long way in the management of ALL, we still have a ways to go if everyone is to be cured.

J. A. Stockman III, MD

Cardiac Failure 30 Years After Treatment Containing Anthracycline for Childhood Acute Lymphoblastic Leukemia
Goldberg JM, Scully RE, Sallan SE, et al (Univ of Miami Leonard M. Miller School of Medicine, FL; Harvard Med School, Boston, MA)
J Pediatr Hematol Oncol 34:395-397, 2012

In 1977, a 5-year-old girl diagnosed with acute lymphoblastic leukemia was treated on Dana-Farber Cancer Institute Childhood Acute Lympho-blastic Leukemia Protocol 77-01, receiving a cumulative doxorubicin dose of 465 mg/m^2, cranial radiation, and other drugs. After being in continuous complete remission for 34 months, she developed heart failure and was treated with digoxin and furosemide. At 16 years of age, she was diagnosed and treated for dilated cardiomyopathy. Over the years, she continued to have bouts of heart failure, which became less responsive to treatment. At 36 years of age, she received a heart transplant. Six months later, she stopped taking her medications and suffered a sudden cardiac death.

▶ The case of this woman who required a heart transplant at age 36 goes back in time to her diagnosis of acute lymphocytic leukemia at age 5, that diagnosis having been made in 1977. The patient received a total dose of doxorubicin of 465 mg/m² as part of her leukemia management. Presumably this drug was the cause of the cardiomyopathy that evolved over a number of years, ultimately leading to the need for a cardiac transplant.

This case is a vivid reminder of the consequences of our successes in the management of a relatively common childhood cancer. Each year about 12 000 children are diagnosed with cancer here in the United States. Fortunately, we are currently seeing an overall 5-year survival across the broad spectrum of pediatric cancers of about 80%. These data translate into the observation that 1 in about 500 adults ages 20 to 34 years in the United States is a survivor of childhood cancer. For this reason, an increasing number of patients treated with anthracyclines, such as doxorubicin, are expected to be at risk for life occurring cardiac morbidity although not every child with cancer is obviously treated with this particular type of drug. Also, with current protocols, the total dose of such drugs has tended to be lower than in the past. As these youngsters transition into adulthood, our adult physician counterparts should be aware of the risks of the early development of heart failure in patients who have been treated with agents that can cause late-term cardiovascular effects, including cardiomyopathy. Cancer survivors do require long-term monitoring of cardiac function as some will develop heart failure and possibly the need for heart transplant.

The authors of this report remind us that we need to find better biomarkers of early signs of cardiac toxicity while we are actively treating these patients. We also need to explore genetic phenotypes that may increase susceptibility to anthracycline toxicity. Cardioprotectant agents have been developed, such as dexrazoxane, that might be helpful in protecting the heart while allowing full chemotherapeutic effects on the types of cancers being treated with this class of cardiotoxic compounds.

J. A. Stockman III, MD

Langerhans Cell Histiocytosis: 40 Years' Experience
Maria Postini A, del Prever AB, Pagano M, et al (Univ of Turin, Italy; et al)
J Pediatr Hematol Oncol 34:353-358, 2012

Objectives.—Our study analyzes 40 years' experience with pediatric Langerhans cell histiocytosis patients.

Materials and Methods.—Between June 1968 and December 2009, 121 patients (79 males, 42 females; median age 4.13 y) were diagnosed at our center (74% monosystemic disease; 26% multisystemic), treated according to current protocols. We evaluated the response, the survival, and the neuro-endocrinological sequelae.

Results.—Overall survival (OS) for all patients was 93% at 10 years from diagnosis, event-free survival (EFS) 77%. OS for patients younger than 2 years and older than or equal to 2 years was 82% and 97% (*P* = 0.003); EFS 48% and 87% (*P* = 0.001). OS for patients diagnosed before and after April 1, 1991 was 84% and 98% (*P* = 0.007), EFS 66% and 85% (*P* = 0.03). OS for monosystemic and multisystemic disease was 100% and 71% (*P* < 0.001); EFS 88% and 45% (*P* < 0.001). OS for "risk" patients (involvement of bone marrow, spleen, liver, lungs) and "low-risk" patients was 50% and 94% (*P* = 0.007), EFS 37% and 54% (*P* = 0.06). Fourteen patients developed diabetes insipidus, 7 patients growth hormone deficiency, 2 hypothyroidism, and 1 neurodegeneration.

Conclusions.—Our study confirms improvement of pathogenetic knowledge and treatment over the last 20 years. Age at diagnosis older than or equal to 2 years and standardized treatment are associated with improved prognoses. Multisystemic involvement, especially with "risk" organs seem to be correlated to a worse outcome.

▶ Certain eponyms remain in use in medicine. One such eponym is the name Langerhans. Dr Langerhans was a German pathologist born in 1847 in Berlin. His full name is Paul Langerhans. He and another German, Friedrich Hoffmann, did extensive explorations of the macrophage system in rabbits and guinea pigs. It was he who described granulomas of what we now call *Langerhans cell histiocytosis*. This is a rare group of disorders with a wide range of clinical presentations. It affects about 5 to 6 per million children per year. The etiology of Langerhans cell histiocytosis remains unknown, and for this reason some still call the disorder *histiocytosis X*. In the last half of the last century, it became convention to divide Langerhans histiocytosis into 3 different entities as they presented clinically: Letterer-Siwe disease, Hand-Schuller-Christian disease, and eosinophilic granuloma. It has been suggested that Langerhans cell histiocytosis is the result of an uncontrolled proliferation of lymphocytes and histiocytes after a viral infection or a gene mutation. Whether the disorder represents a reactive or a neoplastic disease also remains a matter of debate. The disorder may involve bone, skin, lymph nodes, or parenchymal organs, such as liver, spleen, lungs, and bone marrow and may cause endocrinologic disorders, such as diabetes insipidus, growth hormone deficiency, and hypothyroidism, often in association with neurological deficits. Depending on which organs are affected, Langerhans cell histiocytosis may prove rapidly fatal or develop into a chronic reactivating, but therapy-responsive, disorder or may resolve spontaneously.

Postini et al designed a study to review the experience of the last 40 years analyzing improvement in the treatment of Langerhans cell histiocytosis while examining data from 121 affected patients treated from 1968 through 2009 in Turin, Italy. The data confirm a wide range of presentations and a generally good prognosis. All patients who had only one anatomic system affected had a very good outcome with a very low rate of reactivation. No death occurred in such patients. Patients younger than 2 years of age at diagnosis also had the best outcomes. The authors showed that the presence of diabetes insipidus was the most common and significant risk factor for multisystem disease development and was associated with frontal bone, orbital, middle ear, and mastoid involvement. Diabetes insipidus occurred in about 12% of cases.

This study confirms that the prognosis of Langerhans cell histiocytosis has improved over the last 40 years with the greatest improvements seen in patients with monosystemic disease, in particular, bone monofocal lesions. Multisystem disease remains the subgroup with the worst outcomes because of unfavorable localizations and involvement of risk organs. This is a disease that cries out for collaboration and worldwide patient registries.

J. A. Stockman III, MD

Combined BRAF and MEK Inhibition in Melanoma with BRAF V600 Mutations

Flaherty KT, Infante JR, Daud A, et al (Massachusetts General Hosp Cancer Ctr, Boston; Sarah Cannon Res Inst/Tennessee Oncology, Nashville; Univ of California San Francisco; et al)
N Engl J Med 367:1694-1703, 2012

Background.—Resistance to therapy with BRAF kinase inhibitors is associated with reactivation of the mitogen-activated protein kinase (MAPK) pathway. To address this problem, we conducted a phase 1 and 2 trial of combined treatment with dabrafenib, a selective BRAF inhibitor, and trametinib, a selective MAPK kinase (MEK) inhibitor.

Methods.—In this open-label study involving 247 patients with metastatic melanoma and BRAF V600 mutations, we evaluated the pharmacokinetic activity and safety of oral dabrafenib (75 or 150 mg twice daily) and trametinib (1, 1.5, or 2 mg daily) in 85 patients and then randomly assigned 162 patients to receive combination therapy with dabrafenib (150 mg) plus trametinib (1 or 2 mg) or dabrafenib monotherapy. The primary end points were the incidence of cutaneous squamous-cell carcinoma, survival free of melanoma progression, and response. Secondary end points were overall survival and pharmacokinetic activity.

Results.—Dose-limiting toxic effects were infrequently observed in patients receiving combination therapy with 150 mg of dabrafenib and 2 mg of trametinib (combination 150/2). Cutaneous squamous-cell carcinoma was seen in 7% of patients receiving combination 150/2 and in 19% receiving monotherapy ($P = 0.09$), whereas pyrexia was more common in the combination 150/2 group than in the monotherapy group (71% vs. 26%). Median progression-free survival in the combination 150/2 group was 9.4 months, as compared with 5.8 months in the monotherapy group (hazard ratio for progression or death, 0.39; 95% confidence interval, 0.25 to 0.62; $P < 0.001$). The rate of complete or partial response with combination 150/2 therapy was 76%, as compared with 54% with monotherapy ($P = 0.03$).

Conclusions.—Dabrafenib and trametinib were safely combined at full monotherapy doses. The rate of pyrexia was increased with combination therapy, whereas the rate of proliferative skin lesions was nonsignificantly reduced. Progression-free survival was significantly improved. (Funded by GlaxoSmithKline; ClinicalTrials.gov number, NCT01072175.)

▶ This article is included in the YEAR BOOK OF PEDIATRICS to bring the reader up to date with some of the newest developments in the management of melanoma. This study tells us that 2 new drugs, dabrafenib and trametinib, have now been shown to significantly improve progression-free survival in patients with metastatic melanoma who have BRAF V600 mutations.

By way of background, pharmacologic inhibition of the mitogen-activated protein kinase (MAPK) pathways has proven to be a major advance in the treatment of metastatic melanoma. Newly designed recombinant antibodies, such as dabrafenib, that block MAPK signaling in patients with melanoma who have the BRAF V600 E mutation, have been associated with progression-free survival in several studies. In spite of these advances, 50% of patients who are treated with such inhibitors will have disease progression within 6 to 7 months after the initiation of treatment. Resistance to these agents occurs in a number of different ways, but the result is the same, rapid recurrence and death in patients so treated.

The authors of this report in an attempt to delay resistance to BRAF inhibition and to explore the safety of combination therapy with both BRAF and MAPK inhibition conducted a phase I and phase II study to investigate the combination of the BRAF inhibitor dabrafenib and the MEK inhibitor trametinib in patients with metastatic BRAF V600 melanoma. Teenagers were included in this study, although most of the patients were adults ranging from young middle age to older age individuals.

The authors showed that dabrafenib and trametinib could be safely combined when each agent is administered at its full single-agent dose. Indeed the combination of the 2 agents seems to have a lower risk of pyrexia and dose-limiting acneiform dermatitis. The percentage of patients who were alive and progression-free at 1 year was substantially higher in this combined drug therapy arm than those given monotherapy (41% vs 9%). The combination of BRAF-MEK inhibitors represents a successful attempt to combine targeted therapies in an oncogene-defined patient population. Interestingly, as a consequence of unique biochemical effects, this combination appears to be associated with a reduced incidence and severity of some of the toxic effects of monotherapy with either a BRAF or MEK inhibitor. The authors of this report believe that the combination of dabrafenib and trametinib warrants further evaluation as a potential treatment for metastatic melanoma in patients with BRAF V600 mutations and other patients with cancers with these same mutations.

J. A. Stockman III, MD

Radiation exposure from CT scans in childhood and subsequent risk of leukaemia and brain tumours: a retrospective cohort study

Pearce MS, Salotti JA, Little MP, et al (Newcastle Univ, Newcastle upon Tyne, UK; Natl Cancer Inst, Bethesda, MD; et al)
Lancet 380:499-505, 2012

Background.—Although CT scans are very useful clinically, potential cancer risks exist from associated ionising radiation, in particular for children who are more radiosensitive than adults. We aimed to assess the excess risk of leukaemia and brain tumours after CT scans in a cohort of children and young adults.

Methods.—In our retrospective cohort study, we included patients without previous cancer diagnoses who were first examined with CT in National Health Service (NHS) centres in England, Wales, or Scotland (Great Britain) between 1985 and 2002, when they were younger than 22 years of age. We obtained data for cancer incidence, mortality, and loss to follow-up from the NHS Central Registry from Jan 1, 1985, to Dec 31, 2008. We estimated absorbed brain and red bone marrow doses per CT scan in mGy and assessed excess incidence of leukaemia and brain tumours cancer with Poisson relative risk models. To avoid inclusion of CT scans related to cancer diagnosis, follow-up for leukaemia began 2 years after the first CT and for brain tumours 5 years after the first CT.

Findings.—During follow-up, 74 of 178 604 patients were diagnosed with leukaemia and 135 of 176 587 patients were diagnosed with brain tumours. We noted a positive association between radiation dose from CT scans and leukaemia (excess relative risk [ERR] per mGy 0·036, 95% CI 0·005−0·120; $p = 0·0097$) and brain tumours (0·023, 0·010−0·049; $p < 0·0001$). Compared with patients who received a dose of less than 5 mGy, the relative risk of leukaemia for patients who received a cumulative dose of at least 30 mGy (mean dose 51·13 mGy) was 3·18 (95% CI 1·46−6·94) and the relative risk of brain cancer for patients who received a cumulative dose of 50−74 mGy (mean dose 60·42 mGy) was 2·82 (1·33−6·03).

Interpretation.—Use of CT scans in children to deliver cumulative doses of about 50 mGy might almost triple the risk of leukaemia and doses of about 60 mGy might triple the risk of brain cancer. Because these cancers are relatively rare, the cumulative absolute risks are small: in the 10 years after the first scan for patients younger than 10 years, one excess case of leukaemia and one excess case of brain tumour per 10 000 head CT scans is estimated to occur. Nevertheless, although clinical benefits should outweigh the small absolute risks, radiation doses from CT scans ought to be kept as low as possible and alternative procedures, which do not involve ionising radiation, should be considered if appropriate.

▶ The authors of this study examined the question of whether cancer risks are increased after computed tomography (CT) scans in childhood and young adulthood. They assessed the risks of leukemia and brain tumors because these are the endpoints of greatest concern because red bone marrow and brain are highly radiosensitive tissues, especially in childhood. Furthermore, these tissues are also some of the most highly exposed from childhood CT scans, and leukemias and brain tumors are the most common childhood cancers. More than a decade ago, Brenner et al in a landmark report suggested that radiation doses attributed to pediatric CT scans would lead to a significant number of excess cancer deaths. The risk estimates were based on population models of survivors of atomic bombs in Japan. The data from the Brenner et al report were not taken seriously by many because there are differences between CT scan and exposure to an atomic bomb— for example, CT scans are usually focused on a particular part of the body, whereas atomic bomb exposures affect the entire body.[1] The radiologic community has suggested that the risk of medical imaging at effective doses below 50 mSv for single procedures or 100 mSv for multiple procedures over short periods are too low to be detectable and may be nonexistent. This is why the study by Pearce et al is so important.

The authors investigated a cohort of 178 604 children without cancer who underwent CT between 1985 and 2002 in various hospitals in England, Scotland, and Wales. They used state-of-the-art dosimetric methodology to determine radiation doses to individual organs. They identified several subsequent cancers via linkage to the National Health Service Central Registry. The authors were very careful to exclude CT scans undertaken for cancer diagnosis. The authors noted increases in leukemia incidence in children with cumulative bone marrow doses from CT of at least 30 mGy (where 1 mGy = 1 mSv) and increases in brain tumor incidence in children with brain doses of at least 50 mGy. Assuming typical doses used since the start of this past decade, the authors suggest 2 to 3 head CTs could triple the risk of cancer and that 5 to 10 CT scans would triple the risk of leukemia in children younger than 15 years of age.

So what is the implication from this study to clinical practice? It is clear that this study should eliminate any controversy about whether there is a risk related to the development of malignancy from CT scanning. There is. The issue is, is the risk great enough to offset the use of CT scanning for its most common uses for which there is thought to be some clinical benefit? There is evidence to suggest that 20% to 50% of all CT scans could be replaced with some other type of imaging or not done at all.[2]

Pearce et al confirm that CT scans almost certainly produce a small cancer risk. The use of CT scanning continues to rise, almost exponentially, and generally with good reasons. Nonetheless, all of us must redouble our efforts to justify and optimize every CT scan. Elsewhere you will find a report about how low-dose CT scanning may be good enough for many diagnostic purposes. This is an example of wise imaging.

This commentary ends with the observation recently reported that tall people are at greater risk for the development of cancer.[3] Investigators looked at the incidence of 17 cancer types, from breast cancer to leukemia, over 9 years among 1.3 million women in a United Kingdom health study. Cancer was found to rise 16% for every added 10 centimeters in height. Why being taller would increase one's risk of cancer is not known.

J. A. Stockman III, MD

References

1. Brenner D, Elliston C, Hall E, Berdon W. Estimated risks of radiation-induced fatal cancer from pediatric CT. *AJR Am J Roentgenol.* 2001;176:289-296.
2. Malone J, Guleria R, Craven C, et al. Justification of diagnostic medical exposures: some practical issues. Report of an International Atomic Energy Agency Consultation. *Br J Radiol.* 2012;85:523-538.
3. Editorial comment. *Science.* 2011;333:506.

Comparison of a Strategy Favoring Early Surgical Resection vs a Strategy Favoring Watchful Waiting in Low-Grade Gliomas

Jakola AS, Myrmel KS, Kloster R, et al (St Olavs Univ Hosp, Trondheim, Norway; Univ Hosp of Northern Norway, Tromsø, Norway; et al)
JAMA 308:1881-1888, 2012

Context.—There are no controlled studies on surgical treatment of diffuse low-grade gliomas (LGGs), and management is controversial.

Objective.—To examine survival in population-based parallel cohorts of LGGs from 2 Norwegian university hospitals with different surgical treatment strategies.

Design, Setting, and Patients.—Both neurosurgical departments are exclusive providers in adjacent geographical regions with regional referral practices. In hospital A diagnostic biopsies followed by a "wait and scan" approach has been favored (biopsy and watchful waiting), while early resections have been advocated in hospital B (early resection). Thus, the treatment strategy in individual patients has been highly dependent on the patient's residential address. Histopathology specimens from all adult patients diagnosed with LGG from 1998 through 2009 underwent a blinded histopathological review to ensure uniform classification and inclusion. Follow-up ended April 11, 2011. There were 153 patients (66 from the center favoring biopsy and watchful waiting and 87 from the center favoring early resection) with diffuse LGGs included.

Main Outcome Measure.—The prespecified primary end point was overall survival based on regional comparisons without adjusting for administered treatment.

Results.—Initial biopsy alone was carried out in 47 (71%) patients served by the center favoring biopsy and watchful waiting and in 12 (14%) patients served by the center favoring early resection ($P < .001$). Median follow-up was 7.0 years (interquartile range, 4.5-10.9) at the center favoring biopsy and watchful waiting and 7.1 years (interquartile range, 4.2-9.9) at the center favoring early resection ($P = .95$). The 2 groups were comparable with respect to baseline parameters. Overall survival was significantly better with early surgical resection ($P = .01$). Median survival was 5.9 years (95% CI, 4.5-7.3) with the approach favoring biopsy only while median survival was not reached with the approach favoring early resection. Estimated 5-year survival was 60% (95% CI, 48%-72%) and 74% (95% CI, 64%-84%) for biopsy and watchful waiting and early resection, respectively. In an adjusted multivariable analysis the relative hazard ratio was 1.8 (95% CI, 1.1-2.9, $P = .03$) when treated at the center favoring biopsy and watchful waiting.

Conclusions.—For patients in Norway with LGG, treatment at a center that favored early surgical resection was associated with better overall survival than treatment at a center that favored biopsy and watchful waiting. This survival benefit remained after adjusting for validated prognostic factors.

▶ Although this report deals largely with adults, older teenagers were also included in the data analysis, and thus the information probably applies to the pediatric age group as well. Gliomas are classified into grades I to IV, according to histologic criteria. Grades I and II are low-grade gliomas and grades III and IV are considered malignant gliomas. Low-grade gliomas affect both children and adults. The predominant histologic type of glioma found in most children is a grade I tumor, juvenile pilocytic astrocytoma and is curable by complete surgical resection. More problematic are low-grade gliomas that occur in older children, teens, and adults, referred to as grade II gliomas. These tumors are characterized by an entirely different pattern of behavior. They are invasive and cannot be completely resected surgically. Residual tumor cells are almost always present distal to the margin of resection no matter how extensive a surgical procedure is. Commonly the tumors recur, eventually undergo malignant degeneration, and are ultimately fatal.

Controversy has existed in the neurosurgical and neuro-oncology communities regarding the best approach for patients who present with imaging findings supporting a new diagnosis of grade II glioma. Although patients who undergo extensive resections of their tumors in general live longer, there have been no randomized controlled trials of this tumor and its treatment. Overly aggressive attempts at resection can leave a patient with permanent neurologic deficits. Unfortunately, surgical approaches to the management of these patients vary by center. Patients initially may undergo either a period of observation, biopsy, or extended resection. The current treatment for grade II glioma is not uniform and is often center- or surgeon-dependent.

Jakola et al tell us about a study undertaken in Norway comparing 2 hospitals in which treatment philosophies are quite different. One hospital used a biopsy approach followed by a wait-and-see period, whereas the other hospital used an early resection approach. The study findings demonstrate that at the hospital favoring resection, patients had marked improvement in survival over time when compared with patients treated at the hospital favoring biopsy alone (80% vs 70% survival at 3 years). This difference increased over time until at 7-year survival with 68% among patients at the hospital favoring a strategy of resection versus 44% at the institution favoring biopsy.

Generally speaking, in the United States, there has been an increasing trend to maximize the extent of surgical resection in patients with grade II glioma while still maintaining neurologic function. Unfortunately, no clear evidence to support this approach has appeared, at least not until this report by Jakola et al, which does add further evidence to support this approach. Again, most children will have grade I gliomas. These should be surgically resected. For the older pediatric age patient with a grade II glioma, chances are we will see more and more extensive resections taking place to allow longer and better survivorship.

J. A. Stockman III, MD

Thyroid Cancer in Pediatric Age Group: An Institutional Experience and Review of the Literature

Kiratli PÖ, Volkan-Salanci B, Günay EC, et al (Hacettepe Univ Faculty of Medicine, Ankara, Turkey; et al)

J Pediatr Hematol Oncol 35:93-97, 2013

Very few have been reported on children with differentiated thyroid cancer (DTC), although 15% of them are diagnosed below 20 years of age. Children with DTC present with more advanced disease; however, they have a more favorable outcome. In this paper, we aimed to present the data in our institution on pediatric DTC patients, making an emphasis on the risk factors of metastasis and recurrence, as well as to the outcome of treatment. Clinical data of 50 pediatric patients referred to our institution for radioiodine treatment (RAI) between 1976 and 2010 were obtained. Papillary carcinoma was the most common histopathologic diagnosis (36 patients) followed by papillary carcinoma with follicular variant (10 patients). Multifocality was reported in 66% of the pathology reports. At the time of diagnosis 35 patients had regional lymph node metastasis, 18 had local invasion, and 11 had distant metastasis. No distant metastasis was present in patients with unifocal disease ($P = 0.018$). The mean duration of follow-up was 77.6 ± 62.7 months. Patients with local disease had longer disease-free survival than patients with distant metastasis ($P = 0.033$). Despite the small number of patients, the follow-up was relatively long and the presented results confirmed overall good prognosis in children with DTC.

▶ Thyroid cancer is not a common problem in children, but it does occur. Data suggest that thyroid cancer accounts for about 0.7% of all childhood and adolescent cancers. The majority of these cancers are known as differentiated thyroid cancers, whereas medullary thyroid cancer is relatively uncommon, constituting just 5% to 8% of childhood cancers of the thyroid. There has been a renewed interest in thyroid cancer in children since the Chernobyl nuclear accident in 1996. Although it is generally thought that the prognosis for differentiated thyroid cancer is good, most clinical studies have involved very few children. The disease-specific mortality in children seems to be low, but up to 90% of the cancers present with metastatic disease requiring extensive treatment.

This study was designed as a retrospective analysis aimed to review the course of patients treated for differentiated thyroid cancer in children, and it examined whether age, sex, presenting signs and symptoms, tumor characteristics, or method of treatment was related to the risk of recurrence and to overall treatment outcomes. More than 60 pediatric thyroid cancer patients were evaluated over a number of years at a single institution, which constituted the database of this study. The most common presenting symptom in this cluster of children was a thyroid nodule or goiter. The majority of patients had either local lymph node involvement or distant disease. Lymph node and distant metastases at diagnosis were more common in boys (88.2%) vs girls (63%). Treatment was given in almost all cases with surgery and the use of radioiodine. Recurrence rate in this study was high (13 of 20 patients who were followed over a long period of time). Recurrence rates were higher in girls than boys and in those who were younger than 15 years of age at diagnosis. Despite recurrences, all patients except one were alive during follow-up. The one patient who expired actually expired of an unrelated illness, a glioblastoma multiforme.

The results of this study confirm a generally overall good prognosis of differentiated thyroid carcinoma of all types in children and adolescents. Unfortunately, relapse of disease is possible, even after 2 to 3 decades from the time of initial diagnosis, and thus intensive long-term follow-up is needed.

While on the topic of things oncologic, exposure to carcinogenic substances can ultimately result in the development of cancer decades later even if the inciting substance is long removed from an individual's environment. Such is particularly the case with exposure to arsenic. Researchers looking at cancer rates in the Antofagasta region of Chile noted a much higher than anticipated prevalence of bladder cancer as well as lung cancer compared to many other parts of that country. The arsenic in drinking water on Chile's volcanic north coast has a long history. The arsenic that presumably contaminated water supplies came from volcanic ash and has been found in the hair of mummies expiring 7000 years ago. Mining in the area in the 1950s further raised arsenic levels in drinking water. In 1971, water treatment began and quickly lowered arsenic levels. Cancer, however, has developed in those exposed to arsenic some 40 years later. Investigators are attempting to determine whether arsenic exposure is related to the high incidence of testicular cancer. The rates of the latter in Chile are the highest in the world.[1]

J. A. Stockman III, MD

Reference

1. Fraser B. Cancer cluster in Chile linked to arsenic contamination. *Lancet.* 2012; 379:603.

Secondary Gastrointestinal Cancer in Childhood Cancer Survivors: A Cohort Study

Henderson TO, Oeffinger KC, Whitton J, et al (Univ of Chicago, IL; Fred Hutchinson Cancer Res Ctr, Seattle, WA; Univ of Minnesota, Minneapolis; et al)
Ann Intern Med 156:757-766, 2012

Background.—Childhood cancer survivors develop gastrointestinal cancer more frequently and at a younger age than the general population, but the risk factors have not been well-characterized.

Objective.—To determine the risk and associated risk factors for gastrointestinal subsequent malignant neoplasms (SMNs) in childhood cancer survivors.

Design.—Retrospective cohort study.

Setting.—The Childhood Cancer Survivor Study, a multicenter study of childhood cancer survivors diagnosed between 1970 and 1986.

Patients.—14 358 survivors of cancer diagnosed when they were younger than 21 years of age who survived for 5 or more years after the initial diagnosis.

Measurements.—Standardized incidence ratios (SIRs) for gastrointestinal SMNs were calculated by using age-specific population data. Multivariate Cox regression models identified associations between risk factors and gastrointestinal SMN development.

Results.—At median follow-up of 22.8 years (range, 5.5 to 30.2 years), 45 cases of gastrointestinal cancer were identified. The risk for gastrointestinal SMNs was 4.6-fold higher in childhood cancer survivors than in the general population (95% CI, 3.4 to 6.1). The SIR for colorectal cancer was 4.2 (CI, 2.8 to 6.3). The highest risk for gastrointestinal SMNs was associated with abdominal radiation (SIR, 11.2 [CI, 7.6 to 16.4]). However, survivors not exposed to radiation had a significantly increased risk (SIR, 2.4 [CI, 1.4 to 3.9]). In addition to abdominal radiation, high-dose procarbazine (relative risk, 3.2 [CI, 1.1 to 9.4]) and platinum drugs (relative risk, 7.6 [CI, 2.3 to 25.5]) independently increased the risk for gastrointestinal SMNs.

Limitation.—This cohort has not yet attained an age at which risk for gastrointestinal cancer is greatest.

Conclusion.—Childhood cancer survivors, particularly those exposed to abdominal radiation, are at increased risk for gastrointestinal SMNs. These findings suggest that surveillance of at-risk childhood cancer survivors should begin at a younger age than that recommended for the general population.

▶ It is becoming increasingly more common that we see reports appearing in the adult literature regarding secondary malignancies occurring in a childhood cancer survivor. The report by Henderson et al notes that somewhere between 5% and 15% of childhood cancer survivors will develop a subsequent malignant neoplasm in the first 20 to 30 years after diagnosis of a first cancer. Subsequent malignant neoplasms are the second leading cause of premature death in childhood cancer survivors, the first being recurrence of the primary cancer.

The report by Henderson et al tells us that childhood cancer survivors develop gastrointestinal cancers more frequently and at a younger age than the general population. Although prior studies have identified radiation exposure as a risk factor for gastrointestinal malignant neoplasm, no study has assessed the relationship between radiation field and the site of such secondary malignancies or the specific effect of chemotherapy used to treat a primary cancer in childhood. Because of the nature of this problem, the Children's Oncology Group has published guidelines for colorectal cancer surveillance in childhood cancer survivors.

These guidelines recommend that survivors exposed to more than 30 Gy of abdominal radiation undergo colonoscopy at a minimum of every 5 years beginning 10 years after radiation or at age 35 years, whichever is later.

In the report abstracted from the *Annals of Internal Medicine*, the investigators evaluated the risk for gastrointestinal secondary malignant neoplasms and the clinical and pathologic features associated with their development in a large, North American cohort of childhood cancer survivors for whom the investigators had detailed information about the specific therapies received for the primary cancer. They studied information from the Childhood Cancer Survivor Study, a retrospectively assembled and ongoing hospital-based cohort of 14 358 childhood cancer survivors treated at 28 centers in the United States and Canada. This study was established in 1994. Eligibility criteria for the study include a diagnosis of leukemia, central nervous system cancer, Hodgkin lymphoma, non-Hodgkin lymphoma, neuroblastoma, soft-tissue sarcoma, Wilms tumor, or bone cancer. The children in this study were diagnosed with cancer between January 1970 and 1986 and were younger than 21 years at diagnosis and had survived at least 5 years from diagnosis. All patients were followed carefully for the development of a secondary malignancy. Among the 14 337 childhood cancer survivors, 802 secondary malignancies (not including nonmelanoma skin cancer) were identified in 732 individuals. Of these, 45 (5.6%) represented gastrointestinal secondary malignancies. These occurred at a median follow-up of 22.8 years from primary diagnosis. The average age of diagnosis of a secondary gastrointestinal malignancy was 33.5 years (range 9.7—44.8 years). Survivors who developed gastrointestinal secondary malignancies were similar to those who did not in terms of race, sex, family history of gastrointestinal cancer, and smoking history. The most frequent site of secondary gastrointestinal malignancy was the colon, followed by the rectum and anus. Twenty-five (56%) of the 45 gastrointestinal secondary malignancies were adenocarcinomas. Fifty-one percent of those experiencing a secondary malignancy died from the malignancy; of those who developed gastrointestinal secondary malignancy, 65% died. Eighty-seven percent of childhood cancer survivors who developed gastrointestinal secondary malignancies had radiation for their primary cancer. Eighty-two percent of these survivors developed a secondary malignancy in" and/or near their previous radiation field, whereas 15% developed them out of the previous radiation field. The cumulative incidence of persons receiving abdominal radiation developing a secondary malignancy was 1.97%.

This report is the largest study that has focused on the risks for gastrointestinal cancer in childhood cancer survivors and is the only one that has examined detailed treatment information, including chemotherapy exposures and radiation fields. The authors observed that young survivors of childhood cancer, particularly Wilms tumor, Hodgkin lymphoma, and bone and brain cancer tumors are at increased risk for gastrointestinal cancer compared with age-matched general population. Gastrointestinal secondary malignancies can present as young as 9 years, and although all observed secondary malignancies occurred before 45 years of age, the authors expect the incidence to increase as this population ages. Although abdominal radiation appears to be the major culprit in the development of this type of secondary malignancy, survivors not exposed to radiation also had an increased risk for gastrointestinal secondary malignancy. Thirteen of

45 of the gastrointestinal secondary malignancies occurred outside the radiation field or in survivors who did not receive radiation therapy as part of their primary cancer treatment. Two particular cancer drugs were independently associated with an increased risk for secondary gastrointestinal malignancy in those who had radiation. These drugs were procarbazine and platinum. These agents may very well potentiate the carcinogenic effects of radiation.

The authors of this report note that because cure of childhood cancer is the utmost priority when treating newly diagnosed pediatric patients, they do not advocate for modification of the current treatment protocols used for childhood cancer simply to decrease the long-term risk for gastrointestinal secondary malignancies. Nonetheless, pediatric oncologists strive to reduce or eliminate late toxicity without affecting the probability of a cure. For this reason, the necessity for radiation is under constant scrutiny. The data from this report should help pediatric oncologists better identify those who will grow up to be adults with the highest risk for secondary gastrointestinal secondary malignancies, possibly facilitating the implementation of better surveillance in clinical practice. While the Children's Oncology Group currently recommends that survivors exposed to significant amount of abdominal radiation have colonoscopy at a minimum of every 5 years, beginning 10 years after radiation or at age 35, whichever is later, the data from this report suggest that certain forms of chemotherapy exposure should also necessitate very careful surveillance including colonoscopy at more frequent intervals.

The authors of this report are due all of our heartiest congratulations in tackling the problems that long-term survivors of childhood cancer might experience. Every one of the children we treat now must be very carefully followed for the rest of their lives.

J. A. Stockman III, MD

Childhood, Adolescent, and Young Adults (≤ 25 y) Colorectal Cancer: Study of Anatolian Society of Medical Oncology

Kaplan MA, Isikdogan A, Gumus M, et al (Dicle Univ Faculty of Medicine, Diyarbakir, Turkey; Dr Lutfi Kirdar Kartal Training and Res Hosp, Istanbul, Turkey; et al)
J Pediatr Hematol Oncol 35:83-89, 2013

Purpose.—To evaluate the clinicopathologic characteristics and treatment outcomes of young patients with colorectal cancer (CRC).

Methods.—Between May 2003 and June 2010, 76 patients were found eligible for this retrospective study. Age, sex, presenting symptoms, patients with acute presentation, family history, presence of polyps, histologic features, localization and stage of the tumor, treatment outcomes, time and site of recurrence, sites of metastasis, and survival outcomes were recorded from the patient files.

Results.—Seventy-six patients (55.3% male) with a median age of 23 years were evaluated. Patients were evaluated in 2 groups as follows: child-adolescent (0 to 19 y, n = 20) and young adult (20 to 25 y, n = 56).

Sex and symptoms (abdominal pain and rectal bleeding) were significantly differed between the groups and acute presentation was close to statistical significance. Overall survival significantly increased in patients undergoing curative surgery ($P < 0.001$). Other parameters affecting the survival was stage of disease ($P = 0.004$). Response to palliative chemotherapy in metastatic patients ($P = 0.042$) and postoperative adjuvant chemotherapy had a statistically significant survival advantage ($P = 0.028$).

Conclusions.—Diagnosis of CRC should not be excluded solely on the basis of age. CRC features in young-adult patients are more similar to adults compared with that of child-adolescent patients according to the symptoms and presentation. In patients with CRC in this age group, curative surgery, adjuvant chemotherapy, and palliative chemotherapy provide survival advantage.

▶ Colorectal cancer is a common malignancy in adults. It is not a common malignancy in children, adolescents, and young adults. Somewhere between 0.5% and 5% of childhood malignancies arise from the gastrointestinal tract, and the majority of these malignancies originate in the colon. On the other hand, just 1% to 4% of colorectal cancers occur in individuals under the age of 25 to 30 years. This makes our understanding of this particular malignancy particularly difficult, thus the value of this article.

These authors reviewed the records of all patients under the age of 75 who were newly diagnosed with colorectal cancer over a 7-year period between 2003 and 2010. The intent was to characterize the background of this malignancy as it affects young people. Seventy-six such cancers were found in children, adolescents, and the young adult population studied. A sex predominance was noted with a male to female ratio of 1.5 to 2.1. This is different from what is seen in the adult population, where equal ratios are normally found. The most common presentation was that of abdominal pain while changing bowel habits, nausea, vomiting, rectal bleeding, and weight loss were much less frequent. Unfortunately, the symptoms very much overlap common childhood problems associated with abdominal pain. This tended to make a diagnosis of colon cancer delayed.

Colon cancer in the adult population is associated with a small but real association with genetic and family history factors. In this study, 22% of patients had a family history of colon cancer. About 7% of the young adult population had a diagnosis of polyposis coli. Histologically, 45% of pediatric colon cancers were of mucinous carcinomas, unlike adults who have this form of malignancy quite infrequently. One in 4 children presented with metastatic disease and with primary cancers localized more often to the left colon (two-thirds of the malignancies in children). As is true of adults, the best opportunity for cure came with surgical resection. Unfortunately, there were few data in this article or elsewhere to tell us the benefits of combined surgery and chemotherapy.

When colon cancer is seen in a young person, one should always think about the potential for the 2 most common and inherited colorectal cancer syndromes. These are hereditary nonpolyposis colorectal cancer and familial adenomatous polyposis. These affect either sex. The children of people who carry these genes have a 50% chance of inheriting the disease-causing gene. These inherited forms of cancer account for just about 5% of colorectal cancers. Hereditary non-polyposis colorectal cancer is also known as Lynch syndrome. Familial adenomatous polyposis is characterized by the presence of hundreds or even thousands of benign polyps in the large intestine that have an extremely high malignant potential. Fifty percent of individuals develop these polyps by age 15, and if the colon is not surgically removed, there is a 100% chance that these polyps will develop into cancer usually by an average age of 40 years. There are also 2 other relatively rare forms of inherited polyposis syndromes that have a risk of malignancy. One is juvenile polyposis and the other the well-known Peutz-Jeghers syndrome.

J. A. Stockman III, MD

Identification of Lynch Syndrome Among Patients With Colorectal Cancer

Moreira L, for the EPICOLON Consortium (Univ of Barcelona, Spain; et al)
JAMA 308:1555-1565, 2012

Context.—Lynch syndrome is the most common form of hereditary colorectal cancer (CRC) and is caused by germline mutations in DNA mismatch repair (MMR) genes. Identification of gene carriers currently relies on germline analysis in patients with MMR-deficient tumors, but criteria to select individuals in whom tumor MMR testing should be performed are unclear.

Objective.—To establish a highly sensitive and efficient strategy for the identification of MMR gene mutation carriers among CRC probands.

Design, Setting, and Patients.—Pooled-data analysis of 4 large cohorts of newly diagnosed CRC probands recruited between 1994 and 2010 (n = 10 206) from the Colon Cancer Family Registry, the EPICOLON project, the Ohio State University, and the University of Helsinki examining personal, tumor-related, and family characteristics, as well as microsatellite instability, tumor MMR immunostaining, and germline MMR mutational status data.

Main Outcome Measures.—Performance characteristics of selected strategies (Bethesda guidelines, Jerusalem recommendations, and those derived from a bivariate/multivariate analysis of variables associated with Lynch syndrome) were compared with tumor MMR testing of all CRC patients (universal screening).

Results.—Of 10 206 informative, unrelated CRC probands, 312 (3.1%) were MMR gene mutation carriers. In the population-based cohorts (n = 3671 probands), the universal screening approach (sensitivity, 100%; 95% CI, 99.3%-100%; specificity, 93.0%; 95% CI, 92.0%-93.7%; diagnostic yield, 2.2%; 95% CI, 1.7%-2.7%) was superior to the use of Bethesda guidelines (sensitivity, 87.8%; 95% CI, 78.9%-93.2%; specificity, 97.5%; 95% CI, 96.9%-98.0%; diagnostic yield, 2.0%; 95% CI, 1.5%-2.4%; *P* < .001), Jerusalem recommendations (sensitivity, 85.4%; 95% CI, 77.1%-93.6%; specificity, 96.7%; 95% CI, 96.0%-97.2%; diagnostic yield, 1.9%; 95% CI, 1.4%-2.3%; *P* < .001), and a selective strategy based on tumor MMR testing of cases with CRC diagnosed at age 70 years or younger and in older patients fulfilling the

Bethesda guidelines (sensitivity, 95.1%; 95% CI, 89.8%-99.0%; specificity, 95.5%; 95% CI, 94.7%-96.1%; diagnostic yield, 2.1%; 95% CI, 1.6%-2.6%; $P < .001$). This selective strategy missed 4.9% of Lynch syndrome cases but resulted in 34.8% fewer cases requiring tumor MMR testing and 28.6% fewer cases undergoing germline mutational analysis than the universal approach.

Conclusion.—Universal tumor MMR testing among CRC probands had a greater sensitivity for the identification of Lynch syndrome compared with multiple alternative strategies, although the increase in the diagnostic yield was modest.

▶ Although children generally do not manifest hereditary cancer syndromes, they may if they carry the genetic disorder described, thus the importance of this report dealing with the Lynch syndrome. Lynch syndrome refers to one of the most common hereditary cancer syndromes known as the "hereditary nonpolyposis colorectal cancer-related syndrome." Identification of individuals at increased risk of hereditary cancer should allow for the possibility of screening and early cancer detection, possibly relating in decreased disease-specific mortality, and is the justification for germline genetic testing for specific cancer risk alleles. Unfortunately, factors of prevalence and age-specific penetrance, effectiveness and evasiveness of screening procedures, and efficacy of early detection influence the potential benefit of such an approach. With respect to Lynch syndrome, various sets of clinical criteria, combined with pathologic phenotypic characteristics of tumor tissues in carriers, have been used to identify individuals at risk in whom it is important to consider germline genetic testing for deleterious mutations specifically of certain mismatch repair genes.

Lynch syndrome itself was originally defined by the "Amsterdam" clinical criteria as a history of 3 or more family members with histologically confirmed colorectal cancer involving 2 generations with at least 1 person diagnosed before age 50. Although this approach is fairly specific in identifying families with a high penetrance of Lynch syndrome, it is overly restrictive and does not consider the possibility of later-onset variants of the disease, the implications of extracolonic tumors, or limitations imposed by small family size. For these reasons, many families with known Lynch syndrome do not meet the original Amsterdam criteria. The Amsterdam criteria therefore miss many families because of its poor sensitivity. For this reason, it has been suggested that all colorectal cancers should be examined for mismatch gene repair or that all cancers in individuals below a certain age cutoff be so screened. However, the effectiveness of such a "universal" approach to screening for Lynch syndrome has not been tested in a population-based manner, thus the importance of the report of Moreira et al.

Moreira et al address the question of screening for Lynch syndrome by performing a pooled-data analysis of a large set of population-based patient cohorts from around the world to determine the sensitivity and efficiency of several different strategies for Lynch syndrome screening, including the "universal" approach. Using more than 10 000 histologically confirmed specimens from patients with colorectal cancer, the authors found that universal tumor screening for mismatch repair deficiency was superior in sensitivity than any of the current standard guidelines. The data from this report confirm that the prevalence of Lynch syndrome is high enough among patients with colorectal cancer (3.1%) that screening all colorectal cancers should be considered.

Clearly the majority of patients with colorectal cancer do not have Lynch syndrome, and their families are off the hook for this hereditary form of cancer. Nonetheless, in an editorial that accompanied this report, it was noted that in the haystack of patients with colorectal cancer, those with Lynch syndrome are more like large knitting needles than tiny sewing needles—and that a systematic search can find them and help their families know their risk of the development of one hereditary form of cancer.[1]

J. A. Stockman III, MD

Reference

1. Ladabaum U, Ford JM. Lynch syndrome in patients with colorectal cancer: finding the needle in the haystack. *JAMA.* 2012;308:1581-1583.

Cancer in Children with Nonchromosomal Birth Defects
Fisher PG, Reynolds P, Von Behren J, et al (Stanford Univ, Palo Alto, CA; et al)
J Pediatr 160:978-983, 2012

Objective.—To examine whether the incidence of childhood cancer is elevated in children with birth defects but no chromosomal anomalies.

Study Design.—We examined cancer risk in a population-based cohort of children with and without major birth defects born between 1988 and 2004, by linking data from the California Birth Defects Monitoring Program, the California Cancer Registry, and birth certificates. Cox proportional hazards models generated hazard ratios (HRs) and 95% CIs based on person-years at risk. We compared the risk of childhood cancer in infants born with and without specific types of birth defects, excluding infants with chromosomal anomalies.

Results.—Of the 4869 children in the birth cohort with cancer, 222 had a major birth defect. Although the expected elevation in cancer risk was observed in children with chromosomal birth defects (HR, 12.44; 95% CI, 10.10-15.32), especially for the leukemias (HR, 28.99; 95% CI, 23.07-36.42), children with nonchromosomal birth defects also had an increased risk of cancer (HR, 1.58; 95% CI, 1.33-1.87), but instead for brain tumors, lymphomas, neuroblastoma, and germ cell tumors.

Conclusion.—Children with nonchromosomal birth defects are at increased risk for solid tumors, but not leukemias. Dysregulation of early human development likely plays an important role in the etiology of childhood cancer.

▶ It has been known for some time that certain genetic syndromes are associated with an increased risk of childhood malignancy, but less than 5% of such cancers are directly attributable to these genetic syndromes. In most cases of the latter, the resultant cancer is a leukemia seen mostly in children with Down syndrome, bilateral retinoblastomas, tumors associated with neurofibromatosis, and hereditary Wilms tumor. As relatively uncommon as these cancers are, there are other childhood cancers that are likely related to genetic alterations that do not cleanly fit into a syndrome or a specific chromosomal anomaly. Fisher et al have undertaken a study to provide more information on the risk of cancer in children with nonchromosomal birth defects. In examining this relationship, they undertook the largest population-based North American effort to date to examine whether the incidence of childhood cancer is indeed elevated in children with structural birth defects, specifically those birth defects not associated with chromosomal anomalies. They did this by linking three data sources: the California Birth Defects Monitoring Program Registry, the California Cancer Registry, and the live birth death files from the California State Office of Vital Records. Data from these sources include more than 3 million live births between 1988 and 2004 in those California counties covered by the California Birth Defects Monitoring Program.

The results of this study show that of 3.2 million live births, a total of 65 585 infants with structural birth defects (2%) were able to be identified. At the same time, the investigators identified 4869 children with cancer in the birth cohort, representing 81.5% of all cancers occurring in children living in the counties studied. It was concluded that children with nonchromosomal birth defects do indeed have an elevated risk of cancer (odds ratio 1.58), particularly for central nervous system (CNS) tumors, lymphomas, neuroblastomas, and germ cell tumors, but not for leukemia. The investigators observed that the risk for the development of cancer in childhood was substantially increased (2- to 3 fold) in children with nearly every structural birth defect phenotype, with the exception of cleft lip or cleft palate. Interestingly, CNS tumors were more common in children with a history of CNS birth defects and that lymphomas were more common in children with a history of congenital heart defects.

The etiologic link for structural birth defects and childhood cancers remains elusive. The authors of this report hypothesize that dysregulation in human development plays an important role in the etiology of childhood cancer, especially solid tumors. For example, defects in specific homeobox genes might be related to some solid tumors and birth defects, and CNS tumors have been linked to a pathway that is a key regulator of brain development. This is very different from the situation related to the development of leukemia that may hinge on a single gene defect in the clonal proliferation of leukocytes and therefore would be less closely related to aberrant developmental pathways. This report, which identifies the link between structural birth defects and a greater risk of malignancy, should serve to alert pediatricians to the increased risk of cancer in a child with any birth defect.

This commentary closes with information on how a commonly available seasoning may help treat certain malignancies. Best known as a food seasoning and dye, saffron can be effective in controlling hepatic cancers, at least when studied in mice.[1] It appears to suppress a variety of compounds that are cancer related and enhances certain others. Saffron, of course, is an expensive spice made from the flower, *Crocus sativus*. Studies have documented its ability to benefit certain conditions such as depression, inflammatory states, and memory loss. It is also an antioxidant. The exact mechanism as an anti-cancer drug is poorly understood.

J. A. Stockman III, MD

Reference

1. Seppa N. Saffron fights liver cancer. *Science News*. 2011;8.

17 Ophthalmology

Uncorrected Distance Visual Impairment Among Adolescents in the United States
Kemper AR, Wallace DK, Zhang X, et al (Duke Univ, Durham, NC; Ctrs for Disease Control and Prevention, Atlanta, GA; et al)
J Adolesc Health 50:645-647, 2012

Purpose. To describe uncorrected distance visual impairment (VI).

Methods.—We conducted an analysis of the 3,555 adolescents aged 12 through 21 years who participated in the 2005–2008 National Health and Nutrition Examination Survey. Distance VI was defined as 20/40 or worse in the better-seeing eye. Data were weighted to represent the civilian noninstitutionalized population.

Results.—Overall, 12.3% (95% confidence interval [CI]: 10.7%–14.1%) had distance VI, which was correctable to 20/30 or better in both eyes in 86.1% (95% CI: 83.6%–89.5%). The prevalence was higher among those who reported not having corrective lenses available (44.3%) compared with those who reported that they did not need them (8.5%) or who had them available (5.2%; $p < .001$). After adjusting for potential confounders, those who were 12 or 13 years of age had 2.27 (95% CI: 1.32–3.90) greater odds of distance VI than older adolescents, and the odds of distance VI were greater among non-Hispanic blacks (1.66 [95% CI: 1.11–2.48]), Hispanics (1.96 [95% CI: 1.35–2.84]), or other race/ethnicities (2.06 [95% CI: 1.19–3.57]) than among non-Hispanic whites.

Conclusions.—More than 1 in 10 adolescents had uncorrected distance VI. To address this, interventions should address case detection, access to eye care, and adherence with corrective lenses.

▶ There is relatively little information in the literature about the vision status of teenagers in the United States. A study of the National Health and Nutrition Examination Survey (NHANES) covering the period 1999 through 2002 estimated that 9% of individuals aged 12 through 19 years had uncorrected distance vision of 20/50 or worse in their better-seeing eye that could be corrected to at least 20/40.[1] This same report suggested that such vision issues in adolescents and young adults is associated with factors related to poor access to health care (eg, nonwhite race, lower income, no private insurance). In a separate report from the NHANES, it was noted that about 25% of adolescents who need corrective lenses did not have them.[2] The authors of the latter report now tell us about a study conducted to describe not only the prevalence but also the characteristics associated with visual issues among adolescents that identify potential opportunities for improving the situation.

In this article, data were obtained from both the 2005 to 2006 and the 2007 to 2008 NHANES, which are representative of the US civilian noninstitutionalized population. A total of 3555 individuals aged 12 through 21 years were included in the analysis. Information was collected on sex, race or ethnicity, household income, the availability of health insurance, and whether the youngsters had corrective lenses for their visual impairments. Overall, 12.3% of the teenagers had 20/50 or worse vision in their better-seeing eye. Those 12 or 13 years of age compared with those age 14 through 21 years had more than a 2-fold increase in the odds of having uncorrected 20/50 or worse vision. There was no difference in the likelihood of uncorrected vision by sex, household income, health insurance, or having a routine place for health care. Nearly half of those with uncorrected vision of this magnitude were non-Hispanic white. However, non-Hispanic blacks, Hispanics, and those of other than white race or ethnicity had greater odds of having uncorrected visual difficulties.

The gist of this article is consistent with prior research showing about 1 in 10 adolescents have correctable visual difficulties in their better-seeing eye. These findings highlight the need for visual screening as part of routine preventive care. The findings also refute the belief among some health care providers that screening is not necessary at this age because those with uncorrected visual difficulties will be identified because they are symptomatic. This study clearly showed that about half of those with uncorrected visual difficulties reported they had no need for corrective lenses. We should be grateful to the investigators at Duke who mined the data from NHANES to document how poorly we are doing in terms of servicing our teenagers' visual needs.

For who suffer from amblyopia, there may be a simple, and for some a pleasurable, way to help correct the ocular difficulty. Researchers have found that subjects who played video games for 40 hours, while wearing a patch over the good eye, had a 30% improvement in visual acuity. This study was done in adults.[3] No mention was made of whether the study subject got any better at the games they were playing as their vision improved.

J. A. Stockman III, MD

References

1. Vitale S, Cotch MF, Sperduto RD. Prevalence of visual impairment in the United States. *JAMA.* 2006;295:2158-2163.
2. Kemper AR, Gurney JC, Eibschitz-Tsimhoni M, Del Monte M. Corrective lens wear among adolescents: findings from the National Health and Nutrition Examination Survey. *J Pediatr Ophthalmol Strabismus.* 2007;44:356-362.
3. Li R, Ngo C, Nguyen J, et al. Video-Game Play Induces Plasticity in the Visual System of Adults with Amblyopia. *PLoS Biol.* 2011;9:e1001135.

Retinal Hemorrhages in Children: The Role of Intracranial Pressure
Shiau T, Levin AV (Thomas Jefferson Univ, Philadelphia, PA)
Arch Pediatr Adolesc Med 166:623-628, 2012

Objective.—To evaluate the role of intracranial pressure (ICP) in the production of retinal hemorrhage in young children.

Design.—Review of published clinical, postmortem, and experimental research findings worldwide pertinent to our review objective. We used PubMed, MEDLINE, and Ovid Evidence-Based Medicine Reviews as well as references found in other published articles to conduct searches.

Main Exposures.—Increased ICP from various etiologies.

Main Outcome Measure.—Hemorrhagic retinopathy, in particular with extension to the periphery, multiple layers, and too-numerous-to-count hemorrhages. The review also considers additional intraocular findings such as retinoschisis and perimacular folds.

Results.—In general, elevated ICP does not cause extensive hemorrhagic retinopathy. Papilledema may be associated with a small number of hemorrhages on or around the optic disc. There are isolated case reports that severe hyperacute ICP elevation, unlike the subacute pressure increase in abusive head injury, in children may rarely result in extensive retinal hemorrhage. These diagnoses are readily distinguished from child abuse.

Conclusions.—In the absence of the few readily recognizable alternate scenarios, extensive retinal hemorrhage in very young children is not secondary to isolated elevated ICP.

▶ There are many reasons why children develop retinal hemorrhages. The reason that most commonly comes to mind is abusive head trauma secondary to shaken baby syndrome. The authors of this article remind us a little bit about the anatomy of the eye in this regard. The retina is a multilayered organ lining the inside of the eye, extending from the optic nerve to just behind the iris. The interior (peripheral) retinal edge is called the ora serrata. Retina around the optic nerve is called the peripapillary retina. The posterior pole of the retina includes the optic nerve disc, macula (generally defined as posterior retina extending out to the temporal vascular arcades), fovea (center of macula), and peripapillary region (see Fig 1 in the original article). Four vortex veins mark the posterior edge of the peripheral retina. The area between the posterior pole and the peripheral retina is the mid-peripheral retina (see Fig 2 in the original article). Bleeding in front of the retinal hemorrhage is described as preretinal or subhyaloid (underneath the hyaloid [ie, vitreous gel]). Intraretinal hemorrhage encompasses any bleeding within the retinal layers. Bleeding within the superficial nerve fiber layer produces a flame or splinter hemorrhage, whereas hemorrhage into the deeper layers appeared to be and are called dot or blot hemorrhage.

In addition to location, retinal hemorrhages can be characterized by their number. When the number becomes too high to easily count, terms such as confluent, too numerous to count, or rough estimates of number (eg, 50 to 100) are used. Aficionados, however, avoid the terms mild, moderate, severe, or extensive. The reason is obvious. To someone who is naive in terms of never having previously seen a retinal hemorrhage, a severe hemorrhage may in fact be otherwise mild.

These authors have reviewed published clinical, postmortem, and experimental research findings reviewing the world's literature on retinal hemorrhages. They specifically did this to determine whether increased intracranial hemorrhage from various etiologies in and of itself might produce retinal hemorrhages. Their data indicate that the absence of clinical data in children to support the association of extensive retinal hemorrhage with increased intracranial hemorrhage is consistent with both the anatomy and physiology of eye problems. They conclude that intracranial pressure may result in papilledema, with small numbers of intraretinal and preretinal hemorrhage in or about the optic nerve. They did not find data to support the concept that extensive retinal hemorrhage in very young children, in the absence of readily recognizable rare circumstances, is due to increased intracranial pressure. Thus, increased intracranial pressure as a cause of retinal hemorrhages is not supported by peer-reviewed published evidence or empirical experience. If retinal hemorrhages are seen, one should think of trauma as the cause. Retinal hemorrhages occur in approximately 85% of abusive head trauma, and more than 75% of such cases will have bilateral retinal hemorrhages. In such cases, retinal hemorrhages are too numerous to count in two-thirds of cases and generally involve multiple retinal layers covering nearly the entire retinal surface. Retinal hemorrhages from simple accidental trauma rarely reach the periphery, are confined to the posterior pole, and generally are few. The severity of retinal hemorrhage correlates positively with the severity of intracranial trauma. Repetitive acceleration or deceleration produces shearing forces sufficient to allow the vitreous to pull off the retina, leading to splitting of the retinal layers (traumatic retinoschisis); this is found almost exclusively in abusive head trauma arising most often between the superficial internal limiting membrane and nerve fiber layer of the eye. In infants and children, the adherence between the vitreous and the posterior pole and peripheral retina is particularly strong and can be broken generally only by repetitive severe acceleration or deceleration forces. Thus, if one sees the type of retinal hemorrhages described, one should be concerned not about accidental trauma, but rather about abusive head trauma as a cause of significant retinal hemorrhage.

J. A. Stockman III, MD

Treatment with Recombinant Human Growth Hormone during Childhood is Associated with Increased Intraocular Pressure

Youngster I, Rachmiel R, Pinhas-Hamiel O, et al (Assaf Harofeh Med Ctr, Zerifin, Israel; Tel-Aviv Univ, Israel; et al)
J Pediatr 161:1116-1119.e1, 2012

Objective.—To evaluate the association between recombinant human growth hormone (rhGH) treatment and intraocular pressure (IOP) in children.

Study Design.—This is an observational cohort study including comparison between children treated with rhGH for at least 12 months (treatment group), matched children prior to treatment (control group), and population age-adjusted normograms of IOP. All children underwent an ocular slit lamp assessment and Goldmann applanation tonometry. Charts were reviewed for cause of therapy, peak stimulated growth hormone level prior to therapy, treatment duration, insulin-like growth factor 1, and rhGH dosage.

Results.—The treatment group included 55 children and the control group included 24 children. Mean age at examination was comparable at 11.4 ± 3.3 years and 10.3 ± 2.6 years, respectively ($P = .13$). Mean treatment duration was 37.5 ± 22.8 months and mean rhGH dose was 0.04 ± 0.01 mg/kg/d. Mean IOP was significantly increased in the treatment group compared with the control group and compared with age-matched normograms (16.09 ± 2.2 mm Hg, 13.26 ± 1.83 mm Hg and 14.6 ± 1.97 mm Hg, respectively, $P < .001$). IOP was positively correlated with treatment duration ($r = 0.559$, $P < .001$) and rhGH dosage ($r = 0.274$, $P = .043$).

Conclusion.—IOP in children treated with rhGH is increased compared with a similar population without treatment and compared with healthy population normograms. IOP is associated with longer treatment duration and higher dosages.

▶ The world of medical therapies is associated with many unintended consequences. One of the unintended consequences is the development of increased ocular pressure secondary to human growth hormone administration. Although the latter therapy is generally considered safe, side effects can occur with growth hormone therapy. These include headaches, visual problems, nausea and vomiting, fluid retention, arthralgia, myalgia, paresthesia, and local reactions at injection sites. Some children also develop increased intracranial pressure and osseous problems, including Perthes disease and slipped capital femoral epiphysis. Almost 20 years ago, the first case was reported of a 7-year-old boy who had developed severe glaucoma while on human growth hormone treatments, which were given to deal with growth failure secondary to renal disease. In this youngster, cessation of growth hormone therapy and surgical decompression of the optic nerve resulted in resolution of the ocular problem.[1] Glaucoma has also been recognized as a complication of acromegaly with endogenous overproduction of growth hormone.

These authors undertook a study in Israel to determine whether a true association exists between increased ocular pressure in children and the use of recombinant human growth hormone. Children being treated with human growth hormone had determinations performed of intraocular pressure. Data were compared with those for a control group of nontreated children. The mean intraocular pressure in the treatment group was significantly elevated, compared with the control group (16.33 mm Hg vs 13.33 mm Hg for the right eye and 15.85 mm Hg vs 13.20 mm Hg for the left eye) when compared with normal values for the same age group.

A number of prior studies have linked associations between growth hormone levels and ocular difficulties. For example, growth hormone deficiency has previously been implicated in ocular anomalies such as optic nerve hypoplasia and reduced retinal vascularization and hyperopic defects related to a shorter axis of the eye. As noted, acromegaly is commonly associated with increased ocular pressure and glaucoma. It is thought that growth hormone influences the synthesis of extracellular matrix of the sclera, potentially disturbing aqueous humor outflow through the trabecular meshwork of the eye. The study performed in Israel documented a correlation in mean intraocular pressure with the length and dosage of growth hormone treatment. None of the children who had elevated intraocular pressure showed evidence of glaucoma, at least during the period of this study.

Human recombinant growth hormone is increasingly being used in the pediatric population for problems other than idiopathic short stature. In fact, treatment for the latter constitutes the minority of uses of human recombinant growth hormone today. Given its increasing wider application, one must be aware of the possible systemic side effects of long-term growth hormone treatment, including the potential for the development of glaucoma. The data from Israel implied that continuous monitoring of patients for the development of undesirable ocular side effects is essential because once lost, damage to the visual field cannot be recovered. Loss of one's sight for the sake of the development of a centimeter or 2 of growth is a severe price to pay.

J. A. Stockman III, MD

Reference

1. Wingenfeld P, Schmidt B, Hoppe B, et al. Acute glaucoma and intracranial hypertension in a child on long-term peritoneal dialysis treated with growth hormone. *Pediatr Nephrol.* 1995;9:742-745.

Pediatric Eye Injuries Treated in US Emergency Departments, 1990-2009
Pollard KA, Xiang H, Smith GA (The Res Inst at Nationwide Children's Hosp, Columbus, OH)
Clin Pediatr 51:374-381, 2012

This study investigates activity– and consumer product–related eye injuries treated in US hospital emergency departments among children <18 years old using National Electronic Injury Surveillance System data from 1990 through 2009. An estimated 1 406 200 (95% confidence interval = 1 223 409-1 588 992) activity– and consumer product–related pediatric eye injuries occurred during the study period, averaging 70 310 annually. The annual number of injuries declined significantly by 17%. Patients ≤4 years of age accounted for 32% of all injuries and had the highest mean annual eye injury rate (11.31 per 10 000 population). Eye injuries associated with sports and recreation (24%) and chemicals (17%) occurred most frequently. The majority (69%) of eye injuries occurred at home. Opportunities exist to further decrease these injuries. Pediatricians should educate child caregivers and children about risks for

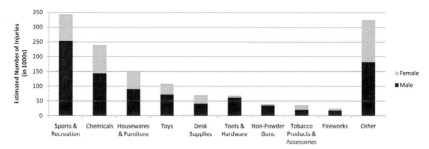

FIGURE 1.—Estimated number of activity— and consumer product—related eye injuries sustained by children <18 years of age who were treated in US hospital emergency departments according to gender and product category, 1990 through 2009. (Reprinted from Pollard KA, Xiang H, Smith GA. Pediatric eye injuries treated in US emergency departments, 1990-2009. *Clin Pediatr.* 2012;51:374-381. © 2012 by Clinical Pediatrics. Reprinted by permission of SAGE Publications.)

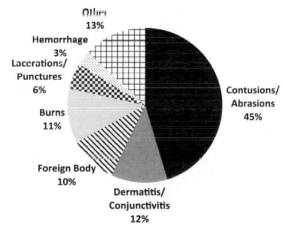

FIGURE 3.—Proportion of activity— and consumer product— related eye injuries sustained by children <18 years of age who were treated in US hospital emergency departments according to type of eye injury, 1990 through 2009. (Reprinted from Pollard KA, Xiang H, Smith GA. Pediatric eye injuries treated in US emergency departments, 1990-2009. *Clin Pediatr.* 2012;51:374-381. © 2012 by Clinical Pediatrics. Reprinted by permission of SAGE Publications.)

eye injuries in the home and about use of appropriate protective eyewear during sports (Figs 1 and 3).

▶ This report from the Center for Injury Research and Policy, the Research Institute at Nationwide Children's Hospital in Columbus, Ohio, reminds us that there are an estimated 2.4 million eye injuries occurring annually in the United States. Nearly 35% of all eye injuries occur in children less than 18 years of age.

Pollard et al tell us a great deal about pediatric eye injuries using information from the National Electronic Injury Surveillance System (NEISS). The US Consumer Product Safety Commission monitors injuries treated in emergency departments here in the United States through NEISS. It does this by obtaining data from a cross sample of 98 hospitals selected from the population of all hospitals with 24-hour emergency departments. Pollard et al were able to calculate injury rates using US census data as a denominator. They also were able to examine the various causes of eye injury.

During the 20-year study period, the annual number of activity and consumer product-related eye injuries in children less than 18 years of age declined over time by 17%. The annual eye injury rate itself declined by 28%. One can assume that these declines are the result of implementation of recommendations and standards regarding eye protection for children, especially while participating in sports. Recommendations have emanated from the American Academy of Pediatrics, which has a policy on protective eyewear for young athletes, and from the US Lacrosse requirement of protective eyewear for women's lacrosse players that was reported back in 2005. As one might suspect, boys account for most (65%) of injuries, likely a reflection of the type of activities that boys become engaged in such as basketball and football. Participation in sports and recreational activities remains the most common cause of eye injury in children, followed by exposure of the eye to chemicals. Patients 4 years and younger were shown in this article to be the most likely to sustain eye injuries associated with chemicals. General purpose household cleaners and nontape adhesives were most frequently associated with chemical-related eye injury. Presumably, the predominance of chemical-related eye injuries among young children is a reflection of their developmental stage characterized by exploration and an inability to recognize potential sources of harm.

In contrast to the trend for eye injuries overall declining, eye injuries associated with nonpowder guns increased during the study period. These were also the injuries most likely to result in hospitalization. The small size and high velocity of projectiles fired from nonpowder guns contribute to their propensity to cause serious eye injury. Most of these nonpowder gun-related eye injuries occur at home, perhaps because of higher exposure or because play in the home environment may be less supervised. Needless to say, children should be old enough to safely handle these guns, be supervised by an adult, and wear appropriate protective eyewear or mask. Nonpowder guns should be stored unloaded in locked locations similar to other firearms.

If there is any good news in this report, it is that eye injuries associated with tobacco products and related accessories decreased by 70% over a 20-year period. This decrease is likely to be associated with a national decline in smoking rates as well as the passage of legislation banning smoking in public places. Children 4 years and younger are the ones most likely to be injured by tobacco products. A cigarette held at or below an adult's waist is at eye level of a young child, making it easy for the child to inadvertently bump into the lit tobacco product and to sustain an eye injury.

This report is the first to provide an in-depth analysis of pediatric activity and consumer product-related eye injuries in children treated in hospital emergency departments in the United States. Figs 1 and 3 tell us a great deal about the types of injuries children sustain as well as their causes. Educating parents, other care providers, and children about the potential risk for eye injuries at home such as those associated with chemicals, tobacco products, and fireworks and promoting the use of appropriate outdoor protective eye gear during sports and recreational activities may help reduce the incidence of eye injuries among children.

This commentary in the Ophthalmology chapter closes with a quiz. Which is mightier, the sword or the pen(cil)? The answer comes from a brief report of the United Kingdom's Home and Leisure Accident Surveillance System.[1] Pens and pencils are often thrown by children and can cause penetrating eye injuries. A review of eye injuries showed that 748 ocular pen injuries and 892 ocular pencil injuries were reported in the United Kingdom between 2001 and 2002 by the Surveillance System data bank. By contrast, no injuries were report as the result of injury by swords or fencing foils, leading the authors to conclude that with regards to eyes, pens are indeed mightier than swords.

J. A. Stockman III, MD

Reference

1. Kelly SP, Reeves GMB. Penetrating eye injuries from writing instruments. *Clin Ophthalmol.* 2012;6:11 14.

Effectiveness of Protective Eyewear in Reducing Eye Injuries Among High School Field Hockey Players

Kriz PK, Comstock RD, Zurakowski D, et al (Brown Univ, Providence, RI; The Res Inst at Nationwide Children's Hosp, Columbus, OH; Boston Children's Hosp, MA; et al)
Pediatrics 130:1069 1075, 2012

Objective.—To determine if injury rates differ among high school field hockey players in states that mandated protective eyewear (MPE) versus states with no protective eyewear mandate (no MPE).

Methods.—We analyzed field hockey exposure and injury data collected over the 2009—2010 and 2010—2011 scholastic seasons from national and regional databases.

Results.—Incidence of all head and face injuries (including eye injuries, concussion) was significantly higher in no-MPE states compared with MPE states, 0.69 vs 0.47 injuries per 1000 athletic exposures (incidence rate ratio [IRR] 1.47; 95% confidence interval [CI]: 1.04—2.15, $P = .048$). Players in the no-MPE group had a 5.33-fold higher risk of eye injury than players in the MPE group (IRR 5.33; 95% CI: 0.71—39.25, $P = .104$). There was no significant difference in concussion rates for the 2 groups (IRR 1.04; 95% CI: 0.63—1.75, $P = .857$). A larger percentage of injuries sustained by athletes in the no-MPE group required >10 days to return to activity (32%) compared with athletes in the MPE group (17%), but this difference did not reach statistical significance ($P = .060$).

Conclusions.—Among high school field hockey players, playing in a no-MPE state results in a statistically significant higher incidence of head and face injuries versus playing in an MPE state. Concussion rates among players in MPE and no-MPE states were similar, indicating that addition of protective eyewear did not result in more player-player contact injuries, challenging a perception in contact/collision sports that increased protective equipment yields increased injury rates.

▶ Over the past 20 years, a number of changes to equipment, playing surfaces, and style of play have taken place in the sport of field hockey. At the same time, advances in stick construction have allowed players to generate much more power and velocity, with ball speeds greater than 50 miles per hour easily achieved by high school girls and nearly 100 miles per hour by elite players. Artificial turf has provided a smoother and faster playing surface, and in recent years the ball is being elevated off the field much more frequently. Field hockey is among the most frequently played team sports in the world, second only to soccer. There has been a 29% increase in participation rates in field hockey at the high school level over the 20-year period from 1990 to 2010.[1]

One of the most important injuries that can be sustained by a field hockey player is damage to the eye. The American Academy of Ophthalmology, American Academy of Pediatrics, International Federation of Sports Medicine, American Optometric Association, and the US Department of Health and Human Services, Prevent Blindness America, and Coalition to Prevent Sports Injury have all recommended protective eyewear use by those participating in field hockey sporting activities. Effective with the 2011 to 2012 scholastic season, the National Federation of High School Associations has mandated that high school field hockey players wear protective eyewear meeting the current American Society for Testing and Material Standards for field hockey.[2]

These authors capitalized on a relatively novel opportunity to investigate whether risk of eye injury for field hockey players differs in states that mandate protective eyewear vs those that do not. Field hockey is a sanctioned high school sport in 19 states, with over 63 000 girls participating annually. At the initiation of this study in the fall of 2009, only 6 state interscholastic athletic associations had mandated protective eyewear for all high school field hockey players (Connecticut, Maine, Massachusetts, New Hampshire, New York, and Rhode Island). The authors initiated their study with the primary objective of examining whether risk of eye or orbital injury during practices and games would differ for high school field hockey players in states with mandated protective eyewear compared with players in states that did not mandate protective eyewear. Secondary objectives included examining differences between cohorts for all head, face, eye or orbital and concussive injuries, concussive injuries only, head and face injuries only (excluding eye or orbital and concussive injury), and all injuries resulting in delayed return to activity.

The results of this study showed that 31 injuries were reported in the mandated protective eyewear group in 66 286 youngsters and 181 injuries were reported in the no-mandated protective eyewear group in 263 episodes of athletic exposure. The incidence of total head and face injuries was 0.69 injuries per 1000 athletic events in the no-mandated protective eye group compared with 0.47 injuries per 1000 athletic events in the mandated protective eyewear group, resulting in a 32% lower injury rate if protective eyewear was worn. There was no difference in concussion rates for the 2 groups. Only 1 eye or orbital injury was recorded in the mandated protective eye group: a corneal abrasion of the right eye in a junior varsity forward that was shooting during practice. This injury resulted from contact with a stick; the injured player was wearing off-the-shelf protective eyewear at the time of injury. The athlete returned to activity within 6 days. In contrast, 21 eye or orbital injuries were recorded in the no-mandated protective eyewear group. Of these injuries, 14% resulted in a time loss greater than 21 days of field playing, none resulted in medical disqualification for the season. The eye or orbital injury rate for the mandated protective eye group compared with the no-mandated protective eyewear group was 0.015 per 1000 athletic episodes vs 0.080 per 1000 athletic episodes, respectively, an 80% lower injury eye rate in the mandated protective eye group.

This article is the first prospective study to use injury surveillance to investigate the effectiveness of mandated protective eyewear in reducing rates and severity of eye injuries in high school field hockey players. The study demonstrates that protective eyewear will confer a reduced risk of total head and face injury by 32% and a reduced eye or orbital rate of injury by 80%. The data indicate that injuries to eye orbits, eye globes, eyebrows, and eyelids are completely eliminated if one wears protective eye gear. The wearing of protective eye gear does not seem to increase the rate of player-to-player contact and injuries caused by the latter. Fortunately, no catastrophic eye injuries were recorded as part of this study in either group of children.

It is very clear from this article that no youngster should enter the hockey field without protective eyewear. The data are quite clear that such eyewear will prevent all types of injury in and about the eye.

This commentary closes with an ocular quiz. You are seeing a young adult male in a clinic that you volunteer your time in. The individual has a history going back a number of years of IV drug abuse. His complaint now is of progressive weight loss. You examine him. The most obvious finding is the presence of long eyelashes. What is your diagnosis for the most likely cause of this finding?

The tip-off here is the the long eyelashes, a condition better known as trichomegaly. Trichomegaly can be congenital or acquired. The differential diagnosis of acquired long eyelashes is fairly short and includes HIV infection, metastatic renal adenocarcinoma, dermatomyositis, and treatment with cyclosporine and interferon alpha 2b and certain other immunomodulators. It has also been described in systemic lupus erythematosus, linear scleroderma and kala-azar, which can lead to severe malnutrition. Given the history presented by this young man, the likely diagnosis is HIV infection.

The topical drug latanoprost, an analogue of prostaglandin F2 analogue, used to treat topically chronic open-angle glaucoma has been shown to cause regional hypertrichosis of the eyelashes and eyelids in approximately 77 percent of the patients treated with this drug. The hypertrichosis is associated with hyperpigmentation of the eyelashes. The new growth of lash-like hair may include extra rows of eyelashes.. This additional growth is typically restricted to the eye under treatment, but a bilateral effect of the treatment of one eye and hypertrichosis of the ipsilateral of the ear lobe has been reported. The hypertrichosis can be persistent even after the medication is discontinued.

Trichomegaly may also be seen in non-acquired (congenital) states. The Oliver-McFarlane syndrome is an extremely rare condition associated with chorioretinal degeneration, dwarfism with growth hormone deficiency, hair abnormalities, and cerebellar dysfunction. Eight cases have been reported since the first report in 1965. All reported cases, although genetic in origin, appear to be sporadic. The genetics of this syndrome remain unclear.[3]

J. A. Stockman III, MD

References

1. National Federation of State High School Associations. Participation figure history. www.nfhs.org/content.aspx?id-3282. Accessed February 9, 2013.
2. National Federation of State High School Associations. NFHS Field Hockey Rules Committee — Eyewear Ruling. www.nfhs.org/content.aspx?id=5117&;terms= field%20hockey%20eyewear. Accessed February 9, 2013.
3. Editorial comment. Trichomegaly as a manifestation of HIV infection. *BMJ*. 2012; 343:964.

18 Respiratory Tract

Improving Detection by Pediatric Residents of Endotracheal Tube Dislodgement with Capnography: A Randomized Controlled Trial
Langhan ML, Auerbach M, Smith AN, et al (Yale Univ School of Medicine, New Haven, CT)
J Pediatr 160:1009-1014.e1, 2012

Objective.—The authors sought to determine if capnography could improve time to correction of a simulated endotracheal tube (ETT) dislodgement by pediatric residents.

Study Design.—Pediatric residents attended a didactic session that included interpretation of capnography. A randomized controlled study was then performed using patient simulators. Residents were randomized to standard monitoring (control group) or standard monitoring plus capnography (intervention group). The primary outcome was time to correction of ETT dislodgement. Correction of dislodgement prior to decline in pulse oximetry was our secondary outcome.

Results.—Twenty-seven subjects completed the simulation. Subjects in the intervention group corrected the ETT dislodgement faster than those in the control group (2.38 minutes vs 3.92 minutes, $P = .02$). There were no differences in time to correction based on postgraduate year, clinical experiences, or comfort with capnography. Two subjects corrected the dislodgement prior to changes in pulse oximetry, both from the intervention group. Fifty-nine percent of subjects had seen capnography used in the past and 82% felt very or somewhat comfortable with capnography.

Conclusion.—Capnography decreased time to correction of ETT dislodgement by pediatric residents. Capnography should be considered as an essential monitoring device for intubated patients to enhance patient safety.

▶ One of the most common problems encountered in neonatal and older child intensive care units is unplanned extubation or dislodgement of a endotracheal tube. This may be the result of inadequate fixation of the tube, patient secretions, patient movement, or procedures that are undertaken that might dislodge the tube. Care providers may fail to properly recognize that an endotracheal tube has come out of its location. It is well known that clinical examination findings such as a rise in the chest wall and auscultation may be unreliable or inaccurate to detect dislodgement of an endotracheal tube, even among experienced care providers. Hypoxia, for example, is not an early finding if a tube comes out of place. Thus, pulse oximetry monitors may be an insensitive indicator of dislodgement.

The authors of this article report on continuous end tidal carbon dioxide monitoring, also known as capnography, as an early indicator of endotracheal tube dislodgement. Capnography tells us about carbon dioxide expired during a respiratory cycle. It can be measured via an inline attachment to an endotracheal tube and is a measure of ventilation that is both continuous and objective. These authors designed a randomized controlled study in which residents were instructed in how to provide care for intubated patients using capnography data. The study demonstrated that pediatric residents were able to detect simulated endotracheal tube dislodgement faster when capnography was used in addition to standard monitoring. This was despite the fact that a large proportion of the residents in this study had never seen capnography used or had personal experience using it for medical decision making. Prior studies have also shown that paramedic students and practicing paramedics correctly detected simulated endotracheal tube dislodgement faster with capnography compared with standard monitoring.

Unplanned extubations and endotracheal tube dislodgement can have serious consequences. Lack of recognition can lead to a poorly reversible clinical cascade that can culminate in death. Capnography offers several advantages in this regard. It has superior sensitivity at detecting endotracheal tube dislodgement or malposition as well as apnea compared to pulse oximetry and clinical examination. Anesthesiologists have documented these advantages multiple times in the literature. It is relatively easily learned by a wide spectrum of care providers. Capnography, based on the data of this report, should be strongly considered when monitoring intubated patients to enhance their safety.

J. A. Stockman III, MD

Pediatric Blast Lung Injury From a Fireworks-Related Explosion
Ratto J, Johnson BK, Condra CS, et al (Univ of Missouri—Kansas City School of Medicine)
Pediatr Emerg Care 28:573-576, 2012

Blast injuries related to explosions have been described in the literature but are uncommon in children. We describe a multisystem blast injury in a child resulting from a commercial firework—related explosion in her home. She presented with respiratory failure, shock, altered level of consciousness, and multiple orthopedic injuries. The patient required immediate stabilization and resuscitation in the emergency department and a prolonged hospitalization. This report reviews the spectrum of injuries that are seen in blast-related trauma and the emergency measures needed for rapid stabilization of these critical patients.

▶ I actually read this report for the first time on Independence Day, which brought into stark contrast how dangerous fireworks can be, even those that most parents might consider to be rather innocuous. The case described was that of a 10-year-old girl who suffered serious injuries resulting from a house explosion. The patient was sitting at a kitchen table unwrapping "Black Eyed Snap Peas," a firework comparable to one that we commonly see both adults and children using, "snappers." A snapper is a small wrapper covered pea-like firework that when thrown to the ground will produce a small "popping" explosion. According to the patient's mother, the family's annual Independence Day routine is to open several cases of this firework to put into the street and then run over them with a car. The patient reported opening approximately 10 to 12 cases (700 individual fireworks) and placing them into a shoebox, which was approximately two-thirds full at the time of the blast. The patient stated she dropped one into the box and then felt an explosion and recalls only being thrown from her chair and hitting the wall at the opposite end of the kitchen. When seen in the emergency room, she was in a critical condition with agonal respirations. She had nonreactive, unequal pupils and extensive burns, and deep ulcerations and lacerations over her entire face and chest. The fourth and fifth digits of her left and the third, fourth, and fifth digits of her right hand were partially amputated. She had an open femur fracture. A chest x-ray showed bilateral pulmonary infiltrates consistent with a blast injury. The patient was in an intensive care unit for 2 weeks, followed by 6 weeks in a burn unit and then was sent to a rehab service.

The type of firework implicated in this patient's injury is generally called adult snappers in the fireworks industry. Adult snappers contain 48 mg of explosive material. This is substantially more than the smaller bang snaps, which contain a minute quantity (approximately 0.08 mg) of silver fulminate. Unfortunately, adult snappers are legal in all states where fireworks are sold.

The case described shows how extensive injuries can be from fireworks related blasts. The severity of such injuries should not be underestimated. Those in clinical practice need to properly counsel families under their care about the dangers of fireworks.

J. A. Stockman III, MD

Fatal and Near-Fatal Asthma in Children: The Critical Care Perspective
Newth CJL, for the *Eunice Kennedy Shriver* National Institute of Child Health and Human Development Collaborative Pediatric Critical Care Research Network (Children's Hosp Los Angeles, CA; et al)
J Pediatr 161:214-221, 2012

Objective.—To characterize the clinical course, therapies, and outcomes of children with fatal and near-fatal asthma admitted to pediatric intensive care units (PICUs).

Study Design.—This was a retrospective chart abstraction across the 8 tertiary care PICUs of the Collaborative Pediatric Critical Care Research Network (CPCCRN). Inclusion criteria were children (aged 1-18 years) admitted between 2005 and 2009 (inclusive) for asthma who received ventilation (near-fatal) or died (fatal). Data collected included medications, ventilator strategies, concomitant therapies, demographic information, and risk variables.

Results.—Of the 261 eligible children, 33 (13%) had no previous history of asthma, 218 (84%) survived with no known complications, and 32 (12%) had complications. Eleven (4%) died, 10 of whom had experienced cardiac arrest before admission. Patients intubated outside the PICU had a shorter duration of ventilation (median, 25 hours vs 84 hours; $P < .001$). African-Americans were disproportionately represented among the intubated children and had a shorter duration of intubation. Barotrauma occurred in 15 children (6%) before admission. Pharmacologic therapy was highly variable, with similar outcomes.

Conclusion.—Of the children ventilated in the CPCCRN PICUs, 96% survived to hospital discharge. Most of the children who died experienced cardiac arrest before admission. Intubation outside the PICU was correlated with shorter duration of ventilation. Complications of barotrauma and neuromyopathy were uncommon. Practice patterns varied widely among the CPCCRN sites.

▶ We should be grateful to the Collaborative Pediatric Critical Care Research Network (CPCCRN) for looking into the issue of fatal and near fatal asthma in children. There has been precious little written about this topic of hospitalized children, critically ill with reactive airway disease. The CPCCRN investigators undertook a retrospective study in 8 children's hospitals of children aged 1 to 18 years admitted with an acute exacerbation of asthma or status asthmaticus who were deemed ill enough to require admission to a pediatric intensive care unit for ongoing therapy. These children were defined as having critical asthma. All children with critical asthma admitted between January 1, 2005, and December 31, 2009, who had received endotracheal intubation and ventilation (near-fatal asthma) or who died (fatal asthma) were included in the study. The authors collected data on age, sex, race or ethnicity, height, weight, primary pair type, asthma history including timing of diagnosis, prior hospitalizations, allergies, psychiatric or behavioral disorders, substance abuse, family history of asthma, chronic asthma medication, and whatever available data there was during hospitalization, including ventilation data, use of extracorporeal membrane oxygenation, and the therapies used prior to intubation. Outcomes including mortality were documented.

The data from this study showed that 11 of 261 children admitted to intensive care units with near fatal or fatal asthma did in fact die. Ten of the 11 children who died experienced cardiac arrest before being admitted to the intensive care unit. Most of the children who were intubated prior to admission to the intensive care unit and these children seemed to do better. A disproportionate number of African American children with asthma ended up being admitted to the pediatric intensive care unit. Most children were treated with pressure ventilators. Extracorporeal membrane oxygenation was used in only 3 children. Ninety-eight percent of the children received steroid therapy, as expected. Although magnesium therapy in children with critical asthma has not been studied, 45% of children in this study were treated with magnesium prior to intubation; 40% were treated with magnesium during mechanical ventilation and 6% after extubation. In contrast, aminophylline was administered to only 4% of children before intubation, 17% during mechanical ventilation, and just 5% after extubation. Ipratropium bromide was used in only 36% of patients before intubation and in 50% during mechanical intubation. Most published guidelines recommend ipratropium bromide for severe asthma. Also, 38% received inhaled helium-oxygen gas mixtures (Heliox) presumably to decrease the work of breathing and to improve the delivery of inhaled drugs in obstructed airways.

This retrospective study of mechanically ventilated patients admitted to critical care units did find significant variability in the types of asthma therapies used and ventilator strategies employed. Despite the disparate therapies applied, patient outcomes were quite similar across the board with most patients ultimately doing well. Unfortunately, there was no use of sensitive tools for grading asthma therapy in these critically ill children. The marked overrepresentation of African American children in this fatal or near-fatal grouping of asthmatics suggests there may be a somewhat different pathophysiology in this subset of children.

J. A. Stockman III, MD

Azithromycin Therapy in Hospitalized Infants with Acute Bronchiolitis is Not Associated with Better Clinical Outcomes: A Randomized, Double-Blinded, and Placebo-Controlled Clinical Trial

Pinto LA, Pitrez PM, Luisi F, et al (Pontifícia Universidade Católica do Rio Grande do Sul, Porto Alegre, Brazil; et al)
J Pediatr 161:1104-1108, 2012

Objective.—To test the hypothesis that azithromycin reduces the length of hospitalization and oxygen requirement in infants with acute viral bronchiolitis (AB).

Study Design.—We performed a randomized, double-blinded, placebo-controlled trial in southern Brazil, from 2009 to 2011. Infants (<12 months of age) hospitalized with AB were recruited in 2 hospitals. Patients were randomized to receive either azithromycin or placebo, administered orally, for 7 days. At enrollment, clinical data were recorded and nasopharyngeal samples were collected for viral identification through immunofluorescence. Main outcomes were duration of oxygen requirement and length of hospitalization.

Results.—One hundred eighty-four patients were included in the study (azithromycin 88 subjects, placebo 96 subjects). Baseline clinical characteristics and viral identification were not different between the groups studied. A virus was detected in 112 (63%) patients, and of those, 92% were positive for respiratory syncytial virus. The use of azithromycin did not reduce the median number of days of either hospitalization ($P = .28$) or oxygen requirement ($P = .47$).

Conclusions.—Azithromycin did not improve major clinical outcomes in a large sample of hospitalized infants with AB, even when restricting the findings to those with positive respiratory syncytial virus samples.

Azithromycin therapy should not be given for AB because it provides no benefit and overuse increases overall antibiotic resistance.

▶ How can one justify the use of azithromycin as part of the management of acute bronchiolitis, a disorder clearly known to be viral in origin? Nonetheless, all too many children take antibiotics as part of the management of acute bronchiolitis without good purpose. On the other hand, it has been suggested that macrolides such as azithromycin might have beneficial effects in the treatment of inflammation, specifically that related to inflammatory lung diseases such as cystic fibrosis and asthma. Macrolides can inhibit interleukin-6 and interleukin-8 production and may reduce overall neutrophilic inflammation. Given the immunomodulatory properties of macrolides, a few studies have in fact confirmed that it is an anti-inflammatory agent of some level, particularly in chronic pulmonary diseases. A few clinical trials have shown benefits in the administration of macrolides in patients with cystic fibrosis.[1] Its use, however, in other respiratory diseases for its anti-inflammatory effects has been quite controversial. Systematic reviews have been inconclusive regarding the benefits of macrolides, for example, in exacerbations of episodes of asthma.

These authors tested the hypothesis that a 7-day course of azithromycin might reduce hospital length of stay and oxygen requirements in patients with acute bronchiolitis. The study was carried out in Brazil, and 184 patients were studied. Patients had typical acute bronchiolitis verified by viral identification. The infants were randomized to receive either a daily oral dose of azithromycin (10 mg/kg/d) or an equivalent volume of placebo for 7 days. Outcome data showed that there was no difference in length of stay in hospital between placebo and treated groups. Subgroup analysis for age and specific viral etiology showed no significant differences. There was no beneficial effect by treatment group in patients who had respiratory syncytial virus infection or among infants stratified by age. Results for other secondary outcomes such as antibiotic or bronchodilator prescription writing did not show significant differences either.

The results of this article support earlier studies indicating that antibiotics are of no benefit among young infants hospitalized with acute bronchiolitis. Unfortunately, antibiotics, particularly azithromycin, are still often prescribed for such children. Considering the published data indicating the overuse of macrolides among preschool-aged children and the results of this study, there seem to be no data at all recommending the routine use of such antibiotics in common conditions such as bronchiolitis, not even if used to theoretically reduce the problems associated with lung inflammation. The data from this report simply reinforce what we already know. It is good to see that investigators are still finding other good reasons to argue against antibiotic overkill.

J. A. Stockman III, MD

Reference

1. Equi A, Balfour-Lynn IM, Bush A, Rosenthal M. Long term azithromycin in children with cystic fibrosis: a randomised, placebo-controlled crossover trial. *Lancet.* 2002;360:978-984.

Should Children Be SCUBA Diving?: Cerebral Arterial Gas Embolism in a Swimming Pool

Johnson V, Adkinson C, Bowen M, et al (Hennepin County Med Ctr, Minneapolis, MN; Children's Hosps and Clinics of Minnesota, Minneapolis)
Pediatr Emerg Care 28:361-362, 2012

Cerebral arterial gas embolism (CAGE) is a well-known serious complication of self-contained breathing apparatus (SCUBA) diving. Most serious complications of SCUBA diving occur in adults because most of SCUBA divers are adults. However, young age is an independent risk factor for injury in SCUBA diving and shallow-water SCUBA diving is the riskiest environment for CAGE. We present a case of a 10-year-old boy who developed CAGE while taking SCUBA diving lessons in a university swimming pool. This case illustrates the potential danger of SCUBA diving for children who lack understanding of the physics of diving as well as the often unappreciated risk of shallow-water SCUBA diving. Our intent is to educate providers of primary care to children, so that they may appropriately advise parents about SCUBA diving, and to educate providers of emergency care to children, so that they will recognize this uncommon but serious emergency condition.

▶ SCUBA diving for sporting purposes is on a rapid increase in those of all ages. The percentage of children diving with SCUBA gear has steadily increased over recent years from about 1% to somewhere between 5% and 10% of all SCUBA divers in the United States.[1] The case of a 10-year-old boy described by Johnson et al tells us one of the hazards of SCUBA diving at a young age. The case was that of a 10-year-old boy who presented to the emergency department complaining of severe headache, dizziness, and weakness. He had just had his first SCUBA diving lesson in a swimming pool. The maximum depth of the pool was 14 feet. For 2 hours, the students were playing games in the pool wearing SCUBA gear. When he emerged from the pool, the boy complained immediately of a bad headache and subsequently of dizziness as well. He was also having difficulty maintaining his balance. He was seen in an emergency room 3 hours after the first onset of symptoms. The initial examination showed an alert interactive and appropriate appearing individual complaining of severe headache and mild nausea stating as though he would fall over if he stood. He denied dizziness or vertigo when lying down. His vital signs were largely unremarkable and his physical examination with the exception of the neurologic system was normal. The neurologic examination showed weakness of the upper and lower extremities and mild truncal weakness when sitting along with an inability to stand or walk without assistance. Suspecting a SCUBA diving-related illness, the National Divers Alert Network was contacted and arrangements were made to transfer the child to the nearest hyperbaric facility, which was approximately 20 minutes away. In the meantime, the child was placed on high-flow oxygen by non-rebreather mask. On arrival to the hyperbaric chamber, he was treated for presumed cerebral arterial gas embolism and after 90 minutes of breathing 100% oxygen, he was able to stand and walk normally in the chamber. After a total of 285 minutes of hyperbaric treatment, he was discharged home symptom-free and neurologically normal.

Cerebral arterial gas embolism is defined as air in the arterial system of the brain. In a SCUBA diver who is breathing compressed air from a tank and who ascends in the water without exhaling or who has some airflow obstruction in the pulmonary tree such as bronchospasm, the conditions are set for the development of an arterial gas embolism. When a diver ascends in the water when the pressure is lower, the volume of air in his lungs expands. If that air is trapped in the lungs, alveoli are overdistended and may rupture. An ascent in water of as little as 2.6 to 3.5 feet at shallow depth can create a pressure differential across the alveolar membrane sufficient to cause rupture and create an air leak into the vasculature. Such leaked air may cause a pneumothorax, mediastinal emphysema, or a cerebral arterial gas embolism. With the latter, the air enters the pulmonary capillaries, travels to the pulmonary vein, to the left side of the heart, and then out with arterial flow to any site in the body. The brain is, understandably, the most sensitive organ to the presence of bubbles blocking arterial flow. There have been several documented cases of cerebral arterial gas embolism occurring in swimming pools, particularly in divers with asthma.[2] National SCUBA diving training courses typically set 12 years as the minimum age for diving instruction and certification. Some believe that this is too young. When injury does occur, whether in an adult or a pediatric patient, rapid diagnosis based on history and physical examination is essential in implementing appropriate therapy. Currently, emergency hyperbaric oxygen therapy is the only effective treatment for cerebral arterial gas embolism. The article by Winkler et al[1] tells us about the contraindications to SCUBA diving in younger individuals.

J. A. Stockman III, MD

References

1. Winkler EE, Muth CM, Tetzlaff K. Should children dive with self-contained underwater breathing apparatus (SCUBA)? *Acta Paediatr.* 2012;101:472-478.
2. Weiss LD, Van Meter KW. Cerebral air embolism in asthmatic SCUBA divers in a swimming pool. *Chest.* 1995;107:1653-1654.

Should children dive with self-contained underwater breathing apparatus (SCUBA)?
Winkler BE, Muth C-M, Tetzlaff K (Univ of Ulm, Germany; Univ of Wuerzburg, Germany; Univ of Tuebingen, Germany)
Acta Paediatr 101:472-478, 2012

Diving with self-contained underwater breathing apparatus (SCUBA) has become a popular recreational activity in children and adolescents. This article provides an extensive review of the current literature.

Conclusions.—Medical contraindications to SCUBA diving for adults apply to children and adolescents, too, but must be adapted. Additional

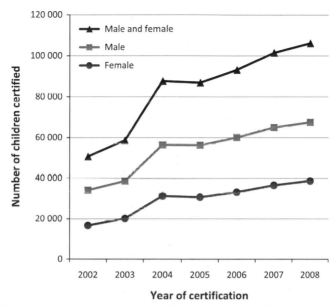

FIGURE 1.—Certifications in 8–14-year-old children by Professional Association of Diving Instructors (PADI). From 2002 till 2008, the numbers of male, female and total certifications per year are presented. (Reprinted from Winkler BE, Muth C-M, Terzlaff K. Should children dive with self-contained underwater breathing apparatus (SCUBA)? *Acta Paediatr.* 2012;101:472-478, with permission from The Author(s)/Acta Pædiatrica and John Wiley and Sons www.interscience.wiley.com.)

restrictions to the fitness to dive must apply to both, children and adolescents. Children should always be accompanied by a trained adult when diving (Fig 1, Table 3).

▶ This report described a 10-year-old who developed an arterial gas embolism while learning to SCUBA dive in a swimming pool [1] Although it is generally advised that SCUBA diving lessons begin only at 12 years of age or older, commercial SCUBA diving associations such as the Professional Association of Diving Instructors (PADI), the world's largest SCUBA diving association, offer special training programs to children starting from 8 years of age. Between 2002 and 2008, 584 680 (377 791 boys, and 206 889 girls) children age 8 to 14 years have been certified by the PADI. Fig 1 shows how rapidly this sport has increased in terms of interest among the young. Unfortunately, although there is a wealth of knowledge about medical risks for SCUBA diving in adults, only scarce data on the consequences and potential hazards from SCUBA diving are available in children and adolescents. This is why the report of Winkler et al is so important. Because of well-known differences in anatomy and physiology, adult fitness to dive recommendations cannot necessarily be transferred to children and adolescents.

Winkler et al searched PubMed for all of the current and historic literature telling us about complications of SCUBA diving in the young. The most comprehensive diving accident statistics are available from the Divers Alert Network

TABLE 3.—Suggested Medical Contraindications to Scuba Diving in Children and Adolescents

Respiratory system
  Absolute contraindications
    Bronchial asthma, history of wheezing
    Cystric fibrosis involving the lung
    Acute upper and lower respiratory tract infections
    Acute pneumonia, interstitial pneumonitis
    Lung cysts and emphysematous lesions
    History of primary pneumothorax
    Interstitial lung diseases including sarcoidosis
    Tuberculosis of the lung
  Relative contraindications
    s/p Thoracotomy
    s/p traumatic pneumothorax
Circulatory contraindications
  Absolute
    Pulmonary arterial hypertension
    Marfan's syndrome
    Hypertrophic/dilatative cardiomyopathy hypertrophe
    Right ventricular dysplasia
    Hemodynamically relevant septal defects arrhythmias (WPW-Syndrome, Long-QT Syndrome, Brugada Syndrome, II° and III° AV Block)
    s/p Implantation of a pacemaker or ICDs/p occlusion of a ASD/VSD (6 months) Syncopes ofunknown primacy
  Relative
    Small persisting Botalli arterial duct
    Aortic valve stenosis with gradient <25 mmHg
    Mild aortic insufficiency (I° and II°)
    Pulmonary valve stenosis with gradient <40 mmHg
    Mild mitral valve insufficiency
    WPW after successful ablation therapy (after 12 months)
Hemodynamically irrelevant ASDs/VSDs
ENT contraindications
  Absolute
    Acute and chronic otitis media
    Acute or chronic limitations in ventilation of the Eustachian tube Acute or chronic limitations in ventilation of the nasal sinus Tracheostoma
  Relative
    Adenoids with recurrent infections of the upper airways without limitation of ventilation
    Chronic sinusitis without limitation of ventilation
    Papillomatosis of the larynx
Psychiatric contraindications
  Absolute
    Attention-Deficit-Hyperactivity-Disorder (ADHD)
    Panic disorder

(DAN). Between 1989 and 2002, DAN documented 1248 fatal diving accidents. A total of 1.9% of these were in those younger than 18 years of age. Drowning and air embolism was the cause of death in most of these cases. A lack of formal training and performing high-risk dives (deep/altitude/cave/wreck) were associated with most of these fatalities. Over a 20-year period, data from the University of Hawaii, where patients are treated for SCUBA-related illnesses, showed 16 cases of decompression sickness occurring in 17 male and 5 female divers younger than 18 years of age. There were also 6 cases of arterial gas embolism, mostly in those who had a history of bronchial asthma or in those who had performed emergency ascents because of panicked reactions underwater.

It is clear that there should be an extensive medical assessment of fitness to dive for young divers. It is probably best not to recommend SCUBA diving to those who are younger than age of 12. Table 3 provides some important health conditions that are potentially associated with adverse events in pediatric SCUBA diving and should therefore conclude from diving. These recommendations are based on varying experts theoretical considerations and are not necessarily supported by evidence-based data from experimental or observational studies. Also, because there are no internationally accepted guidelines on pediatric fitness to dive, consensus to these recommendations may differ between regions and there might be national peculiarities not addressed in the recommendations appearing in Table 3. When it comes to diving at a young age, however, one might best say better safe than sorry and defer this sporting activity until one is grown up.

J. A. Stockman III, MD

Reference

1. Johnson V, Adkinson C, Bowen M, Ortega H. Should children be SCUBA diving? Cerebral arterial gas embolism in a swimming pool. *Pediatr Emerg Care*. 2012;28: 361-362.

Prevalence of Hyponatremia at Diagnosis and Factors Associated with the Longitudinal Variation in Serum Sodium Levels in Infants with Cystic Fibrosis

Guimarães EV, Schettino GC, Camargos PAM, et al (Faculty of Medicine/ Universidade Federal de Minas Gerais, Belo Horizonte, Brazil; Univ Hosp/ Universidade Federal de Minas Gerais, Belo Horizonte, Brazil)
J Pediatr 161:285-289, 2012

Objective.—To determine the prevalence of hyponatremia at diagnosis in patients with cystic fibrosis and identify the factors associated with changes in serum sodium concentration over time.

Study Design.—This longitudinal study investigated whether variations in serum sodium concentration were associated with age, diet, infection status, and climate/temperature. Multivariate analysis was performed using the random-effects model for longitudinal data.

Results.—Hyponatremia at diagnosis was observed in 19 of the 20 patients (95%). Factors identified as associated with variations in serumsodium concentration were diet ($P = .008$) and climate/temperature ($P = .005$). Intake of solid foods appeared to greatly increase the serum sodium concentration (increase of 5 mEq/L after introduction of solid foods); however, a confounding factor between diet and age cannot be definitively ruled out. Climate/temperature contributed in an inverse way; a 1°C-increase in ambient temperature was associated with a 0.5-mEq/L decrease in serum sodium concentration.

Conclusion.—Infants with cystic fibrosis who feed on breast milk or formula and live in a high-temperature environment are at increased risk for hyponatremia, even when receiving a higher salt intake in accordance with recommendations.

▶ Many in practice now are not familiar with the fact that the disorder we call cystic fibrosis was initially detected in the summer of 1948 when a number of children presented to hospitals with dehydration and salt depletion. This was in a particularly hot summer. The patients had what was thought to be "heat prostration." Within half a decade, Di Sant' Agnese et al[1] reported that this condition was caused by the loss of salt through the sweat glands. The sweat was of normal volume, but it had increased electrolyte content. Salt depletion is recognized as a relatively important and often common effect of having cystic fibrosis. This occurs often in periods of high ambient temperature and may occur at any age, but mainly in young children. A chronic course is associated with metabolic alkalosis in infants who may also exhibit anorexia and poor weight gain.

These authors report on infants with cystic fibrosis presenting with hypernatremia at diagnosis and the clinical and environmental factors that influence their serum sodium values. The study was conducted in the southeast region of Brazil, a part of the country with tropical and semiarid climates. For newly diagnosed children with cystic fibrosis, hyponatremia was observed at diagnosis in 95% of the newly diagnosed patients. Hyponatremia was defined as a serum sodium level less than 135 mEq/L. In this article, severe hyponatremia was defined as a serum sodium less than 120 mEq/L. The mean age of diagnosis was 45 plus or minus 18 days. All patients in this study were ultimately found to have pancreatic insufficiency.

In this study, high ambient temperature and wearing excessively warm clothing in the winter did appear to be precipitating factors to the electrolyte disorders found. The humidity itself had little effect on serum sodium measurements, but the ambient temperature itself had a major impact. Every 1°C increase in ambient temperature was associated with a 0.53 mmol/L decrease in serum sodium level. Breastfeeding and formula feeding were equally associated with hyponatremia in infants living in high temperature environments.

If there is a lesson to be learned from this study it is that if you are unaware of the results of newborn screening for cystic fibrosis and it is an extremely warm day (or days) in summer, when newborns present with hyponatremia, think cystic fibrosis. Although this is not a new piece of information, this article does vividly remind us that significant hyponatremia can signal the presence of cystic fibrosis.

J. A. Stockman III, MD

Reference

1. Di Sant' Agnese PA, Darling RC, Perera GA, Shea E. Abnormal electrolyte composition of sweat in cystic fibrosis of the pancreas; clinical significance and relationship to the disease. *Pediatrics.* 1953;12:549-563.

Inhaled Hypertonic Saline in Infants and Children Younger Than 6 Years With Cystic Fibrosis: The ISIS Randomized Controlled Trial

Rosenfeld M, for the ISIS Study Group (Seattle Children's Hosp, WA; et al)
JAMA 307:2269-2277, 2012

Context.—Inhaled hypertonic saline is recommended as therapy for patients 6 years or older with cystic fibrosis (CF), but its efficacy has never been evaluated in patients younger than 6 years with CF.

Objective.—To determine if hypertonic saline reduces the rate of protocol-defined pulmonary exacerbations in patients younger than 6 years with CF.

Design, Setting, and Participants.—The Infant Study of Inhaled Saline in Cystic Fibrosis (ISIS), a multicenter, randomized, double-blind, placebo-controlled trial conducted from April 2009 to October 2011 at 30 CF care centers in the United States and Canada. Participants were aged 4 to 60 months and had an established diagnosis of CF. A total of 344 patients were assessed for eligibility; 321 participants were randomized; 29 (9%) withdrew prematurely.

Intervention.—The active treatment group (n = 158) received 7% hypertonic saline and the control group (n = 163) received 0.9% isotonic saline, nebulized twice daily for 48 weeks. Both groups received albuterol or levalbuterol prior to each study drug dose.

Main Outcome Measures.—Rate during the 48-week treatment period of protocol-defined pulmonary exacerbations treated with oral, inhaled, or intravenous antibiotics.

Results.—The mean pulmonary exacerbation rate (events per person-year) was 2.3 (95% CI, 2.0-2.5) in the active treatment group and 2.3 (95% CI, 2.1-2.6) in the control group; the adjusted rate ratio was 0.98 (95% CI, 0.84-1.15). Among participants with pulmonary exacerbations, the mean number of total antibiotic treatment days for a pulmonary exacerbation was 60 (95% CI, 49-70) in the active treatment group and 52 (95% CI, 43-61) in the control group. There was no significant difference in secondary end points including height, weight, respiratory rate, oxygen saturation, cough, or respiratory symptom scores. Infant pulmonary function testing performed as an exploratory outcome in a subgroup (n = 73, with acceptable measurements at 2 visits in 45 participants) did not demonstrate significant differences between groups except for the mean change in forced expiratory volume in 0.5 seconds, which was 38 mL (95% CI, 1-76) greater in the active treatment group. Adherence determined by returned study drug ampoules was at least 75% in each group. Adverse event profiles were also similar, with the most common adverse event of moderate or severe severity in each group being cough (39% of active treatment group, 38% of control group).

Conclusion.—Among infants and children younger than 6 years with cystic fibrosis, the use of inhaled hypertonic saline compared with isotonic saline did not reduce the rate of pulmonary exacerbations over the course of 48 weeks of treatment.

Trial Registration.—clinicaltrials.gov Identifier: NCT00709280.

▶ It is well known that the absence of functional cystic fibrosis transmembrane conductance regulator (CFTR) protein, caused by a mutation in the gene that encodes this protein in patients with cystic fibrosis, results in decreased chloride secretion and increased sodium absorption, causing depletion of water from the airway surface. This results in decreased mucociliary clearance, leading to an environment for infection and inflammation to occur, problems that ultimately lead to destruction of the lungs. For some time now, treatment strategies to manage cystic fibrosis have targeted restoring salt and water balance in the airways of affected individuals. One particular agent, ivacaftor, a potentiator of CFTR, has been shown to improve lung function and decrease pulmonary exacerbations. Although this agent targets a specific mutation affecting only 4% to 5% of patients with cystic fibrosis worldwide, other CFTR-specific investigational agents that have the potential to affect nearly all patients with cystic fibrosis are currently being studied. While these studies are under way, adding salt directly to the airway may be of some benefit, and several studies have suggested this approach in patients older than 6 years of age with cystic fibrosis.

These authors report on results from a multicenter trial comparing inhaled 7% hypertonic saline with 0.9% isotonic saline as a control, both given twice daily for 48 weeks in 321 infants and young children with cystic fibrosis. During the 48-week treatment period analyzed, the study did not achieve its primary endpoint, that being reduction in the rate of pulmonary exacerbations. In addition, there were no significant differences among participants receiving hypertonic and isotonic saline for the secondary endpoints, including height, weight, respiratory rate, oxygen saturation, cough, or respiratory symptom score. As bad as this news is, the study results are important since it identifies a treatment that should *not* be routinely used. The endpoints looked for here in a sense are quite crude, and an editorial that accompanied this article suggests that other potential endpoints might be looked for to determine subtle beneficial effects of new or emerging treatments.[1] Other potential endpoints might include imaging and other modalities assessing lung function. This theoretically could include chest computed tomography, which is sensitive for detecting early lung disease because of its ability to detect regional disease. Magnetic resonance imaging is a potential alternative without the adverse effects of ionizing radiation and has been tested in patients with cystic fibrosis. Lung clearance index could also be used, which is a measure of ventilation inhomogeneity.

Despite the crudeness of the outcomes examined in this article, it does assist clinicians and researchers in that it demonstrates that inhaled hypertonic saline does not offer an advantage over isotonic saline in decreasing pulmonary exacerbations in infants and children with cystic fibrosis. The current Cystic Fibrosis Foundation guidelines recommend the use of inhaled hypertonic saline only for patients 6 years of age or older. However, although the results of this study suggest that inhaled hypertonic saline should not be used routinely in young children, the final verdict on its use for infants and young children has not yet been established. The goal for infants and young children with no apparent or minimal cystic fibrosis associated lung disease, as opposed to older patients with established disease, should focus on prevention of disease progression rather than treatment of existing disease. The article demonstrates that testing therapeutic agents in infants and young children may very well require different endpoints capable of assessing onset and progression of disease.

J. A. Stockman III, MD

Reference

1. Dasenbrook EC, Konstan MW. Inhaled hypertonic saline in infants and young children with cystic fibrosis. *JAMA*. 2012;307:2316-2317.

Effect of Estrogen on Pseudomonas Mucoidy and Exacerbations in Cystic Fibrosis

Chotirmall SH, Smith SG, Gunaratnam C, et al (Royal College of Surgeons in Ireland, Dublin; Trinity College Dublin, Ireland; et al)
N Engl J Med 366:1978-1986, 2012

Background.—Women with cystic fibrosis are at increased risk for mucoid conversion of *Pseudomonas aeruginosa*, which contributes to a sexual dichotomy in disease severity.

Methods.—We evaluated the effects of estradiol and its metabolite estriol on *P. aeruginosa* in vitro and in vivo and determined the effect of estradiol on disease exacerbations in women with cystic fibrosis.

Results.—Estradiol and estriol induced alginate production in *P. aeruginosa* strain 01 and in clinical isolates obtained from patients with and those without cystic fibrosis. After prolonged exposure to estradiol, *P. aeruginosa* adopted early mucoid morphology, whereas short-term exposure inhibited bacterial catalase activity and increased levels of hydrogen peroxide, which is potentially damaging to DNA. Consequently, a frameshift mutation was identified in *mucA*, a key regulator of alginate biosynthesis in *P. aeruginosa*. In vivo levels of estradiol correlated with infective exacerbations in women with cystic fibrosis, with the majority occurring during the follicular phase ($P < 0.05$). A review of the Cystic Fibrosis Registry of Ireland revealed that the use of oral contraceptives was associated with a decreased need for antibiotics. Predominantly nonmucoid *P. aeruginosa* was isolated from sputum during exacerbations in the luteal phase (low estradiol). Increased proportions of mucoid bacteria were isolated during exacerbations occurring in the follicular phase (high estradiol), with a variable *P. aeruginosa* phenotype evident in vivo during the course of the menstrual cycle corresponding to fluctuating estradiol levels.

Conclusions.—Estradiol and estriol induced mucoid conversion of *P. aeruginosa* in women with cystic fibrosis through a mutation of *mucA* in vitro and were associated with selectivity for mucoid isolation, increased exacerbations, and mucoid conversion in vivo. (Funded by the Molecular Medicine Ireland Clinician—Scientist Fellowship Programme.)

▶ Until this article appeared, I did not know that there was a sex difference in the survival rate in patients with cystic fibrosis. Although the median overall survival among patients with cystic fibrosis in the United States is 39 years, there is a sexual dichotomy that has persisted over time in disease severity, with women having a survival disadvantage and poorer lung function. It is well known that patients with cystic fibrosis become colonized and infected with nonmucoid *Pseudomonas aeruginosa*, and that these strains convert over time to a more virulent mucoid strains. This phenomenon occurs at a younger age in women than in men.

Investigators from Dublin, Ireland, have studied the effects of the female sex hormone estradiol on airway biology. They have shown that women with cystic fibrosis appear to be at greater risk for exacerbations during periods of high circulating levels of estradiol, when airway-surface liquid is diminished and antimicrobial peptides are scarce and there is a blunted inflammatory response to microbial agonists. These observations, however, have not been confirmed in vivo. In this abstracted article, the same investigators have evaluated the effect of estradiol and its metabolite estriol on laboratory and clinical isolates of *P aeruginosa* and have also assessed the effect of estradiol on infective exacerbations in women with cystic fibrosis. They showed that estradiol and estriol will induce the conversion of nonmucoid to mucoid forms of *P aeruginosa* in women with cystic fibrosis and will stimulate mutations in the gene *mucA*, a negative regulator of the substance that defines the mucoid conversion of *P aeruginosa*. They also showed that in vivo estradiol levels correlate with infective exacerbations among menstruating women with cystic fibrosis, and that during such periods it was much easier to culture the presence of mucoid *P aeruginosa*.

The data from this article provide support for historical information indicating that the median age of chronic infection with mucoid *P aeruginosa* occurs some 1.7 years earlier in women and that this change accelerates the rate of decline in pulmonary function. It has now been shown that a significant relationship exists between exacerbations and estradiol levels, with the majority of exacerbations occurring during the follicular phase, a stage with the highest estradiol levels. It is also apparent that women with cystic fibrosis who are taking oral contraceptives have lower rates of exacerbation. Although oral contraceptives may be protective against exacerbations, a double-blind, placebo-controlled study of the use of oral contraceptives in women with cystic fibrosis would be necessary to provide proof that oral contraceptives might be useful in the management of women with this genetic disorder.

Although much has been learned about the role of estradiol within the airways of patients with cystic fibrosis, further work is necessary, particularly in the assessment of the use of oral contraceptives and their potential effect on exacerbations and the microbiologic or endocrine effects of estradiol on *P aeruginosa*. We are grateful to these investigators from Dublin who carried out this important study.

Curiously, the Republic of Ireland has the highest incidence and carrier rate of cystic fibrosis worldwide.[1]

J. A. Stockman III, MD

Reference

1. Farrell PM. The prevalence of cystic fibrosis in the European Union. *J Cyst Fibros.* 2008;7:450-453.

Influence of Smoking Cues in Movies on Children's Beliefs About Smoking

Lochbuehler K, Sargent JD, Scholte RHJ, et al (Radboud Univ Nijmegen, Netherlands; Dartmouth Med School, Lebanon, NH)
Pediatrics 130:221-227, 2012

Objective.—Experimental research has revealed that short exposure to movie smoking affects beliefs about smoking in adolescents. In this study, we tested that association in children.

Methods.—In 2 experiments, participants were exposed to either a cartoon or family-oriented movie and randomly assigned to 20-minute segments with or without smoking characters. Data collection took place at elementary schools. A total of 101 children (8—10 years; 47.5% boys) were exposed to a cartoon, and in a second experiment, 105 children (8—11 years; 56.2% boys) were exposed to a family-oriented movie. Beliefs about smoking (assessed by questionnaire) and implicit associations toward smoking (single target implicit association task) were assessed after watching the movie.

Results.—The majority of both samples of children viewed smoking unfavorably. Exposure to movie smoking had no effect on implicit associations toward smoking when experiments were analyzed separately or if the results were combined. For smoking beliefs, effects were again small and only statistically significant for social norms regarding smoking.

Conclusions.—Short-term exposure to smoking in cartoon and family-oriented movies had little immediate impact on beliefs about smoking in preadolescent children, but a significant cumulative impact on norms cannot be ruled out.

▶ There is much that is unknown about movie exposure to tobacco and the uptake of tobacco smoking by youngsters. Because movie smoking exposure begins well before adolescents start to smoke, it is quite important to clarify whether and how depictions of smoking in movies affect children who have not yet experimented with smoking and who are in the process of developing beliefs about smoking. The question that the authors of this report raise is whether brief exposure to movie smoking affects beliefs about smoking in 8- to 11-year-old children. Forty-eight boys and 53 girls were requested to watch a segment of 1 or 2 movies with smoking scenes with a control condition in which there was exposure to a similar segment of the movie, but without any portrayal of smoking.

The movies chosen were considered otherwise suitable for all ages. The studies were conducted in 5 elementary schools in different regions of the Netherlands. Before and after watching the films, the children were surveyed in various ways.

This study revealed that a 20-minute segment of smoking from a family-related film entertainment had no effect on implicit associations toward smoking and only a small effect on smoking-related cognition, antismoking norms. Thus a significant effect was found only for antismoking norms. This study did not answer the question whether cumulative exposure to movies with smoking would influence smoking experimentation among adolescents so future research is needed. The current study suggests that prevention and policy initiatives would best focus on the effect of smoking in family-oriented movies and that tobacco control initiatives in the United States should pay attention to adjusting the rating system to address smoking in PG-13 films as well as R-rated films.

The Centers for Disease Control and Prevention tells us that from 2000 to 2011, total cigarette consumption in the United States underwent a 32.8% decrease.[1] That is the good news. The bad news is that the consumption of pipe tobacco and large cigars has increased substantially during the same period. The Federal Tobacco Excise Tax change has made pipe tobacco significantly less expensive than roll-your-own tobacco and manufactured cigarettes. Manufacturers have relabeled roll-your-own tobacco as pipe tobacco for marketing purposes to take advantage of the tax "loop holes." Needless to say, smoke from pipes and cigars contain the same toxic chemicals as cigarette smoke. The percentage of combustible tobacco consumption composed of loose tobacco and cigars more than doubled in the past decade.

While on the topic of smoking, it is clear that at least in some countries, bans on smoking in public do result in fewer people smoking.[2] In the first year after Spain introduced its ban on smoking in public places, 569 million fewer packs of cigarettes were sold and some 600,000 individuals stopped smoking. Also, hospital admissions for heart attacks at the La Paz Hospital in Madrid fell by some 10%, and children's admissions for asthma fell by 15%. The ban did not adversely affect business in bars and restaurants, a finding similar to what has been seen in the US.

J. A. Stockman III, MD

References

1. Centers for Disease Control and Prevention (CDC). Consumption of cigarettes and combustible tobacco — United States, 2000–2011. *MMWR Morb Mortal Wkly Rep.* 2012;61:565-570.
2. Editorial Comment. Spain sees 600,000 fewer smokers after smoking ban. *BMJ.* 2012;344:4.

19 Therapeutics and Toxicology

Unfilled Prescriptions in Pediatric Primary Care

Zweigoron RT, Binns HJ, Tanz RR (Ann and Robert H. Lurie Children's Hosp of Chicago, IL)
Pediatrics 130:620-626, 2012

Background and Objectives.—Filling a prescription is the important first step in medication adherence, but has not been studied in pediatric primary care. The objective of this study was to use claims data to determine the rate of unfilled prescriptions in pediatric primary care and examine factors associated with prescription filling.

Methods.—This retrospective observational study of pediatric primary care patients compares prescription data from an electronic medical record with insurance claims data. Illinois Medicaid provided claims data for 4833 patients who received 16 953 prescriptions during visits at 2 primary care sites over 26 months. Prescriptions were compared with claims to determine filling within 1 day and 60 days. Clinical and demographic variables significant in univariate analysis were included in logistic regression models.

Results.—Patients were 51% male; most (84%) spoke English and were African American (38.7%) or Hispanic (39.1%). Seventy-eight percent of all prescriptions were filled. Among filled prescriptions, 69% were filled within 1 day. African American, Hispanic, and male patients were significantly more likely to have filled prescriptions. Younger age was associated with filling within 1 day but not with filling within 60 days. Prescriptions for antibiotics, from one of the clinic sites, from sick/follow-up visits, and electronic prescriptions were significantly more likely to be filled.

Conclusions.—More than 20% of prescriptions in a pediatric primary care setting were never filled. The significant associations with clinical site, visit type, and electronic prescribing suggest system-level factors that affect prescription filling. Development of interventions to increase adherence should account for the factors that affect primary adherence.

▶ There has been much written about the problem of unfilled prescriptions given to adult patients. Up to 22% of adults do not fill their prescriptions after hospital discharge.[1] What little data there are suggest that when children are discharged from hospital with a prescription as many as 25% of prescriptions are not filled.[2] The authors of this report designed a study to determine the rate of nonadherence

511

in an outpatient pediatric setting. They analyzed electronic medical record prescription data matched to claims data and reported the proportion of prescriptions written to pediatric primary care patients that went unfilled. The study included all Medicaid-insured patients with a primary care encounter between October 1, 2008, and December 1, 2010, at either of 2 primary care sites that treat only children. The data from this report represent the first study to evaluate primary care medication adherence exclusively among pediatric primary care patients. A total of 78% of all prescriptions were filled. There was no association between the age of a child and a prescription being filled. Electronic prescribing increased the likelihood that a prescription would be filled. We already know that electronic prescribing reduces prescription errors and costs. It is suggested that electronic prescriptions are more often filled on the basis of convenience. Also, there was variation in rates of the filling of a prescription, depending on why the prescription was written. For example, there is a much higher rate of filled prescriptions for antibiotics in comparison to other drugs. This study was carried out in a population of patients insured through the Medicaid program. It might be difficult, therefore, to extrapolate the data to the pediatric population as a whole.

The reasons for not filling prescriptions are multifold including distance from home, clinic, and pharmacy as well as nondemographic factors such as the method of prescribing (electronic vs paper), clinic site, medication type, and type of visit. Patient factors may promote prescription filling such as race and ethnicity.

J. A. Stockman III, MD

References

1. Kripalani S, Price M, Vigil V, Epstein KR. Frequency and predictors of prescription-related issues after hospital discharge. *J Hosp Med.* 2008;3:12-19.
2. Wright H, Forbes D, Graham H. Primary compliance with medication prescribed for pediatric patients discharged from a regional hospital. *J Paediatr Child Health.* 2003;39:611-612.

Out-of-Pocket Medication Costs and Use of Medications and Health Care Services Among Children With Asthma

Karaca-Mandic P, Jena AB, Joyce GF, et al (Univ of Minnesota, Minneapolis; Massachusetts General Hosp, Boston; Univ of Southern California, Los Angeles)
JAMA 307:1284-1291, 2012

Context.—Health plans have implemented policies to restrain prescription medication spending by shifting costs toward patients. It is unknown how these policies have affected children with chronic illness.

Objective.—To analyze the association of medication cost sharing with medication and hospital services utilization among children with asthma, the most prevalent chronic disease of childhood.

Design, Setting, and Patients.—Retrospective study of insurance claims for 8834 US children with asthma who initiated asthma control therapy between 1997 and 2007. Using variation in out-of-pocket costs for a fixed "basket" of asthma medications across 37 employers, we estimated multivariate models of asthma medication use, asthmarelated hospitalization, and emergency department (ED) visits with respect to out-of-pocket costs and child and family characteristics.

Main Outcome Measures.—Asthma medication use, asthma-related hospitalizations, and ED visits during 1-year follow-up.

Results.—The mean annual out-of-pocket asthma medication cost was $154 (95% CI, $152-$156) among children aged 5 to 18 years and $151 (95% CI, $148-$153) among those younger than 5 years. Among 5913 children aged 5 to 18 years, filled asthma prescriptions covered a mean of 40.9% of days (95% CI, 40.2%-41.5%). During 1-year follow-up, 121 children (2.1%) had an asthma-related hospitalization and 220 (3.7%) had an ED visit. Among 2921 children younger than 5 years, mean medication use was 46.2% of days (95% CI, 45.2%-47.1%); 136 children (4.7%) had an asthma-related hospitalization and 231 (7.9%) had an ED visit. An increase in out-of-pocket medication costs from the 25th to the 75th percentile was associated with a reduction in adjusted medication use among children aged 5 to 18 years (41.7% [95% CI, 40.7%-42.7%] vs 40.3% [95% CI, 39.4%-41.3%] of days; P =.02) but no change among younger children. Adjusted rates of asthma-related hospitalization were higher for children aged 5 to 18 years in the top quartile of out-of-pocket costs (2.4 [95% CI, 1.9-2.8] hospitalizations per 100 children vs 1.7 [95% CI, 1.3-2.1] per 100 in bottom quartile; P =.004) but not for younger children. Annual adjusted rates of ED use did not vary across out-of-pocket quartiles for either age group.

Conclusion.—Greater cost sharing for asthma medications was associated with a slight reduction in medication use and higher rates of asthma hospitalization among children aged 5 years or older.

▶ This article from the University of Minnesota, Massachusetts General Hospital, and the University of Southern California examines cost sharing for treatments of asthma, now the most common chronic childhood health condition. The investigators looked at the association of cost sharing for asthma medication in children with medication use, asthma-related hospital admissions, and emergency department visits. To adapt to increasing economic pressures, insurance providers and programs that cover drug costs have moved to medication cost sharing. This involves the sharing of the cost of medications with patients through copayments, coinsurance, and deductibles. The intent is to reduce overall medication cost. The theory is based on studies performed more than 20 years ago that showed that patients will reduce consumption of unnecessary health services when faced with cost sharing.[1] This effect of medication cost sharing on health resource use has been extensively studied for adult chronic diseases. Information on its application to the care of children, however, has been quite limited.

These authors found that greater out-of-pocket asthma medication cost was associated with a small but statistically significant reduction in medication use and total (patients plus health care plan) asthma medication expenditures among children aged 5 years or older with asthma. No such association was found for children younger than 5 years. However, these investigators found no statistically significant associations with emergency department visits or with asthma-related hospitalization expenditures.

The Affordable Care Act required insurance plans to cover preventative health services such as vaccines as well as well-child visits at no cost to families. This is in addition to prohibiting health plans from limiting coverage of children with preexisting health conditions. The study reported suggests that medication generosity mandates have small effects on asthma-related hospitalizations, but other strategies to improve medication use, such as routine access to primary care and pulmonary specialists, written plans of care for families, and regularly scheduled follow-up appointments, may be important in improving medication use as opposed to providing medications more liberally with fewer restrictions. This article suggests that greater prescription medication cost sharing among children with asthma could lead to small reductions in the use of important medications with the unintended consequence, however, of more frequent asthma-related hospitalizations.

To read more about this important topic, see the excellent commentary by Ungar.[2]

J. A. Stockman III, MD

References

1. Manning WG, Newhouse JP, Duan N, Keeler EB, Leibowitz A, Marquis MS. Health insurance and the demand for medical care: evidence from a randomized experiment. *Am Econ Rev.* 1987;77:251-277.
2. Ungar WJ. Medication cost sharing and health outcomes in children with asthma. *JAMA.* 2012;307:1316-1318.

Ondansetron in Pregnancy and Risk of Adverse Fetal Outcomes
Pasternak B, Svanström H, Hviid A (Statens Serum Institut, Copenhagen, Denmark)
N Engl J Med 368:814-823, 2013

Background.—Ondansetron is frequently used to treat nausea and vomiting during pregnancy, but the safety of this drug for the fetus has not been well studied.

Methods.—We investigated the risk of adverse fetal outcomes associated with ondansetron administered during pregnancy. From a historical cohort of 608,385 pregnancies in Denmark, women who were exposed to ondansetron and those who were not exposed were included, in a 1:4 ratio, in propensity-score—matched analyses of spontaneous abortion (1849 exposed women vs. 7396 unexposed women), stillbirth (1915 vs. 7660), any major birth defect (1233 vs. 4932), preterm delivery (1792 vs. 7168), and birth of infants at low birth weight and small for gestational age (1784 vs. 7136). In addition, estimates were adjusted for hospitalization for nausea and vomiting during pregnancy (as a proxy for severity) and the use of other antiemetics.

Results.—Receipt of ondansetron was not associated with a significantly increased risk of spontaneous abortion, which occurred in 1.1% of exposed women and 3.7% of unexposed women during gestational weeks 7 to 12 (hazard ratio, 0.49; 95% confidence interval [CI], 0.27 to 0.91) and in 1.0% and 2.1%, respectively, during weeks 13 to 22 (hazard ratio, 0.60; 95% CI, 0.29 to 1.21). Ondansetron also conferred no significantly increased risk of stillbirth (0.3% for exposed women and 0.4% for unexposed women; hazard ratio, 0.42; 95% CI, 0.10 to 1.73), any major birth defect (2.9% and 2.9%, respectively; prevalence odds ratio, 1.12; 95% CI, 0.69 to 1.82), preterm delivery (6.2% and 5.2%; prevalence odds ratio, 0.90; 95% CI, 0.66 to 1.25), delivery of a low-birth-weight infant (4.1% and 3.7%; prevalence odds ratio, 0.76; 95% CI, 0.51 to 1.13), or delivery of a small-for-gestational-age infant (10.4% and 9.2%; prevalence odds ratio, 1.13; 95% CI, 0.89 to 1.44).

Conclusions.—Ondansetron taken during pregnancy was not associated with a significantly increased risk of adverse fetal outcomes. (Funded by the Danish Medical Research Council.)

▶ It is important for those caring for newborns to know a significant amount about drugs that may be given to a woman during pregnancy. One such class of drugs includes those that control nausea and vomiting, an all too common problem affecting more than half of all pregnant women. Because nausea and vomiting generally present early during pregnancy (onset between 3 and 8 weeks of gestation with peak symptoms in weeks 7 to 12 in most cases), drug treatment often coincides with the interval within which a fetus is most susceptible to teratogenic effects. The most frequently used prescription antiemetic here in the United States is 5-hydroxytryptamine type 3 receptor antagonist, ondansetron. It is estimated that somewhere between 3% and 5% of all pregnancies have been exposed to this antiemetic, despite limited information regarding safety for the fetus. This is where the report of Pasternak et al becomes important. These investigators conducted a historical cohort study to investigate whether receiving ondansetron during pregnancy is associated with an increased risk of fetal outcomes defined as spontaneous abortion, stillbirth, any major birth defect, preterm delivery, low birth weight, or small size for gestational age. This birth registry contains extensive information about outcomes of pregnancy, use of various drugs, and other related factors. It also documents any cases of major birth defects through one year of follow-up after birth. Spontaneous abortions through 22 gestational weeks are recorded.

In this nationwide study from Denmark, the antiemetic ondansetron was not associated with a significantly increased risk of major adverse fetal outcomes. In most pregnancies with exposure to the antiemetic, exposure occurred in the second half of the first trimester. This pattern of exposure probably reflects the fact that nausea and vomiting peak during this period. It also implies that the results from this study of birth defects primarily apply to the second half of the first trimester. Thus, the data would be insufficient to definitively say that the use of this agent does not cause problems very early in pregnancy, although from what information is available, this seems unlikely. This large study found that exposure to ondansetron in pregnancy is not associated with a significant increase in the risk of spontaneous abortion, stillbirth or any major birth defect, preterm delivery, low birth weight, or being small for gestational age. The results cannot definitively rule out the possibility of adverse effects in association with use of this antiemetic; however, the results do provide reassurance regarding the use of an agent for control of nausea and vomiting in pregnancy.

J. A. Stockman III, MD

Defining Risk Factors for Red Man Syndrome in Children and Adults

Myers AL, Gaedigk A, Dai H, et al (Univ of Missouri—Kansas City, MO; et al)
Pediatr Infect Dis J 31:464-468, 2012

Background.—Red man syndrome (RMS) is a well-known adverse reaction that occurs in pediatric patients receiving vancomycin, yet reported prevalence is varied, and characteristics and risk factors are not well understood. Our objective was to determine the prevalence, characteristics and risk factors for RMS in pediatric patients receiving vancomycin, including contributing genetic factors.

Methods.—A multicenter retrospective study of 546 subjects (0.5–21 years) who received at least 1 dose of intravenous vancomycin was conducted. Demographic and symptom data were collected through chart review and parent/nurse report. Genotype analysis included 10 single nucleotide polymorphisms in the histamine pathway.

Results.—RMS was observed in 77 (14%) subjects receiving vancomycin. Forty percent of subjects with RMS symptoms developed rash, pruritis and flushing, without hypotension. Antecedent antihistamine use was identified as a risk factor for RMS ($P < 0.001$). Multivariate regression analysis identified age > 2 years ($P = 0.008$), previous RMS ($P < 0.001$), vancomycin dose ($P = 0.02$) and vancomycin concentration ($P = 0.017$) as RMS risk factors, whereas African American race was protective ($P = 0.011$). We observed an apparent association between RMS and a single nucleotide polymorphism in the diamine oxidasegene ($P = 0.044$); however, no associations were revealed by multifactor dimensionality reduction analysis.

Conclusions.—RMS is a common adverse event in children receiving vancomycin. Identified risk factors are Caucasian ethnicity, age ≥ 2 years, previous RMS history, vancomycin dose ≥ 10 mg/kg, vancomycin concentration ≥ 5 mg/mL and antecedent antihistamine use. Known genetic variants in histamine metabolism or receptors do not appear to be substantial contributors to risk of RMS.

▶ If you are not familiar with red man syndrome, it is the most common adverse drug reaction that occurs when vancomycin is given. About 5% to 10% of hospitalized patients and up to 90% of control subjects have been reported to have developed red man syndrome. Its true incidence, however, remains unknown, and previous studies of red man syndrome in children have described widely varying clinical features. Vancomycin is an antibiotic widely used in children for the treatment of severe gram-positive infections. Most literature recommends vancomycin as a first-line agent in the setting of serious or invasive methicillin-resistant *Staphylococcus aureus* infections. In patients receiving vancomycin, red man syndrome is believed to be an anaphylactoid type of reaction due to vancomycin-induced direct mast cell degranulation. It has been shown to be associated with a rise in blood histamine level in some studies. The syndrome encompasses a spectrum of symptoms that range from a mild reaction such as flushing, urticarial rash, or pruritus to a severe reaction that includes a generalized erythema, intense itching, and even hypotension. Unfortunately, there is no standard definition of red man syndrome, and lack of a precise phenotype may account for the widely reported estimates of incidence in the literature.

This article was designed to precisely describe the clinical syndrome, further characterize the epidemiology of the syndrome, and identify risk factors for its development in pediatric patients. In this study, the prevalence of the syndrome was consistent with the ranges noted in prior studies. The data from the report indicate that vancomycin dose, concentration, prior red man syndrome history, age, and ethnicity all are risk factors for red man syndrome. It is unclear why patients of African American ethnicity are less likely to develop red man syndrome, although it is possible that rash and flushing may be harder to determine in this patient population. Also observed in this article was the fact that antihistamines, commonly used before giving vancomycin, were not found to protect against red man syndrome or to ameliorate rash or pruritus. Not only are antihistamines not protected for red man syndrome, but administration of an antihistamine for any reason before receiving vancomycin was associated with increased risk of red man syndrome.

Some of the key information from this report included the fact that the risk of red man syndrome in hospitalized children runs about 14%. This article is the first to note that dose and concentration of infused vancomycin do play a key role in the development of red man syndrome. Clearly vancomycin should be infused slowly. Known genetic polymorphisms of histamine pathway and histamine receptor genes have little influence on risk of the syndrome. What was unexpected in this article was that pretreatment with an antihistamine did not prevent red man syndrome from developing and did not ameliorate most symptoms once present.

Be aware of this disorder. Chances are you will see it a fair amount of time in patients who are receiving vancomycin.

J. A. Stockman III, MD

Oral Dimenhydrinate Versus Placebo in Children With Gastroenteritis: A Randomized Controlled Trial
Gouin S, Vo T-T, Roy M, et al (Université de Montréal, Quebec, Canada)
Pediatrics 129:1050-1055, 2012

Objective.—To evaluate the efficacy and safety of oral dimenhydrinate in the treatment of acute gastroenteritis.

Methods.—This was a randomized, double-blind, placebo-controlled trial conducted in the emergency department of a pediatric university-affiliated center. Children 1 to 12 years old who presented to the emergency department with at least 5 episodes of vomiting in the previous 12 hours and diagnosed with acute gastroenteritis were block-randomized to receive oral dimenhydrinate (1 mg/kg; maximum: 50 mg) every 6 hours for 4 doses or placebo for 4 doses. The primary outcome measure was treatment failure as defined by the occurrence of ≥ 2 episodes of vomiting in the 24 hours after administration of the first dose of the study medication.

Results.—During the study period, 209 patients met inclusion criteria, but 50 refused to participate and 7 were missed. Eight participants were lost to follow-up, and 144 were thus included in the primary analysis. Of these patients, 74 were randomized to receive dimenhydrinate and 70 placebo. The proportions of patients showing failure of treatment were similar for both treatment groups: dimenhydrinate, 31% (23 of 74); placebo, 29% (20 of 70) (difference: 0.02 [95% confidence interval: −0.12 to 0.17]). There were no differences between the 2 groups in rates of intravenous cathether insertion, mean number of episodes of vomiting or diarrhea, abdominal pain, nausea, duration of symptoms, revisit rates, or parental absenteeism. The proportions of adverse effects were similar in both groups (53% vs 54%).

Conclusions.—The prescription of oral dimenhydrinate did not significantly decrease the frequency of vomiting in children with acute gastroenteritis compared with placebo.

▶ No data have been previously published on the efficacy of oral dimenhydrinate to control vomiting in children with acute gastroenteritis. Dimenhydrinate, an over-the-counter agent widely used in Canada and Europe, is an ethanolamine derivative antihistamine. It limits stimulation of the vomiting center by the vestibular system, which is rich in histamine receptors. Multiple studies over the years have shown dimenhydrinate's effectiveness in the treatment of postoperative nausea and vomiting in children. It is also used for the treatment of vertigo in children. It is inexpensive. In the United States, the cost per dose runs $0.30. The principal adverse effects of dimenhydrinate are drowsiness, dizziness, and anticholinergic symptoms. Restlessness and insomnia have also been described in children.

Given the lack of data on the efficacy of dimenhydrinate to control vomiting in children with acute gastroenteritis, these authors conducted a randomized, double-blind, placebo-controlled clinical trial in a pediatric university-affiliated hospital emergency department to determine the benefits, or lack of benefits, of this drug as part of the management of gastroenteritis. The intervention consisted of the administration of oral dimenhydrinate or placebo at a dosage of 1 mg/kg per dose every 6 hours for 4 doses, with a maximum dose of 200 mg/day. The first dose was administered in the emergency department by nurses and the patients were kept under observation. If the patient vomited within 5 minutes after drug ingestion, a second dose was administered. The drug is absorbed rapidly and produces an initial response within 15 minutes. Fifteen minutes after drug administration, oral rehydration was offered with a standardized rehydration solution at a rate of 0.2 mL/kg/minute. During the emergency department stay, the number of episodes of emesis and diarrhea, quantity of fluids consumed, need for intravenous rehydration, and length of stay were recorded. After discharge from the emergency department, parents were instructed to give the medication every 6 hours for an additional 3 doses and to continue oral rehydration. Telephone follow-up was then conducted. A total of 209 patients were evaluated.

This study found that oral dimenhydrinate did not significantly decrease the frequency of vomiting in children with acute gastroenteritis compared with placebo. Similar adverse effects were found with dimenhydrinate and placebo, suggesting that dimenhydrinate is a safe medication, albeit an ineffective one.

Despite the many antiemetic drugs available in pediatrics, their use in gastroenteritis remains controversial. Although widely used, there is no study documenting the effectiveness of these drugs In the management of children with acute gastroenteritis. Recently, randomized clinical trials and meta-analyses have studied the efficacy and safety of ondansetron, a selective serotonin receptor blocking agent in decreasing emesis in the emergency department.[1] This agent has shown promising results in alleviating the frequency of vomiting in acute gastroenteritis. However, studies have not shown a reduction in the rate of hospitalizations as a result of using this drug.

The bottom line is that prescribing oral dimenhydrinate cannot be expected to significantly reduce the proportion of children experiencing recurrent vomiting as part of the management of acute gastroenteritis when compared with placebo. As of now, the search continues for the perfect antiemetic. Chances are it will not be found anytime soon.

J. A. Stockman III, MD

Reference

1. DeCamp LR, Byerley JS, Doshi N, Steiner MJ. Use of antiemetic agents in acute gastroenteritis: a systematic review and meta-analysis. *Arch Pediatr Adolesc Med.* 2008;162:858-865.

Chest Wall Rigidity in Two Infants After Low-Dose Fentanyl Administration
Dewhirst E, Naguib A, Tobias JD (Nationwide Children's Hosp and the Ohio State Univ, Columbus)
Pediatr Emerg Care 28:465-468, 2012

Since its introduction into clinical practice, it has been known that fentanyl and other synthetic opioids may cause skeletal muscle rigidity. Involvement of the respiratory musculature, laryngeal structures, or the chest wall may impair ventilation, resulting in hypercarbia and hypoxemia. Although most common with the rapid administration of large doses, this rare adverse effect may occur with small doses especially in neonates and infants. We present 2 infants who developed chest wall rigidity, requiring the administration of neuromuscular blocking agents and controlled ventilation after analgesic doses of fentanyl. Previous reports regarding chest wall rigidity after the administration of low-dose fentanyl in infants and children are reviewed, the pathogenesis of the disorder is discussed, and treatment options offered.

▶ All pediatricians should be aware of side effects of fentanyl. Fentanyl use for analgesia, sedation, and anesthesia has spread widely in the past 2 decades. We are seeing increasing numbers of reports of unintentional exposure to children, particularly from fentanyl patches. Such exposure can cause life-threatening harm. The US Food and Drug Administration (FDA) issued a warning in this regard in April 2012.[1] The agency analyzed 26 cases of such unintentional exposures over a 15-year period, many of which ended in hospitalization or death. More than half the cases involved children 2 years old or younger. Such very young children are at particular risk of exposure because they are mobile and curious and may find lost, discarded, or improperly stored patches and put them in their mouths or on their skin. Children may also be exposed to a patch being worn by an adult that is inadvertently transferred to the child. The amount of fentanyl in transdermal patches, even those that have been discarded after use, is sufficient to cause serious harm to children. The FDA has stressed the importance of proper use and storage of fentanyl patches by patients, their caregivers, and health professionals to prevent such unintentional exposures.

This article reminds us that fentanyl and other synthetic opioids may cause skeletal muscle rigidity. When this involves the respiratory musculature, laryngeal structures, or the chest wall, clinical manifestations range from mild coughing to severe chest wall and laryngeal rigidity, which may impair ventilation. Although extensively mentioned in the adult literature, there have been a limited number of chest wall rigidity cases resulting from fentanyl in the pediatric population since its first description about 30 years ago.

These authors describe a 2-month-old infant who received fentanyl for the placement of a percutaneous intravenous central catheter. During the procedure, no air exchange was noted in association with an obstructed, asynchronous breathing pattern. Breath sounds could not be heard. The patient had to be mechanically ventilated. The second case was that of a newborn with congenital heart disease who received fentanyl postcorrective surgery. Again, oxygen tensions dropped rapidly after fentanyl administration. Fentanyl immediately induced chest wall rigidity in both patients after its administration, even at the low doses that were being used.

Chances are that most in pediatric practice will not be directly using fentanyl. One should be aware of the complications of its use, however. Chest wall rigidity can be treated with naloxone, which should be immediately available whenever fentanyl is administered to newborns and infants. Airway management equipment and neuromuscular blocking agents should also be readily available should severe hypoxemia and the inability to ventilate not be reversed by naloxone administration.

One other comment about fentanyl. Recently a 15-year-old adolescent girl with depression applied 5 fentanyl patches to her body. These were obtained from her stepfather's supply without his knowledge. He had used fentanyl patches for management of pain due to osteoporosis of the spine. The girl did this with the intention of committing suicide. Within an hour of placement of the fentanyl patches, she had severe respiratory depression and when taken to an emergency room had a Glasgow coma score of 14 (of 15) with pinpoint pupils. Fortunately, with multiple doses of naloxone, she recovered.[2]

J. A. Stockman III, MD

References

1. Kuehn BM. Fentanyl patch warning. *JAMA*. 2012;307:2139.
2. Lyttle MD, Verma S, Isaac R. Transdermal fentanyl in deliberate overdose in pediatrics. *Pediatr Emerg Care*. 2012;28:463-466.

Apixaban for Extended Treatment of Venous Thromboembolism

Agnelli G, for the AMPLIFY-EXT Investigators (Univ of Perugia, Italy; et al)
N Engl J Med 368:699-708, 2013

Background.—Apixaban, an oral factor Xa inhibitor that can be administered in a simple, fixed-dose regimen, may be an option for the extended treatment of venous thromboembolism.

Methods.—In this randomized, double-blind study, we compared two doses of apixaban (2.5 mg and 5 mg, twice daily) with placebo in patients with venous thromboembolism who had completed 6 to 12 months of anticoagulation therapy and for whom there was clinical equipoise regarding the continuation or cessation of anticoagulation therapy. The study drugs were administered for 12 months.

Results.—A total of 2486 patients underwent randomization, of whom 2482 were included in the intention-to-treat analyses. Symptomatic recurrent venous thromboembolism or death from venous thromboembolism occurred in 73 of the 829 patients (8.8%) who were receiving placebo, as compared with 14 of the 840 patients (1.7%) who were receiving 2.5 mg of apixaban (a difference of 7.2 percentage points; 95% confidence interval [CI], 5.0 to 9.3) and 14 of the 813 patients (1.7%) who were receiving 5 mg of apixaban (a difference of 7.0 percentage points; 95% CI, 4.9 to 9.1) ($P < 0.001$ for both comparisons). The rates of major bleeding were 0.5% in the placebo group, 0.2% in the 2.5-mg apixaban group, and 0.1% in the 5-mg apixaban group. The rates of clinically relevant nonmajor bleeding were 2.3% in the placebo group, 3.0% in the 2.5-mg apixaban group, and 4.2% in the 5-mg apixaban group. The rate of death from any cause was 1.7% in the placebo group, as compared with 0.8% in the 2.5-mg apixaban group and 0.5% in the 5-mg apixaban group.

Conclusions.—Extended anticoagulation with apixaban at either a treatment dose (5 mg) or a thromboprophylactic dose (2.5 mg) reduced the risk of recurrent venous thromboembolism without increasing the rate of major bleeding. (Funded by Bristol-Myers Squibb and Pfizer; AMPLIFY-EXT ClinicalTrials.gov number, NCT00633893.)

▶ Anyone caring for a pediatric-age patient or an adult patient with venous thromboembolism should read this article in detail and also an accompanying report by Schulman et al.[1] It is well known that the standard management of venous thromboembolism is the use of warfarin, which has a high degree of efficacy (90%) in preventing recurrent thromboembolism. Unfortunately, it is also associated with the major side effect of bleeding, which occurs in 1% to 2% of patients for each year of use. Warfarin requires fairly close laboratory monitoring.

This article explains an important alternative to the use of warfarin. Data are presented about apixaban, an orally administered factor-Xa inhibitor that is administered in fixed doses without the need for laboratory monitoring. At a dose of 5 mg daily, apixaban has been shown to be effective for the prevention of stroke in patients with atrial fibrillation, and at a dose of 2.5 mg twice daily, it has been shown to be effective for prevention of recurrent venous thromboembolism after orthopedic surgery.[2,3] This study compared 2 levels of dosing of apixaban (2.5 mg vs 5.0 mg twice daily) with placebo in patients with venous embolism who previously had completed between 6 and 12 months of anticoagulation therapy for recurrent thromboembolism. The data from this study show that both doses significantly reduce the risk of recurrent venous thrombosis and do so with the ease of oral medication use, lack of need for laboratory monitoring, and without increasing the risk of major bleeding. Similar findings were reported in the study by Schulman et al[1] using dabigatran, a direct thrombin inhibitor, which also does not require frequent monitoring or dose adjustments and can be given orally. It should be noted that neither dabigatran nor apixaban had been approved for short-term or extended-term use treatment of venous thromboembolism at the time of the publication of these reports. A similar orally administered drug has, however. Rivaroxaban is the first anticoagulant of this type approved for use in the United States and Europe. It has been shown to be more effective than placebo for extended treatment of venous thromboembolism (82% reduction in relative risk), albeit with some increased risk of bleeding.[4]

With the potential for lower bleeding rates, earlier administration, and similar efficacy, the new targeted anticoagulants are a much more attractive alternative to warfarin, which has to be given parenterally and requires frequent monitoring with laboratory studies. The finding that a low prophylactic dose of apixaban has the same efficacy as the full therapeutic dose, with no increased risk for major bleeding, may tip the risk-to-benefit ratio in favor of extended treatment for patients requiring long-term anticoagulation. Which patients would benefit most with these new agents has yet to be determined. Currently, the patients who seem to stand the greatest benefit from extended anticoagulant treatment are those who have had a first unprovoked episode of venous thromboembolism.

To read more about the extended treatment of venous thromboembolism, see the excellent editorial by Connors.[5]

J. A. Stockman III, MD

References

1. Schulman S, Kearon C, Kakkar AK, et al. Extended use of dabigatran, warfarin, or placebo in venous thromboembolism. *N Engl J Med.* 2013;368:709-718.
2. Granger CB, Alexander JH, McMurray JJ, et al. Apixaban versus warfarin in patients with atrial fibrillation. *N Engl J Med.* 2011;365:981-982.
3. Raskob GE, Gallus AS, Pineo GF, et al. Apixaban versus enoxaparin for thromboprophylaxis after hip or knee replacement: pooled analysis of major venous thromboembolism and bleeding in 8464 patients from the ADVANCE-2 and ADVANCE-3 trials. *J Bone Joint Surg Br.* 2012;94:257-264.
4. EINSTEIN Investigators; Bauersachs R, Berkowitz SD, Brenner B, et al. Oral rivaroxaban for symptomatic venous thromboembolism. *N Engl J Med.* 2010;363:2499-2510.
5. Connors JM. Extended treatment of venous thromboembolism. *N Engl J Med.* 2013;368:767-769.

Effective Analgesia Using Physical Interventions for Infant Immunizations

Harrington JW, Logan S, Harwell C, et al (Eastern Virginia Med School, Norfolk, VA)

Pediatrics 129:815-822, 2012

Background.—To measure the analgesic effectiveness of the 5 S's (swaddling, side/stomach position, shushing, swinging, and sucking) alone and combined with sucrose, during routine immunizations at 2 and 4 months.

Methods.—We conducted a prospective, randomized, placebo-controlled trial with 2- and 4-month-old infants during well-child visits. Patients were assigned into 4 groups (2×2) receiving either 2 mL of water or 2 mL of 24% oral sucrose and then either standard-of-care comfort measures by parents or intervention with the 5 S's immediately postvaccination. The Modified Riley Pain Score was used to score the infants' pain at 15-second intervals for 2 minutes, then every 30 seconds up to 5 minutes postvaccination. Repeated-measures analysis of variance examined between group differences and within-subject variability of treatment effect on overall pain scores and length of crying.

Results.—Two hundred thirty infants were enrolled. Results revealed significantly different mean pain scores between study groups with the exception of the 5S's and 5S's with sucrose groups. These 2 groups had lower similar mean scores over time, followed by sucrose alone, then control. The same trend was found with the proportion of children crying as with the mean pain score outcome measure.

Conclusions.—Physical intervention of the 5 S's (swaddling, side/stomach position, shushing, swinging, and sucking) provided decreased pain scores on a validated pain scale and decreased crying time among 2- and 4-month-old infants during routine vaccinations. The use of 5S's did not differ from 5S's and sucrose.

▶ With all the stuff in the literature about how to provide effective analgesia as part of infant immunization, you would think there is nothing left to write about. Well, there is—and there probably is a lot more to learn. This article reminds us that nonpharmacologic pain relief prior to or at the time of immunization is coming into increasing favor. The interest in nonpharmacologic pain relief has increased largely because 1 study found that acetaminophen, the most commonly used pain relief at the time of vaccination, significantly reduces antibody levels to several vaccine antigens.[1] The literature is ripe with nonpharmacologic pain reduction alternatives including nonnutritive sucking, breastfeeding, skin-to-skin contact, swaddling, oral glucose, distraction techniques, and combinations of all these.

Dr Harvey Karp, in his book *The Happiest Baby on the Block*, has described 5 pain relievers, the 5 Ss: swaddling, side/stomach position, shushing, swinging, and sucking. He also describes how these interventions trigger an infant's calming reflex. Harrington et al undertook a study to identify whether the 5 Ss could be used as a physical intervention to provide analgesia to infants receiving immunizations. A prospective, randomized, placebo-controlled trial with 2- and 4-month-old infants during well-child visits was undertaken. Infants were assigned into several groups receiving either physical intervention to relieve pain or oral sucrose (24%). The physical interventions included the 5 Ss. You will need to read this article in detail to see exactly how the 5 Ss were applied and in what sequence.

The study of Harrington et al demonstrated that physical intervention using the 5 Ss did result in decreased pain scores and less crying time during routine vaccination. The authors concluded that the 5 Ss appear to be a viable nonpharmacologic option for clinics to implement when providing analgesia during vaccinations. The use of the 5 Ss alone did not differ from the 5 Ss and sucrose. It was also clear that parents could be taught the 5 Ss so they could use the various maneuvers on their own at the time of the next immunization. It is fairly easy to teach parents how to swaddle, place a baby in the side/stomach position, shush, swing, and institute sucking. Karp's book is one that is heavily read by parents, so you may wish to be familiar with its content if you are not already.[2]

J. A. Stockman III, MD

References

1. Prymula R, Siegrist CA, Chlibek R, et al. Effect of prophylactic paracetamol administration at time of vaccination on febrile reactions and antibody responses in children: Two open-label randomized controlled trials. *Lancet.* 2009;374: 1339-1350.
2. Karp H. *The Happiest Baby on the Block.* New York, NY: Bantam Books; 2003.

Effect of Intravenous Paracetamol on Postoperative Morphine Requirements in Neonates and Infants Undergoing Major Noncardiac Surgery: A Randomized Controlled Trial

Ceelie I, de Wildt SN, van Dijk M, et al (Erasmus MC—Sophia Children's Hosp, Rotterdam, the Netherlands; et al)
JAMA 309:149-154, 2013

Importance.—Continuous morphine infusion as standard postoperative analgesic therapy in young infants is associated with unwanted adverse effects such as respiratory depression.

Objective.—To determine whether intravenous paracetamol (acetaminophen) would significantly (>30%) reduce morphine requirements in neonates and infants after major surgery.

Design, Setting, and Patients.—Single-center, randomized, double-blind study conducted in a level 3 pediatric intensive care unit in Rotterdam, the Netherlands. Patients were 71 neonates or infants younger than 1 year undergoing major thoracic (noncardiac) or abdominal surgery between March 2008 and July 2010, with follow-up of 48 hours.

Interventions.—All patients received a loading dose of morphine 30 minutes before the end of surgery, followed by continuous morphine or intermittent intravenous paracetamol up to 48 hours postsurgery. Infants in both study groups received morphine (boluses and/or continuous infusion) as rescue medication on the guidance of the validated pain assessment instruments.

Main Outcome Measures.—Primary outcome was cumulative morphine dose (study and rescue dose). Secondary outcomes were pain scores and morphine-related adverse effects.

Results.—The cumulative median morphine dose in the first 48 hours postoperatively was 121 (interquartile range, 99-264) µg/kg in the paracetamol group (n = 33) and 357 (interquartile range, 220-605) µg/kg in the morphine group (n = 38), $P < .001$, with a between-group difference that was 66% (95% CI, 34%-109%) lower in the paracetamol group. Pain scores and adverse effects were not significantly different between groups.

Conclusion and Relevance.—Among infants undergoing major surgery, postoperative use of intermittent intravenous paracetamol compared with continuous morphine resulted in a lower cumulative morphine dose over 48 hours.

Trial Registration.—trialregister.nl Identifier: NTR1438.

▶ We have come a long way in recognizing that infants experience significant pain, and we must be aware of that every time we undertake a procedure that could induce pain. It became clear in studies as early as 1987 that neonates have a well-developed nociceptive pathway and therefore are capable of experiencing pain, the consequences of which are significant even for simple procedures such as neonatal circumcision.[1,2] For these reasons, it has become commonplace to use opioids for management of induced pain, but it is well known that such therapies are associated with significant side effects, particularly respiratory depression. As a result, investigators have been looking for the benefits of other commonly used analgesics such as paracetamol (acetaminophen).

These authors designed a randomized, controlled, double-blinded trial in infants younger than 1 year old who had undergone major abdominal and thoracic (noncardiac) surgery to determine if intravenous acetaminophen would reduce the cumulative morphine dose needed to provide adequate analgesia. The study was performed in Rotterdam, the Netherlands. The trial was designed to address the gap in evidence about the use of acetaminophen as an opioid-sparing analgesic. Among patients randomized to receive acetaminophen or morphine postoperatively, the cumulative morphine dose during the first 48 hours following surgery was 121 µg/kg versus 357 µg/kg, respectively, a 66% relative reduction between groups. It should be noted that all patients received morphine in this analysis before leaving the operating room.

In an editorial that accompanied this report by Anand,[3] it was suggested that opiophobia in infants is an outmoded fallacy. The data from this study suggest that among infants undergoing major surgery, postoperative use of intermittent intravenous acetaminophen compared with continuous morphine will result in lower cumulative morphine dosing, at least in the first 48 hours following surgery. When it comes to drugs such as morphine that can produce respiratory suppression, less is more now that we know that acetaminophen in combination with morphine can be sparing of the use of a narcotic.

J. A. Stockman III, MD

References

1. Anand KJ, Hickey PR. Pain and its effects in the human neonate and fetus. *N Engl J Med.* 1987;317:1321-1329.
2. Taddio A, Katz J, Ilersich AL, Koren G. Effect of neonatal circumcision on pain response during subsequent routine vaccination. *Lancet.* 1997;349:599-603.
3. Anand KJ. Pain panacea for opiophobia in infants? *JAMA.* 2013;309:183-184.

Association Between Urinary Bisphenol A Concentration and Obesity Prevalence in Children and Adolescents
Trasande L, Attina TM, Blustein J (New York Univ School of Medicine)
JAMA 308:1113-1121, 2012

Context.—Bisphenol A (BPA), a manufactured chemical, is found in canned food, polycarbonate-bottled liquids, and other consumer products. In adults, elevated urinary BPA concentrations are associated with obesity and incident coronary artery disease. BPA exposure is plausibly linked to childhood obesity, but evidence is lacking to date.

Objective.—To examine associations between urinary BPA concentration and body mass outcomes in children.

Design, Setting, and Participants.—Cross-sectional analysis of a nationally representative subsample of 2838 participants aged 6 through 19 years randomly selected for measurement of urinary BPA concentration in the 2003-2008 National Health and Nutrition Examination Surveys.

Main Outcome Measures.—Body mass index (BMI), converted to sex- and age-standardized z scores and used to classify participants as overweight (BMI $\geq$ 85th percentile for age/sex) or obese (BMI $\geq$ 95th percentile).

Results.—Median urinary BPA concentration was 2.8 ng/mL (interquartile range, 1.5-5.6). Of the participants, 1047 (34.1% [SE, 1.5%]) were overweight and 590 (17.8% [SE, 1.3%]) were obese. Controlling for race/ethnicity, age, caregiver education, poverty to income ratio, sex, serum cotinine level, caloric intake, television watching, and urinary creatinine level, children in the lowest urinary BPA quartile had a lower estimated prevalence of obesity (10.3% [95% CI, 7.5%-13.1%]) than those in quartiles 2 (20.1% [95% CI, 14.5%-25.6%]), 3 (19.0% [95% CI, 13.7%-24.2%]), and 4 (22.3% [95% CI, 16.6%-27.9%]). Similar patterns of association were found in multivariable analyses examining the association between quartiled urinary BPA concentration and BMI z score and in analyses that examined the logarithm of urinary BPA concentration and the prevalence of obesity. Obesity was not associated with exposure to other environmental phenols commonly used in other consumer products, such as sunscreens and soaps. In stratified analysis, significant associations between urinary BPA concentrations and obesity were found among whites ($P < .001$) but not among blacks or Hispanics.

Conclusions.—Urinary BPA concentration was significantly associated with obesity in this cross-sectional study of children and adolescents. Explanations of the association cannot rule out the possibility that obese children ingest food with higher BPA content or have greater adipose stores of BPA.

▶ Much has been written about bisphenol A (BPA). BPA is used in the manufacturing of polycarbonate resins. It is also a breakdown product of coatings that prevent metal corrosion of food and beverage containers. Everyone in the United States is exposed to this substance on a daily basis. One study showed that 93% of people 6 years of age or older have detectable BPA levels in their urine.[1] BPA is literally in the air around us. Fortunately, it is rapidly excreted in urine and has a half-life in the range of 4 to 43 hours. It does get into fat, and it has been suggested that it can accumulate in fat.

It has also been suggested that BPAs increase body mass index in environmentally irrelevant doses by disrupting various metabolic mechanisms and thereby contributing to obesity in humans. There is a study that examined this possibility in adults. It did show a relationship.[2] Trasande et al now tell us about urinary BPA concentrations and body mass issues in a pediatric population aged 6 to 19 years old. The investigators compared urinary BPA concentrations obtained in the 2003 to 2008 National Health and Nutrition Examination Survey with information provided on participants' body mass index. More than 1000 obese and overweight individuals were studied and compared with normal body mass index subjects. It was clear that urinary BPA concentration was significantly associated with obesity in this cross-sectional study of children and adolescents.

The report of Trasande et al is the first study of an association of an environmental chemical exposure with childhood obesity using a wide national representative sample. Policy makers have been concerned about BPA exposure for some time. The Food and Drug Administration has banned BPA in baby bottles and sippy cups. Unfortunately the Food and Drug Administration declined to ban BPA in aluminum cans and other food packaging. In a country where one state's motto is live free or die, one will likely not see regulatory oversight of much of what makes us fat.

This commentary closes with mention of a new form of intoxication resulting from the abuse of psychoactive bath salts (PABS).[3] The primary ingredient in PABS is methylenedioxypyrovalerone (MDPV). MDPV inhibits norepinephrine-dopamine reuptake and thus acts as a central nervous system stimulant. PABS are readily available via the internet under such names as Ivory Wave and Vanilla Sky. They are sometimes referred to as "legal cocaine." PABS are abused via oral, intranasal, intravenous, and rectal routes. Orally, PABS are rapidly absorbed, reaching a peak in 1.5 hours. Effects last up to 8 hours. PABS causes extreme sympathetic stimulation and a profoundly altered mental status. Tachycardia, hypertension, hyperthermia, and seizures can result. Deaths have been reported. Routine drug screening will not detect PABS. Treatment is largely supportive, typically with intravenous benzodiazepines and intravenous fluids.

J. A. Stockman III, MD

References

1. Calafat AM, Ye X, Wong LY, Reidy JA, Needham LL. Exposure of the US population to BPA and 4-tertiary-octylphenol: 2003–2004. *Environ Health Perspect.* 2008;116:39-44.
2. Carwile JL, Michels KB. Urinary bisphenol A and obesity: NHANES 2003–2006. *Environ Res.* 2011;111:825-830.
3. Ross EA, Watson M, Goldberger B. "Bath Salts" intoxication. *N Eng J Med.* 2011; 365:967.

Prenatal Exposure to Mercury and Fish Consumption During Pregnancy and Attention-Deficit/Hyperactivity Disorder–Related Behavior in Children

Sagiv SK, Thurston SW, Bellinger DC, et al (Boston Univ School of Public Health, MA; Univ of Rochester School of Medicine and Dentistry, NY; Children's Hosp, Boston, MA; et al)

Arch Pediatr Adolesc Med 166:1123-1131, 2012

Objective.—To investigate the association of prenatal mercury exposure and fish intake with attention-deficit/hyperactivity disorder (ADHD)–related behavior.

Methods.—For a population-based prospective birth cohort recruited in New Bedford, Massachusetts (1993-1998), we analyzed data for children examined at age 8 years with peripartum maternal hair mercury measures (n = 421) or maternal report of fish consumption during pregnancy (n = 515). Inattentive and impulsive/hyperactive behaviors were assessed using a teacher rating scale and neuropsychological testing.

Results.—The median maternal hair mercury level was 0.45 µg/g (range, 0.03-5.14 µg/g), and 52% of mothers consumed more than 2 fish servings weekly. In multivariable regression models, mercury exposure was associated with inattention and impulsivity/hyperactivity; some outcomes had an apparent threshold with associations at 1 µg/g or greater of mercury. For example, at 1 µg/g or greater, the adjusted risk ratios for mild/markedly atypical inattentive and impulsive/hyperactive behaviors were 1.4 (95% CI, 1.0-1.8) and 1.7 (95% CI, 1.2-2.4), respectively, for an interquartile range (0.5 µg/g) mercury increase; there was no confounding by fish consumption. For neuropsychological assessments, mercury and behavior associations were detected primarily for boys. There was a protective association for fish consumption (>2 servings per week) with ADHD-related behaviors, particularly impulsive/hyperactive behaviors (relative risk = 0.4; 95% CI, 0.2-0.6).

Conclusions.—Low-level prenatal mercury exposure is associated with a greater risk of ADHD-related behaviors, and fish consumption during pregnancy is protective of these behaviors. These findings underscore the difficulties of balancing the benefits of fish intake with the detriments of low level mercury exposure in developing dietary recommendations in pregnancy.

▶ Everyone knows that mercury is a neurotoxin, as demonstrated by the effects of mass poisoning in Japan and Iraq, both having occurred during our lifetime.[1,2] What we do not know much about are the effects of lower-dose mercury exposures common in the population. The latter, nonoccupational exposure largely results from fish consumption. This is particularly problematic during pregnancy. The US Environmental Protection Agency and the US Food and Drug Administration have issued a joint federal advisory recommending that pregnant women, for example, limit their total fish intake to no more than 2 6-ounce servings per week, but at the same time, fish is also a source of nutrients such as omega-3 fatty acids, which have been shown to benefit brain development, potentially confounding mercury-related risk estimates.

These authors have studied the association of peripartum maternal hair mercury levels and prenatal fish intake with attention-deficit/hyperactivity disorder (ADHD)-related behaviors at 8 years of age in a prospective birth cohort to determine whether the mercury ingested by pregnant women from the consumption of fish might in any way relate to the development of ADHD-type behaviors in children. This population-based prospective cohort study found that hair mercury levels were consistently associated with ADHD-related behaviors, including inattention and hyperactivity or impulsivity. The investigators also found that higher levels of prenatal fish consumption were protective for these behaviors.

Again, we see some inconsistency in the pros and cons of eating fish. One explanation for the inconsistency is that nutrients in fish that promote neurodevelopment, such as omega-3 fatty acids, may offset the neurotoxicant effects of mercury exposure. In addition, the degree of confounding by fish consumption is likely a function of the fish species consumed in various study populations. The results of this study do suggest that prenatal mercury exposure is associated with a higher risk of ADHD-related behaviors, but that fish consumption by itself during pregnancy is associated with a lower risk of these behaviors. A single estimate combining these beneficial versus detrimental effects of fish intake is not possible from these data, although these data are consistent with the growing literature showing a risk of mercury exposure and a benefit of the consumption of fish on fetal brain development. The ideal would be to eat fish that is mercury-free if at all possible—neat trick!

J. A. Stockman III, MD

References

1. Harada M. Congenital Minamata disease: intrauterine methylmercury poisoning. *Teratology.* 1978;18:285-288.
2. Bakir F, Damluji SF, Amin-Zaki L, et al. Methylmercury poisoning in Iraq. *Science.* 1973;181:230-241.

Low-Level Lead Exposure and the Prevalence of Gout: An Observational Study
Krishnan E, Lingala B, Bhalla V (Stanford Univ School of Medicine, Palo Alto, CA)
Ann Intern Med 157:233-241, 2012

Background.—Blood lead levels (BLLs) less than 1.21 μmol/L (<25 μg/dL) among adults are considered acceptable by current national standards. Lead toxicity can lead to gouty arthritis (gout), but whether the low lead exposure in the contemporary general population confers risk for gout is not known.

Objective.—To determine whether BLLs within the range currently considered acceptable are associated with gout.

Design.—Population-based cross-sectional study.

Setting.—The National Health and Nutrition Examination Survey for 2005 through 2008.

Patients.—6153 civilians aged 40 years or older with an estimated glomerular filtration rate greater than 10 mL/min per 1.73 m^2.

Measurements.—Outcome variables were self-reported physician diagnosis of gout and serum urate level. Blood lead level was the principal exposure variable. Additional data collected were anthropometric measures, blood pressure, dietary purine intake, medication use, medical history, and serum creatinine concentration.

Results.—The prevalence of gout was 6.05% (95% CI, 4.49% to 7.62%) among patients in the highest BLL quartile (mean, 0.19 μmol/L [3.95 μg/dL]) compared with 1.76% (CI, 1.10% to 2.42%) among those in the lowest quartile (mean, 0.04 μmol/L [0.89 μg/dL]). Each doubling of BLL was associated with an unadjusted odds ratio of 1.74 (CI, 1.47 to 2.05) for gout and 1.25 (CI, 1.12 to 1.40) for hyperuricemia. After adjustment for renal function, diabetes, diuretic use, hypertension, race, body mass index, income, and education level, the highest BLL quartile was associated with a 3.6-fold higher risk for gout and a 1.9-fold higher risk for hyperuricemia compared with the lowest quartile.

Limitation.—Blood lead level does not necessarily reflect the total body lead burden.

Conclusion.—Blood lead levels in the range currently considered acceptable are associated with increased prevalence of gout and hyperuricemia.

▶ Who would have thought we would still be learning more about which blood concentrations of lead at its lowest levels would still be capable of doing the body harm? Even the ancient Greeks and Romans eventually recognized the adverse effects related to exposure to lead. Lead was largely smelted to separate the lead from the more valuable silver. Civilizations actually rose and fell depending on their access to silver-containing lead ore. It was only later in recognition of lead's malleability and density that myriad other uses were found for it, including weaponry, weights, and plumbing. Moreover, lead, in its carbonate form, which has a pure white color, was used extensively in pigments and paints. Most exposure to lead in children still comes from exposure to lead-based paints that are no longer used in new home construction but may be present in homes built more than 40 years ago.

For the last 2 decades, the Centers for Disease Control and Prevention specified that blood lead concentrations greater than 0.48 μmol/L (10 μg/dL) were unacceptable and potentially harmful to children. However, a growing body of scientific evidence indicates that even lower levels of lead exposures can harm children, impairing intellectual ability. In response to such evidence and stakeholder activism, the Centers for Disease Control and Prevention have decreased the maximum acceptable blood level among children to 0.24 μmol/L (5 μg/dL). Here in the United States, blood lead levels greater than 1.21 μmol/L (> 25 μg/dL) are considered potentially harmful to adults. There are studies, however, showing adverse effects at significantly lower levels of blood lead (< 0.24 μmol/L) (< 5 μg/dL). Krishnan et al designed a study to determine whether blood lead levels within the range currently considered to be acceptable for adults are independently associated with the development of gout. Using a cross-sectional study design, the authors examined adult participants from 2 cycles of the National Health and Nutrition Examination Survey. They found that participants in the highest quartile of blood lead level were nearly 4 times as likely to have a self-reported physician diagnosis of gout compared with those in the lowest quartile. Moreover, there was a strong dose-response relationship, and even participants in the second quartile (with blood lead levels of 0.06–0.09 μmol/L and 1.2–1.8 μg/dL) were at elevated risk. Results were similar when objective measures of serum urate were examined.

These adult data do warn us that it is entirely possible that any exposure to lead can theoretically produce harm. Lower thresholds for toxic lead levels that are both desirable and feasible have appeared. For example, Germany's Human Biomonitoring Commission uses levels of 0.17 μmol/L (3.5 μg/dL), 0.34 μmol/L (7 μg/dL), and 0.43 μmol/L (9 μg/dL) as reference values for children, women, and men, respectively. According to the Commission, levels greater than these should be assumed to come from a specific lead source, one that should be sought out.

Thus, currently accepted blood lead levels may in fact not be safe. Even low, nonelevated levels of lead, for example, have been clearly documented to be associated with an elevated prevalence of gout. If you encounter a youngster with an elevated uric acid level, it might even be wise to measure blood lead concentrations to determine secondary causes of high urate levels. Children rarely get gout, but every now and then you will find a child with a high uric acid level. The authors of this report suggest that anyone who has symptoms of gout should have a blood lead level measured. It has been known for years that high concentrations of lead affect tubular urate transport, causing decreased urate excretion, thus, the term *saturnine gout*. In cases of lead intoxication, these effects are often associated with renal failure but may occur without clinical features of lead toxicity and renal damage.

While on the topic of lead poisoning, the past several years have seen the largest outbreak of lead poisoning ever recorded. This was in the Zamfara state of northwest Nigeria. In 2010, villages in Zamfara experienced a child mortality rate of 40% largely the result of lead poisoning.[1] The culprit was artisanal gold mining. Miners, some of whom included children, hit upon a vein of gold heavily contaminated with lead. The miners would return home covered in lead-contaminated dust. The mining process — dry milling intended for grain — exacerbated the problem, throwing up thick clouds of dust contaminating food, soil and children, particularly those crawling. More than 400 children expired from lead poisoning and several thousand have been under treatment.

J. A. Stockman III, MD

Reference

1. Burki TK. Nigeria's lead poisoning crisis could leave long legacy. *Lancet.* 2012; 379:732.

Regional Brain Morphometry and Impulsivity in Adolescents Following Prenatal Exposure to Cocaine and Tobacco

Liu J, Lester BM, Neyzi N, et al (Women & Infants Hosp, Providence, RI; Weill Cornell Med College, NY)
JAMA Pediatr 167:348-354, 2013

Importance.—Animal studies have suggested that prenatal cocaine exposure (PCE) deleteriously influences the developing nervous system, in part attributable to its site of action in blocking the function of monoamine reuptake transporters, increasing synaptic levels of serotonin and dopamine.

Objective.—To examine the brain morphologic features and associated impulsive behaviors in adolescents following prenatal exposure to cocaine and/or tobacco.

Design.—Magnetic resonance imaging data and behavioral measures were collected from adolescents followed up longitudinally in the Maternal Lifestyle Study.

Setting.—A hospital-based research center.

Participants.—A total of 40 adolescent participants aged 13 to 15 years were recruited, 20 without PCE and 20 with PCE; a subset of each group additionally had tobacco exposure. Participants were selected and matched based on head circumference at birth, gestational age, maternal alcohol use, age, sex, race/ethnicity, IQ, family poverty, and socioeconomic status.

Main Outcome Measures.—Subcortical volumetric measures of the thalamus, caudate, putamen, pallidum, hippocampus, amygdala, and nucleus accumbens; cortical thickness measures of the dorsolateral prefrontal cortex and ventral medial prefrontal cortex; and impulsivity assessed by Conners' Continuous Performance Test and the Sensation Seeking Scale for Children.

Results.—After controlling for covariates, cortical thickness of the right dorsolateral prefrontal cortex was significantly thinner in adolescents following PCE ($P = .03$), whereas the pallidum volume was smaller in adolescents following prenatal tobacco exposure ($P = .03$). Impulsivity was correlated with thalamic volume following either PCE ($P = .05$) or prenatal tobacco exposure ($P = .04$).

Conclusions and Relevance.—Prenatal cocaine or tobacco exposure can differentially affect structural brain maturation during adolescence and underlie enhanced susceptibility to impulsivity. Additional studies with larger sample sizes are warranted.

▶ There is a fair amount of information about prenatal exposure to illicit drugs and tobacco effects on newborns and young children. For example, one study reported that cocaine-exposed boys who were studied at an average age of 4.5 years are more likely to express frustration and had more difficulty in controlling their frustration in problem-solving tasks.[1] There are a number of ways in which drugs affect the fetus either by causing the placenta to alter its nutrient supply or through immediate and direct effects on fetal growth. The study by Liu et al takes us well into the adolescent period by telling us about brain imaging technologies that are on the cutting edge and by examining cognitive assessment in a prospective cohort of 40 adolescents age 13 years to 15 years who were born to mothers who had used tobacco or cocaine or both during pregnancy. Using magnetic resonance imaging, the study documented specific brain morphologic effects for these 2 drugs. There was decreased cortical thickness in the right dorsolateral prefrontal cortex of adolescents exposed to cocaine and decreased volumes in the globus pallidus in those exposed to nicotine. Reported also was that larger volumes of the thalamus were associated with greater impulsivity both in adolescents exposed to cocaine and in those exposed to nicotine. These findings seem to be consistent with an increased risk for externalizing disorders in those adolescents exposed to cocaine and nicotine during pregnancy because impaired prefrontal cortex is associated with low self control and impulsivity. If the data from this report are accurate, smoking during pregnancy could theoretically account for up to one-quarter of all externalizing behaviors.

An editorial that accompanied this report by Volkow reminds us that it is not possible to separate all the factors that are related to fetal drug exposures from those that relate to genetic factors that are well known to modulate brain development and function.[2] Additionally, genetic factors in the mother may determine whether a woman continues to take drugs during pregnancy. It is almost impossible to control for drug exposure during versus after pregnancy. Women who take drugs while pregnant are likely to have difficult interactions with their infants as that child grows.

It is clear from the findings of Liu et al that a legal drug such as the nicotine in tobacco and illegal drugs taken during pregnancy will affect fetal development and modify brain structure during adolescence, a period marked with remarkable plasticity and a period that, if fouled up, will result in lifelong consequences.

As an aside, recent information has appeared to document that smoking bans actually reduce preterm births. Since Belgium instituted a phased-in ban on smoking in public places, a steady decline in preterm births has been noted. Belgium halted smoking in most public places in 2006 then extended the ban to restaurants in 2007 and to bars serving food in 2010. A research team has found a 3.1% decline in preterm births in 2007 and a further decrease of 2.7% in 2010.[3] The research that found this accounted for other factors that might influence preterm birth, such as age of the mother, her national origin, and even local air pollution. Whether this is cause and effect or an "epi" phenomenon remains to be seen.

J. A. Stockman III, MD

References

1. Dennis T, Bendersky M, Ramsay D, Lewis M. Reactivity and regulation in children prenatally exposed to cocaine. *Dev Psychol.* 2006;42:688-697.
2. Volkow ND. Impact of fetal drug exposures on the adolescent brain. *JAMA Pediatr.* 2013;167:390-391.
3. Editorial comment Smoking ban cuts preterm births. *Science News.* March 23, 2013:18.

Association of Coffee Drinking with Total and Cause-Specific Mortality

Freedman ND, Park Y, Abnet CC, et al (Natl Insts of Health, Rockville, MD; et al)

N Engl J Med 366:1891-1904, 2012

Background.—Coffee is one of the most widely consumed beverages, but the association between coffee consumption and the risk of death remains unclear.

Methods.—We examined the association of coffee drinking with subsequent total and cause-specific mortality among 229,119 men and 173,141 women in the National Institutes of Health—AARP Diet and Health Study who were 50 to 71 years of age at baseline. Participants with cancer, heart disease, and stroke were excluded. Coffee consumption was assessed once at baseline.

Results.—During 5,148,760 person-years of follow-up between 1995 and 2008, a total of 33,731 men and 18,784 women died. In age-adjusted models, the risk of death was increased among coffee drinkers. However, coffee drinkers were also more likely to smoke, and, after adjustment for tobacco-smoking status and other potential confounders, there was a significant inverse association between coffee consumption and mortality. Adjusted hazard ratios for death among men who drank coffee as compared with those who did not were as follows: 0.99 (95% confidence interval [CI], 0.95 to 1.04) for drinking less than 1 cup per day, 0.94 (95% CI, 0.90 to 0.99) for 1 cup, 0.90 (95% CI, 0.86 to 0.93) for 2 or 3 cups, 0.88 (95% CI, 0.84 to 0.93) for 4 or 5 cups, and 0.90 (95% CI, 0.85 to 0.96) for 6 or more cups of coffee per day ($P < 0.001$ for trend); the respective hazard ratios among women were 1.01 (95% CI, 0.96 to 1.07), 0.95 (95% CI, 0.90 to 1.01), 0.87 (95% CI, 0.83 to 0.92), 0.84 (95% CI, 0.79 to 0.90), and 0.85 (95% CI, 0.78 to 0.93) ($P < 0.001$ for trend). Inverse associations were observed for deaths due to heart disease, respiratory disease, stroke, injuries and accidents, diabetes, and infections, but not for deaths due to cancer. Results were similar in subgroups, including persons who had never smoked and persons who reported very good to excellent health at baseline.

Conclusions.—In this large prospective study, coffee consumption was inversely associated with total and cause-specific mortality. Whether this was a causal or associational finding cannot be determined from our data. (Funded by the Intramural Research Program of the National Institutes of Health, National Cancer Institute, Division of Cancer Epidemiology and Genetics.)

▶ A discussion regarding coffee drinking may seem out of place but children eventually will grow into teens and young adults who, like many of us, are addicted to their morning (or more often than that) coffee. Coffee is indeed one of the most widely consumed beverages, not just in the United States, but elsewhere throughout the world where it is not at all uncommon for the underaged to partake of the dark brown nectar. Since coffee contains caffeine, a stimulant, coffee drinking is generally not considered part of a healthy lifestyle. On the other hand, coffee is a rich source of antioxidants and other bioactive chemicals, and studies have shown inverse associations between coffee consumption and serum biomarkers of inflammation and insulin resistance. Coffee contains more than 1000 compounds that might affect the risk of death. Considerable attention has focused on the possibility that coffee may increase the risk of heart disease, particularly since drinking coffee has been associated with increased low-density lipoprotein cholesterol levels and short-term increases in blood pressure. Large cohort studies, however, do not support a positive association between coffee drinking and mortality. Nonetheless, quality data are lacking to clarify the association between coffee drinking and mortality.

In order to examine the issue of the relation of coffee with mortality, investigators from the National Institutes of Health examined data from a very large study, the National Institutes of Health Diet and Health Study, to determine whether coffee consumption is associated with total or cause-specific mortality. The analysis involved more than 400 000 participants and 52 000 deaths and therefore had adequate sample size to detect even modest associations between coffee drinking and risk factors for mortality. The study observed a dose-dependent inverse association between coffee drinking and total mortality, after adjusting for potential confounders (smoking status in particular). Compared with men who did not drink coffee, men who drank 6 or more cups of coffee per day had a 10% lower risk of death, whereas women at this level of consumption had a 15% lower risk. Similar associations were observed whether participants drank predominantly caffeinated or decaffeinated coffee. These same inverse associations persisted among many subgroups, including participants who had never smoked and those who were former smokers and participants with a normal body mass index and those with a high body mass index. The investigators noted inverse associations between coffee drinking and most major causes of death, with the exception of cancer. The results are consistent with previous studies showing inverse associations between coffee consumption and diabetes, stroke, and death due to inflammatory diseases.

This was an extremely well-done study. As in all observational studies, associations could possibly reflect confounding by unmeasured or poorly measured variables. It is also possible that the data from this report merely represent reverse causality (eg, those with chronic disease and poor health might abstain from coffee drinking). The authors of this article, while recognizing these disclaimers, believe that reverse causality is not likely to be a major factor in discrediting the strong association between heavy coffee drinking and decreased mortality.

The obvious question is what is in coffee that may be protective to a person's health? The authors speculate that it is some combination of antioxidants, including polyphenol. In any event, this large prospective cohort study does show significant inverse associations of coffee consumption with deaths from all causes and especially with deaths due to heart disease, a respiratory disease, stroke, injuries, in addition to accidents, diabetes, and infections.

Drink coffee to your heart's desire, and if you do not like the jitters of regular coffee, all the benefits also come with decaf!

This is the last entry in the Therapeutics and Toxicology chapter, so we will end with a quiz. You are a toxicologist on a summer vacation in Europe and are visiting Brittany. You read about the death of 36 wild boar at a picturesque beach where there is also a strong smell of hydrogen sulfide. You offer your expert services to town officials who are anxious to determine the cause of the demise of the boar. You inspect the beach and find the presence of algae common to the area, but this particular algae has a bright green color to it. You make a diagnosis.

If you made a diagnosis of death as the result of hydrogen sulfide inhalation from gases produced by rotting green algae, you would be correct. This was the exact situation that occurred in Brittany as reported in July 2011, when it is claimed that nitrate runoff entering the shore line from excessive fertilizer use by local farmers was the cause.[1] The farmers in the region suggested that activists had poisoned the boar in protest of the use of fertilizers. It turns out that autopsy of the animals did prove that hydrogen sulfide inhalation was the cause of the boars' deaths. It is believed that two years earlier a horse had met a similar end as did a local man who died trying to remove algae from the beach in front of his home.

Beware of green algae, particularly if it smells of rotten eggs.

J. A. Stockman III, MD

Reference

1. Editorial comment. Green Algae pose mortal danger. *Science*. 2011;333:922.

Article Index

Chapter 1: Adolescent Medicine

Chapter 2: Allergy and Dermatology

Chapter 3: Blood

Chapter 4: Child Development/Behavior

Chapter 5: Dentistry and Otolaryngology (ENT)

Chapter 6: Endocrinology

Chapter 7: Gastroenterology

Chapter 10: Infectious Diseases and Immunology

Chapter 11: Miscellaneous

Chapter 12: Musculoskeletal

Chapter 13: Neurology Psychiatry

Chapter 14. Newborn

Chapter 15: Nutrition and Metabolism

Chapter 16: Oncology

Chapter 17: Ophthalmology

Chapter 18: Respiratory Tract

Chapter 19: Therapeutics and Toxicology

Author Index

Edwards Brothers Malloy
Thorofare, NJ USA
January 10, 2014